Prevention of Diseases in Populations

From Biology to Policy

Thomas Farley, MD, MPH

Adjunct Professor of Sociomedical Sciences,
Columbia University Mailman School of Public Health
Adjunct Professor, Celia Scott Weatherhead School of
Public Health and Tropical Medicine, Tulane University

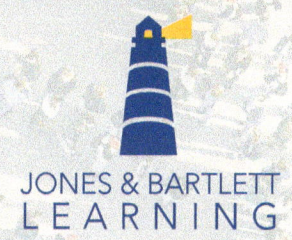

JONES & BARTLETT
LEARNING

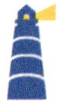

World Headquarters
Jones & Bartlett Learning
25 Mall Road
Burlington, MA 01803
978-443-5000
info@jblearning.com
www.jblearning.com

Jones & Bartlett Learning books and products are available through most bookstores and online booksellers. To contact Jones & Bartlett Learning directly, call 800-832-0034, fax 978-443-8000, or visit our website, www.jblearning.com.

Substantial discounts on bulk quantities of Jones & Bartlett Learning publications are available to corporations, professional associations, and other qualified organizations. For details and specific discount information, contact the special sales department at Jones & Bartlett Learning via the above contact information or send an email to specialsales@jblearning.com.

Production Credits

Vice President, Innovative Learning and Assessment Solutions: Ada Woo
Senior Director, Content Production and Delivery: Christine Emerton
Director, Product Management: Melissa Kleeman Moy
Manager, Content Development: Bill Lawrensen
Product Manager: Sophie Fleck Teague
Content Manager: Jessica Covert
Content Coordinator: Samantha Gillespie
Manager, Intellectual Properties and Content Production: Kristen Rogers
Content Production Manager: Madelene Nieman

Senior Product Marketing Manager: Susanne Walker
Director, Product Fulfillment: Aaron McKinzie
Purchasing Manager: Wendy Kilborn
Composition and Project Management: Exela Technologies
Cover and Text Design: MPS Limited
Intellectual Property Specialist: Faith Brosnan
Intellectual Property Specialist: Maria Leon Maimone
Cover Image (Title Page, Part Opener, Chapter Opener): © Boris SV/Moment/Getty Images
Printing and Binding: Lakeside Book Company

29716-4

Library of Congress Cataloging-in-Publication Data

Library of Congress Cataloging-in-Publication Data unavailable at time of printing.

LCCN: 2025009725

6048

Printed in the United States of America
29 28 27 26 25   10 9 8 7 6 5 4 3 2 1

To everyone who works to protect
the health of others.

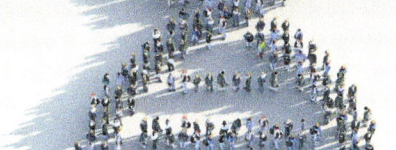

Brief Contents

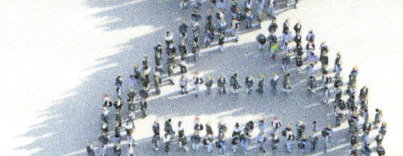

Contents

PART I Public Health Strategy — 1

CHAPTER 1 Disease Prevention and Populations 3

PART II Diseases, Injuries, and Disabling Conditions — 17

CHAPTER 2 Heart Disease and Stroke 19

CHAPTER 3 Cancer 43

PART III Behavioral and Social Risks   317

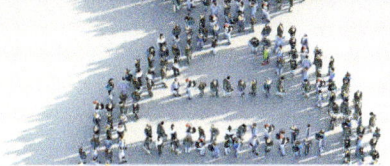

Preface

Success in public health, like success in medical care, requires both art and science.

Practicing the art of medical care requires listening to patients and working with them as partners in solving their health problems. Practicing the art of public health requires communicating with populations about health risks, working with communities, managing a team within a nonprofit or government organization, and maintaining a focus on health in a political environment.

To its credit, the field of public health has taken these skills seriously in recent years. Students are taught health communications, program planning, and organizational management. Practitioners of public health attend workshops on risk communication, community engagement, and strategic planning. But I worry that with this emphasis on the art of public health, training in the science of public health has become outdated.

A century ago, the science of public health had a clear focus: infectious diseases. Health departments were led by doctors and nurses, the leading causes of death featured tuberculosis, diarrheal diseases, and diphtheria, and the tools of public health were the bacteriology laboratory, sanitary regulations, and public vaccination clinics. All that has since changed. The leading health problems today, in the United States and increasingly around the globe, are chronic diseases, injuries, mental illnesses, and musculoskeletal problems. Those health problems are heavily influenced by behaviors like unhealthy diets, physical inactivity, and use of tobacco, alcohol, and other drugs. And both the leading health problems and the key health-related behaviors are shaped by our modern physical and social environment, including traffic-clogged streets, handheld digital devices, the marketing of junk food and addictive drugs, and the gap between the rich and the poor. Public health students and workers today are mostly not doctors or nurses; they are more likely to have degrees in fields like psychology or communications. I believe that our training of students and practitioners in public health

science has not kept up with these tectonic shifts in our health risks and workforce.

I also worry that the gap left in that training has been filled by the science of medicine. Too often, public health students and workers assume that the solution to public health problems is to give people more medical care. Too often, they see only drug-centered strategies to address problems like hypertension (antihypertensives), diabetes (hypoglycemics), asthma (inhaled steroids), and depression (antidepressants).

The science of medical care overlaps with but is different from the science of public health. Doctors' goal is to cure; they need to know diseases' symptoms, diagnostic tests, and the pros and cons of different drugs or types of surgery. Public health practitioners' goal is to prevent; they need to know diseases' biologic, behavioral, and social causes, and where the chain of cause-and-effect can be interrupted to prevent diseases. One cannot substitute for the other.

Medical care is focused on individuals, while public health concerns itself with populations. As Geoffrey Rose taught us, a risk factor that may be of trivial importance to any individual, if widely prevalent, can have a great impact on the health of a population. Conversely, a risk factor that may be of major importance to an individual—a genetic risk, for example—can be irrelevant to improving the health of populations.

Over-reliance on the science of medical care is dangerous. If a governor, whose son just went into renal failure, asks for a plan to address chronic kidney disease, it would be a grave mistake for the plan to just request more dialysis machines and pig-kidney transplants. We know much about the causes and prevention of kidney disease, and if we miss opportunities to prevent it, we fail the people whose lives might have been saved. Similarly, we fail if we overlook primary prevention of other high-burden health problems like breast cancer, depression, and alcohol addiction.

The science of population-based prevention is distinct. It integrates the physiology of organ systems, the pathophysiology of high-burden diseases, the patterns and trends in disease rates in populations, the factors that increase the risk of disease, and the evaluations of prevention initiatives. In the internet age, these scientific facts and findings are just a few mouse clicks away. But they are widely scattered, often in obscure journals and government reports, and frequently described using intimidating vocabulary. Much of this crucial information does not appear in books for public health students or in trainings for public health workers.

This book is an attempt to synthesize the public health science of today's leading causes of death and disability. It is meant to lay a foundation of concepts and vocabulary for these health problems—a foundation upon which public health strategies can be built. It is directed toward students and practitioners of public health who may have either very much or little biomedical training and who may be working (or plan to work) either in the United States or overseas. It is my hope that this attempt to refocus on the science of public health will help practitioners do better what they already do—protect large numbers of people from avoidable illness and needless death.

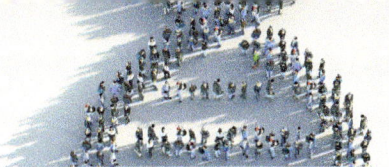

Learning and Teaching Resources

Instructor Resources

Qualified instructors can receive the full suite of Instructor Resources, including the following:

- Slides in PowerPoint format
- Test Bank, including in LMS-compatible formats
- Instructor Manual
- Case Studies
- Image Bank

Student Resources

Each new purchase of the print textbook or Navigate Advantage course includes:

- Navigate eBook chapter review slides, animations, and interactive glossary
- Flashcards

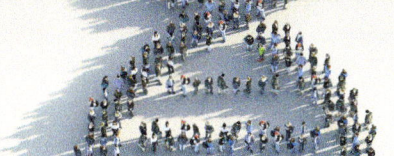

Acknowledgments

The author thanks the many experts who reviewed and gave helpful comments on early versions of chapter sections, including Jay Varma (HIV infection), Matthew Ippolito (malaria), Tom Frieden (tuberculosis), Adam Karpati (mental illnesses and use of addictive drugs), Matthew Freeman (diarrheal diseases), and Jennyfer Wolf (diarrheal diseases and lower respiratory infections).

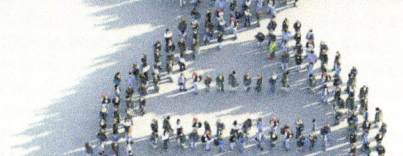

Reviewers

Oyindamola Akinso, DrPH, MPH, MCHES®
Assistant Professor
Wingate University

Hilary Aquino, PhD
Assistant Professor
Albright College

Nesta Bortey Sam, PhD
Assistant Professor
University of Pittsburgh

Stefanie G. Brown, DHA, MS
Dean, Health Sciences
Orangeburg-Calhoun Technical College

Jessica Camp, DNP, MSN, APRN, RN, AGCNS-BC, NE-BC, CDP
Assistant Professor
Arkansas State University

Kruti S. Chaliawala, PhD, MS, MA, CHES
Assistant Professor
Boise State University

Mark Dal Corso, MD, MPH
Clinical Associate Professor
Tulane University, Celia Scott Weatherhead School of Public Health & Tropical Medicine

Susan Dobson, MPH, CHES
Lecturer/Teaching Professor
University of Southern Mississippi

Amy Estlund, PhD, MPH
Associate Professor
Lindenwood University

Audrey Folsom, DHSc, MSHS, MLS (ASCP)
Assistant Professor of Clinical Lab Sciences
Arkansas State University

Kim Garcia, MEd, RRT-NPS
Senior Lecturer
The University of Texas Rio Grande Valley

Jake Goering, EdD, MPH, LNHA, LALD
Assistant Professor of Healthcare Leadership and Director of Long-Term Care Program
Concordia College – Moorhead, MN

Kelli J. Jones, PhD, RN
Clinical Assistant Professor
Marquette University

JoAnn L. Jordan, PhD, MPH, CHES
Department Chair
Franklin University

Alyssa Lee, MPH
Associate Professor
University of South Alabama

Ying Li, PhD
Professor
Western Washington University

Humberto López Castillo, MD, PhD, CPH, CMI-Spanish
Assistant Professor
Department of Health Sciences, University of Central Florida

Javier Lopez-Rios, PhD, MPH
Assistant Teaching Professor
Drexel University

Tawanda M. McNair, MSN, RN
Assistant Professor
The University of Mississippi Medical Center, School of Health Related Professions

Brittani Moberly, MBA, RHIA, CCS
Assistant Professor
Eastern Kentucky University

Wynette Mockler, DNP, MPH, RN
Instructor
University of South Dakota

Kim Mossburg, MS, RD, LDN, ATC
Senior Lecturer/Dietitian/Athletic Trainer
Indiana University Kokomo

Benito Moya, PhD, MPH, BAT-MHSM, LVN
Lecturer I
The University of Texas Rio Grande Valley

Vicki Perrine, RN, BSN, MBA, MHA, LNHA, FACHE
Assistant Professor
SUNY Canton

Jan Reichard-Brown, PhD
Associate Professor of Health Care Studies and
Biology
Susquehanna University

**Jason Robertson, DHSc, MPH, MS, MCHES, RHEd,
CPH, PAPHS, CCWS**
Associate Professor/Program Director, Public Health
and Health Science
Salem College

Andrea Rossin, CHES, MPH, EdD
Associate Professor
Winona State University

Lauren Savaglio, EdD, MS, EMT
Associate Teaching Professor, Degree Director
Arizona State University

**Peter Sayles, PhD - Immunology of Infectious
Diseases**
Professor Emeritus
North Country Community College

Mary Ellen R. Stewart, PhD, RN
Assistant Professor, Department Chair of Public
Health
Mississippi College

Lisa M. Taylor, DNP, RN, FNP-BC, CDCES, BC-ADM
Assistant Clinical Professor
University of New Mexico College of Nursing

Daniel D. White, PhD, MPH
Assistant Professor
Siena College

Michael Wiblishauser, PhD
Associate Professor of Health Studies
University of Houston-Victoria

Lisa M. Wisniewski, PhD
Assistant Professor
Saint Francis University

Shauna Zorich, MD, MPH
Clinical Assistant Professor
University at Buffalo

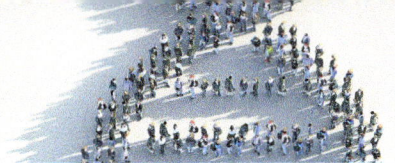

About the Author

Thomas A. Farley, MD, MPH has been a public health educator, researcher, and practitioner for more than three decades. He has served as a professor of public health and held positions in health agencies at the federal, state, and big city levels.

Dr. Farley is trained in pediatrics and in epidemiology, and he served on CDC's Epidemic Intelligence Service. In the Louisiana Office of Public Health, he led prevention programs for HIV/AIDS, other sexually transmitted diseases, tuberculosis, and vaccine-preventable diseases. At the Tulane University School of Public Health and Tropical Medicine, Dr. Farley was Professor and Chair of the Department of Community Health Sciences, where he focused on the promotion of physical activity, healthy eating, and the prevention of obesity. He served as Commissioner of Health for the New York City Department of Health and Mental Hygiene, where he led initiatives on obesity and smoking prevention. He later served as Commissioner of Health for the City of Philadelphia, where he directed efforts to address the crisis in opioid addiction and the COVID-19 pandemic. He was the Principal Senior Deputy Director for the Washington, D.C. Department of Health, where he focused on the health of children. Dr. Farley has authored or co-authored more than 100 peer-reviewed scientific publications, coauthored of *Prescription for a Healthy Nation,* and is the author of *Saving Gotham: A Billionaire Mayor, Activist Doctors, and the Fight for 8 Million Lives.* He is currently an Adjunct Professor at the Columbia University Mailman School of Public Health and an Adjunct Professor at the Celia Scott Weatherhead School of Public Health and Tropical Medicine at Tulane University.

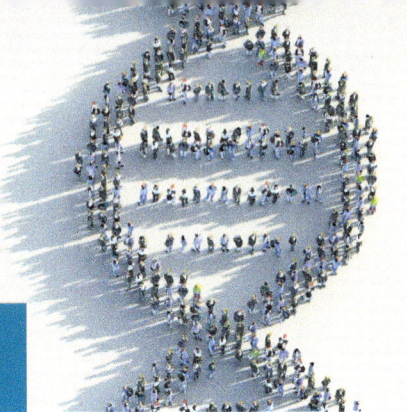

PART I

Public Health Strategy

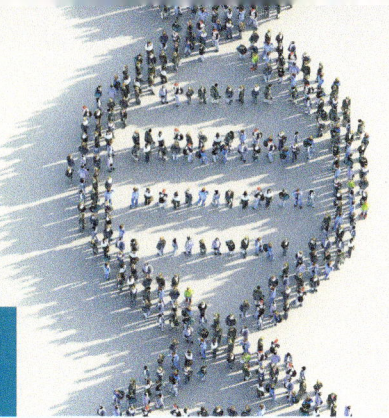

CHAPTER 1

Disease Prevention and Populations

"When a population is sick, it is a superficial and symptomatic response simply to treat the cases and the conspicuously vulnerable individuals; they represent the manifestation of the problem, not its roots. We need to ask why cases occur, and then to seek a remedy for their underlying determinants."

–Geoffrey Rose, The Strategy of Preventive Medicine

This book is based on three ideas. First, prevention of diseases is better than cure. Second, diseases can be prevented at the population level. And third, the best way to prevent diseases is with a strategy that first identifies and then eliminates or mitigates the underlying causes.

Why Prevention?

Preventing disease, when it is possible, is better than medical treatment because it avoids the suffering of illness. That is true for every disease, but it is especially meaningful for diseases that are not curable.

And prevention is often possible. While mortality rates have fallen dramatically in the past 100 years, there is still great potential for improvement. Humans do not vary much in their innate capability to live long and healthy lives, so when children in Zambia are nearly 10 times as likely as children in Uruguay to die before age 5, and when adults in Serbia are more than twice as likely as adults in Sweden to die of chronic diseases before age 70, most of those deaths must be preventable.[1]

Even in the United States, a relatively healthy country, the fraction of deaths that can be prevented is surprisingly large. The American Cancer Society estimates that 45% of cancer deaths are preventable by changes in just a few risk factors.[2] The Centers for Disease Control and Prevention (CDC) estimates that 25% of deaths from the five leading killers in America could be prevented if all U.S. states were only as healthy as the three healthiest ones.[3]

Another reason to focus on prevention is because our political systems typically do *not* focus on it. People suffering the symptoms of illness demand medical treatment. That demand, summed up across entire nations, creates a powerful political force. Our systems of government respond to that force by delivering medical care—roughly $5 trillion per year worth in the United States. People do not demand prevention in the same way. If more people understand the potential for prevention, though, maybe more will work to achieve it.

Opportunities for prevention appear at different stages of disease. **Primary prevention** involves reducing exposures or behaviors before any signs of disease appear, such as reducing air pollution or smoking, or vaccinating healthy persons. **Secondary prevention** involves detecting early signs of biologic damage and then taking actions to prevent diseases from progressing. Examples are treating high blood pressure to prevent stroke or removing polyps to prevent colon cancer. **Tertiary prevention** involves taking actions on persons who have already suffered an illness or injury to prevent additional illness or injuries from piling on. For example, treating a person who has had a stroke with anticoagulants to prevent a second stroke.

Health advocacy organizations often emphasize secondary prevention and tend to pay less attention to primary prevention. For example, breast cancer groups advocate for mammograms but speak much less about reducing the risk factors of obesity and alcohol use. This book will instead mostly emphasize primary prevention and will include discussions of secondary prevention only when it has the potential to reduce disease rates at the population level.

Why Populations?

Diseases can be understood at different levels of biologic organization, or how much you "zoom" in or out, from the sub-microscopic to the global level (**Figure 1.1**). An individual can be understood as sick because of sick **macromolecules**, such as having a DNA mutation or the faulty hemoglobin of sickle cell disease. Or because of sick **cells** or **tissues**, as in cancer cells growing in the colon. Or because of sick **organs** or **organ systems**, as in cirrhosis of the liver. Or because the individual's entire **organism** is sick, as in type 2 diabetes mellitus. But groups or populations can also be viewed as being sick, as in a village suffering from a cholera outbreak, or an entire nation struggling with extraordinarily high rates of drug overdose deaths. With the advent of global warming, sickness can even be assigned to entire **ecosystems** or the **biosphere**.

The field of medicine tends to measure its progress by understanding diseases at smaller and smaller levels. The field of public health looks for prevention opportunities at the level of groups and populations.

Groups and populations are not just collections of disconnected individuals. They each have their own characteristics—characteristics that can make individuals within the groups and populations more or less likely to become ill. Why?

First, groups and populations inhabit environments that can promote or prevent illness, regardless of the actions of individuals. For example, a group living in a refugee camp without sanitation will have high rates of diarrheal diseases, no matter how often individuals wash their hands. A population in a city with heavily polluted air will have high rates of heart and lung disease, no matter how motivated individual members are to stay healthy.

Second, for contagious diseases, the vulnerability of a group affects the risk of every individual within it. For example, tuberculosis is more common in low-income communities, increasing the risk even to individuals in those communities who do not themselves have low incomes. And measles outbreaks occur in populations when a high fraction of people within them are unvaccinated—posing a risk to both people who are vaccinated and those who are not.[4]

And third, people within groups and populations influence each other, in ways that establish **behavioral norms** that can increase or decrease everyone's

	Macromolecule	Cell or tissue	Organ or organ system	Organism	Group or population	Ecosystem or biosphere
Level of biologic organization	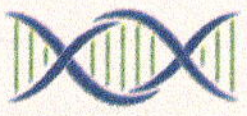 DNA	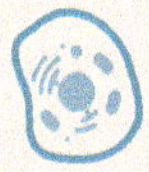 Human Cell	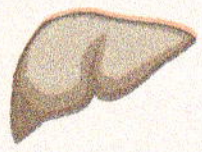 Liver	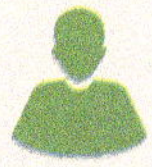 Person	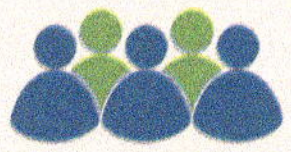 Group of people	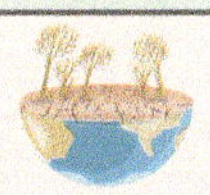 Region
Examples of disease	Sickle cell disease	Breast cancer	Liver cirrhosis	Type 2 diabetes	Cholera, drug overdose deaths	Injuries from severe weather events
Diagnostic tools	DNA probe, polymerase chain reaction test, biochemical test	Microscope	Medical imaging	Physical examination	Vital statistics, surveys, and other population datasets	Measures of the local or global ecosystem
Prevention tools	Gene therapy	Drugs	Surgery	Patient education and counseling	Policies, environmental change, information, and communication	Laws and international agreements

Figure 1.1 Levels of Biologic Organization and Disease Examples. Human diseases can be understood at many different levels of biologic organization. Here are examples of diseases, diagnostic tools, and prevention tools for diseases at each level.

disease risk. More than most of us are willing to admit, behavior itself is contagious. For example, smoking is more socially acceptable in France than in the United States, so an individual French person is more likely to take up smoking than an American.[5] During the COVID-19 pandemic, behavioral norms around wearing face masks varied markedly across regions of the United States and sometimes between urban and rural locations. The behavioral norms around mask-wearing of any community affected the mask-wearing behavior and thus the COVID-19 risk for every member.

Preventing disease at the population level is *not* the same as preventing it in individuals many times over. It represents a fundamentally different approach. That is because the risks for disease differ between the individual level and the population level. To an individual, the greatest risk of lung cancer is smoking, and the best way to prevent it is to quit. At the population level, key risks for lung cancer may be the marketing activities of tobacco companies, such as price discounts advertised behind the cash register, and the best ways to prevent it may be raising the price of a pack of cigarettes through taxes. The most important determinant of whether an individual dies of heart disease may be the foods that person chooses to eat, but the most important determinant of heart disease rates for a population may be the food options at neighborhood stores.

Population-level prevention takes advantage of what British epidemiologist Geoffrey Rose called the **prevention paradox**.[6] That is, the observation that a small change in the risk of disease of individuals, if broadly shared, can amount to a very large change in the disease rate of an entire population. For example, many years ago, researchers estimated that if every member of a population were to lower their blood pressure by only 5 mm Hg (through reducing the amount of sodium in food), it would prevent 22% of deaths from stroke—more than could be prevented by medical treatment of every member of that population who has hypertension.[7] A population-based approach to prevention seeks "nudges" like this; that is, interventions that may have small effects on individuals but lead to large reductions in population-level rates of disease.

In the media messages that we all consume today, prevention is usually framed as solely an individual choice. Advice on how you personally can eat right, stay fit, avoid catching COVID-19, and otherwise stay free of disease fills the "wellness" sections of news outlets and bookstores. This book will not recap that advice. Instead, it will focus on the actions that organizations or society can take to prevent disease in entire populations.

Why Do We Need a Strategy?

It is fair to ask why a strategy for prevention of specific diseases is needed. Isn't it enough to speak up about heart disease, HIV/AIDS, and breast cancer, figuring that whatever must be done to prevent them is either obvious or will be worked out by others?

Unfortunately, no. As the chapters in this book show, the actions to prevent our most important health problems are not obvious. And unless people put forward a clear prevention strategy, the gravitational pull will be toward medical care and research for cures.

While medical care has elements of prevention built into it, medicine is still fundamentally designed to give people treatment after they become sick. People seek medical care because they want relief from symptoms.[8] Because it typically occurs after the fact, medical care is about as effective at preventing diseases as automobile repair shops are at preventing car crashes—useful, but without much overall benefit.

Even when medical care has clear value in prevention, for example, in treatment of high blood pressure or early detection of colon cancer, many steps must take place to realize that value. Patients must get health insurance, schedule appointments, attend those appointments, undergo tests, and fill and take prescriptions. Healthcare providers must order tests, check the results, prescribe the correct treatments, and remind patients to return for follow-up visits. Each of those steps is a potential failure point, so the entire process fails frustratingly often. For example, despite enormous efforts by healthcare systems today, only about half of people with hypertension have their blood pressure adequately controlled.[9]

Also, a strategy is needed because even with the best thinking, public health initiatives often fail. When they fail, people must learn why so the approach can be revised. Without a clearly articulated strategy and a paired evaluation plan, no one can learn what went wrong.

Causes and Risk Factors

Any strategy for prevention at the population level involves first identifying what is causing disease. That raises the question of what we mean when we say something "causes" a disease.

With infectious diseases, the answer may seem obvious. Many people would state that SARS-CoV-2 causes COVID-19 and *Mycobacterium tuberculosis* causes tuberculosis. But what causes a heart attack? Clogged arteries or physical inactivity? Or, if a person who loses their romantic partner becomes depressed, drinks several shots of whiskey, finds a gun at home, and then shoot themselves, what caused their suicide? Was it losing their former partner, depression, alcohol, or the gun? Or the combination?

The most useful way to think about this is that *disease is caused by the presence of a combination of factors, each of which increases the risk of illness.* Epidemiologists refer to the combination of factors that produces a disease as a **sufficient cause** and the individual factors as **component causes** (**Figure 1.2**).[10] In the suicide example, availability of a gun would be considered a component cause. Alcohol consumption would be another component cause. The sufficient cause would be the combination of depression, alcohol consumption, availability of a gun, and many other risk factors that we are unaware of.

More than one combination of component causes can create sufficient causes. Suicide for this person has a sufficient cause of depression, alcohol consumption, and gun availability, but for another person, suicide might have a sufficient cause of schizophrenia, social isolation, and alcohol consumption. And one component cause (in these examples, alcohol consumption) can be part of more than one sufficient cause.

This book will refer to these component causes as **risk factors** (or sometimes using the synonym **determinants**). *A risk factor is a characteristic of an individual, group, or environment that increases the likelihood that a specific disease or injury will occur.* (If a factor makes a disease *less* likely to occur, it is called a **protective factor**.) For example, smoking is a risk factor for lung cancer, alcohol consumption is a risk factor for suicide, unprotected sex is a risk factor for HIV infection, and lack of vaccination is a risk factor for COVID-19. A risk factor is not just statistically associated with disease. For example, a habit of carrying matches is probably statistically associated with lung cancer, but match-carrying is not a risk factor for lung cancer; smoking is. Factors that are statistically associated with but do not cause disease are called **risk markers**. To be a risk factor, a characteristic must have a statistical association with disease and have a cause-and-effect relationship.

With this fuller understanding, it is not correct to state that SARS-CoV-2 causes COVID-19 or that *Mycobacterium tuberculosis* causes tuberculosis. Exposure to these pathogens certainly increases the likelihood that the diseases will occur, so these exposures are risk factors or component causes. But the chance that persons will develop these illnesses after these exposures also depends on other risk factors,

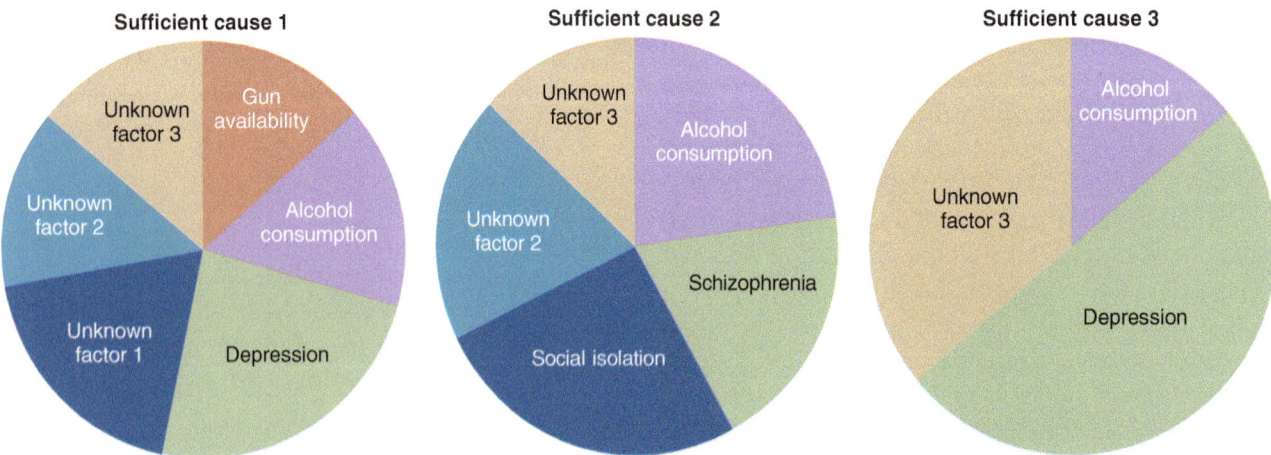

Figure 1.2 Sufficient Causes and Component Causes for Disease, Using Example of Suicide. Diseases result from a combination of several factors coming together in one person. Each individual factor that increases the risk of disease is called a component cause. The combination of component causes that results in disease is called a sufficient cause. There may be many sufficient causes. The example above shows three different sufficient causes for suicide. The combination of alcohol consumption, gun availability, depression, and three unknown factors makes up sufficient cause 1. Other component causes (some known, some unknown) make up sufficient cause 2 and 3. Individual component causes may appear in more than one sufficient cause. For example, the component cause of alcohol consumption appears in all three of these sufficient causes. This book will refer to component causes as risk factors.

like their age, whether they have chronic illnesses or deficient immune systems, whether they have been vaccinated, the amount of ventilation in the site where they are exposed, and poverty. That means that these diseases can be prevented either by reducing exposure to the pathogens or by mitigating these other risk factors.

Some risk factors are well known. For example, risk factors for heart attacks include smoking, an unhealthy diet, and physical inactivity. Risk factors for suicide include social isolation, depression, and access to guns. Many risk factors, though, will be discovered in the future or may never be known. That should not stop us from preventing disease today, though. There are many opportunities to prevent major causes of death by mitigating risk factors that are already known.

The chapters in this book show our current understanding of risk factors for selected diseases with cause-and-effect diagrams like that in **Figure 1.3**. A potential risk factor is included in these diagrams if most experts would consider it to be a risk factor (and not just a risk marker), and if it is *modifiable*—that is, the risk factor can be eliminated or mitigated—in theory, even if not easily in practice. Demographic risk factors like age, race, sex, and genetic factors may be strongly linked to disease and have a cause-and-effect relationship, but they are not modifiable, so they are not included. On the other hand, exposure to mosquitos, risky sexual behavior, and unhealthy diets are modifiable, so they are included.

Risk factors can exert their effect on disease risk directly or indirectly—that is, through other risk factors (as in Risk Factor 1 in Figure 1.3). Their impact may be through a gradual accumulation of damage over years (for example, red meat consumption leading to colon cancer) or through a sudden event

(e.g., failure to wear a seatbelt at the time of a crash). Some risk factors matter only when other risk factors are present (e. g., lack of vaccination posing a risk only to persons exposed to an infectious agent). Some risk factors (like Risk Factors 3, 4, 5, and 6 in Figure 1.3) initiate a disease process, and others (like Risk Factor 7 in Figure 1.3) take that process to completion.

Risk factors can be classified as metabolic (such as high blood pressure, high blood cholesterol, or obesity), behavioral (such as smoking or physical inactivity), or environmental (such as air pollution or occupational hazards). **Metabolic risk factors** may be very important to doctors treating patients, but they cannot be changed directly at the population level. **Behavioral risk factors** cannot be changed directly at the population level but can be influenced by policies and rules, such as smoke-free air laws. **Environmental risk factors**, on the other hand, can be changed directly at the population level, for example, reducing air pollution.

Some risk factors cause many diseases. For example, alcohol consumption is a risk factor for liver disease, colon cancer, and falls, among many other health problems. Smoking is a risk factor for a large fraction of the diseases in this book. Prevention strategies can be built for these common risk factors too. Part II of this book covers specific diseases and Part III covers the most important common risk factors.

Social disadvantage—particularly poverty or membership in a racial group that has experienced discrimination—is distinct because it is a risk factor for nearly all diseases. The impact of social disadvantage on health is deep, complex and not fully understood, but it is very important to the health of populations. This broad risk factor and the **social determinants of health** are discussed later in this book in Chapter 16.

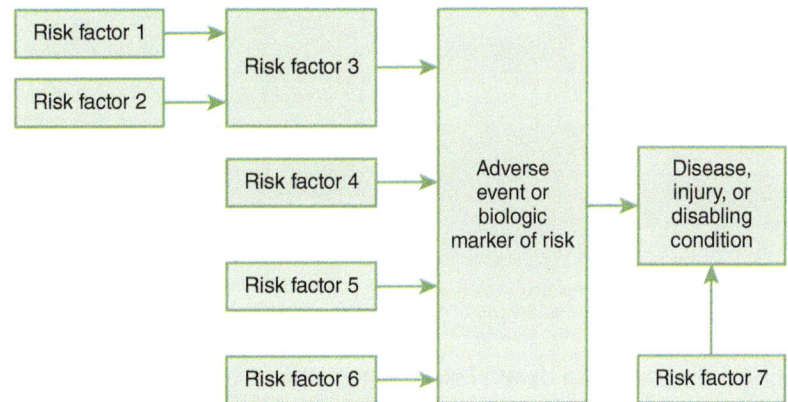

Figure 1.3 Cause-and-Effect Diagram for a Health Problem. Diseases are caused not by a single exposure or event, but instead by a combination of risk factors that relate to each other and to the disease in webs and chains.

Deciding what risk factors to include in the cause-and-effect diagrams requires judgement. No two experts will completely agree on which risk factors to include, whether to lump or split potential risk factors, the labels to use for risk factors, or the structure of the diagrams. The risk factors and diagrams that are included in this book represent the author's attempt to fairly represent today's scientific knowledge. In the future, as knowledge grows, the lists and diagrams can be revised.

Preventive Interventions and Strategies

Once risk factors are established, the job of public health workers is to develop, test, implement, and evaluate preventive **interventions**, that is, actions that either eliminate, reduce the frequency of, or otherwise mitigate risk factors (**Figure 1.4**). Interventions to prevent disease can involve the following:

- *Environmental change*, in which the "environment" is defined very broadly. Examples include improvements in ventilation, greater access to healthy food, and provision of clean water and sanitation.
- *Policies*, that is, rules that prohibit, allow, discourage, or encourage actions of individuals or organizations. Examples include mask mandates during the COVID-19 pandemic, smoke-free air policies, and tobacco taxes.

- *Information, education, and communication*, that is, distributing information in a way that may reduce unhealthy behaviors or exposures.
- *Programs*, which involve delivery of services to members of a population. Examples include vaccination, Vitamin A supplementation, and screen-and-treat programs for high blood pressure.

Programs can accomplish either primary prevention (e.g., vaccination), or secondary prevention (e. g., treatment of high blood pressure). In Figure 1.4, Intervention 5 is designed for primary prevention of Risk Factor 5, but Intervention 8 is designed for secondary prevention by treating an adverse event or biologic marker of risk.

Public health strategies represent combinations of preventive interventions, interrupting the chain of cause-and-effect in as many places as possible. The big public health problems are big because they are difficult to prevent, so no opportunity for prevention should be overlooked. For example, prevention of malaria involves disruption of mosquito breeding sites *and* insecticide-treated bed nets *and* preventive use of antimalarial drugs. Likewise, prevention of injuries from motor vehicle crashes involves safer cars *and* safer roadways *and* reduction in alcohol use *and* mandatory seat belt laws.

Some preventive interventions may be very difficult to put in place for some populations due to practical, financial, or political reasons. It may be nearly impossible today to prevent malaria in East Africa by building mosquito-proof housing or car crashes in

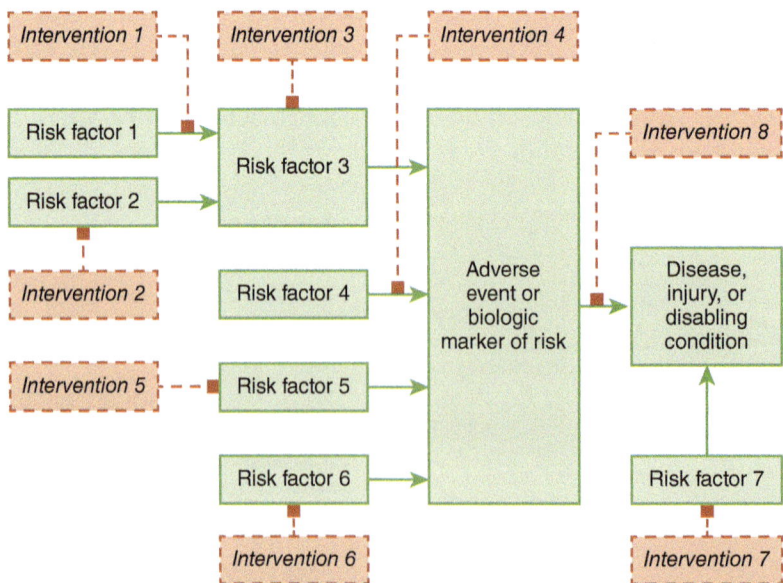

Figure 1.4 Cause-and-Effect Diagram for a Health Problem, with Preventive Interventions. Preventive interventions can be designed to eliminate, reduce the frequency of, or mitigate risk factors. They can accomplish primary prevention (for example, Intervention 5 eliminating Risk Factor 5) or secondary prevention (for example, Intervention 8, which prevents a disease or injury by treating an adverse event or biologic marker of risk).

the United States by raising the liquor tax. But interventions that may be impossible in one population may be embraced in another. As the world changes; with those changes, ideas can quickly change from unthinkable to inevitable. (Even tobacco-growing North Carolina now has smoke-free restaurants.) Instead of choosing interventions based on their feasibility in any specific place or time, this book provides a menu of options for preventive interventions, allowing others to decide which are politically or practically feasible.

What Health Problems Should We Prevent?

Preventing diseases in populations requires time, money and political will, all of which are in short supply. People working in public health are usually forced to choose which health problems they can take on. Too often, these choices are based solely on political pressures, tradition or inertia. But more lives can be saved and more suffering prevented if priorities were instead based on the problems creating the greatest health burden.

The list of major health problems includes diseases (like HIV/AIDS or lung cancer), injuries (like firearm suicides or motor vehicle crashes), and disabling conditions (like arthritis or low back pain). For simplicity, this book will often refer to all of these as "diseases." Ideally, these diverse health problems should be ranked in their public health burden using a common metric.

The Global Burden of Disease project involves a large collaboration of epidemiologists who create estimates of disease burden globally and for each nation in the world.[13] Because data often are missing, their estimates have plenty of uncertainty, but they are the best available sources of data to rank public health problems around the globe. (The experts continually refine their methods, so the numbers that they publish change periodically.)

The simplest measure of public health burden of a disease on a population is the number of deaths that disease causes—the **mortality**. For comparison of populations of different sizes, this is usually divided by the number of people in the population, producing the **mortality rate** (**Table 1.1**). **Figure 1.5** shows estimates by the Global Burden of Disease group for the 15 diseases with highest mortality rates worldwide. The most recent year available for these estimates as of this writing are for 2021, in the middle of the COVID-19 pandemic. By this metric, other than COVID-19, the leading public health problems are chronic diseases, like ischemic heart disease, stroke, chronic obstructive pulmonary disease, and cancers.

As a way to rank health problems, the mortality rate has a disadvantage of assigning equal importance to deaths that occur in younger and older people. Most of us feel that more is lost when someone dies at age 25 than at age 80.

A metric designed to address this weakness is the **years of (potential) life lost**, usually abbreviated **YLL**. This measure accounts for the age at which each death occurs (Table 1.1). For example, if optimal life expectancy were 92 years of age, then a person dying at age 25 would lose 67 years of life, while a person dying at age 80 would lose only 12. To compare populations, YLL is also usually divided by the size of the population to produce a **YLL rate**.

Estimates of the top 15 causes of years of life lost worldwide are in **Figure 1.6**. The leading causes of YLL are similar to the leading causes of mortality, with (after COVID-19) ischemic heart disease and stroke still at the top. But lower respiratory infections and neonatal disorders—health problems related to low birth weight and prematurity—rank among them. Also appearing on the list are other major infectious diseases, including malaria, tuberculosis, and HIV/AIDS, which often lead to the deaths of children or younger adults. And road injuries, which tend to kill younger people, rise in these rankings.

If these graphs are limited to the United States, the rankings change, but not by as much as many people would think.

What about diseases that do not kill people directly but instead cause people to suffer—like depression? For these, the experts have developed another metric called the **Disability-Adjusted Life Years (DALYs)** lost (Table 1.1). This metric includes not just how many years of life are lost by premature death but also the years of suffering these diseases cause, assigning a "disability weight" to each disease. This is the best available measure of disease burden that combines **morbidity** (the suffering from nonfatal diseases) with mortality. Like the other measures, it is usually divided by the population size to compare populations.

The top causes of DALYs lost, worldwide and in the United States, are in Figures 1.7 and 1.8. Appearing in these rankings are mental illnesses like depressive disorders and anxiety. Also appearing on the list are some common disabling conditions, including low back pain and osteoarthritis.

Table 1.1 Metrics to Measure the Health Burden of Diseases In Populations

The impact of a disease on a population can be expressed using different metrics. Three metrics that will be used in this book are mortality, years of life lost (YLL), and Disability-Adjusted Life Years (DALYs). Each metric has its strengths and weaknesses.

Metric	Mortality	Years of Life Lost (YLLs)	Disability-Adjusted Life Years (DALYs)
Calculation	The number of deaths in a population	Life expectancy minus age of death, summed across all deaths in a population	The sum of YLLs and years lived with disability, where years lived with disability is the prevalence of a disabling condition multiplied by the disability weight for that condition
Strengths	■ Simple to calculate; intuitive; easy to communicate	■ Gives more weight to diseases that kill younger people	■ Gives more weight to diseases that kill younger people ■ Includes diseases that cause disability but not death
Weaknesses	■ Gives equal weight to the deaths in young and old persons ■ Does not consider diseases that cause disability but not death	■ Difficult to calculate ■ Less intuitive; harder to communicate ■ Does not consider diseases that cause disability but not death	■ Depends on disability weights, which are subjective and may vary between populations ■ Very difficult to calculate ■ Not intuitive; difficult to communicate

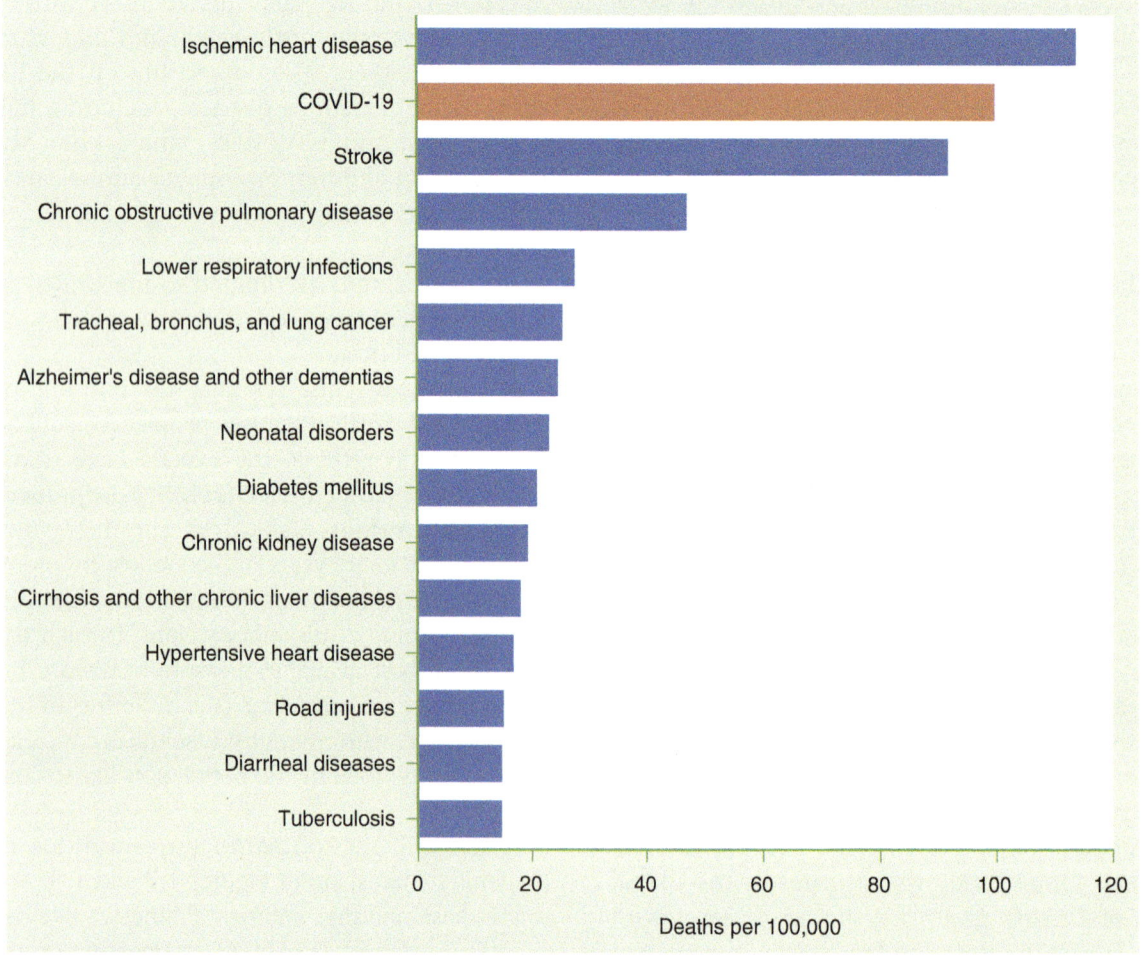

Figure 1.5 Leading Causes of Mortality Worldwide, 2021.

Data from Global Burden of Disease Collaboration. Global Burden of Disease tool - GBD Results. Published 2024. Accessed August 7, 2024. https://vizhub.healthdata.org/gbd-results

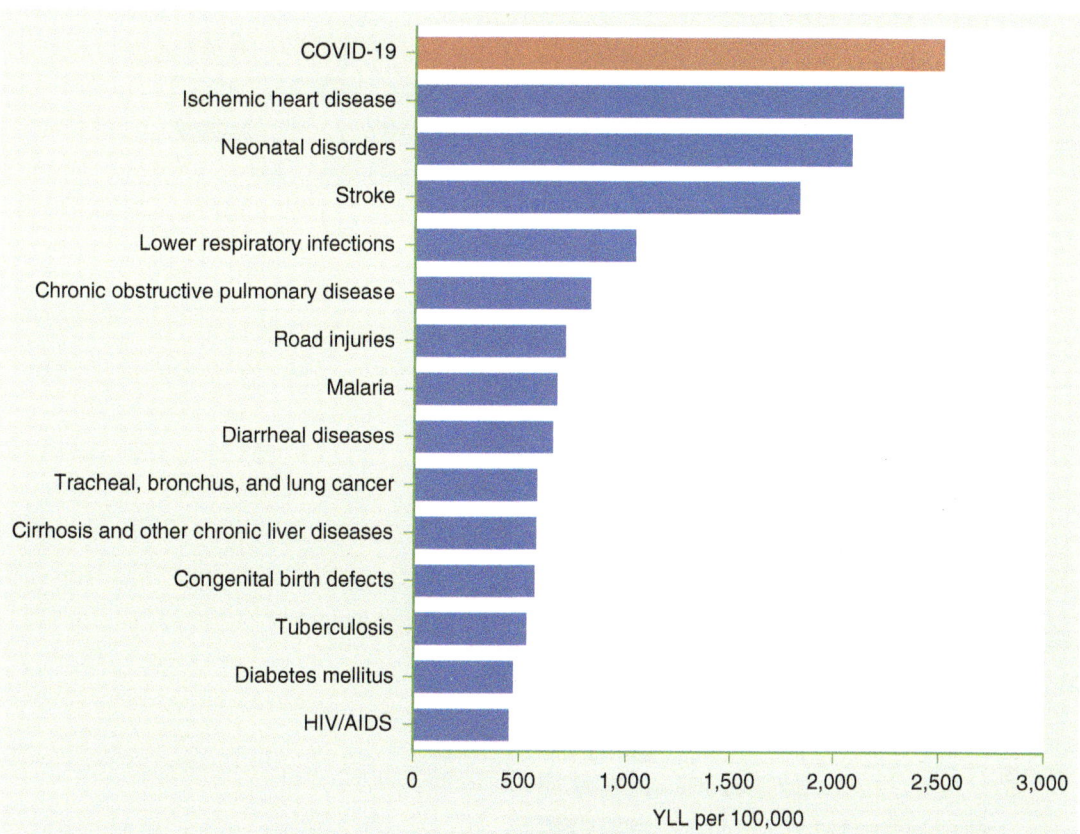

Figure 1.6 Leading Causes of Years of Life Lost (YLL) Worldwide, 2021.

Data from Global Burden of Disease Collaboration. Global Burden of Disease tool - GBD Results. Published 2024. Accessed August 7, 2024. https://vizhub.healthdata.org/gbd-results

There are a few key differences between **Figure 1.7** and **Figure 1.8**. Neonatal disorders appear near the top of the global graph but are low on the U.S. graph. Diarrheal diseases, malaria, and tuberculosis are in the middle of the global graph but do not appear on the U.S. graph. Otherwise, there is a large overlap between the biggest public health problems in the United States and globally. The overlap is mainly in **non-communicable diseases** (NCDs), in particular, heart disease, stroke, cancer, chronic respiratory disease, and diabetes. According to the World Health Organization, NCDs grew from causing 47% of DALYs globally in 2000 to 63% in 2019.[1] Increasingly, then, the issues faced by those working in global health and U.S. health are the same.

Public health programs are often organized not on diseases by instead on common risk factors, like smoking or obesity. How can these risk factors be ranked in public health importance?

The Global Burden of Disease group also estimates how many deaths, YLL, and DALYs are caused by common risk factors. These are called **attributable risk** calculations. They are mathematically designed to estimate how many deaths, YLL, or DALYs would not occur if the risk factors were not present at all. The calculations for attributable risk are complex and incorporate a great deal of uncertainty, so the numbers they generate should never be considered anything close to precise, but they are still useful in ranking risk factors. The risk factors to which the Global Burden of Disease experts attribute the most DALYs are shown in **Figure 1.9** and **Figure 1.10**. In the United States, the most important behavioral risk factors are tobacco use, dietary risks, drug use, and alcohol use, in that order. (Metabolic risk factors are shown in light blue.) Globally, the most important risk factors are child and maternal undernutrition, air pollution, tobacco use, and dietary risks, with alcohol use not far behind.

These graphs are the basis for the table of contents of this book. The ranking of the diseases causing the most DALYs lost in the United States and globally (Figure 1.7 and Figure 1.8) guided the diseases covered in Part II, and the ranking of risk factors causing the most DALYs lost in the United States and globally (Figures 1.9 and 1.10) guided the risk factors covered in Part III. To prevent the greatest amount of avoidable illness, rankings like these should also guide people in setting priorities for public health initiatives.

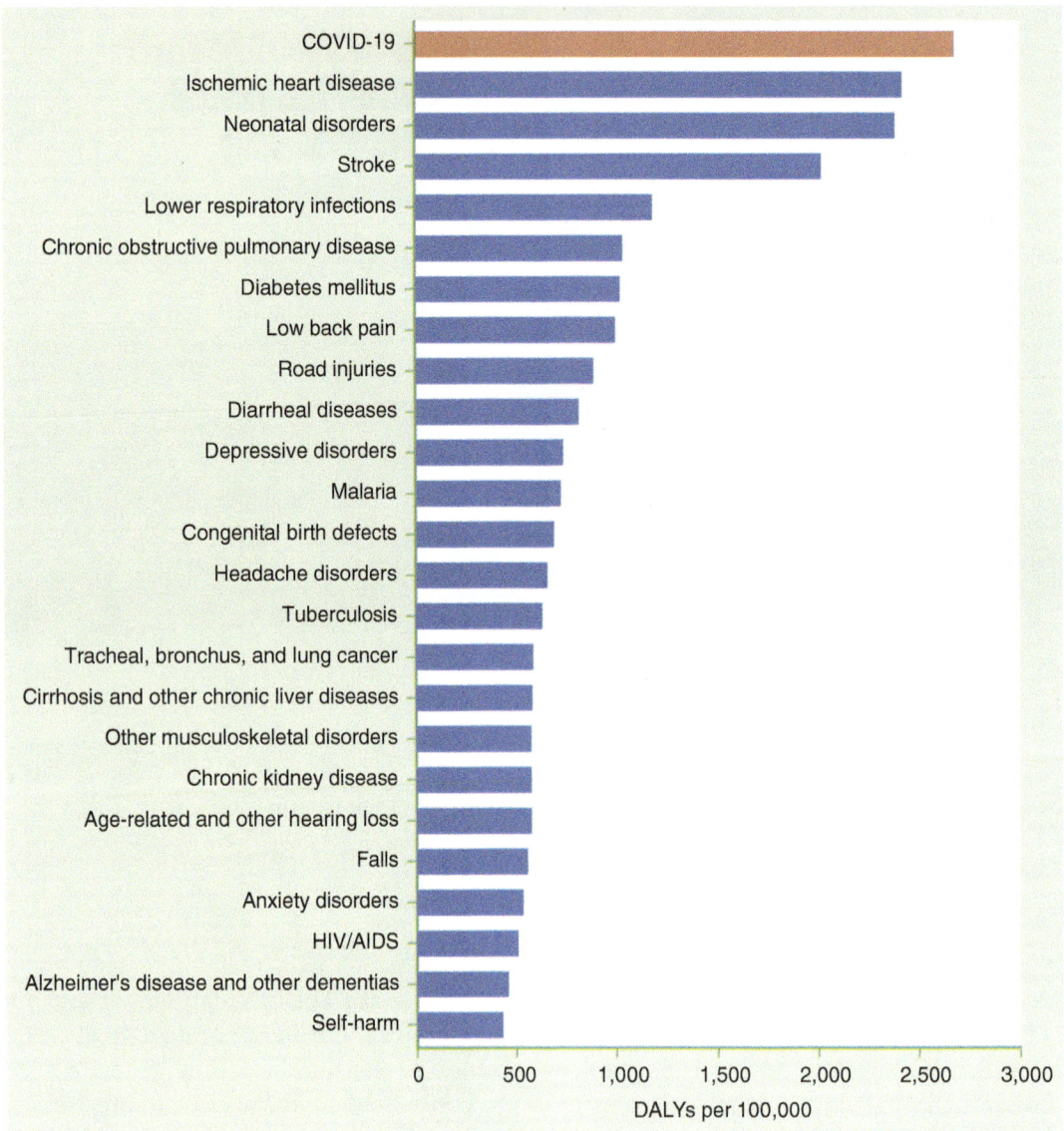

Figure 1.7 Leading Causes of DALYs Lost Worldwide, 2021.

Data from Global Burden of Disease Collaboration. Global Burden of Disease tool - GBD Results. Published 2024. Accessed August 7, 2024. https://vizhub.healthdata.org/gbd-results

---

Box 1.1 Key Words–Disease Prevention and Populations

Attributable risk
Behavioral norm
Behavioral risk factor
Biosphere
Cell
Component cause
Determinant
Disability-adjusted life years (DALYs)
Ecosystem
Environmental risk factor
Intervention
Macromolecule
Metabolic risk factor
Morbidity
Mortality
Mortality rate

Non-communicable disease
Organ
Organ system
Organism
Prevention paradox
Primary prevention
Protective factor
Risk factor
Risk marker
Secondary prevention
Social determinants of health
Sufficient cause
Tertiary prevention
Tissue
Years of (potential) life lost (YLL)
YLL rate

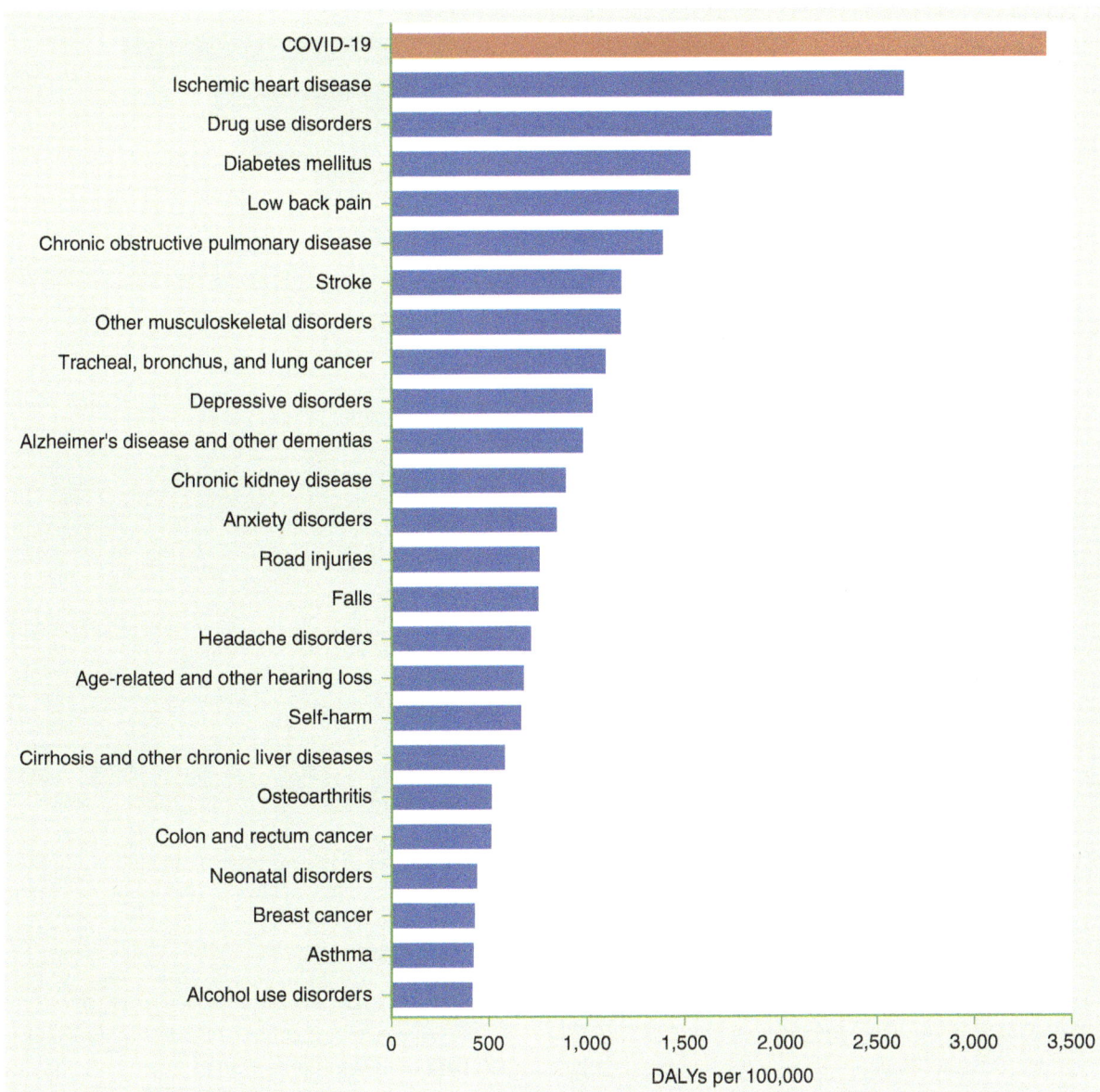

Figure 1.8 **Leading Causes of DALYs Lost in the United States, 2021.**

Data from Global Burden of Disease Collaboration. Global Burden of Disease tool - GBD Results. Published 2024. Accessed August 7, 2024. https://vizhub.healthdata.org/gbd-results

Resources—Disease Prevention and Populations

- Islami F, Goding Sauer A, Miller KD, et al. Proportion and number of cancer cases and deaths attributable to potentially modifiable risk factors in the United States. *CA Cancer J Clin.* 2018;68(1). doi:10.3322/caac.21440. Estimates of the potential for primary prevention of cancer by experts at the American Cancer Society.
- García MC, Bastian B, Rossen LM, et al. Potentially Preventable Deaths Among the Five Leading Causes of Death—United States, 2010 and 2014. *MMWR Morb Mortal Wkly Rep.* 2016;65(45). doi:10.15585/mmwr.mm6545a1. This paper shows

one way to estimate the potential for disease prevention in the United States.

- Institute for Health Metrics and Evaluation. Global Burden of Disease. www.healthdata.org. This website provides detailed estimates of disease patterns and trends at the global and national level, together with a rich set of tools to analyze and display these patterns and trends.
- Rose G. *The Strategy of Preventive Medicine.* Oxford: Oxford University Press; 1992. This classic book explains the prevention paradox, the difference between sick individuals and sick populations, and the concept of population-based approaches to prevention.

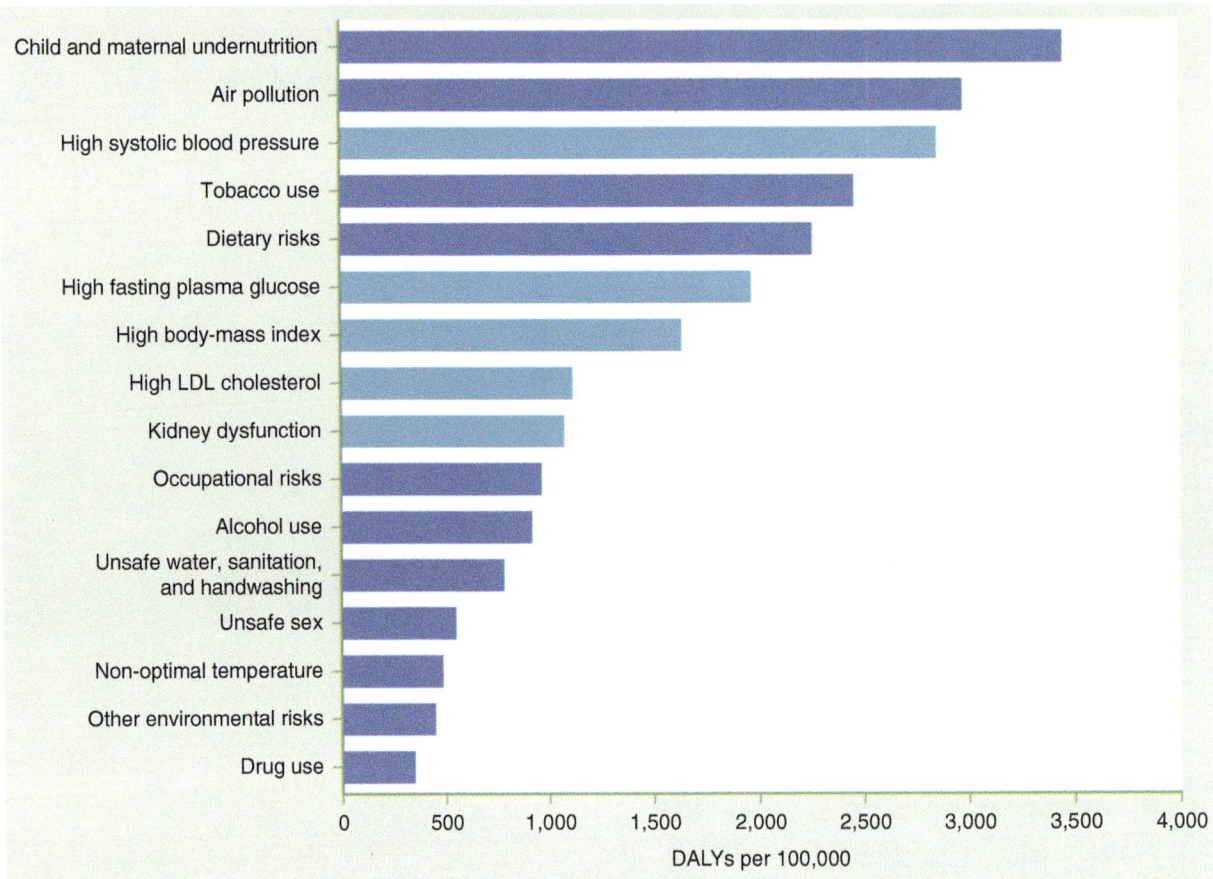

Figure 1.9 **Leading Risk Factors for DALYs Lost Worldwide, 2021.** Estimates of the number of disability-adjusted life years lost (per 100,000 persons) attributable to the leading risk factors for disease worldwide. Metabolic risk factors are in light blue; behavioral and environmental risk factors are in dark blue.

Data from Global Burden of Disease Collaboration. Global Burden of Disease tool - GBD Results. Published 2024. Accessed August 7, 2024. https://vizhub.healthdata.org/gbd-results

- Farley T, Cohen DA. *Prescription for a Healthy Nation*. Boston: Beacon Press; 2005. This book presents to general readers the rationale for population-based disease prevention, as well as environmental or structural approaches to prevention.
- World Health Organization. *World Health Statistics 2023: Monitoring Health for the SDGs Sustainable Development Goals*. http://www.who.int/publications. This is an annual compilation of global health and health-related indicators.
- World Health Organization. Global Health Estimates. https://www.who.int/data/global-health-estimates. This provides estimates of global, regional, and national health trends.

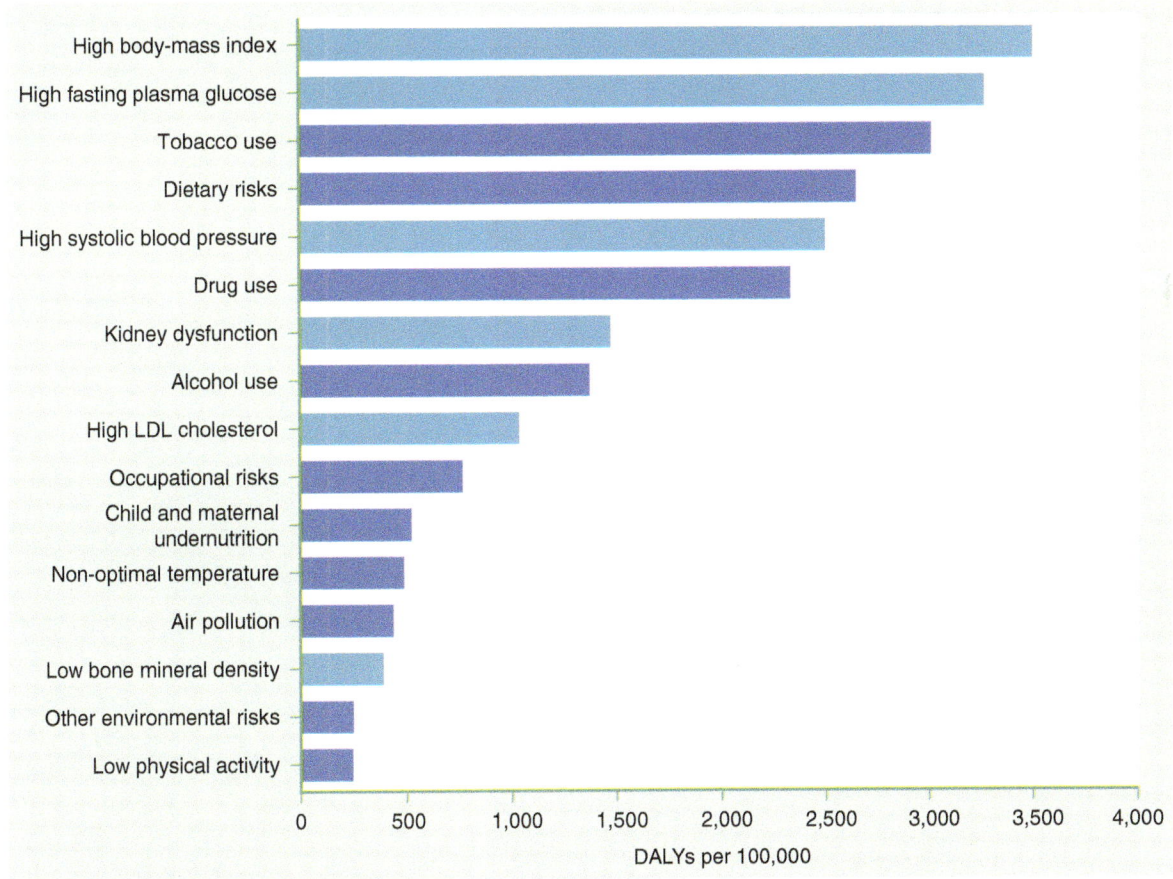

Figure 1.10 Leading Risk Factors for DALYs Lost in the United States, 2021. Estimates of the number of disability-adjusted life years lost (per 100,000 persons) attributable to the leading risk factors for disease in the United States. Metabolic risk factors are in light blue; behavioral and environmental risk factors are in dark blue.

Data from Global Burden of Disease Collaboration. Global Burden of Disease tool - GBD Results. Published 2024. Accessed August 7, 2024. https://vizhub.healthdata.org/gbd-results

References

1. World Health Organization. *World Health Statistics 2023: Monitoring Health for the SDGs, Sustainable Development Goals.* Geneva; 2023. Accessed July 23, 2024. Available at: https://www.who.int/publications/i/item/9789240074323

2. Islami F, Goding Sauer A, Miller KD, et al. Proportion and number of cancer cases and deaths attributable to potentially modifiable risk factors in the United States. *CA Cancer J Clin.* 2018;68:31-54. doi:10.3322/caac.21440

3. García MC, Bastian B, Rossen LM, et al. Potentially Preventable Deaths Among the Five Leading Causes of Death—United States, 2010 and 2014. *MMWR Morb Mortal Wkly Rep.* 2016;65(45):1245-1255. doi:10.15585/mmwr.mm6545a1

4. Phadke VK, Bednarczyk RA, Salmon DA, Omer SB. Association between vaccine refusal and vaccine-preventable diseases in the United States: A review of measles and pertussis. *JAMA - Journal of the American Medical Association.* 2016;315(11):1149-1158. doi:10.1001/jama.2016.1353

5. World Health Organization. Noncommunicable Diseases Data Portal. NCD Data Portal. Published 2023. Accessed July 23, 2023. https://ncdportal.org

6. Rose G. Sick individuals and sick populations. *Int J Epidemiol.* 2001;30:427-432.

7. Law MR, Frost CD, Wald NJ. By how much does dietary salt reduction lower blood pressure? III—Analysis of data from trials of salt reduction. *BMJ.* 1991;302(6780):819-824. doi:10.1136/bmj.302.6780.819

8. Liss DT, Uchida T, Wilkes CL, Radakrishnan A, Linder JA. General Health Checks in Adult Primary Care: A Review. *JAMA.* 2021;325(22):2294-2306. doi:10.1001/jama.2021.6524

9. Muntner P, Miles MA, Jaeger BC, et al. Blood pressure control among US adults, 2009 to 2012 through 2017 to 2020. *Hypertension.* 2022;79(9):1971-1980. doi:10.1161/HYPERTENSIONAHA.122.19222

10. Rothman KJ, Greenland S. Causation and causal inference in epidemiology. *Am J Public Health.* 2005;95(Suppl 1):S144-S150. doi:10.2105/AJPH.2004.059204

11. Bradford Hill A. The environment and disease: association or causation? *Proc R Soc Med.* 1965;58:295-300.

12. Office of Assistant Secretary for Health. Social Determinants of Health. *Healthy People 2030.* Published 2023. Accessed October 3, 2024. Available at: https://health.gov/healthypeople/priority-areas/social-determinants-health

13. Institute for Health Metrics and Evaluation. Global Burden of Disease. *Global Burden of Disease.* Published 2024. Accessed August 6, 2024. Available at: https://vizhub.healthdata.org/gbd-results/

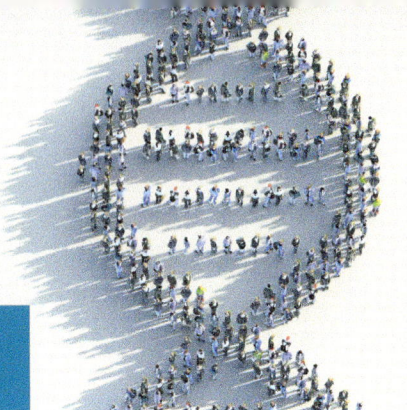

PART II

Diseases, Injuries, and Disabling Conditions

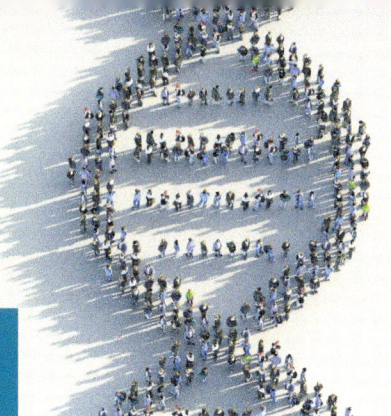

CHAPTER 2

Heart Disease and Stroke

Heart disease is the number one killer of humans, and **stroke**, which causes damage to the brain, is not far behind.[1] This is true not just in the United States, and not just in the world as a whole, but also in most individual countries in the world.[1] Of course, everyone dies eventually, and when they die their hearts stop beating, but the major types of heart disease are not inevitable features of aging. They are preventable by changing just a few well-established risk factors. This chapter covers the two most common types of heart disease and stroke. First, we will present an overview and definitions of some key terms.

The Cardiovascular System

The heart and the blood vessels make up the **cardiovascular** system (**Figure 2.1**). The heart pumps blood through the blood vessels. The blood vessels distribute blood containing oxygen and nutrients to tissues throughout the body and then return blood containing carbon dioxide to the lungs and the waste products of metabolism to the kidneys.

The cardiovascular system is composed of two connected circuits. The left side of the heart pushes blood full of oxygen through **arteries** in the **systemic circuit** to most of the body's organs and tissues; that blood is returned to the right side of the heart through **veins**. The right side of the heart pushes blood low in oxygen through **pulmonary arteries** in the **pulmonary circuit** to the lungs, where the blood picks up oxygen. That blood is then returned to the left side of the heart through the **pulmonary veins**.

Overview of Ischemic and Hypertensive Cardiovascular Disease

Diseases frequently involve both the heart and the blood vessels, so they are often grouped as **cardiovascular disease**. The two responsible for the most deaths are **ischemic cardiovascular disease** and **hypertensive cardiovascular disease**.

For blood to flow into tissues, the arteries maintain a **blood pressure**—the force of blood pressing against the arteries' walls—within a certain range. If the pressure in an artery is too low, blood will not flow into tissues and those tissues will be damaged from lack of oxygen. That condition is called **ischemia**. When this happens in arteries supplying blood to the heart muscle itself, it is called **ischemic heart disease**. When this happens in the brain it causes an **ischemic stroke** (**Figure 2.2**). Either of these conditions qualifies as ischemic cardiovascular disease.

If the blood pressure is too high, the condition is called **hypertension**. Hypertension can cause an artery to burst, spilling blood into tissues and shutting off the oxygen supply to those tissues. The leaking of blood is called a **hemorrhage**. When an artery supplying the brain bursts, it causes a **hemorrhagic stroke** (Figure 2.2). Over many years, hypertension puts a strain on the heart, which weakens it in what is called **hypertensive heart disease** or **hypertensive cardiovascular disease**.

These types of heart disease and stroke are caused by a group of risk factors that are intertwined, so the

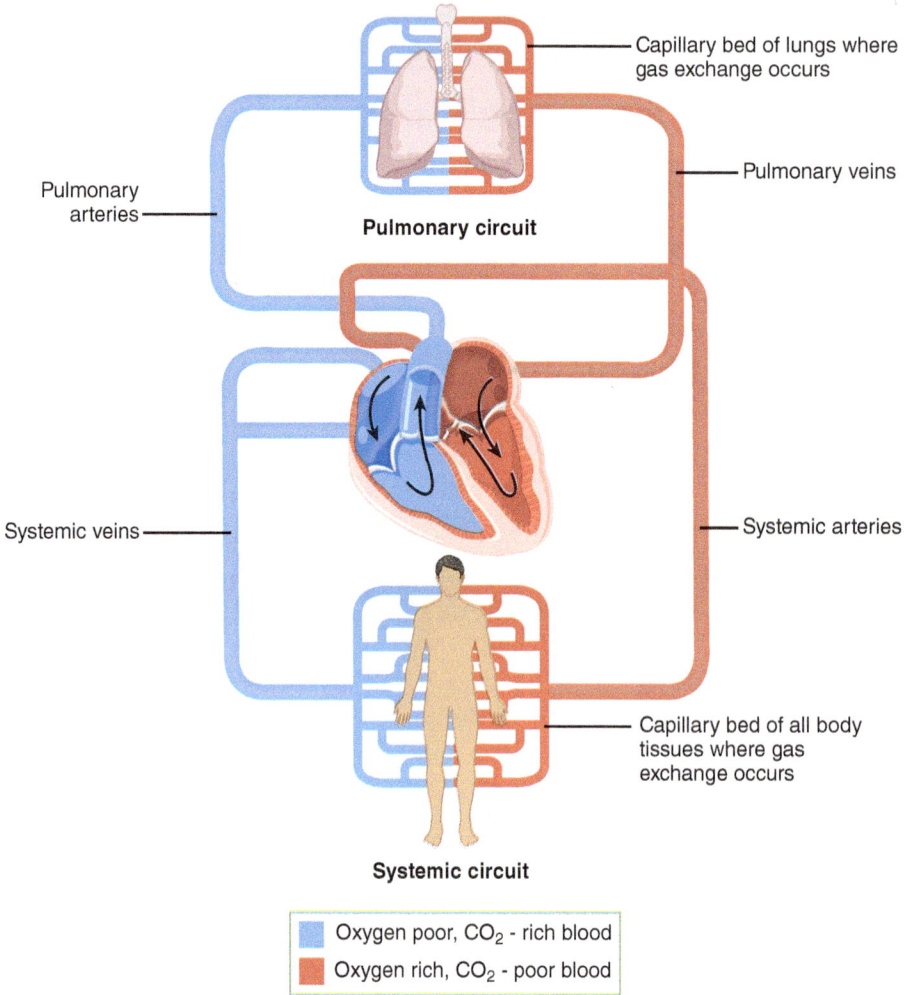

Capillary bed of lungs where gas exchange occurs

Pulmonary veins

Pulmonary arteries

Pulmonary circuit

Systemic veins

Systemic arteries

Capillary bed of all body tissues where gas exchange occurs

Systemic circuit

■ Oxygen poor, CO_2 - rich blood
■ Oxygen rich, CO_2 - poor blood

Figure 2.1 The Cardiovascular System. The cardiovascular system is composed of two connected circuits: the systemic circuit, which supplies oxygen to most of the body's organs, and the pulmonary circuit, which moves blood through the lungs to pick up oxygen.

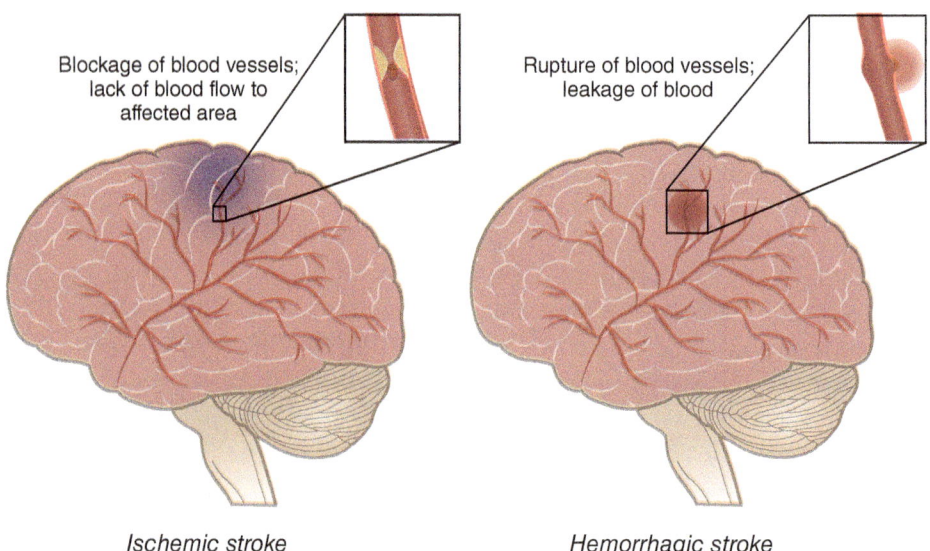

Blockage of blood vessels; lack of blood flow to affected area

Rupture of blood vessels; leakage of blood

Ischemic stroke

Hemorrhagic stroke

Figure 2.2 Ischemic Stroke vs. Hemorrhagic Stroke. A stroke is a sudden loss of brain function due to an interruption in the supply of oxygen and other nutrients to brain tissue. There are two main types of strokes. In an ischemic stroke, an artery supplying the brain becomes narrowed or obstructed, interrupting blood flow. In a hemorrhagic stroke, an artery supplying the brain ruptures, spilling blood into tissues and shutting off the oxygen supply to those tissues.

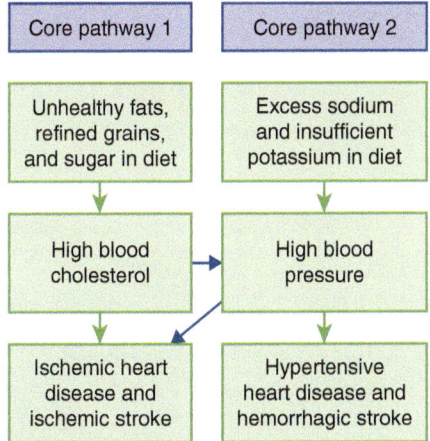

Figure 2.3 Core Pathways Leading to Heart Disease and Stroke. Cardiovascular disease can occur through two core pathways, one involving high blood cholesterol, ischemic heart disease, and ischemic stroke, and the other involving high blood pressure, hypertensive heart disease, and hemorrhagic stroke. These pathways connect to each other.

chains of cause-and-effect can be confusing. A useful way to think about these two types of cardiovascular disease is through two core pathways, each of which starts with different aspects of an unhealthy diet (**Figure 2.3**). In Core Pathway 1, a diet that contains an unhealthy mix of fats, refined grains, and sugar causes high blood **cholesterol**, which leads to ischemic heart disease and ischemic stroke. In Core

Box 2.1 Key Words–Heart Disease and Stroke

Artery
Blood pressure
Cardiovascular
Cardiovascular disease
Cholesterol
Hemorrhage
Hemorrhagic stroke
Hypertension
Hypertensive cardiovascular disease
Hypertensive heart disease
Ischemia
Ischemic cardiovascular disease
Ischemic heart disease
Ischemic stroke
Potassium
Pulmonary artery
Pulmonary circuit
Pulmonary vein
Sodium
Stroke
Systemic circuit
Vein

Pathway 2, a diet that contains too much **sodium** and not enough **potassium** causes high blood pressure, which leads to hypertensive heart disease and hemorrhagic stroke.

These two core pathways connect to each other: high blood cholesterol indirectly increases blood pressure and high blood pressure indirectly increases the risk of ischemic heart disease and stroke. In addition, there are several other very important risk factors involved, including smoking, insufficient physical activity, obesity, alcohol consumption, and air pollution. The next two sections explain each of these two core pathways in more detail and the role of the additional risk factors.

Ischemic Heart Disease and Ischemic Stroke

Pathophysiology of Ischemic Cardiovascular Disease

Ischemic heart disease and ischemic stroke are caused by **plaques** that narrow or block arteries. Plaques are swellings that develop just under the interior lining of the arteries. When a person has many of these plaques in many arteries, the condition is called **atherosclerosis**.[2]

Plaques can gradually grow large enough to close off an artery. And blood clots can form on plaques, causing a sudden complete blockage of an artery.

Each organ in the body is supplied by its own arteries, and plaques can occur in any of these arteries. The heart muscle itself needs a constant supply of oxygen and nutrients to keep pumping; it is supplied by arteries called **coronary arteries** because they wrap around the heart like a crown. When plaques form in these coronary arteries, they reduce blood flow to the heart muscle (**Figure 2.4**).

After many years, this reduction in blood to the heart can weaken the heart muscle. That can leave the heart unable to pump enough blood for the body, a condition called **congestive heart failure**. Alternatively, the coronary artery can suddenly become completely blocked by a blood clot forming on a plaque. This causes immediate, severe damage to the heart muscle and is called a **myocardial infarction**, also known as a heart attack. Either of these conditions qualifies as ischemic heart disease, which is also called **atherosclerotic heart disease**.

Other arteries supply blood to the brain. Plaques that narrow these arteries can gradually lead to **dementia**. Or if a blood clot forms on a plaque in

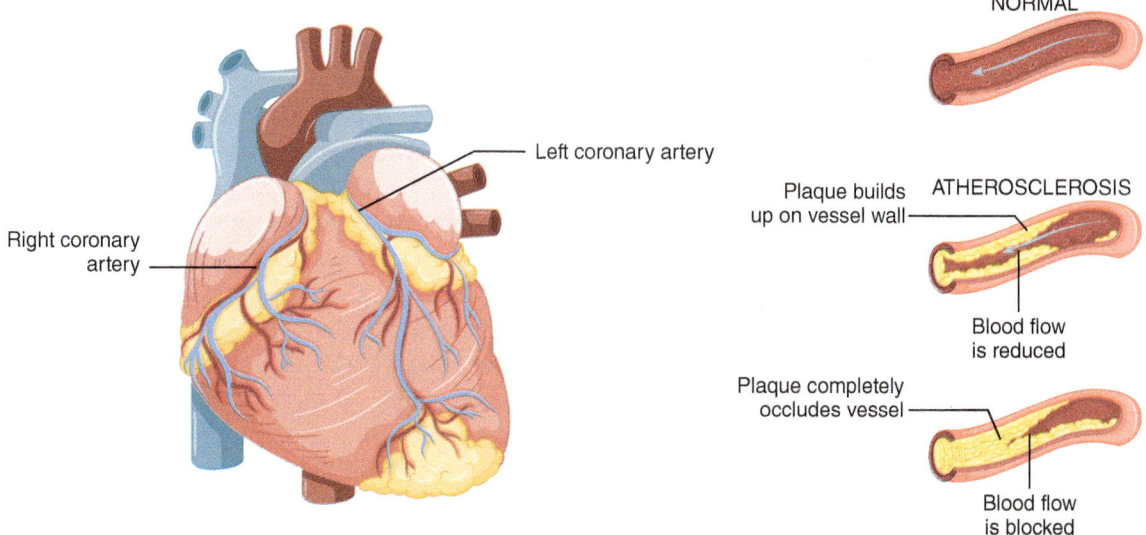

Figure 2.4 Coronary Arteries and Plaques of Atherosclerosis. The coronary arteries supply blood to the heart muscle itself. If plaques form in these coronary arteries, they make the arteries narrower, which reduces the flow of blood to the heart muscle, weakening the muscle. If they grow large enough, plaques can completely block the flow of blood to the heart muscle. Also, blood clots can form on plaques, reducing or blocking the flow of blood. If the blood flow in the coronary arteries is blocked completely, it can cause severe (and sometimes sudden) damage to the heart muscle, commonly called a heart attack.

one of these arteries, it causes a sudden damage to the brain called an ischemic stroke (see Figure 2.2).

Atherosclerosis and the tissue damage resulting from blocked arteries can also occur throughout the body. When it occurs in arms or legs, it is called **peripheral artery disease**.

Any of these conditions reflecting tissue damage from atherosclerosis is considered **atherosclerotic cardiovascular disease (ASCVD)**.

The Development of Plaques and Atherosclerosis

Plaques are composed mainly of an organic compound called **cholesterol**.[2] They develop when there are high levels of cholesterol circulating in the blood, and they are much more likely to develop when the lining of the arteries has been injured.[2] That could be the physical injury resulting from a blood pressure that is too high, a chemical injury from toxins circulating in the blood (particularly the chemicals in tobacco smoke), or even injury from the body's immune response to infections (**Figure 2.5**). This injury to the lining of the arteries is very important to the development of atherosclerosis, and it explains many of the risk factors for ischemic cardiovascular disease beyond an unhealthy diet, like smoking and high blood pressure.

Although atherosclerosis usually causes overt disease only in the later adult years, the condition begins

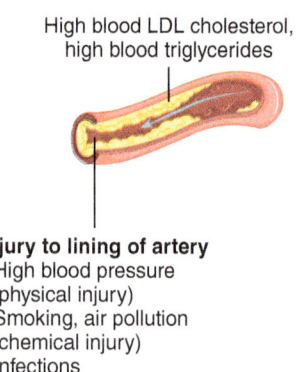

Figure 2.5 Causes of Plaques in Atherosclerosis. Plaques of atherosclerosis develop when there are high levels of cholesterol and triglycerides in the blood and are much more likely to develop if the lining of arteries has been injured in some way.

in early childhood. One study found plaques in children under age 10 and plaques in the coronary arteries in one-third of teenagers.[3]

The Role of Cholesterol and Fats

Because cholesterol is so central to ischemic heart disease and ischemic stroke, researchers have spent decades studying why blood cholesterol levels become too high and how to lower them.

Cholesterol is a normal, healthy component of cell membranes that is stored mainly in the liver and that helps the body function in many ways. It circulates in the blood in different clumps called **lipopro-teins**, some of which are denser than others. Most cholesterol in the blood is in **low-density lipopro-teins (LDL)** and **very low-density lipoproteins (VLDL)**.[4] People with high levels of cholesterol in LDL and VLDL are more likely to develop atherosclerosis (Figure 2.5).[2] In contrast, people with higher levels of cholesterol in **high-density lipoproteins (HDL)** have a lower risk of atherosclerosis, which is why some people call HDL "good cholesterol."[2] A useful way to think of this is that LDL and VLDL transport cholesterol *to* blood vessels, causing plaques, while HDL transport cholesterol *from* blood vessels back to the liver, shrinking plaques.

It is natural to assume that people get high levels of cholesterol in their blood by eating foods containing cholesterol. But most of the cholesterol circulating in the blood does not come from food; it is produced by the liver.[4] Instead, different types of **fats** in the diet, as well as other food components, appear more important in raising or lowering blood cholesterol levels.[4]

Fats, also known as **triglycerides**, are large organic molecules in which three different **fatty acids** are connected to a backbone of a small molecule called **glycerol** (Figure 2.6). These triglycerides circulate in the blood like cholesterol does, and higher levels of triglycerides in the blood, like higher levels of cholesterol, promote the formation of plaques.

There are different types of triglycerides, though, and their effects in the diet vary. Any of the three fatty acids in triglycerides can be **saturated, monounsaturated** or **polyunsaturated**. When a high percentage of a triglyceride is composed of saturated fatty acids, it is called a **saturated fat**. When a triglyceride is made up mainly of monounsaturated and polyunsaturated fatty acids, it is called **unsaturated fat**. The most important finding from decades of research on the connection between diet and heart disease is this: *people consuming high levels of saturated fatty acids have high blood cholesterol levels and a high risk of atherosclerosis, but substituting polyunsaturated fatty acids for these saturated fatty acids lowers blood cholesterol levels and these risks.*[5] Monounsaturated fatty acids also seem to lower risk, but to a lesser degree than polyunsaturated fatty acids do.[5]

Fats are found naturally in animals, fish, and plants, where they contain different mixtures of fatty acids (**Figure 2.7**). At room temperature, saturated fats are typically waxy solids and unsaturated fats are typically oily liquids. Fats from warm-blooded animals have more saturated fatty acids, so they are more solid than liquid. For example, lard—a fat separated from pork—contains 41% saturated fatty acids and 12% polyunsaturated fatty acids and is mainly solid at room temperature.[6] On the other hand, fats from fish (which live in colder temperatures) are typically about equal parts saturated, mono-unsaturated, and polyunsaturated fatty acids, and are more likely to be oils.[6] And fats found in plants are richer in monounsaturated and polyunsaturated fatty acids and are also typically oils. For example, corn oil and olive oil each contain only about 15% saturated fatty acids, with different splits of the monounsaturated and polyunsaturated fatty acids.[6] Eating seafood and plant-based foods like fruits, vegetables, legumes, nuts, and seeds[7]

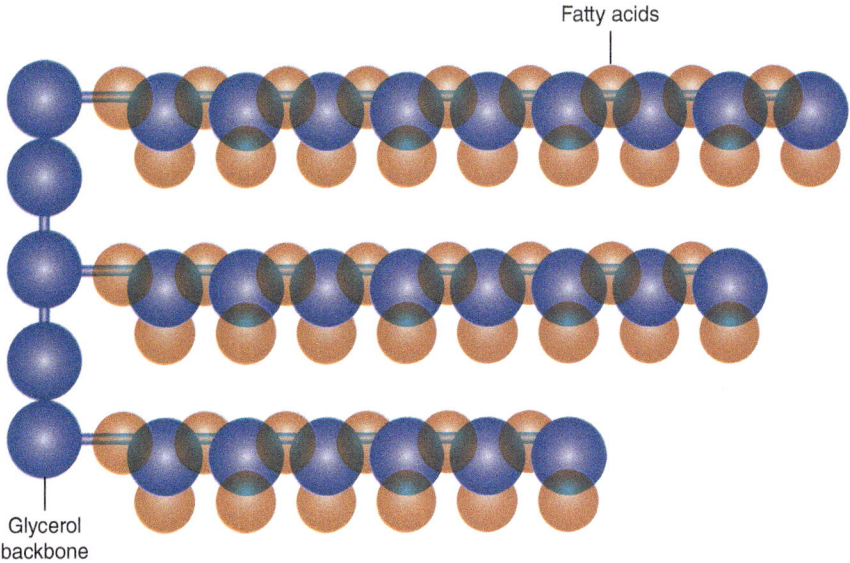

Fatty acids

Glycerol backbone

Figure 2.6 Triglycerides and Fatty Acids. Triglycerides, also known as fats, are molecules composed of three fatty acids connected to a molecule called glycerol.

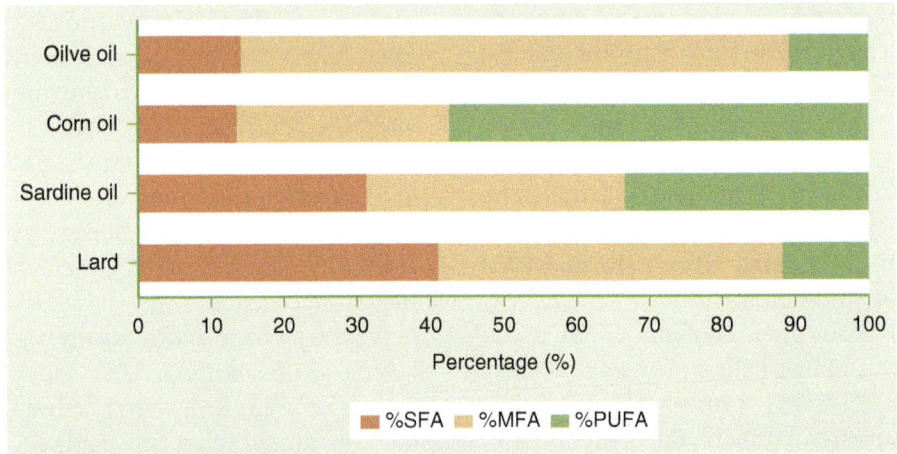

Figure 2.7 **Fatty Acid Composition of Fats from Animals, Fish, and Plants.** Fats from warm-blooded animals (like lard) have more saturated fatty acids and are solid at room temperature. Fats from fish, which live in colder temperatures, and from plants are richer in monounsaturated and polyunsaturated fatty acids and are typically oils. SFA—saturated fatty acids, MFA—monounsaturated fatty acids, PUFA—polyunsaturated fatty acids.

Data from Agricultural Research Service, United States Department of Agriculture. FoodData Central at https://fdc.nal.usda.gov

containing unsaturated fats reduces the risk of atherosclerosis compared to eating animal fats.[8,9]

About a century ago, industrial chemists learned how to make soybean oil and corn oil more shelf-stable and less likely to burn through a process called hydrogenation. This created "partially hydrogenated vegetable oil," which they called "oleomargarine" and sold as a cheaper substitute for butter. This hydrogenation process creates fats called **trans fats**. Many years after the introduction of oleomargarine to the market, studies showed that these *trans* fats increased LDL cholesterol and the risk of ischemic heart disease.[5]

Other Dietary Factors

Some components of food other than fats are now thought to also have an important impact on blood cholesterol levels or atherosclerosis.

Consumption of red meat and processed meat promotes atherosclerosis. This may be because these meats contain more saturated fats or because meats include a compound in the blood of animals called **heme**. Heme may cause inflammation in the blood vessels, damaging the lining and promoting atherosclerosis.[10]

Added sugars and refined grains like white flour also promote atherosclerosis. When people eat these foods, they get a quick rise in their blood sugar. The body responds to this rise in blood sugar by secreting the hormone **insulin**.[11-15] (Insulin and its effects are discussed more in Chapter 7 Chronic Metabolic Diseases.) A high level of insulin in the blood leads to an increase in blood cholesterol and triglycerides, which

results in atherosclerosis. In contrast, whole grains are thought to have the opposite effect, reducing insulin levels and the risk of atherosclerosis. And foods containing fiber, like fruits, vegetables, nuts, and seeds are thought to reduce the atherosclerosis risk in part by similarly helping prevent a spike in insulin levels.[7,12,16]

Physical Inactivity

Exercise and other forms of physical activity have long been known to greatly reduce the risk of ischemic heart disease—or to put it another way, physical inactivity promotes atherosclerosis. It is not fully clear why exercise is so beneficial, but we know that exercise: 1) increases the body's sensitivity to insulin and the body's metabolism of triglycerides, which in turn reduces triglycerides circulating in the blood, 2) improves the health of the cells that line the arteries, making them less susceptible to the injuries that produce plaques, 3) reduces blood pressure, and 4) expands the network of very small arteries, which helps the flow of oxygen to tissues.[17-19]

Epidemiology: Patterns and Trends

Because atherosclerosis produces damage gradually over many years, mortality rates from ischemic heart disease increase sharply with age (**Figure 2.8**). Rates are twice as high in men as in women, most likely because the female hormone estrogen slows the development of atherosclerosis (**Figure 2.9**).[20,21]

In the United States, age-adjusted ischemic heart disease mortality rates are much higher in African

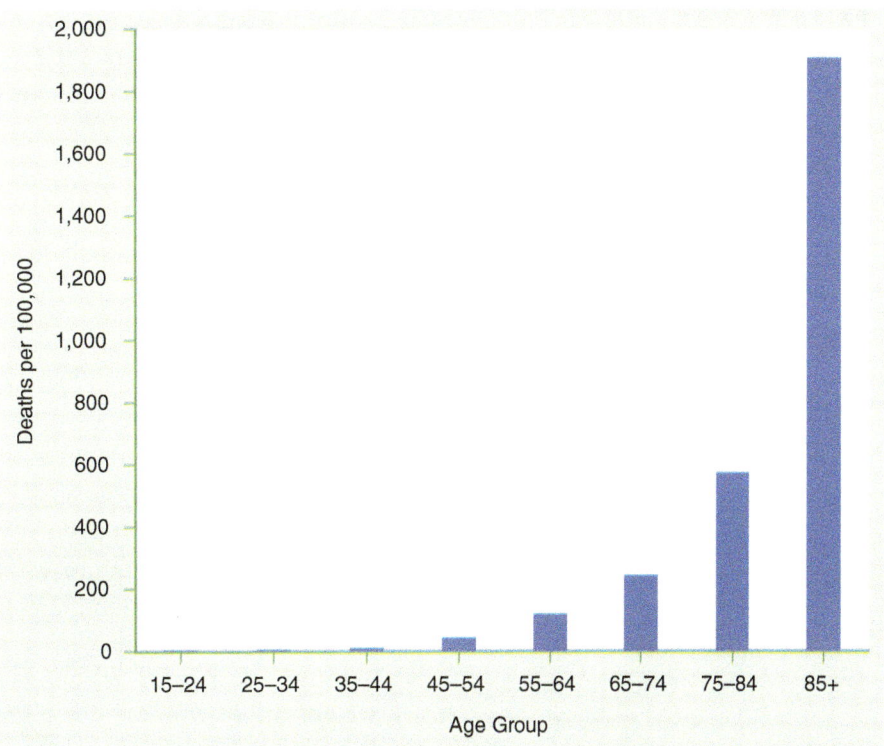

Figure 2.8 **Mortality Rates from Ischemic Heart Disease in the United States by Age Group, 2018–2022.**

Data from National Center for Health Statistics, Centers for Disease Control and Prevention. Underlying Cause of Death Data on CDC WONDER. Published 2023. Accessed June 12, 2024. https://wonder.cdc.gov/Deaths-by-Underlying-Cause.html

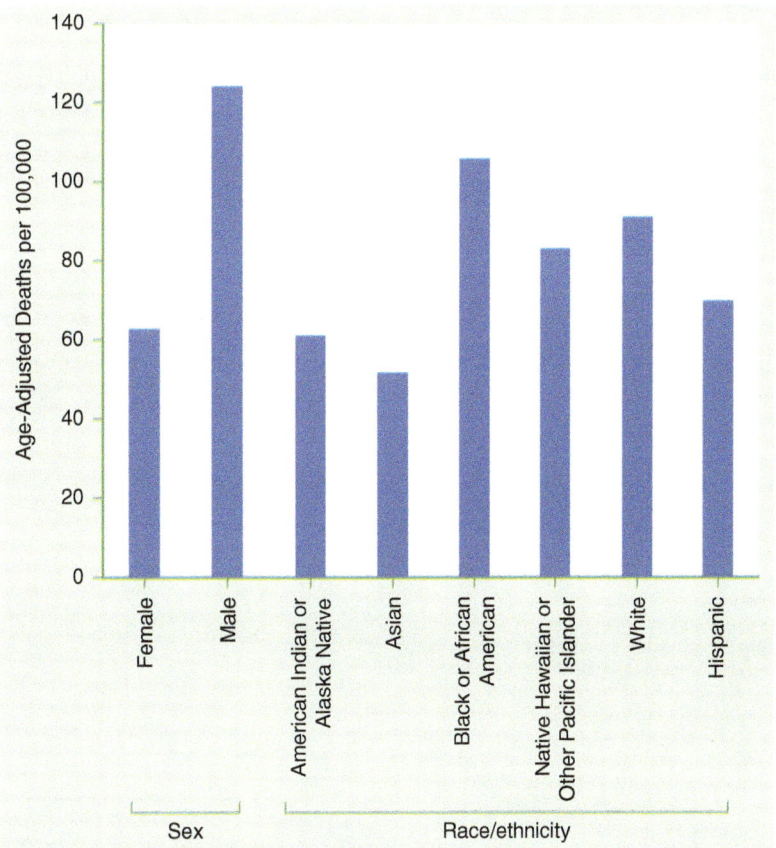

Figure 2.9 **Mortality Rates from Ischemic Heart Disease in the United States by Race/Ethnicity and Sex, 2018–2022.**

Data from National Center for Health Statistics, Centers for Disease Control and Prevention. Underlying Cause of Death Data on CDC WONDER. Published 2023. Accessed June 12, 2024. https://wonder.cdc.gov/Deaths-by-Underlying-Cause.html

Americans and Whites than Asians, American Indians and Alaskan Natives (Figure 2.9).[21] These racial differences in mortality rates are not well understood, but they may be caused by the indirect health effects of social disadvantage (discussed in Chapter 16 Social Disadvantage), higher levels of behavioral risk factors, such as smoking, unhealthy diet, or physical inactivity (which are themselves related to social disadvantage), or a combination.[22] Ischemic heart disease mortality rates are also higher in persons with lower incomes and are nearly twice as high in the southern states as they are in the northeastern and northwestern states.[21,23] Likewise, these differences are not fully explained but probably are related to some combination of social disadvantage and behavioral risk factors.

Globally, ischemic heart disease is common everywhere, but rates still vary. Mortality rates for ischemic heart disease are highest in the former Soviet Union countries and lowest in southern Europe (data are not available for most African countries).[24] The differences are stark: the ischemic heart disease mortality rate in Russia is nearly three times that of the United States and seven times that of Spain.[24] Rates are falling in the United States (**Figure 2.10**) and in most high-income countries as a result of a combination of reductions in risk factors (smoking, unhealthy diet, and physical inactivity) and medical treatment for hypertension and high blood cholesterol.[25,26] At the same time,

ischemic heart disease mortality rates are rising in many low- and middle-income countries as they pick up unhealthy habits of Western countries.[24]

Risk Factors

Researchers have identified many metabolic, behavioral, and environmental risk factors for ischemic heart disease and stroke.

Metabolic Risk Factors

The metabolic factors that increase the risk of ischemic heart disease and ischemic stroke include:

- *High levels of LDL cholesterol and triglycerides in the blood.*[5,27]
- *High blood pressure.* Injury to the lining of the arteries from high blood pressure leads to the development of plaques.[27]
- *Obesity.*[27] Compared to people with a healthy weight, those who are obese are nearly twice as likely to develop ischemic heart disease.[28] In part, this is because both obesity and atherosclerosis can be caused by an unhealthy diet and physical inactivity. But in addition, people with obesity tend to have higher levels of insulin in their blood, which increases blood cholesterol and triglyceride levels.
- *Type 2 diabetes mellitus.* People with diabetes tend to have high levels of cholesterol and triglycerides

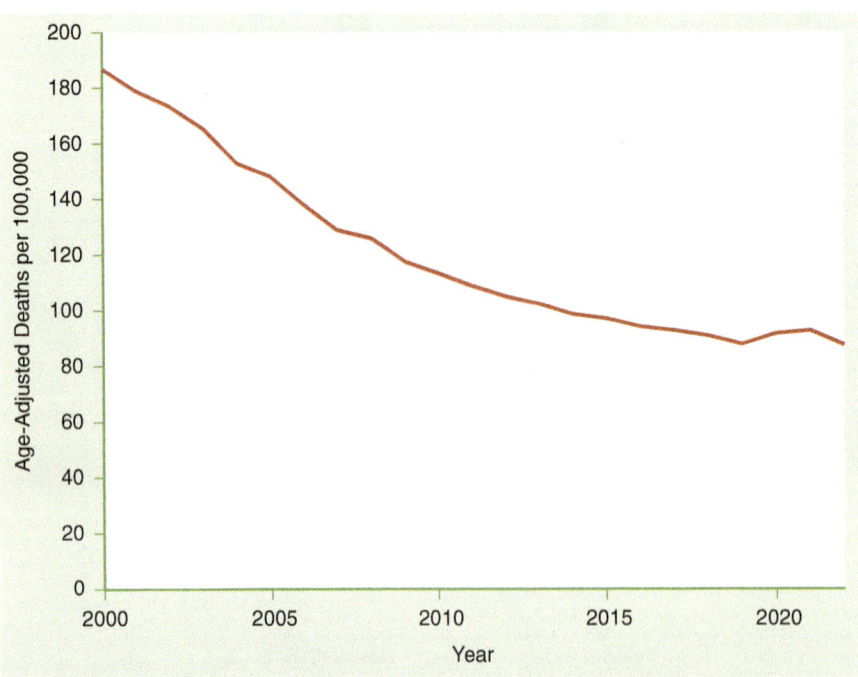

Figure 2.10 **Mortality Rates from Ischemic Heart Disease in the United States, 2000–2022.**

Data from National Center for Health Statistics, Centers for Disease Control and Prevention. Underlying Cause of Death Data on CDC WONDER. Published 2023. Accessed June 12, 2024. https://wonder.cdc.gov/Deaths-by-Underlying-Cause.html

in their blood, and the high blood sugars that occur in diabetes injure the lining of arteries.[27,29,30] Having diabetes roughly doubles the risk of ischemic heart disease and ischemic stroke.

Many of these metabolic risk factors travel together. In recent years, experts have named a group of them the **Metabolic Syndrome** (formerly *Syndrome X*). People are considered to have the Metabolic Syndrome if they have any three of the following: central obesity (measured by high waist circumference), high blood sugar, high blood triglycerides, low HDL cholesterol, and high blood pressure.[27]

Behaviors and Exposures

Figure 2.11 shows the key behavioral and environmental risk factors for atherosclerosis.

- *Unhealthy diet* has long been recognized as a key risk factor for ischemic heart disease or stroke. Our knowledge now about what is harmful and beneficial involves a mix of foods and food components, as shown in **Table 2.1**.[13,16,27,31] Most of the items that increase risk are those that contain saturated fats (such as red meat and processed meat) or that provoke high levels of insulin (such as sugar-sweetened beverages, refined grains, and added sugars). Most of the items that reduce risk contain unsaturated fats (including seafood, fruits, and vegetables). In addition, sodium in the diet increases the risk of

atherosclerosis while potassium lowers it, most likely because of their effects on blood pressure. Sodium, potassium, and blood pressure are part of the Core Pathway 2 discussed later in this chapter.

In recent years, researchers have turned to studying dietary patterns—that is, combinations of foods that people often eat together. One pattern linked to an increased risk of ischemic heart disease is the "Southern" dietary pattern, which is heavy in fried foods, added fats, processed meats, and sugar-sweetened beverages.[27] A pattern that reduces risk is the "Mediterranean diet," which emphasizes olive oil, nuts, fresh fruits, vegetables, fish, legumes, and white meat instead of red meat.[27,32] Other dietary patterns linked to a reduced risk are vegetarian and plant-based diets, which rely on nuts, seeds, and vegetables instead of meats.[27,33]

- *Physical inactivity and sedentary behavior.* The less active people are, the greater their risk. The most inactive people are about 40%–100% more likely to develop ischemic heart disease than those who are most active.[34,35] There is no lower limit to the benefit of physical activity—that is, any amount reduces the risk of ischemic heart disease compared to none.[36] Walking is an excellent form of exercise, and even small amounts of walking can have big health benefits. For those counting steps, the optimal daily step

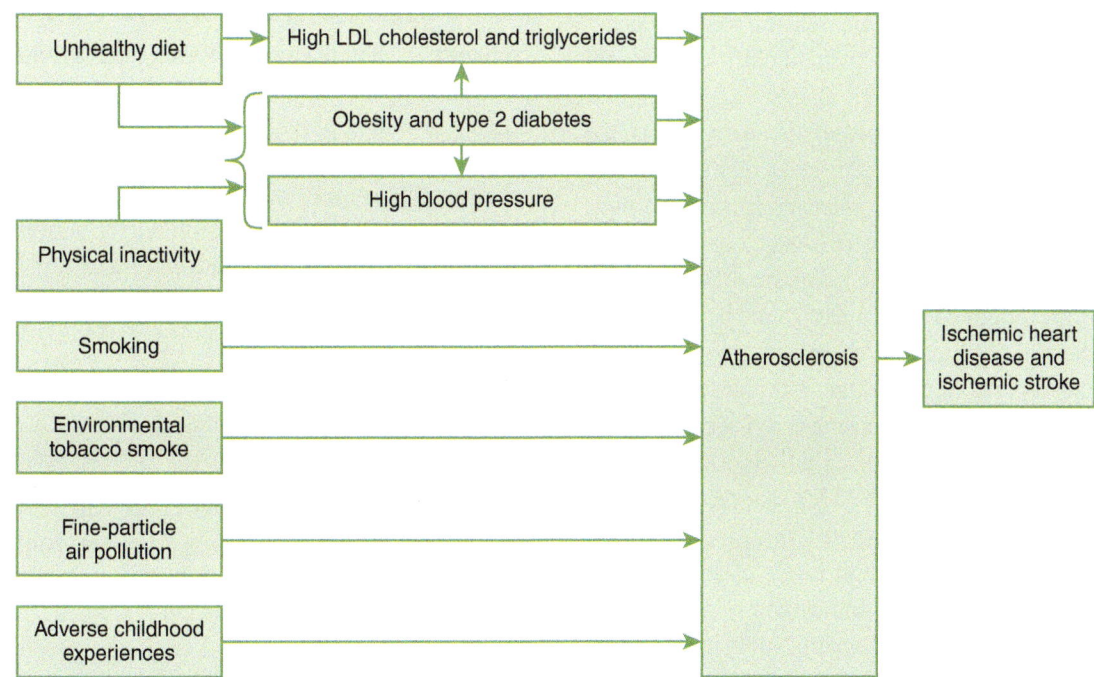

Figure 2.11 **Cause-and-Effect Diagram for Ischemic Heart Disease and Ischemic Stroke.**

Table 2.1 Dietary Risks for Atherosclerosis, Ischemic Heart Disease, and Ischemic Stroke

	Increase Risk	Reduce Risk
Foods	Processed meat	Fish and other seafood
	Red meat	Fruits, vegetables, legumes, nuts, and seeds
	Refined grains	Whole grains
	Sugar-sweetened beverages	Low-fat dairy products
Food Components	Saturated fats, cholesterol, trans fats	Unsaturated fats
	Added sugar	Fiber

Data from Arnett DK, Blumenthal RS, Albert MA, et al. 2019 ACC/AHA Guideline on the Primary Prevention of Cardiovascular Disease: A Report of the American College of Cardiology/American Heart Association Task Force on Clinical Practice Guidelines. Circulation. 2019;140(11):e596-e646 and Dietary Guidelines Advisory Committee. Scientific Report of the 2020 Dietary Guidelines Advisory Committee Advisory Report to the Secretary of Agriculture and Secretary of Health and Human Services. Washington, DC; 2020.

count is about 10,000—the faster the better.[36] At the same time, exercise is not an antidote to an unhealthy diet; atherosclerosis is common even in marathon runners.[37] Separately, **sedentary behavior**, such as watching television, working at a computer, or just sitting increases the risk for ischemic heart disease.[27,38,39] Exercise helps reduce the risk of sedentary behavior but does not eliminate it.[39,40]

- *Smoking* is a powerful risk factor for ischemic heart disease.[24,38] The toxic chemicals in tobacco smoke injure the lining of arteries, leading to plaques, and also increase the likelihood that blood clots will form on plaques.

- *Environmental tobacco smoke*, also known as second-hand smoke, increases the risk of people who do not smoke, most likely by the same mechanism.[41-43]

- ***Fine-particle air pollution*** also increases ischemic heart disease risk. Particles floating in the air that are less than 2.5 microns in size, known as **particulate matter** or **PM$_{2.5}$**, are just the right size to travel into the lung's smallest airways, where the chemicals they carry can be absorbed into the blood. Inhaling these fine particles, like inhaling second-hand smoke, damages the lining of the blood vessels, increasing the risk of plaques, and also increases the risk that blood clots will form on those plaques.[44,45] This risk factor is particularly important in some low- and middle-income countries with high levels of ambient air pollution (e. g., cities in India) where many people like using smoke-producing fuels indoors for heat and cooking. Air pollution is discussed more in Chapter 8 Chronic Respiratory Diseases.

- *Adverse childhood experiences*. Many studies have found a higher risk of ischemic heart disease in adults who had adverse family experiences when they were children (e. g., abuse, neglect, or parents with alcohol or drug addiction[46,47]). These same adverse childhood experiences increase the risk of mental illness in adults, as discussed in Chapter 5. Mental Illness. The biologic connection to ischemic heart disease is not clear, but it may involve the body's response to stress, which causes the release of hormones and inflammation that can promote atherosclerosis.[47] Stress in adults may also increase the risk of ischemic heart disease, but to a lesser extent.[47,48]

Preventive Interventions

Ischemic heart disease and ischemic stroke can be prevented by reducing high-risk behaviors and exposures (primary prevention) or by identifying and treating high LDL cholesterol (secondary prevention), as shown in **Figure 2.12**. Because plaques begin to develop early in life, these preventive actions should be directed to entire populations, including children, not just those showing signs of atherosclerosis.

Primary Prevention

Primary prevention for ischemic heart disease and ischemic stroke includes:

- *Promotion of healthy diets*. This can be achieved by reducing the promotion of unhealthy foods and increasing the availability, accessibility, and promotion of healthy foods shown in Table 2.1. Promotion of healthier diets is discussed more in Chapter 14. Nutrition. One policy that specifically prevents heart disease is banning *trans* fats

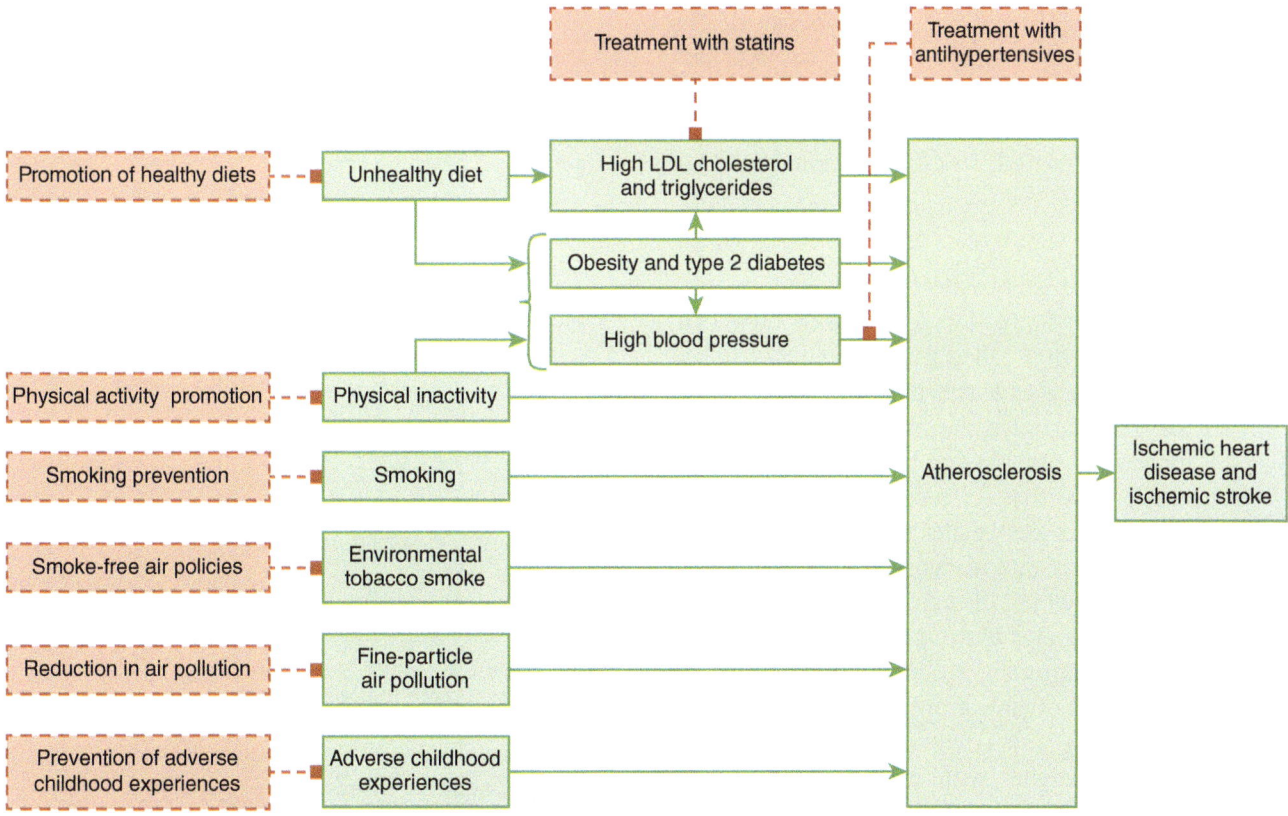

Figure 2.12 **Cause-and-Effect Diagram for Ischemic Heart Disease and Ischemic Stroke, with Preventive Interventions.**

in foods. *Trans* fats are artificial and increase the rates of the world's number one killer, so there is no justification for allowing them in the food supply. Fortunately, the FDA now prohibits artificial *trans* fats in foods in the United States,[49] and many other countries are taking similar actions.

- *Promotion of physical activity.* Two interventions can help here: increasing exercise (or more precisely, moderate-to-vigorous physical activity) and reducing sedentary behavior, such as watching television or sitting at a computer. See Chapter 15. Physical Inactivity for more on this.
- *Prevention of smoking* and *enactment of smoke-free policies.* Prevention of smoking is discussed in Chapter 11. Tobacco Use. Smoke-free policies help in two ways: they prompt many people to quit smoking and they protect those who do not from second-hand smoke. One review found that prohibitions on smoking in public places led to a 17% reduction in myocardial infarctions.[50]
- *Reduction in air pollution.* Air pollution can be reduced by use of cleaner energy sources or by emission control systems.
- *Prevention of adverse childhood experiences.* Protecting children from adverse experiences in entire populations is not easy, but to the extent that it is

possible it should reduce rates of ischemic heart disease in the future. The work involves both supporting families that are experiencing high levels of stress and at times intervening to shield children from abusive parents.

Table 2.2 shows estimates by the Global Burden of Disease project of the percentage of ischemic heart disease deaths attributable to behavioral and environmental risk factors.[1] These estimates suggest

Table 2.2 **Estimated Percentage of Ischemic Heart Disease Deaths Attributable to Key Risk Factors**

	United States	World
Unhealthy diet	53%	53%
Smoking	19%	18%
Air pollution	3%	20%
Physical inactivity	4%	5%
Environmental tobacco smoke	2%	5%

Data from Global Burden of Disease Project, available through GDB Results tool. Accessed August 22, 2023. https://vizhub.healthdata.org/gbd-results/

that the majority of ischemic heart disease deaths could be avoided by changes in a few key risk factors, with the most important being diet and smoking.[1] Air pollution is a particularly important (and often under-appreciated) risk for ischemic heart disease worldwide.

Secondary Prevention

- *Treatment with statins* for people with high LDL cholesterol. Drugs called **statins** reduce cholesterol and the risk of ischemic heart disease and stroke.[51] Statins have the unfortunate side effect of increasing the risk of type 2 diabetes, but experts believe that for most people the benefit of these drugs outweighs their risks.[51] Experts have published algorithms that guide healthcare providers on which of their patients should take these medications.[51] Only about 60% of Americans for whom statins are recommended are taking them.[52] Health organizations are trying to respond by simplifying and streamlining the process of identifying patients with high LDL cholesterol and helping them get these medications. These streamlined approaches are often integrated with similar approaches to streamlining the treatment of hypertension, which is discussed in the next section of this chapter.[53]

- *Treatment with antihypertensives.* High blood pressure can be reduced by medications called **antihypertensives**, and treatment with these drugs reduces the risk of ischemic heart disease and ischemic stroke.[53] Prevention and treatment of high blood pressure are discussed in depth in the next section.

Box 2.2 Summary–Prevention of Ischemic Heart Disease and Ischemic Stroke

- Primary prevention
  - Promotion of healthy diets
  - Promotion of physical activity
  - Prevention of smoking and enactment of smoke-free air policies
  - Reduction in air pollution
  - Prevention of adverse childhood experiences
- Secondary prevention
  - Treatment with statins for people with high LDL cholesterol
  - Treatment with antihypertensives for people with high blood pressure

---

Box 2.3 Key Words–Ischemic Heart Disease and Ischemic Stroke

Antihypertensive
Atherosclerosis
Atherosclerotic cardiovascular disease
Atherosclerotic heart disease
Cholesterol
Congestive heart failure
Coronary arteries
Dementia
Fats
Fatty acids
Fine particle air pollution
Glycerol
Heme
High-density lipoproteins (HDL)
Insulin
Lipoproteins
Low-density lipoproteins (LDL)
Metabolic Syndrome
Monounsaturated fatty acids
Myocardial infarction
Particulate matter
Peripheral artery disease
Plaque
$PM_{2.5}$
Polyunsaturated fatty acids
Saturated fats
Saturated fatty acids
Sedentary behavior
Statin
Trans fats
Triglycerides
Unsaturated fat
Very low-density lipoproteins (VLDL)

Resources–Ischemic Heart Disease and Ischemic Stroke

- Sacks FM, Lichtenstein AH, Wu JHY, et al. Dietary fats and cardiovascular disease: A presidential advisory from the American Heart Association. *Circulation.* 2017;136(3): e1-e23. doi:10.1161/CIR.0000000000000510. This provides detail on the research relating dietary fats and grains to ischemic heart disease.

- *Scientific Report of the 2020 Dietary Guidelines Advisory Committee: Advisory Report to the Secretary of Agriculture and Secretary of Health and Human Services.* This contains a detailed review of the dietary factors that increase or reduce the risk of ischemic heart disease.

- Lichtenstein AH, Appel LJ, Vadiveloo M, et al. 2021 Dietary Guidance to Improve Cardiovascular Health: A Scientific Statement from the American

Heart Association. *Circulation.* 2021;144(23): E472-E487. doi:10.1161/CIR.0000000000001031

- Arnett DK, Blumenthal RS, Albert MA, et al. 2019 ACC/AHA Guideline on the Primary Prevention of Cardiovascular Disease: A Report of the American College of Cardiology/American Heart Association Task Force on Clinical Practice Guidelines. *Circulation.* 2019;140(11): e596-e646. doi:10.1161/CIR.0000000000000678. This is a highly detailed set of recommendations designed for physicians on how to assess and treat patients at risk for ischemic heart disease, together with detailed summaries of the research supporting these recommendations.

Hypertension and Hypertensive Cardiovascular Disease

Introduction

High blood pressure increases the risk of heart disease, stroke, and kidney disease. Unfortunately, modern diets and physical inactivity cause blood pressure to rise to risky levels in most people. Because of its severe consequences and because it is so common, hypertension is responsible for more deaths than any other metabolic risk factor.[1] In the United States, more than 400,000 deaths per year are attributed to high blood pressure.[1] This section will discuss what blood pressure is, how the body regulates it, and the causes, consequences, and prevention of high blood pressure.

Physiology: Regulation of Blood Pressure

Blood pressure rises and falls with each contraction of the heart. It is this quick rise and fall in pressure that you feel when you take your pulse. The maximum pressure in this cycle is called the **systolic blood pressure**, and the minimum is called the **diastolic blood pressure** (**Figure 2.13**). A blood pressure reported as "140 over 90," typically written 140/90, indicates a systolic pressure of 140 millimeters of mercury (or mm Hg) and a diastolic pressure of 90 mm Hg. The average blood pressure through the cycle is called the mean arterial pressure.

The mean arterial pressure is the product of two factors: the amount of blood that the heart is pushing (called the **cardiac output**) and the amount of resistance to blood flow created by the arteries (called the

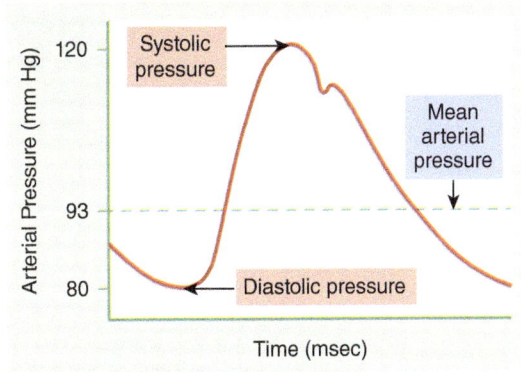

Figure 2.13 **Blood Pressure Through the Heartbeat Cycle.** Blood pressure rises and falls with each contraction of the heart. The maximum pressure in this cycle is called the systolic blood pressure, and the minimum is called the diastolic blood pressure.

vascular resistance). If either of those increases, the blood pressure rises (**Figure 2.14**).

The kidneys sense the body's blood pressure and constantly take actions to keep the pressure in a healthy range. If the blood pressure drops too low, the kidneys (working with other organs) release hormones that cause the small arteries to become narrower (constrict), which raises the vascular resistance. At the same time, the kidneys, which

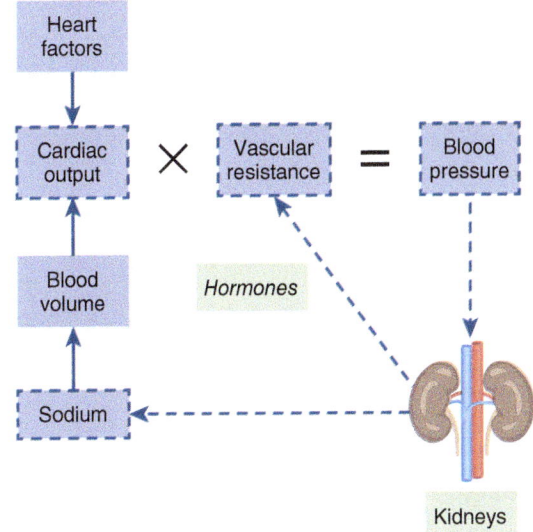

Figure 2.14 **Regulation of Blood Pressure by the Kidneys.** Blood pressure is a product of two factors: the amount of blood that the heart is pushing (cardiac output) and the resistance in the arteries (vascular resistance). The kidneys sense the blood pressure and regulate it by: 1) retaining more or less sodium, which increases or decreases the blood volume, and 2) secreting hormones that increase or decrease the vascular resistance.

Modified from Mitchell RN, Halushka MK. Blood Pressure Regulation. In: Kumar V, Abbas AK, Aster JC, Turner JR, eds. Robbins & Cotran Pathologic Basis of Disease. 10th Edition. Philadelphia: Elsevier; 2021:490–492.

filter the blood and make urine, retain more **sodium** in the blood. When the body retains sodium, it retains fluid with it. That increases the volume of blood in the body and the cardiac output.[54] With a higher vascular resistance and a higher cardiac output, the blood pressure rises (Figure 2.14).

If the blood pressure becomes too high, the reverse occurs. Under the influence of various hormones released by the kidneys, the small arteries become larger ("dilate"). At the same time, the kidneys allow more sodium to flow from the blood into the urine. This both reduces the systemic vascular resistance and reduces blood volume and cardiac output, which reduces blood pressure.[54]

Unfortunately, for most of us, over many years these regulatory mechanisms gradually fail, and blood pressure rises to unhealthy levels.

Pathophysiology of High Blood Pressure

Sodium and Potassium

While high blood pressure can be a consequence of other diseases, for nearly everyone with the condition, there is no obvious individual cause.[53] How is it possible that a near majority of the world's population develops such a dangerous condition? It is now clear that an unhealthy diet is the primary cause of high blood pressure, particularly an excessive intake of sodium.[53,55] While some people are more sensitive to sodium than others, consuming too much sodium tends to raise blood pressure in everyone.[53,56,57]

In the short term, taking in too much sodium increases blood volume, which raises the blood pressure.[58] Over a few days, the kidney can handle that by disposing the excess sodium and lowering the pressure. But over years and decades, this unrelenting excessive intake of sodium gradually overwhelms the kidney's ability to dispose of it, and the blood pressure stays high. High blood pressure then damages arteries and kidneys in ways that raise blood pressure even further.[58]

The fundamental problem is that the human body is not adapted to take in nearly as much sodium as people do today. Humans consume sodium mainly as **sodium chloride**, which is the salt used in food. This salt is dug up from mines or produced through the evaporation of seawater—processes that were developed after humans evolved to what we are today. Until commerce and industry started, salt was difficult to find, so humans and their hominid ancestors consumed very little sodium. (It is probably *because*

salt was so difficult to find but necessary for life that humans evolved a craving for food that tastes salty.) People in ancient hunter-gatherer societies are believed to have consumed less than 1,000 mg of sodium per day, and isolated hunter-gatherer societies today take in less than 400 mg sodium per day, which is less than a third of what Americans consume.[59] People in today's isolated societies have much lower blood pressure than other people, with systolic pressures averaging about 105 mm Hg and diastolic pressures averaging about 70 mm Hg.[60,61] Tellingly, their blood pressures do not rise with age, and for them strokes are rare.[59,61]

Today, sodium appears in large amounts in nearly all of the processed foods that Americans eat, including not only pizza, chips, and hot dogs but also cheese, bread, soups, cookies, muffins, breakfast cereal, condiments, and canned vegetables.[62] An estimated 71% of the sodium in Americans' diets is added during commercial food processing, only an estimated 11% comes from salt added during home cooking or at the table, and 14% is inherently in the food (**Figure 2.15**).[63] Because of the high levels in processed food, American adults take in about 3,400 mg of sodium per day.[64] It should not be surprising, then, that the body's regulatory systems are overwhelmed.

Other dietary factors can also raise blood pressure. Most importantly, the inadequate consumption of potassium raises blood pressure.[16,53] Exactly why is unclear, but it appears that low levels of potassium prompt the kidneys to retain more sodium.[65] Potassium and sodium, which are chemically similar positive ions, play opposing roles in many areas of biology. In particular, potassium is the major positive ion in fluids inside of cells, but sodium is the major positive ion in fluids outside of cells. Americans take in an average of 2,500 mg of potassium per day, and the World Health Organization recommends at least 3,500 mg.[31,53] Experts do not recommend that people take dietary supplements of potassium. Instead, they recommend that people eat foods that are naturally rich in potassium, such as greens, legumes, fruit, potatoes, tomatoes, and fish.[31,53]

Definition of Hypertension

The distribution of systolic blood pressure among American adults is shown in **Figure 2.16**. There is no natural cut point that distinguishes high from normal blood pressure. For many years, a person was labelled as having **hypertension** if that person had a systolic blood pressure above 140 mm Hg or a diastolic blood pressure above 90 mm Hg. An estimated

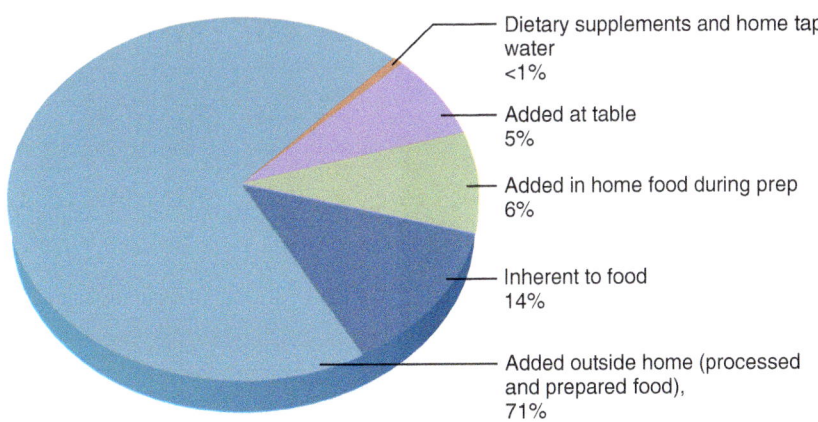

Figure 2.15 Sources of Sodium in Americans' Diet. More than 70% of the sodium in Americans' diet is added outside the home, appearing in in processed and prepared food. Only about 11% is added in the home during food preparation or at the table.

Data from Harnack JL et al. Sources of Sodium in US Adults from 3 Geographic Regions. Circulation 2017; 135:1775-1783.

32% of American adults are either already taking medicine for hypertension or have blood pressure above those cutpoints.[53]

In the 2010s, it became increasingly clear that this old definition of hypertension did not adequately describe the risks of different levels of blood pressure. Even people with "normal" blood pressure were shown to have higher rates of cardiovascular disease than people with blood pressures lower than theirs. Starting at a systolic blood pressure as low as 115 mm Hg, every increase of 20 mm Hg roughly doubles the risk of death from heart disease or stroke.[53,66] With that in mind, in 2017 experts in the United States redefined the labels they use (**Table 2.3**).[53]

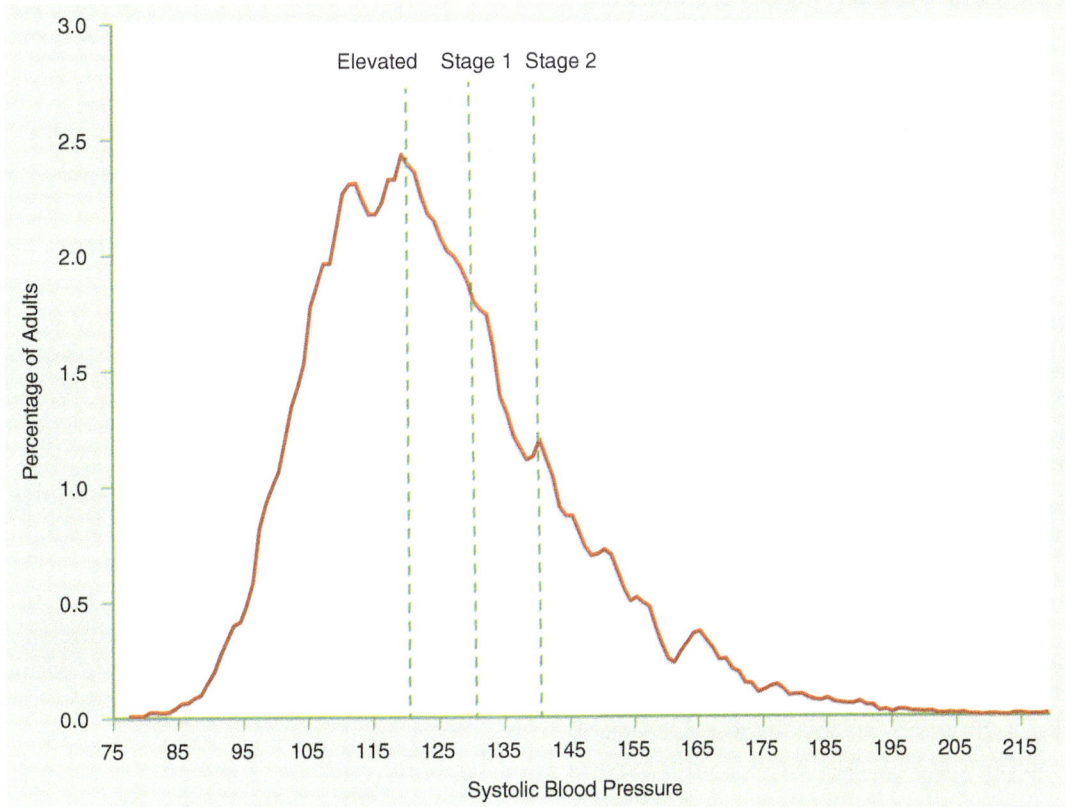

Figure 2.16 Distribution of Systolic Blood Pressure in American Adults. Systolic blood pressure in American adults ranges from about 85 to more than 190 mm Hg. Approximately half have systolic blood pressures that are now considered elevated or in the hypertension Stage 1 or Stage 2 range.

Data from National Health and Nutrition Examination Survey 2017-2020. National Center for Health Statistics, Centers for Disease Control and Prevention. Accessed July 27, 2023. https://wwwn.cdc.gov/nchs/nhanes/continuousnhanes/default.aspx?Cycle=2017-2020

Table 2.3 Categories of Blood Pressure in Adults

Blood Pressure (mm Hg)			
Systolic		**Diastolic**	**Category**
<120	and	<80	Normal
120–129	and	<80	Elevated
130–139	or	80–89	Hypertension Stage 1
>140	or	>90	Hypertension Stage 2

Reproduced from Whelton PK, Carey RM, Aronow WS, et al. 2017 Guideline for the Prevention, Detection, Evaluation, and Management of High Blood Pressure in Adults. J Am Coll Cardiol. 2018;71(19). doi:10.1016/j.jacc.2017.11.006

Persons are now considered to have **normal blood pressure** if their measurements are below 120/80, **elevated blood pressure** if they are between 120/80 mm Hg and 130/80 mm Hg, and **hypertension** if their systolic blood pressure is above 130 mm Hg or their diastolic blood pressure is above 80 mm Hg. The experts then divided hypertension into two categories—the lower-risk **Stage 1** and the higher-risk **Stage 2**—with the cut point between them the previous definition of hypertension, that is, a systolic blood pressure above 140 mm Hg or a diastolic above 90 mm Hg. The revision increased the percentage of American adults labelled as having hypertension from 32% to 46%.[53]

Consequences of Hypertension

Blood pressure that is too high causes damage to organs throughout the body.

First, high blood pressure damages small arteries by putting more stress on their interior walls, as forcing more air into a balloon puts more stress on the rubber. That damage to the walls of the arteries increases the vascular resistance, raising blood pressure further. That makes high blood pressure a self-reinforcing problem which, without treatment, will continue to worsen. As blood pressure rises, it can lead to:

- *Stroke.* A stroke is a sudden loss of brain function caused by lack of blood flow. Different areas of the brain control different parts of the body, so a stroke's symptoms can include a sudden paralysis of an arm or leg, difficulty speaking, loss of vision, or loss of coordination. As discussed in the first section of this chapter, an **ischemic stroke** is caused by a blockage of blood flow from atherosclerosis, and a **hemorrhagic stroke** is caused by the bursting of an artery under high

pressure. Ischemic strokes are more common than hemorrhagic strokes.[67] High blood pressure increases the risk of both types.

- *Congestive heart failure.* High blood pressure puts a strain on the heart muscle, which gradually weakens the heart, to the point where it cannot pump enough blood to meet the body's needs. When a person has congestive heart failure from longstanding hypertension, he or she is said to have **hypertensive heart disease** or **hypertensive cardiovascular disease**.

- *Atherosclerosis and ischemic heart disease.* Atherosclerosis is more likely to develop if the lining of arteries is injured (see Figure 2.5). Like toxic chemicals in the blood, high blood pressure also injures the lining of arteries. This means atherosclerosis and high blood pressure reinforce each other: the plaques of atherosclerosis make arteries stiffer and increase blood pressure, and high blood pressure damages the lining of arteries and promotes development of plaques.

- *Chronic kidney disease.* Damage to small arteries in the kidneys from high blood pressure gradually harms the kidney tissue itself.[68] Because the kidneys play a key role in regulating blood pressure, damage to them raises blood pressure further, setting up another self-reinforcing mechanism. Hypertension is the second most important cause of kidney failure in the United States, after diabetes. Chronic kidney disease is discussed in Chapter 7. Chronic Metabolic Diseases.

Epidemiology of Hypertension: Patterns and Trends

The prevalence of hypertension in the United States has not changed much since the early 2000s.[69]

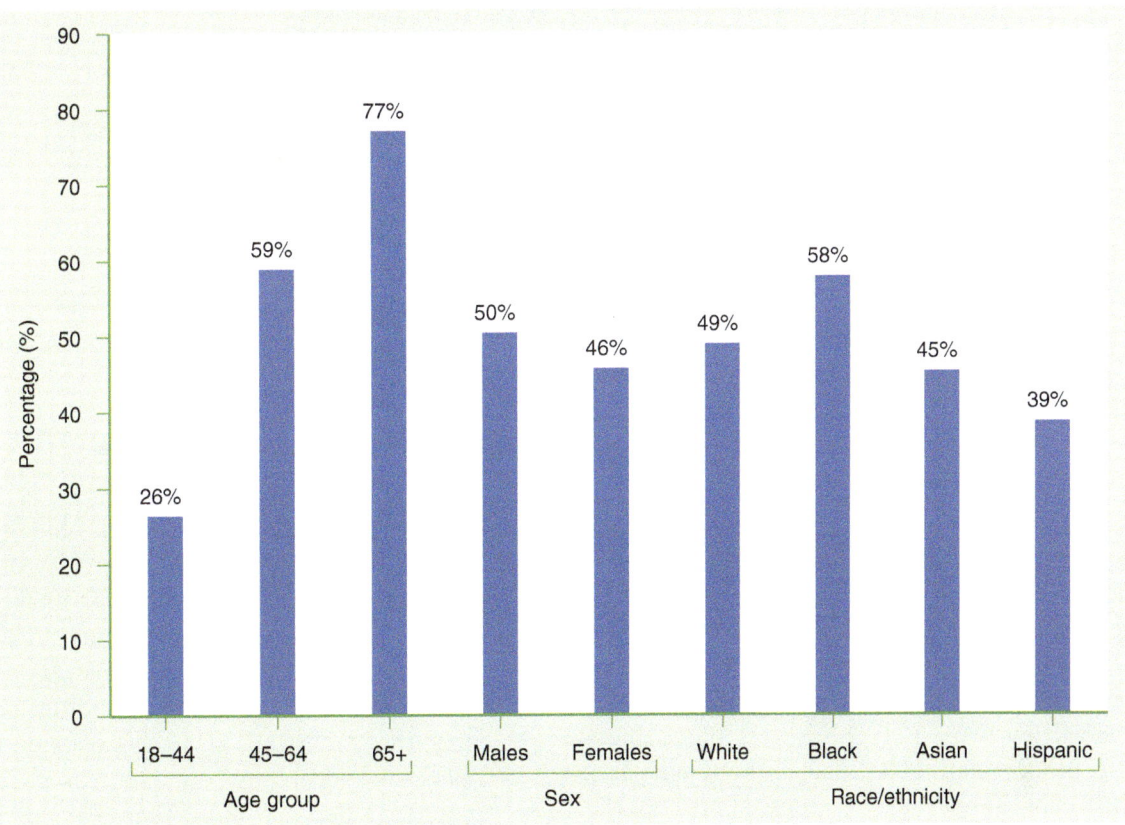

Figure 2.17 Prevalence of Hypertension in U.S. Adults, 2017–2020.

Data from Centers for Disease Control and Prevention. Estimated Hypertension Prevalence, Treatment, and Control Among US Adults: Tables. Accessed July 24, 2025. https://millionhearts.hhs.gov/files/Estimated-Hypertension-Prevalence-tables-508.pdf

The percent of people with hypertension (Stage 1 or Stage 2) rises as people age (**Figure 2.17**). Among adults 45–64, nearly 60% have hypertension.[70] The prevalence is high in every racial and ethnic group but it is more common in Black adults (Figure 2.16).[70] Hypertension is also more common in people with lower incomes and those living in low-income neighborhoods, regardless of race.[71,72] As with ischemic heart disease, these racial and income-based differences in hypertension are not well understood, but they may be caused by the indirect health effects of social disadvantage (discussed in Chapter 16. Social Disadvantage) unhealthy diet or physical inactivity (which are themselves related to social disadvantage), genetic differences in sensitivity to sodium, or a combination of the three.[22]

The health consequences of hypertension follow similar racial and economic patterns. For example, Black adults have a mortality rate from hypertension-related heart and kidney disease that is twice that of White adults.[21]

Globally, about one-third of adults have hypertension as it was previously defined (above 140/90 mm Hg).[73] In recent decades, rates of hypertension have been falling somewhat in high-income countries and rising in low-income countries.[73]

Risk Factors

Key modifiable risk factors for high blood pressure are the following (see **Figure 2.18**):

- *Excess sodium intake*, as discussed above.
- *Insufficient potassium intake*, as discussed above.
- *Unhealthy diet.* More than 20 years ago, researchers showed that when people who switched from their typical American eating pattern to a healthier diet, their blood pressure fell. The healthier diet was called the Dietary Approach to Stopping Hypertension (DASH), and the fall in blood pressure was independent of the effect of sodium.[74] Dietary patterns linked to higher blood pressure emphasize red meat, processed meat, sugar-sweetened foods and drinks, saturated fat, and cholesterol.[75] The DASH diet that lowered blood pressure emphasizes fruits, vegetables, low-fat dairy, whole grains, poultry, fish, and nuts.[74] The biologic mechanism for the benefit of the DASH diet on blood pressure is still unclear, but the DASH diet closely matches the dietary patterns that increase or decrease the risk of atherosclerosis, as shown in Table 2.1.
- *Overweight and obesity.* Obesity increases blood pressure in ways not caused directly by diet.

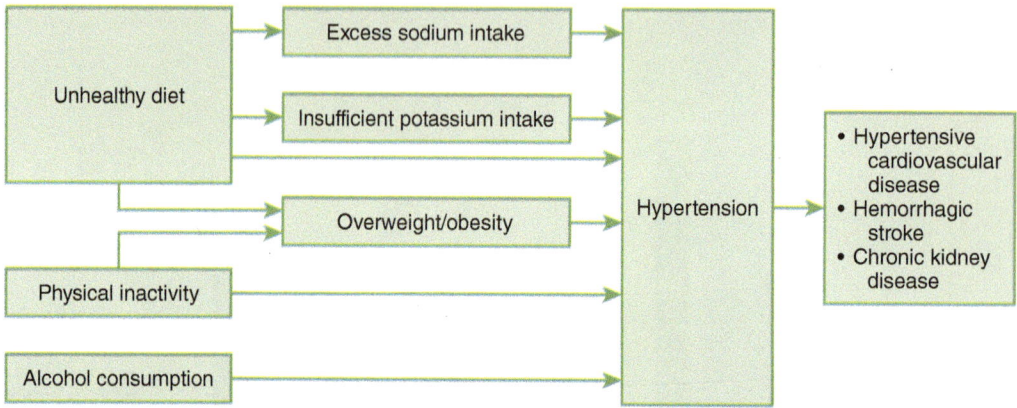

Figure 2.18 **Cause-and-Effect Diagram for Hypertension and Hypertensive Cardiovascular Disease.**

The reason is not fully clear, but obesity increases the kidneys' sodium retention, cardiac output, and the hormone released by the kidneys that increase vascular resistance—all of which raise blood pressure.[76] When overweight people lose weight, their blood pressures tend to fall.[53]

- *Physical inactivity.* Exercise lowers blood pressure, independent of its effect on body weight.[53] This may be because exercise increases the diameter of small arteries, which reduces vascular resistance.[77]

- *Alcohol consumption.* Drinking alcohol increases blood pressure, hypertension, and the risk of hemorrhagic stroke.[78,79] The mechanism for this effect is not fully understood, but it is reversible— that is, people who quit or reduce their drinking experience a reduction in their blood pressure.[79] It is estimated that about 10% of the hypertension in the United States is attributable to alcohol consumption.[53]

There is evidence that psychological stress is linked to high blood pressure.[53,80] It is possible that psychological stress may partially explain the higher rates of hypertension in low-income people and African-Americans. However, it is unclear whether this psychological stress is a risk factor that is modifiable at the population level.[53] The relationship between stress and social disadvantage is discussed in Chapter 16 Social Disadvantage.

Preventive Interventions

Primary Prevention

Hypertension can be prevented by the following (see **Figure 2.19**):

- *Reduction of sodium in processed foods.* People who take in less sodium have lower blood pressures, and when people with hypertension

reduce their sodium intake, their blood pressure falls.[58] The Dietary Guidelines for Americans recommend that adults cut their intake to less than 2,300 mg of sodium per day.[64] The World Health Organization recommends reducing intake to below 2,000 mg of sodium per day[81] and the American Heart Association recommends an "ideal limit" of no more than 1,500 mg per day.[82] Because more than 70% of people's sodium intake comes from processed and restaurants foods,[63] almost no one can cut their sodium intake below these level on their own. For people to achieve this much sodium reduction, food companies need to add less sodium during processing. The FDA has announced voluntary guidance for food companies on how they can gradually reduce the amount of sodium they put into processed food with the goal of reducing American's sodium consumption from 3,400 mg/day to 2,750 mg/day.[83,84] The World Health Organization has adopted sodium reduction "benchmarks" to help other countries put similar policies in place.[85]

- *Promotion of healthy diets.* Hypertension can be partially prevented by making it easier for people to shift their diets away from processed food. Unprocessed fruits, vegetables, and legumes are very low in sodium and rich in potassium, as are unprocessed meat and fresh fish. Processed and canned versions of these foods typically have much added sodium. Separate from sodium and potassium, hypertension can be reduced by encouraging and facilitating people to shift from the unhealthy to the healthy foods listed in Table 2.1. This would also reduce obesity. Because hypertension is a population-wide problem, everyone should emphasize these healthier foods, including people who do not

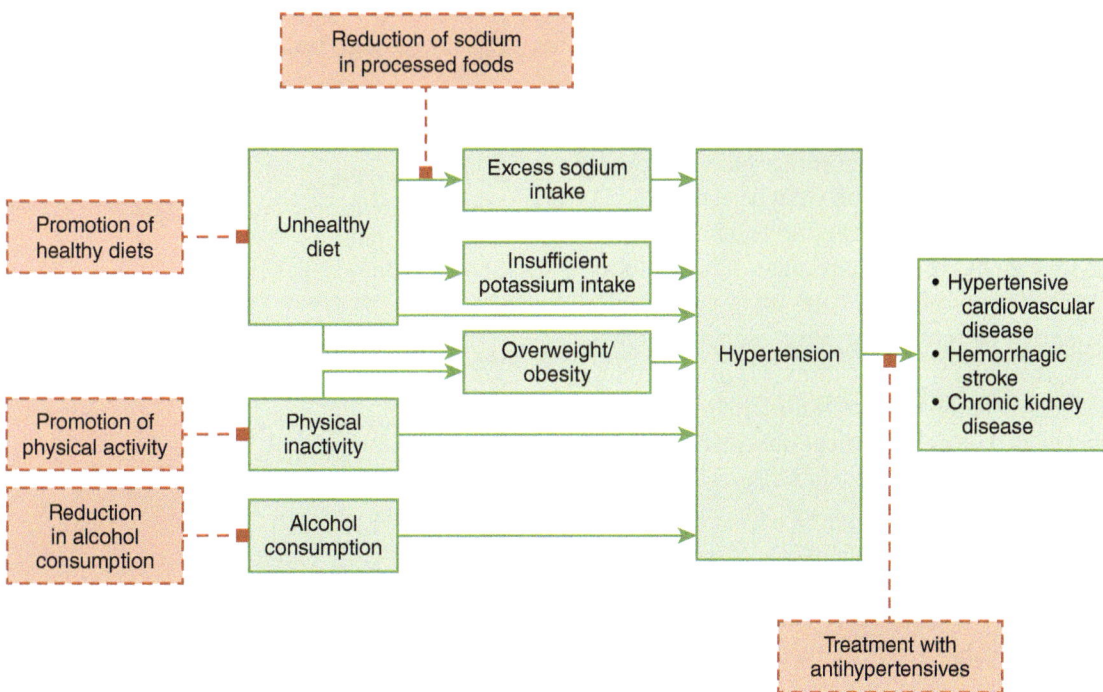

Figure 2.19 **Cause-and-Effect Diagram for Hypertension and Hypertensive Cardiovascular Disease, with Preventive Interventions.**

(yet) have high blood pressure and certainly children. See Chapter 12. Nutrition for strategies to promote healthy foods and limit the promotion of unhealthy foods.

- *Promotion of physical activity.* See Chapter 15. Physical Inactivity.
- *Reduction of alcohol consumption.* See Chapter 14. Alcohol Use.

Secondary Prevention

While primary prevention has great potential over the long term, a huge proportion of nearly every population will have hypertension for the foreseeable future. That makes it essential to expand secondary prevention—that is, medical treatment of hypertension. Fortunately, today medical providers can prescribe many different **antihypertensives** that lower blood pressure and reduce the risk of heart attacks and strokes. For every drop in systolic blood pressure of 10 mm Hg, people's risk of ischemic heart disease falls by 20–25% and their risk of death from all causes falls by 13%.[86]

Experts have developed algorithms to help primary care providers decide whether patients should take antihypertensives and if so, which drugs are best for them. These algorithms consider a person's age, sex, race, blood pressure, cholesterol levels, smoking, use of statins, and presence of diabetes. From these factors

they estimate the chances that the patient will have a heart attack, stroke, or other dangerous cardiovascular event within the next 10 years. This estimate is called the **atherosclerotic cardiovascular risk or ASCVD** risk.

Experts recommend only "lifestyle modification" for people whose blood pressure is classified as "elevated" or Stage 1 hypertension and who have an ASCVD risk of less than 10%.[53] In this context, lifestyle modification means losing weight if overweight, reducing sodium intake, increasing potassium intake, eating healthier (and unprocessed) foods, increasing physical activity, and reducing alcohol consumption.[53]

However, experts recommend *antihypertensive treatment* for people who have Stage 1 or 2 hypertension and an ASCVD risk of more than 10%, with the goal to reduce blood pressure to below 130/80 mm Hg. Some of the most effective antihypertensive drugs have been available for decades and are safe and inexpensive.[53]

While treatment of high blood pressure is medically very simple, it involves many steps. Providers must take patients' blood pressure, diagnose their condition, and prescribe the appropriate medications. Patients must then take the prescribed medications and then return to follow-up appointments in order to determine if the drugs are working. At any step, the process can fail. Because of that, even using the old definition of hypertension above 140/90 mm Hg, only 80% of American adults with hypertension are aware that they have it, 72% are taking antihypertensives, and just less than 50% have their blood pressure adequately controlled.[87] Those percentages are far lower when using the newer definition of hypertension.

This has prompted innovations to simplify the diagnosis, treatment, and management of high blood pressure. These innovations are also commonly used to identify patients who have high LDL cholesterol and treat them with statins.[88] For example, electronic health records have built-in *clinical decision support tools* that help medical providers identify patients who need testing, medications, or follow-up appointments. Through *team-based care*, physicians delegate the job of tracking patients to nurses and paraprofessionals in order to make sure they are taking their medications. *Continuous quality improvement* approaches establish treatment metrics for populations of patients and involve the entire care team in redesigning clinic systems to improve those metrics. These metrics are sometimes tied to *financial incentives for providers* who hit high marks. *Pharmacy-based interventions* allow pharmacists to check patients' blood pressures and adjust medications so that fewer medical appointments are needed. Other streamlining approaches include patients' *self-monitoring of blood pressure* and use of digital devices that allow medical providers to observe these blood pressure results remotely. Finally, since patients often must pay for these appointments, tests, and medicines, other approaches to promote blood pressure control are policies that *reduce out-of-pocket costs*.[88]

Box 2.4 Summary–Prevention of Hypertension and Hypertensive Cardiovascular Disease

- Primary Prevention
  - Reduction of sodium in processed foods
  - Promotion of healthy diets
  - Promotion of physical activity
  - Reduction of alcohol consumption
- Secondary Prevention
  - Antihypertensive treatment
    - Clinical decision support tools
    - Team-based care
    - Continuous quality improvement
    - Financial incentives for providers
    - Pharmacy-based interventions
    - Self-monitoring of blood pressure
    - Policies to reduce out-of-pocket costs

Box 2.5 Key Words–Hypertension and Hypertensive Cardiovascular Disease

Antihypertensive
Atherosclerotic cardiovascular risk (ASCVD risk)
Cardiac output
Chronic kidney disease
Diastolic blood pressure
Elevated blood pressure
Hypertension
Hypertensive cardiovascular disease
Hypertensive heart disease
Normal blood pressure
Sodium
Sodium chloride
Stage 1 hypertension
Stage 2 hypertension
Systolic blood pressure
Vascular resistance

Resources–Hypertension and Hypertensive Cardiovascular Disease

- Hypertension and Hypertensive Cardiovascular Disease
- Community Preventive Services Task Force. *CPTSF Findings for Heart Disease and Stroke Prevention* at www.communityguide.org describes proven interventions to streamline and improve treatment of high cholesterol and high blood pressure in populations.
- Whelton PK, Carey RM, Aronow WS, et al. 2017 Guideline for the Prevention, Detection, Evaluation, and Management of High Blood Pressure in Adults. *J Am Coll Cardiol.* 2018;71(19). doi:10.1016/j.jacc.2017.11.006. This is a detailed set of recommendations for medical providers on blood pressure, which includes background on the causes and consequences of high blood pressure.
- Zhou B, Carrillo-Larco RM, Danaei G, et al. Worldwide trends in hypertension prevalence and progress in treatment and control from 1990 to 2019: a pooled analysis of 1201 population-representative studies with 104 million participants. *The Lancet.* 2021;398(10304):957-980. doi:10.1016/S0140-6736(21)01330-1. This is a detailed description of the global problem of hypertension and responses to it.
- He FJ, Tan M, Ma Y, et al. Salt Reduction to Prevent Hypertension and Cardiovascular Disease: JACC State-of-the-Art Review. *J Am Coll*

Cardiol. 2020;75(6):632-647. doi: 10.1016/j.jacc.2019.11.055. This provides detailed background on the relationship between sodium and high blood pressure.

- Ahmed M, Ng A, Christoforou A, et al. Top Sodium Food Sources in the American Diet—Using National Health and Nutrition Examination Survey. *Nutrients.* 2023;15(4):831. doi: 10.3390/nu15040831. By providing information on sodium intake by food sources and by demographic groups, this report identifies the foods most important in causing hypertension.

References

1. Global Burden of Disease Collaboration. Global Burden of Disease tool - GBD Results. Published 2023. Accessed August 21, 2023. Available at: https://vizhub.healthdata.org/gbd-results

2. Mitchell RN, Halushka MN. Atherosclerosis. In: Kumar V, Abbas AK, Aster JC, Turner JR, eds. *Robbins & Cotran Pathologic Basis of Disease.* 10th ed. Elsevier; 2021:493-504.

3. Berenson GS, Wattigney WA, Tracy RE, et al. Atherosclerosis of the aorta and coronary arteries and cardiovascular risk factors in persons aged 6 to 30 years and studied at necropsy (The Bogalusa Heart Study). *Am J Cardiol.* 1992;70(9):851-858. doi:10.1016/0002-9149(92)90726-F.

4. Hall JE, Hall ME. Phospholipids and cholesterol. In: *Guyton and Hall Textbook of Medical Physiology.* 14th ed. Elsevier; 2021:860-864.

5. Sacks FM, Lichtenstein AH, Wu JHY, et al. Dietary fats and cardiovascular disease: A presidential advisory from the American Heart Association. *Circulation.* 2017;136(3):e1-e23. doi:10.1161/CIR.0000000000000510.

6. US Department of Agriculture. FoodData Central. Published 2024. Accessed June 4, 2024. Available at: https://fdc.nal.usda.gov/

7. Kim Y, Keogh JB, Clifton PM. Benefits of nut consumption on insulin resistance and cardiovascular risk factors: Multiple potential mechanisms of actions. *Nutrients.* 2017;9(11):1271. doi:10.3390/nu9111271.

8. Rimm EB, Appel LJ, Chiuve SE, et al. Seafood long-chain n-3 polyunsaturated fatty acids and cardiovascular disease: A science advisory from the American Heart Association. *Circulation.* 2018;138(1):e35-e47. doi:10.1161/CIR.0000000000000574.

9. Lichtenstein AH, Appel LJ, Vadiveloo M, et al. 2021 dietary guidance to improve cardiovascular health: A scientific statement from the American Heart Association. *Circulation.* 2021;144(23):E472-E487. doi:10.1161/CIR.0000000000001031.

10. Rohrmann S, Linseisen J. Processed meat: The real villain? *Proc Nutr Soc.* 2016;75(3):233-241. doi:10.1017/S0029665115004255.

11. Ludwig DS, Ebbeling CB. The carbohydrate-insulin model of obesity: Beyond "calories in, calories out." *JAMA Intern Med.* 2018;178(8):1098-1103. doi:10.1001/jamainternmed.2018.2933.

12. Mozaffarian D. Dietary and policy priorities for cardiovascular disease, diabetes, and obesity. *Circulation.* 2016;133(2):187-225. doi:10.1161/CIRCULATIONAHA.115.018585.

13. Swaminathan S, Dehghan M, Raj JM, et al. Associations of cereal grains intake with cardiovascular disease and mortality across 21 countries in prospective urban and rural epidemiology study: Prospective cohort study. *BMJ.* 2021;372:m4948. doi:10.1136/bmj.m4948.

14. Lichtenstein AH. Last nail in the coffin for sugar-sweetened beverages: Now let's focus on the hard part. *Circulation.* 2019;139(18):2126-2128. doi:10.1161/CIRCULATIONAHA.119.040245.

15. Johnson RK, Appel LJ, Brands M, et al. Dietary sugars intake and cardiovascular health a scientific statement from the American Heart Association. *Circulation.* 2009;120(11):1011-1020. doi:10.1161/CIRCULATIONAHA.109.192627

16. Miller V, Mente A, Dehghan M, et al. Fruit, vegetable, and legume intake, and cardiovascular disease and deaths in 18 countries (PURE): A prospective cohort study. *Lancet.* 2017;390(10107):2037-2049. doi:10.1016/S0140-6736(17)32253-5

17. Tucker WJ, Fegers-Wustrow I, Halle M, Haykowsky MJ, Chung EH, Kovacic JC. Exercise for primary and secondary prevention of cardiovascular disease: JACC Focus Seminar 1/4. *J Am Coll Cardiol.* 2022;80(11). doi:10.1016/j.jacc.2022.07.004

18. Neufer PD, Bamman MM, Muoio DM, et al. Understanding the Cellular and Molecular Mechanisms of Physical Activity-Induced Health Benefits. *Cell Metab.* 2015;22(1):4-11. doi:10.1016/j.cmet.2015.05.011

19. Pierce GL, Donato AJ, Larocca TJ, Eskurza I, Silver AE, Seals DR. Habitually exercising older men do not demonstrate age-associated vascular endothelial oxidative stress. *Aging Cell.* 2011;10(6):1032-1037. doi:10.1111/j.14749726.2011.00748.x

20. Hakamaa E, Goebeler S, Martiskainen M, et al. Sex differences in coronary atherosclerosis during the pre- and postmenopausal period: The Tampere Sudden Death Study. *Atherosclerosis.* 2024;390:117459. doi:10.1016/j.atherosclerosis.2024.117459

21. National Center for Health Statistics, Centers for Disease Control and Prevention. Underlying Cause of Death Data on CDC WONDER. CDC. Published 2023. Accessed June 12, 2024. Available at: https://wonder.cdc.gov/Deaths-by-Underlying-Cause.html

22. Carnethon MR, Pu J, Howard G, et al. Cardiovascular health in African Americans: A scientific statement from the American Heart Association. *Circulation.* 2017;136(21):e393-e423. doi:10.1161/CIR.0000000000000534

23. Steenland K, Hu S, Walker J. All-cause and cause-specific mortality by socioeconomic status among employed persons in 27 US states, 1984–1997. *Am J Public Health.* 2004;94(6):1037-1042. doi:10.2105/AJPH.94.6.1037

24. World Health Organization. WHO Mortality Database. Published 2020. Accessed August 22, 2023. Available at: https://platform.who.int/mortality

25. Tuppo EE, Trivedi MP, Kostis JB, Daevmer J, Cabrera J, Kostis WJ. The role of public health versus invasive coronary interventions in the decline of coronary heart disease mortality. *Ann Epidemiol.* 2021;55:91-97. doi:10.1016/j.annepidem.2020.10.005

26. Ford ES, Capewell S. Proportion of the decline in cardiovascular mortality disease due to prevention versus treatment: Public health versus clinical care. *Annu Rev Public Health.* 2011;32:5-22. doi:10.1146/annurev-publhealth-031210-101211

27. Arnett DK, Blumenthal RS, Albert MA, et al. 2019 ACC/AHA guideline on the primary prevention of cardiovascular disease: A report of the American College of Cardiology/American Heart Association Task Force on Clinical Practice Guidelines. *Circulation.* 2019;140(11):e596-e646. doi:10.1161/CIR.0000000000000678

28. Flint AJ, Rexrode KM, Hu FB, et al. Body mass index, waist circumference, and risk of coronary heart disease: A prospective study among men and women. *Obes Res Clin Pract.* 2010;4(3):e171-e181. doi:10.1016/j.orcp.2010.01.001

29. Rosengren A, Dikaiou P, Se AR. Cardiovascular outcomes in type 1 and type 2 diabetes. *Diabetologia.* 2023;66:425-437. doi:10.1007/s00125-022-05857-5

30. Rosengren A. Cardiovascular disease in diabetes type 2: current concepts. *J Intern Med.* 2018;284(3):240-253. doi:10.1111/joim.12804

31. Dietary Guidelines Advisory Committee. *Scientific Report of the 2020 Dietary Guidelines Advisory Committee Advisory Report to the Secretary of Agriculture and Secretary of Health and Human Services.* Published 2020. Accessed June 12, 2024. Available at: https://www.dietaryguidelines.gov/2020-advisory-committee-report

32. Estruch R, Ros E, Salas-Salvadó J, et al. Primary prevention of cardiovascular disease with a Mediterranean diet supplemented with extra-virgin olive oil or nuts. *N Engl J Med.* 2018;378(25):e34. doi:10.1056/nejmoa1800389

33. Tharrey M, Mariotti F, Mashchak A, Barbillon P, Delattre M, Fraser GE. Patterns of plant and animal protein intake are strongly associated with cardiovascular mortality: The Adventist Health Study-2 cohort. *Int J Epidemiol.* 2018;47(5):1603-1612. doi:10.1093/ije/dyy030

34. Ramakrishnan R, Doherty A, Smith-Byrne K, et al. Accelerometer measured physical activity and the incidence of cardiovascular disease: Evidence from the UK Biobank Cohort study. *PLoS Med.* 2021;18(1). doi:10.1371/journal.pmed.1003487

35. Wahid A, Manek N, Nichols M, et al. Quantifying the association between physical activity and cardiovascular disease and diabetes: A systematic review and meta-analysis. *J Am Heart Assoc.* 2016;5:e002495. doi:10.1161/JAHA.115.002495

36. Del Pozo Cruz B, Ahmadi MN, Lee IM, Stamatakis E. Prospective associations of daily step counts and intensity with cancer and cardiovascular disease incidence and mortality and all-cause mortality. *JAMA Intern Med.* 2022;182(11):1139-1148. doi:10.1001/jamainternmed.2022.4000

37. Merghani A, Maestrini V, Rosmini S, et al. Prevalence of subclinical coronary artery disease in masters endurance athletes with a low atherosclerotic risk profile. *Circulation.* 2017;136(2):126-137. doi:10.1161/CIRCULATIONAHA.116.026964

38. Young DR, Hivert MF, Alhassan S, et al. Sedentary behavior and cardiovascular morbidity and mortality: A science advisory from the American Heart Association. *Circulation.* 2016;134(13):e262–e279. doi:10.1161/CIR.0000000000000440

39. Lavie CJ, Ozemek C, Carbone S, Katzmarzyk PT, Blair SN. Sedentary behavior, exercise, and cardiovascular health. *Circ Res.* 2019;124(5):799-815. doi:10.1161/CIRCRESAHA.118.312669

40. Ekelund U, Steene-Johannessen J, Brown WJ, et al. Does physical activity attenuate, or even eliminate, the detrimental association of sitting time with mortality? A harmonised meta-analysis of data from more than 1 million men and women. *Lancet.* 2016;388:1302-1310. doi:10.1016/S0140-6736(16)30370-1

41. Barnoya J, Glantz SA. Cardiovascular effects of secondhand smoke: Nearly as large as smoking. *Circulation.* 2005;111:2684-2698. doi:10.1161/CIRCULATIONAHA.104.492215

42. Meyers DG, Neuberger JS, He J. Cardiovascular effect of bans on smoking in public places. *J Am Coll Cardiol.* 2009;54:1249-1255. doi:10.1016/j.jacc.2009.07.022

43. Lv X, Sun J, Bi Y, et al. Risk of all-cause mortality and cardiovascular disease associated with secondhand smoke exposure: A systematic review and meta-analysis. *Int J Cardiol.* 2015;199:106-115. doi:10.1016/j.ijcard.2015.07.011

44. Lechner K, von Schacky C, McKenzie AL, et al. Lifestyle factors and high-risk atherosclerosis: Pathways and mechanisms beyond traditional risk factors. *Eur J Prev Cardiol.* 2020;27(4):394-406. doi:10.1177/2047487319869400

45. Münzel T, Miller MR, Sørensen M, Lelieveld J, Daiber A, Rajagopalan S. Reduction of environmental pollutants for prevention of cardiovascular disease: it's time to act. *Eur Heart J.* 2020;41(41):3989-3997. doi:10.1093/eurheartj/ehaa745

46. Pierce JB, Kershaw KN, Kiefe CI, et al. Association of childhood psychosocial environment with 30-year cardiovascular disease incidence and mortality in middle age. *J Am Heart Assoc.* 2020;9:e015326. doi:10.1161/JAHA.119.015326

47. Kivimäki M, Steptoe A. Effects of stress on the development and progression of cardiovascular disease. *Nat Rev Cardiol.* 2018;15(4):215-229. doi:10.1038/nrcardio.2017.189

48. Al Rifai M, Greenland P, Blaha MJ, et al. Factors of health in the protection against death and cardiovascular disease among adults with subclinical atherosclerosis. *Am Heart J.* 2018;198:180-188. doi:10.1016/j.ahj.2017.10.026

49. Food and Drug Administration. Trans Fat. Published 2024. Accessed October 8, 2024. Available at: https://www.fda.gov/food/food-additives-petitions/trans-fat

50. Meyers DG, Neuberger JS, He J. Cardiovascular effect of bans on smoking in public places. A systematic review and meta-analysis. *J Am Coll Cardiol.* 2009;54(14):1249-1255. doi:10.1016/j.jacc.2009.07.022

51. Grundy SM, Stone NJ, Bailey AL, et al. Guidelines on the management of blood cholesterol: A report of the American College of Cardiology/American Heart Association Task Force on Clinical Practice Guidelines. *Circulation.* 2019;139(25):e1082-e1143. doi:10.1161/CIR.0000000000000625

52. Centers for Disease Control and Prevention. *Million Hearts: Meaningful Progress 2012-2016—A Final Report.* Published

2016. Accessed June 12, 2024. Available at: https://millionhearts.hhs.gov/data-reports/reports.html

53. Whelton PK, Carey RM, Aronow WS, et al. 2017 guideline for the prevention, detection, evaluation, and management of high blood pressure in adults. *J Am Coll Cardiol.* 2018;71(19):e127-e248. doi:10.1016/j.jacc.2017.11.006

54. Mitchell RN, Halushka MK. Hypertensive vascular disease. In: Kumar V, Abbas AK, Aster JC, Turner JR, eds. *Robbins & Cotran Pathologic Basis of Disease.* 10th ed. Elsevier; 2021:489-493.

55. Appel LJ, Frohlich ED, Hall JE, et al. The importance of population-wide sodium reduction as a means to prevent cardiovascular disease and stroke: A call to action from the American Heart Association. *Circulation.* 2011;123(10):1138-1143. doi:10.1161/CIR.0b013e31820d0793

56. Razavi MA, Bazzano LA, Nierenberg J, et al. Advances in genomics research of blood pressure responses to dietary sodium and potassium intakes. *Hypertension.* 2021;78(1):4-15. doi:10.1161/HYPERTENSIONAHA.121.16509

57. Elijovich F, Weinberger MH, Anderson CAM, et al. Salt sensitivity of blood pressure : A scientific statement from the American Heart Association. *Hypertension.* 2016;68(3):e7-e46. doi:10.1161/HYP.0000000000000047

58. He FJ, Tan M, Ma Y, MacGregor GA. Salt reduction to prevent hypertension and cardiovascular disease: JACC State-of-the-Art Review. *J Am Coll Cardiol.* 2020;75(6):632-647. doi:10.1016/j.jacc.2019.11.055

59. Cappuccio FP, Campbell NRC, He FJ, et al. Sodium and health: Old myths and a controversy based on denial. *Curr Nutr Rep.* 2022;11(2):172-184. doi:10.1007/s13668-021-00383-z

60. Lemogoum D, Ngatchou W, Bika Lele C, et al. Association of urinary sodium excretion with blood pressure and risk factors associated with hypertension among Cameroonian pygmies and bantus: A cross-sectional study. *BMC Cardiovasc Disord.* 2018;18(1):49. doi:10.1186/s12872-018-0787-3

61. Mueller NT, Noya-Alarcon O, Contreras M, Appel LJ, Dominguez-Bello MG. Association of age with blood pressure across the lifespan in isolated Yanomami and Yekwana Villages. *JAMA Cardiol.* 2018;3(12):1247-1249. doi:10.1001/jamacardio.2018.3676

62. Ahmed M, Ng A, Christoforou A, Mulligan C, L'Abbé MR. Top sodium food sources in the American diet—Using National Health and Nutrition Examination Survey. *Nutrients.* 2023;15(4):831. doi:10.3390/nu15040831

63. Harnack LJ, Cogswell ME, Shikany JM, et al. Sources of sodium in US adults from 3 geographic regions. *Circulation.* 2017;135(19):1775-1783. doi:10.1161/CIRCULATIONAHA.116.024446

64. United States Department of Agriculture, United States Department of Health and Human Services. *Dietary Guidelines for Americans 2020-2025.* Published 2020. Accessed September 19, 2023. Available at: https://www.dietaryguidelines.gov

65. Nomura N, Shoda W, Uchida S. Clinical importance of potassium intake and molecular mechanism of potassium regulation. *Clin Exp Nephrol.* 2019;23(10):1175-1180. doi:10.1007/s10157-019-01766-x

66. Lewington S, Clarke R, Qizilbash N, Peto R, Collins R. Age-specific relevance of usual blood pressure to vascular mortality: A meta-analysis of individual data for one million adults in 61 prospective studies. *Lancet.* 2002;360 (9349):1903-1913. doi:10.1016/S0140-6736(02)11911-8

67. Go AS, Mozaffarian D, Roger VL, et al. Heart disease and stroke statistics—2013 update: A report from the American Heart Association. *Circulation.* 2013;127:e6-e245. doi:10.1161/CIR.0b013e31828124ad

68. Ono H, Ono Y. Nephrosclerosis and hypertension. *Medical Clinics of North America.* 1997;81(6):1273-1288. doi:10.1016/S0025-7125(05)70582-4

69. Kibria GM Al, Crispen R. Prevalence and trends of chronic kidney disease and its risk factors among US adults: An analysis of NHANES 2003-18. *Prev Med Rep.* 2020;20:101193. doi:10.1016/j.pmedr.2020.101193

70. Centers for Disease Control and Prevention. *Estimated Hypertension Prevalence, Treatment, and Control Among US Adults: Tables.* Published 2021. Accessed March 5, 2025. https://wwwn.cdc.gov/nchs/nhanes/ResponseRates.aspx#population-totals

71. Xu J, Lawrence KG, O'Brien KM, Jackson CL, Sandler DP. Association between neighbourhood deprivation and hypertension in a US-wide Cohort. *J Epidemiol Community Health (1978).* 2022;76(3):268-273. doi:10.1136/jech-2021-216445

72. Leng B, Jin Y, Li G, Chen L, Jin N. Socioeconomic status and hypertension: A meta-analysis. *J Hypertens.* 2015;33(2):221-229. doi:10.1097/HJH.0000000000000428

73. Zhou B, Carrillo-Larco RM, Danaei G, et al. Worldwide trends in hypertension prevalence and progress in treatment and control from 1990 to 2019: A pooled analysis of 1201 population-representative studies with 104 million participants. *Lancet.* 2021;398(10304):957-980. doi:10.1016/S0140-6736(21)01330-1

74. Sacks FM, Svetkey LP, Vollmer WM, et al. Effects on blood pressure of reduced dietary sodium and the Dietary Approaches to Stop Hypertension (DASH) diet. *New England Journal of Medicine.* 2001;344(1):3-10. doi:10.1056/nejm200101043440101

75. Center for Nutrition Policy and Promotion, Department of Agriculture. *A Series of Systematic Reviews on the Relationship Between Dietary Patterns and Health Outcomes.* Published 2014. Accessed July 24, 2024. Available at: https://nesr.usda.gov/sites/default/files/2019-06/DietaryPatternsReport-FullFinal2.pdf

76. Hall JE, Do Carmo JM, Da Silva AA, Wang Z, Hall ME. Obesity-induced hypertension: Interaction of neurohumoral and renal mechanisms. *Circ Res.* 2015;116(6):991-1006. doi:10.1161/CIRCRESAHA.116.305697

77. Sabbahi A, Arena R, Elokda A, Phillips SA. Exercise and hypertension: Uncovering the mechanisms of vascular control. *Prog Cardiovasc Dis.* 2016;59(3):226-234. doi:10.1016/j.pcad.2016.09.006

78. Roerecke M, Tobe SW, Kaczorowski J, et al. Sex-specific associations between alcohol consumption and incidence of hypertension: A systematic review and meta-analysis of cohort studies. *J Am Heart Assoc.* 2018;7:e008202. doi:10.1161/JAHA.117.008202

79. Roerecke M. Alcohol's impact on the cardiovascular system. *Nutrients.* 2021;13(10):3419. doi:10.3390/nu13103419

80. Marwaha K. Examining the role of psychosocial stressors in hypertension. *Journal of Preventive Medicine and Public Health.* 2022;55(6):499-505. doi:10.3961/jpmph.21.266

81. World Health Organization. *Guideline: Sodium Intake for Adults and Children.* Published 2012. Accessed June 12, 2024. Available at: https://www.who.int/publications/i/item/9789241504836

82. American Heart Association. How much sodium should I eat per day? Published January 5, 2024. Accessed June 5, 2024. Available at: https://www.heart.org/en/healthy-living/healthy-eating/eat-smart/sodium/how-much-sodium-should-i-eat-per-day

83. Moran AJ, Wang J, Sharkey AL, Dowling EA, Curtis CJ, Kessler KA. US food industry progress toward salt reduction, 2009-2018. *Am J Public Health*. 2022;112(2):325-333. doi:10.2105/AJPH.2021.306571

84. Center for Food Safety and Applied Nutrition, Food and Drug Administration. *Voluntary Sodium Reduction Goals: Target Mean and Upper Bound Concentrations for Sodium in Commercially Processed, Packaged, and Prepared Foods (Edition 2)*. US Food and Drug Administration; 2024.

85. World Health Organization. *WHO Global Sodium Benchmarks for Different Food Categories*. Published 2021. Accessed December 11, 2024. Available at: https://www.who.int/publications/i/item/9789240025097

86. Ettehad D, Emdin CA, Kiran A, et al. Blood pressure lowering for prevention of cardiovascular disease and death: A systematic review and meta-analysis. *Lancet*. 2016;387(10022):957-967. doi:10.1016/S0140-6736(15)01225-8

87. Muntner P, Miles MA, Jaeger BC, et al. Blood pressure control among US adults, 2009 to 2012 through 2017 to 2020. *Hypertension*. 2022;79(9):1971-1980. doi:10.1161/HYPERTENSIONAHA.122.19222

88. Community Preventive Services Task Force. *CPTSF Findings for Heart Disease and Stroke Prevention*. Published 2023. Accessed August 21, 2023. Available at: https://www.thecommunityguide.org/pages/task-force-findings-heart-disease-stroke-prevention.html

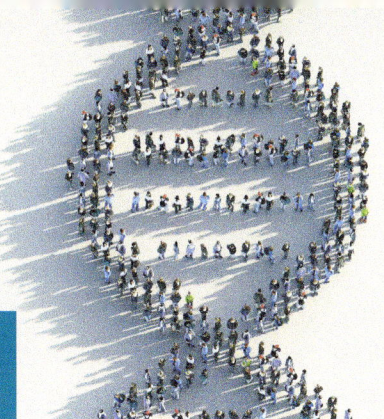

CHAPTER 3

Cancer

More than one in three people will develop cancer at some point in their lives. The disease is often but not always, fatal. If you group all types together, cancer is the second leading cause of death (after cardiovascular disease) in the United States and globally. As undernutrition and infectious diseases become less common and people live longer, cancer is becoming even more prominent as a cause of death.

A few key terms: a **tumor**, also called a **neoplasm**, is an abnormal growth arising from a single cell that has acquired damage to its genes.[1] Tumors can be either **benign** or **malignant**. The difference is that benign tumors' cells do not invade other tissues, even if the tumors become very large. In contrast, cells in a malignant tumor do invade the tissues surrounding them or at distant sites in the body. **Cancer** is another word for a malignant tumor.

Overview of Cancer and Its Causes

Cancer is not a single disease but instead encompasses hundreds of diseases, each involving a different cell line. Cancers are named for the type of cells from which they arise. Cells that make up the lining of organs are called **epithelial cells**, and the lining tissue is called **epithelium**. Cancers that arise from epithelial cells are called **carcinomas**. Cells that produce and secrete a substance are called **gland** cells. Many epithelial cells are also gland cells because they secrete mucus or other fluids. A benign tumor of gland cells is called an **adenoma**. A malignant tumor that arises from epithelial gland cells is called an **adenocarcinoma**. All the cancers discussed in this chapter are carcinomas and most are adenocarcinomas.

When cancer cells invade distant sites, they are said to **metastasize** those cell colonies are called **metastases**, and the cancer is called **metastatic**.

Common Mechanisms of Cancer Development

One biologic mechanism underlies all types of cancer: **mutations**. Mutations are alterations of a cell's normal DNA. They can result from the DNA being exposed to chemicals or radiation. But more often, mutations leading to cancer result from errors in the copying of DNA when individual cells divide (undergo **mitosis**).[2]

The copying of DNA during mitosis is called DNA **replication**. Humans' DNA is composed of some 3 billion "base pairs"—molecules that carry the genetic code. Imagine if you had to copy, by hand, the letters in one thousand bibles. You would undoubtedly make mistakes. Likewise, when cells copy their DNA, they make errors; these errors are mutations.

Most mutations, regardless of whether they appear during mitosis or in a cell at rest, make very little difference in how the cell works. Those mutations are then just copied when that cell undergoes mitosis, and they become permanently part of that cell line's DNA. However, some mutations change how a cell operates, and those mutations are likewise passed to the cells' daughters. With the enormous amount of DNA and potential errors involved, there are billions of changes in cell function that can result from mutations. Among them, some can make it easier for additional mutations to occur in subsequent cell divisions. *A normal cell line becomes transformed into a cancer cell line through a series of mutations, each of which increases the likelihood of subsequent mutations, ultimately producing a profoundly altered cell that grows in an uncontrolled way* (**Figure 3.1**). As cells in a transformed cell line divide repeatedly, different daughter cells acquire different additional mutations, so by the time a cancer is diagnosed, even though it has begun as a single cell line, it appears as a heterogenous group of cancerous cells.

The transformation of a normal cell line into cancer may take as few as 10 mutations or as many as thousands. Some common cancers are caused by sequences of mutations that happen the same way in many different people. Other cancers are the result of many quite-varied, unique mutations.[1]

Mutations of a few key types of genes are often involved in the transformation of a normal cell into a cancer cell.[1]

- *Tumor suppressor genes.* All cells contain the potential to **proliferate**—that is, to make many copies of themselves by dividing repeatedly. But because most cell proliferation is not healthy for multi-celled organisms like humans, those organisms have mechanisms to block proliferation, including specific genes that suppress mitosis called **tumor suppressor genes**. If mutations disable any tumor suppressor genes, the cells involved (and their daughters) will undergo inappropriate proliferation.
- *DNA repair genes.* Some genes are responsible for identifying and repairing DNA that has become defective. If those DNA repair genes are themselves damaged by mutations, defective DNA in any gene will be more likely to be passed to daughter cells.
- *Apoptosis genes.* It is not normal for most human cell lines to keep dividing indefinitely. Normal cells are programmed to die after their daughter cells undergo a certain number of divisions, such as 40 or 60. This programmed cell death is called **apoptosis**. There are genes within cells responsible for apoptosis. If these genes become defective because of mutations, the cells in that cell line will divide indefinitely, making the cell line immortal.[1]
- *Immune recognition genes.* A key line of an organism's defense against cancer is the **immune system**, which is a network of cells that kills off viruses, bacteria, and other foreign agents that are trying to cause an infection. The immune system can also recognize cancer cells as abnormal or "foreign" and then kill them. It is common for cancerous cell lines to develop but be killed by the immune system before they do damage. However, if cancer cells mutate in ways that prevent them from being recognized by the immune system as foreign, they can evade the immune system and thrive.

The final result of the series of mutations that transform normal cells is a line of cells that grows uncontrollably, is immortal, can resist the body's immune system, and invades other tissues, that is, cancer.[1]

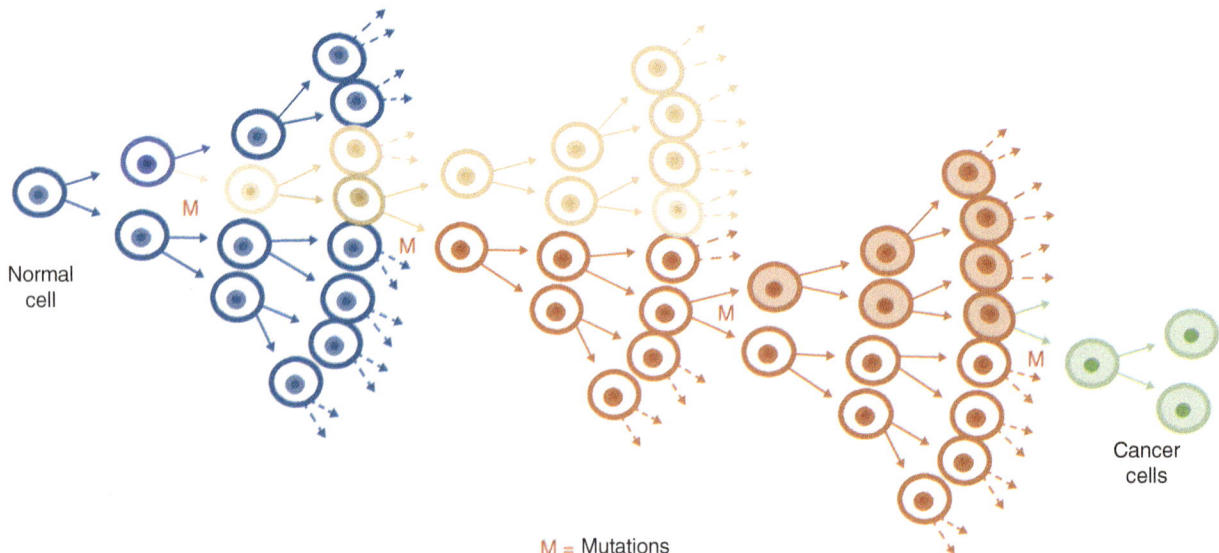

M = Mutations

Figure 3.1 **Stepwise Transformation of Normal Cells into Cancer Cells.** A normal cell line is transformed into a cancer cell line through a series of mutations, which are errors in DNA replication. Mutations commonly occur when cells make copies of themselves, i.e., they undergo mitosis. Each mutation increases the chances of a cell acquiring more mutations in later cell mitoses. This diagram shows just four mutations, but the transformation from a normal cell line into a cancer cell line actually requires between 10 and many thousands of mutations.

One way to view cancer is that it is just individual cells reverting to the normal behavior of single-cell organisms, breaking free of the constraints imposed on them by the multi-celled organism of which they are part. Unfortunately for the human involved, those liberated single-cell organisms "succeed" by making copies of themselves in an aggressive and destructive way.

Common Causes of Cancer

Because errors of DNA replication are bound to happen, cancer can occur without any cause other than bad luck. The older people are, the more likely that their luck will run out and the mutations they have acquired will result in cancer.

But certain exposures change the odds. A cell line is more likely to be transformed into cancer if:

- *The cell line is exposed to agents that damage DNA or interfere with DNA replication.*[1] Many chemicals, such as those in tobacco smoke, produce this damage to DNA, leading to mutations. When chemicals cause cancer, they are called **carcinogens**. Radiation likewise damages DNA and can lead to cancer, as do some viruses, such as the human papillomavirus (HPV).

- *The cell line undergoes frequent cell division.* Some types of cells in the body, such as the epithelial cells in the colon or the female breast, are regularly lost, so they must be constantly replaced. Replacing cells involves cell divisions, with more copying of DNA taking place. The more times a cell makes copies of its DNA, the more mutations are bound to occur. In addition, some hormones stimulate cells to divide. Most important is estrogen, a female hormone that stimulates epithelial cells in the breast to divide and that increases the risk of breast cancer.[3] The hormone insulin also promotes cell division and may be a link between obesity and cancer.[4]

- *The organism's immune system is weakened or activated.* Cancer is more common in people who are born with defective immune systems or who develop ineffective immune systems from AIDS or chemotherapy for a previous cancer. The defective immune systems allow early cancers that might otherwise be killed to grow. [1] Also, strangely, some cancers are more likely to develop when a normal immune system is activated to fight a perceived invader. When the immune system is activated, it puts in place a complex response called **inflammation**. Although researchers have known for decades that inflammation can promote

the development of cancer, they still do not fully understand why.[1] We do know, though, that the complex response in inflammation involves both cells that activate other immune cells and cells that suppress other immune cells. It may be that during the complex response of active inflammation, new cancer cells can more easily take advantage of the immune suppressors to survive.

The amount of time a cell line or a person is exposed to carcinogens matters. An exposure of a single day is much less likely to induce the series of mutations needed to cause cancer than daily exposure for years. That is one reason that regular smoking is much more likely to cause cancer than, for example, a single chemical spill. And that is why people who smoke increase their risk of cancer with each month that they smoke.

The carcinogenic chemicals that matter most, then, are those that humans encounter regularly over years. Humans are mostly exposed to chemicals regularly by ingesting or inhaling them, that is, from eating, drinking, or breathing. That is why, as the rest of this chapter shows, the most important common risk factors for cancer are smoking, drinking alcohol, eating certain foods, and breathing air that contains carcinogens.

When cancer strikes, people tend to look for a single cause, and they often suspect unfamiliar chemicals in their environment, such as food additives with unpronounceable names or a chemical factory nearby. They are right to suspect their environment, and it is possible that these exposures could trigger cancer. But the odds of getting cancer are tilted most by the familiar chemicals in the environment that people are exposed to heavily and regularly, such as those in cigarette smoke, alcohol, automobile exhaust, and processed meat. Prevention of cancer in populations depends in large part on communicating the risks of those familiar exposures clearly.

Common Sites of Cancer

This chapter covers the four sites of cancer with the highest **mortality rates** (deaths per 100,000 persons per year) in the United States: cancers of the lung, breast, colon, and pancreas. These sites have high mortality rates for different reasons (**Table 3.1**). Breast cancer has a very high **incidence rate** (130 new cancer cases per 100,000 persons per year) but fortunately has a very high relative **survival rate** (91% five years after the diagnosis).[5] In contrast, cancer of the pancreas has a relatively low incidence rate (14 cases per 100,000) but a very low survival rate after diagnosis (13%). Lung cancer has both a high incidence rate and a low survival rate, so it has the

Table 3.1 Incidence, Survival, and Mortality of Four Key Cancer Sites in the United States

Cancer Site	Incidence Rate*	5-Year Relative Survival**	Mortality Rate***
Lung	53	28%	29.9
Breast (female)	130	91%	18.7
Colon and Rectum	36	64%	12.6
Pancreas	14	13%	11.1

* Cases per 100,000 persons, 2017-2021

**Percentage of people with cancer alive 5 years after diagnosis (in 2014-2020), relative to expected survival of persons without cancer

***Deaths per 100,000 persons, 2018-2022

Data from U.S. Cancer Statistics Working Group. U.S. Cancer Statistics Data Visualizations Tool. U.S. Department of Health and Human Services, Centers for Disease Control and Prevention and National Cancer Institute, released in June 2024. https://www.cdc.gov/cancer/dataviz

highest mortality rate of any cancer type. Compared to these other cancer sites, colorectal cancer has moderate incidence and mortality rates, leading to a mortality rate similar to that of cancer of the pancreas.

Some risk factors (e.g., smoking) are shared by these cancer types, while others (such as radon gas) are unique to specific sites.

The sections that follow have more information on the pathophysiology, risk factors, and prevention of these types of cancer.

Box 3.1 Key Words–Cancer

Adenocarcinoma
Adenoma
Apoptosis
Benign (neoplasm)
Cancer
Carcinogen
Carcinoma
Epithelium, epithelial cells
Gland
Incidence, incidence rate
Immune system
Inflammation
Malignant (neoplasm)
Metastasize, metastasis, metastatic
Mitosis
Mortality, mortality rate
Mutation
Neoplasm
Proliferate
Replication (of DNA)
Survival rate
Tumor
Tumor suppressor gene

Resources–Cancer

- The National Cancer Institute maintains web pages with easy-to-understand information for patients about common causes of cancer, prevention, and treatment. https://www.cancer.gov/
- The Centers for Disease Control and Prevention maintain an interactive database that calculates and displays cancer incidence, mortality, and survival in the United States, at https://gis.cdc.gov/Cancer/USCS/#/AtAGlance/
- Sung H, Ferlay J, Siegel RL, et al. Global Cancer Statistics 2020: GLOBOCAN Estimates of Incidence and Mortality Worldwide for 36 Cancers in 185 Countries. *CA Cancer J Clin*. 2021;71(3): 209-249. doi:10.3322/caac.21660
- Islami F, Goding Sauer A, Miller KD, et al. Proportion and number of cancer cases and deaths attributable to potentially modifiable risk factors in the United States. *CA Cancer J Clin*. 2018;68(1). doi:10.3322/caac.21440

Cancer of the Lung

Introduction

The leading cause of cancer death in the United States and globally is cancer of the lung.[6] Lung cancer was once rare, but since the early 20th century it has undergone a massive, global, slow-moving epidemic, driven by smoking. The effort to prevent lung cancer is mostly a continuing battle against tobacco companies to reduce smoking. However, there are other exposures to lung tissue known to increase the risk of lung cancer that can also be prevented or reduced.

Physiology of the Lung

The job of the lung is to supply oxygen to the blood and remove carbon dioxide from it. To do this, the lungs move oxygen and carbon dioxide through an extensive branching network of large airways called **bronchi** and small airways called **bronchioles** that end in air sacs called **alveoli**. The alveoli are where the gas exchange takes place (**Figure 3.2**). These alveoli are wrapped in **capillaries**, through which the blood moves. Gases diffuse across the thin membranes between capillaries and the alveoli (**Figure 3.3**). One of the flaws of this system is that drugs like nicotine that are inhaled can also quickly diffuse across these membranes and into the blood.

Pathophysiology of Lung Cancer

More than 90% of lung cancers are carcinomas, arising from the epithelial cells lining the bronchi, bronchioles, or alveoli (**Figure 3.4**).[7] These cells are susceptible to cancer-causing mutations because they have a high turnover and they are directly exposed to carcinogenic chemicals or inflammation-causing particles in the air.

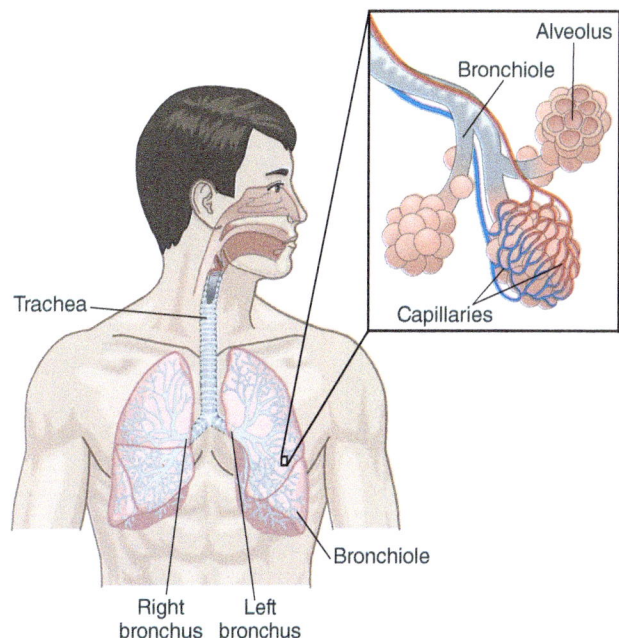

Figure 3.2 The Lung, Airways and Alveoli. The lung is composed of a branching network of large airways called bronchi and small airways called bronchioles, which end in tiny air sacs called alveoli.

© MAYO FOUNDATION FOR MEDICAL EDUCATION & RESEARCH

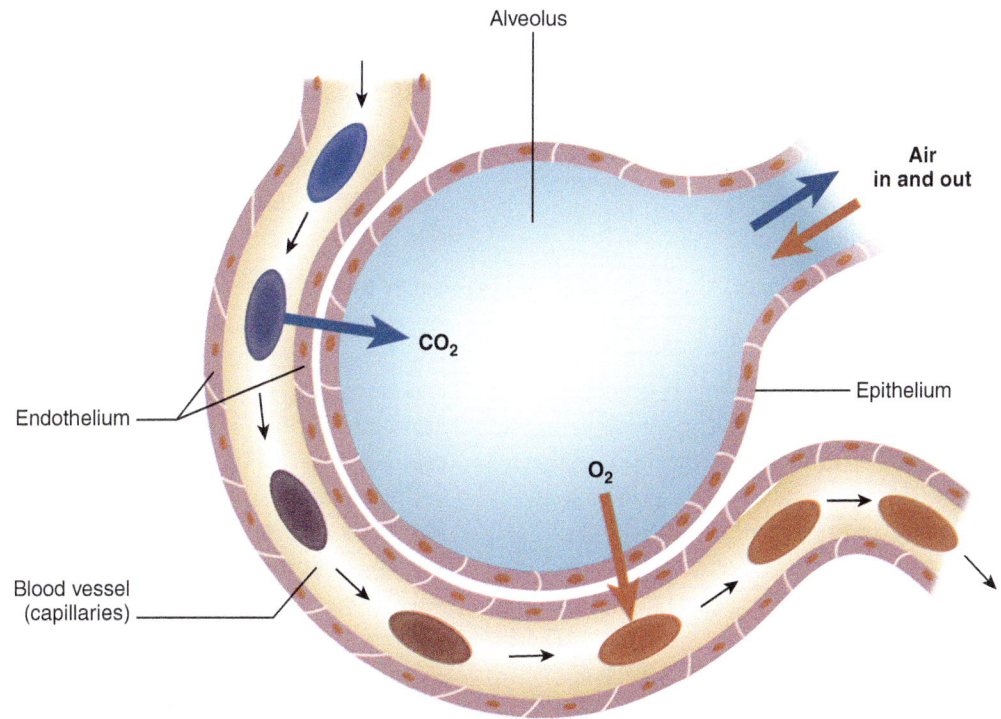

Figure 3.3 How Lung Alveoli Remove Carbon Dioxide and Supply Oxygen. The airways supply fresh air to the alveoli. Blood that is full of carbon dioxide and depleted of oxygen enters capillaries that wrap around the alveoli. As the blood passes the alveoli, carbon dioxide diffuses across the lining of the capillaries (endothelium) and the lining of the alveoli (epithelium) into the alveoli. At the same time, oxygen diffuses across the epithelium and endothelium in the opposite direction. This leaves the blood exiting the lungs full of oxygen and depleted of carbon dioxide.

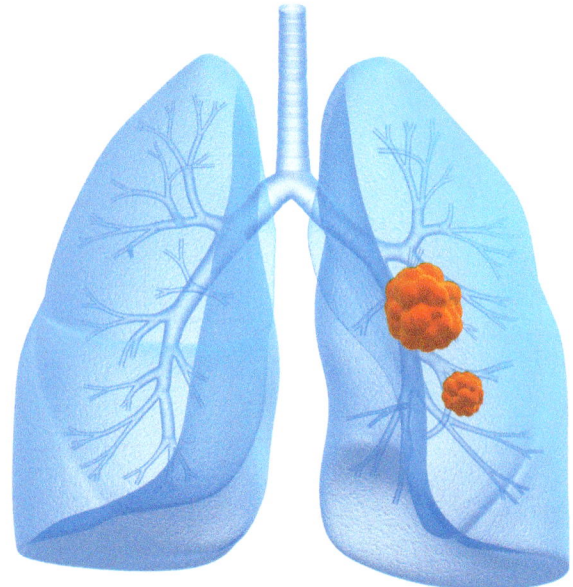

Figure 3.4 **Lung Cancer.** Most lung cancers arise from the epithelial cells lining the bronchi, bronchioles, or alveoli. These cells are directly exposed to cancer-causing chemicals in tobacco smoke.

© Sebastian Kaulitzki/Shutterstock

Smokers get an extraordinary dose of chemicals and particles in the lining of their airways. But tobacco smoke is not the only trigger for lung cancer. Carcinogen-containing smoke from burning wood, coal or diesel fuel likewise lands on lung epithelial cells. Industrial exposure to some metals, including arsenic, can cause lung cancer, as can inhaling asbestos fibers. And radiation exposure, from inhaling radioactive gases such as radon, can likewise induce cancer-causing mutations.[7]

The early mutations that ultimately lead to lung cancer involve deletions of tumor suppressor genes. That gets the epithelial cells dividing at an abnormal rate. With additional mutations, the cell lines show characteristic changes that an expert can recognize under a microscope. For example, experts can detect signs that cells are dividing quickly and in a disorganized way. While many areas of the lung in smokers show early changes, only some develop the right combination of mutations to become cancer.[7] The process is slow, taking 10 to 30 years.[7]

The slow development of lung cancer provides a theoretical opportunity to diagnose and remove lung cancers early. However, by the time lung cancer is recognized, for about 80% of affected people, the cancer has already spread within the lung or to other areas of the body, which makes it very difficult to remove.[8] While treatments for lung cancer are improving, only 28% of people with the disease survive for five years after the diagnosis.[5]

Epidemiology: Patterns and Trends

In 2020, about 136,000 people died of lung cancer in the United States.[5] That's roughly equal to the number of deaths from colon, breast, and pancreatic cancer combined.[5] Over the past century, the number of deaths from lung cancer skyrocketed, but fortunately, it is now falling. The rise and fall are similar to the rise and fall in smoking rates about 25 years earlier.[5] **Figure 3.5** shows the delayed but enormous impact of public health efforts to reduce smoking on lung cancer.

Figures 3.6 and **3.7** show lung cancer incidence rates by demographic group in the United States. Because of the long time it takes lung cancer to develop, the disease mainly occurs in older adults. Case rates are currently higher in men than in women (although that is changing) and are lower in Asians than other racial and ethnic groups.[5] People with low incomes are about twice as likely to develop lung cancer as those with higher incomes;[9] some but not all that difference is due to higher smoking rates in low-income populations.[10]

Across the globe, more than 2 million people develop lung cancer and 1.8 million die from it each year.[11,12] The incidence of lung cancer is highest in Europe, North America, and East Asia because there were high smoking rates in these regions in the past. However, lung cancer rates are rising in many other parts of the world due to recent increased rates of smoking.[6,11]

Risk Factors

Modifiable risk factors for lung cancer include (**Figure 3.8**):

- *Smoking.* While there are many known risk factors for lung cancer, smoking is by far the most important because of the heavy, constant, years-long exposure of the epithelial cells to tobacco smoke. Tobacco smoke contains thousands of chemicals, dozens of which are known carcinogens, including some particularly potent ones, such as **N-nitrosamines** and **polycyclic aromatic hydrocarbons**.[13] An estimated one in six people who smoke eventually develops lung cancer.[8] The relative risk of lung cancer in people who smoke is 10 to 30 times that of those who do not, with those who smoke more cigarettes per day or for more years having higher risks.[12] Current estimates are that about 80% of lung cancer deaths (or roughly 110,000 people per year) in the United States are attributable to smoking.[14] While cigarette smoking is by far the most important culprit, smoking pipes and cigars (which involves inhaling less smoke into the lungs) somewhat increases risk.[7]

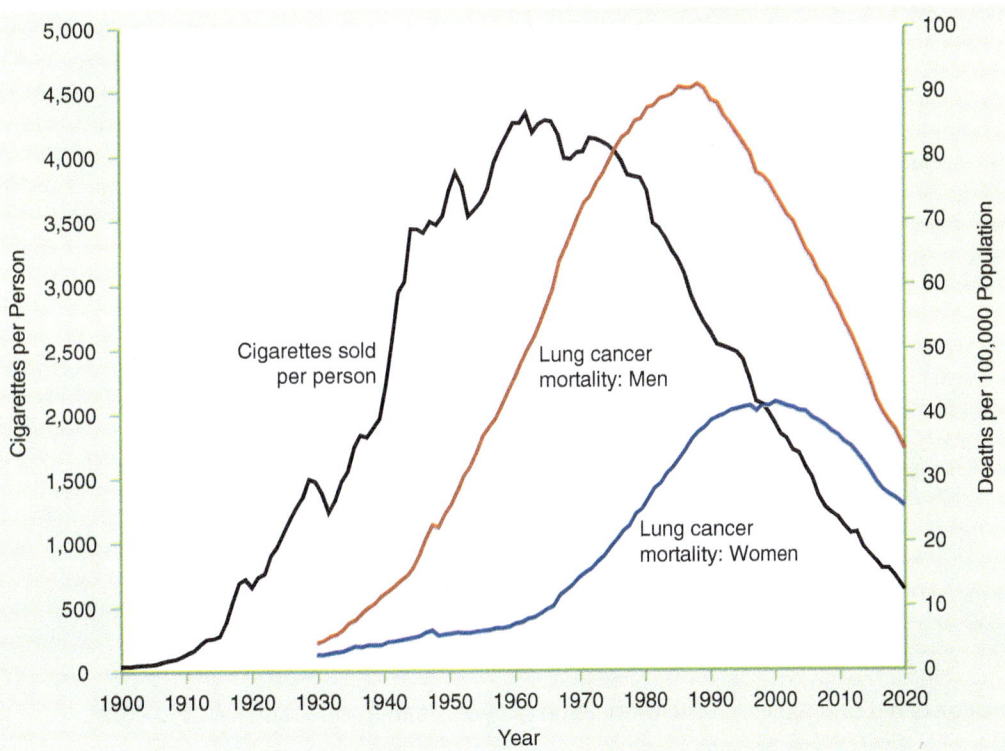

Figure 3.5 **Trends in Smoking and Lung Cancer Mortality in the United States.** Lung cancer rates rose and fell about 20 years after the rise and fall in cigarette consumption

- *Environmental tobacco smoke.* People who do not smoke still breathe in tobacco smoke if they are near smokers indoors. Those who live with people who smoke have about a 25% increase in risk of developing lung cancer.[8,12] That is far below the risk for people who actively smoke, but so many people are exposed that an estimated 4,400 lung cancer deaths in the United States annually are attributable to second-hand smoke.[14]

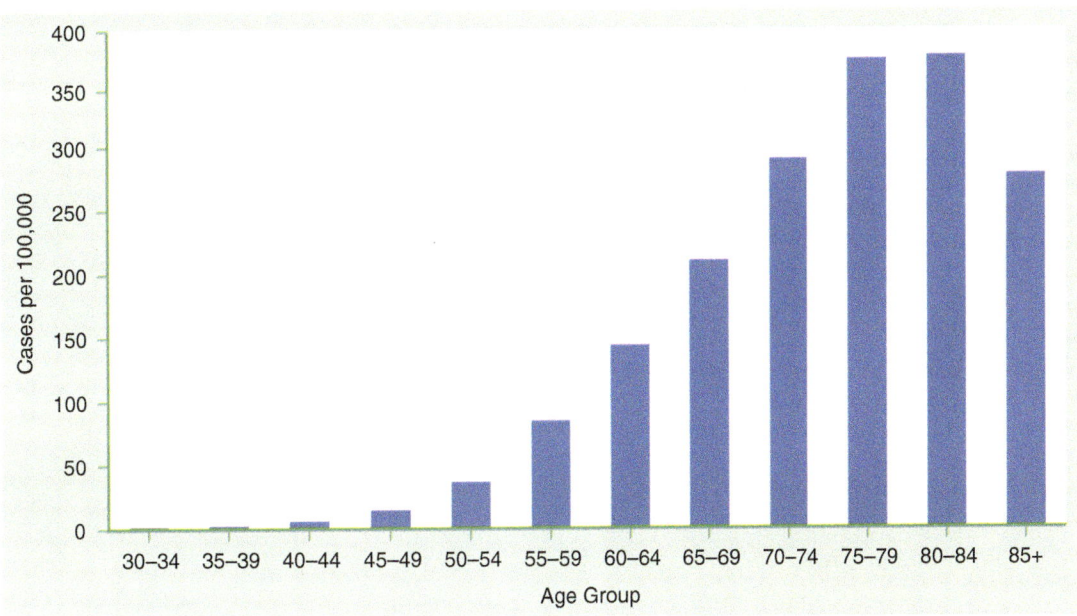

Figure 3.6 **Incidence of Lung Cancer in the United States by Age Group, 2017–2021.**

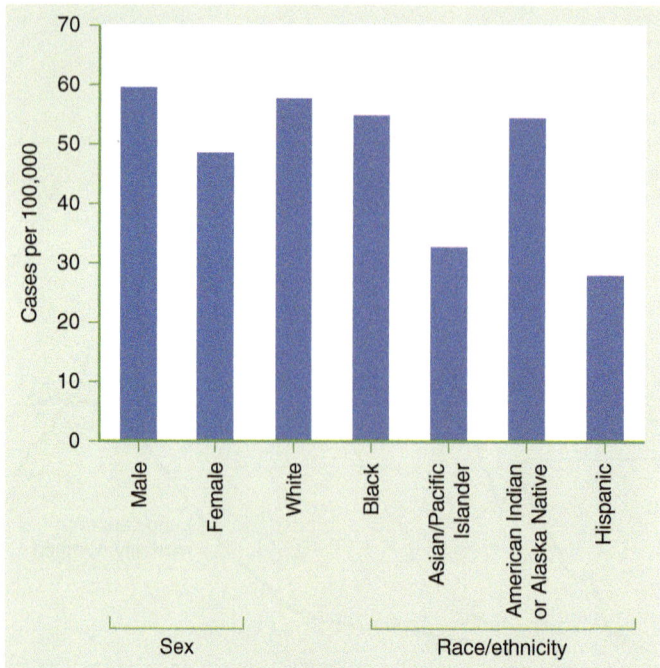

Figure 3.7 **Incidence of Lung Cancer in the United States by Sex and Race/Ethnicity, 2017–2021.**

Data from U.S. Cancer Statistics Working Group. U.S. Cancer Statistics Data Visualizations Tool. U.S. Department of Health and Human Services, Centers for Disease Control and Prevention and National Cancer Institute, released in June 2024. https://www.cdc.gov/cancer/dataviz

- *Household air pollution* from fuel burning. In low-income countries people often burn wood, sticks, leftovers from crops (referred to as **biomass**) or coal indoors for heat and cooking. The smoke from these

fires contains many carcinogens, and regular exposure substantially increases the risk of lung cancer.[8,12]

- *Ambient particulate air pollution.*[7] **Ambient** (or outdoor) air pollution is produced by sources outside

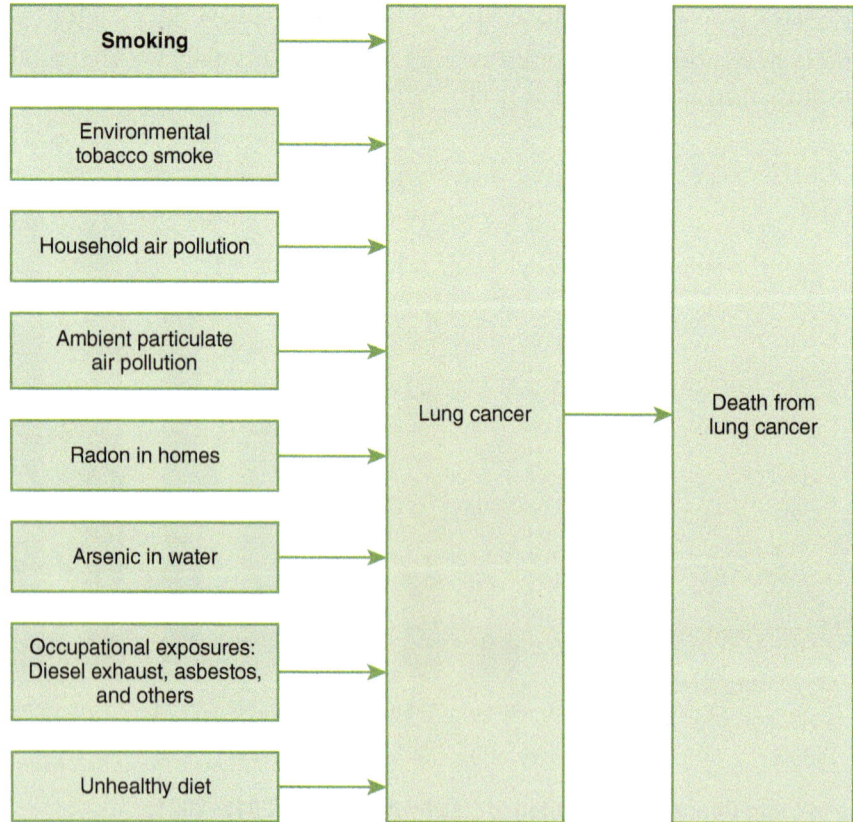

Figure 3.8 **Cause-and-Effect Diagram for Lung Cancer.**

of the home and exposes people outdoors, such as particles and gases emitted by coal-burning power plants or motor vehicles. The particles in air pollution are called **particulate matter (PM)** or particulate air pollution. The particles that do the most damage to health are those below 2.5 microns in size, called **PM$_{2.5}$**. These particles are small enough to be inhaled into the small airways and alveoli. Particulate air pollution increases the risk of lung cancer in the same way that environmental tobacco smoke does.[8] Although exposure to particulate air pollution outdoors is far less intense than exposure to smoke indoors, the number of people exposed (in mega-cities in Asia, for example) is many millions. Air pollution is discussed more in Chapter 8. Chronic Respiratory Diseases.

- *Radon.*[7] **Radon** is a radioactive gas that is naturally present underground in rock and soil. The gas seeps into houses and other buildings through cracks in the foundations, walls, and joints. People who live in homes where radon gas intrudes can get radioactivity into their lungs, increasing their risk of developing lung cancer by about 15%.[8,12] Because so many people are exposed, at a population level, the risk of radon is significant. One estimate is that 9% of lung cancer cases in Europe are attributable to radon.[15]
- *Arsenic in drinking water.* Arsenic is a carcinogenic mineral present naturally in the soil that can contaminate drinking water. While high levels of arsenic can cause arsenic poisoning, low levels of arsenic in drinking water can cause lung cancer.[12]
- *Occupational exposure to carcinogens.*[7]
  - *Diesel exhaust* causes lung cancer in people who regularly breathe in air near equipment with diesel engines, such as miners, truck drivers, railroad workers, farm workers, machine operators, mechanics, filling station attendants, and parking lot attendants.[12]
  - Several chemicals and minerals used in industrial processes are known to increase the risk of lung cancer in workers exposed to them. Among them are *asbestos, silica, nickel, cadmium, chromium,* and *arsenic.*[12] By one estimate, 10% of lung cancer deaths in men and 5% in women are attributable to these industrial exposures.[8]
- *Unhealthy diet.* Some foods that increase or decrease the risk of other cancers also have a meaningful impact on lung cancer. Specifically, red meat and processed meat have been linked to an increase in risk and fruits and vegetables to a decrease in risk.[8,12,14]

Preventive Interventions

Primary Prevention

The following are preventive interventions addressing these risk factors (**Figure 3.9**):

- *Smoking prevention.* Refer to Chapter 11. Tobacco Use for a full discussion of policies to reduce smoking.
- *Smoke-free policies* in public places like bars and restaurants greatly reduce people's exposure to second-hand smoke. Also, tobacco smoke can travel between adjacent apartments and through ventilation systems, so apartment buildings should likewise be smoke-free.
- *Substitution of biomass fuels.* Several low- and middle-income countries operate programs to help people switch from biomass fuels or coal to safer household fuels. These programs can reduce their carcinogen exposure indoors.[16]
- *Air pollution regulation and reduction in fossil fuel use* can reduce ambient particulate air pollution. Airborne fine particles are produced by coal-burning power plants, other industrial sources, vehicles, and wildfires.[17] Emission-control equipment has reduced levels of PM$_{2.5}$ in the United States over many years, but levels are still extremely high in some cities in Asia and other areas in the world that rely on coal for energy.[18] Particulate air pollution can also be reduced by changing from combustion to electric vehicles and shifting from fossil fuels to renewable energy sources.[17]
- *Radon-resistant construction* techniques reduce people's exposure to radon in homes and other buildings. These techniques create a better seal around the underground portions of buildings and redirect underground gases outdoors. The Environmental Protection Agency (EPA) has a plan to reduce the risk of radon, including detailed recommendations for new construction, and testing and mitigation of existing buildings.[19]
- Exposure to arsenic in water can be reduced by *systems that remove arsenic* from water or by *substituting other sources of water for drinking.*[20]
- *Replacement of diesel engines* with those that use cleaner fuels is the best solution to the risk of diesel exhaust. If that is not possible, diesel engines can be retrofitted to reduce emissions.[12]
- *Occupational respiratory protection standards* can protect workers from industrial exposures to carcinogens in the air. These standards require companies to reduce emissions of harmful chemicals and particles, or if that is not possible, to protect workers with **respirators** that prevent them from

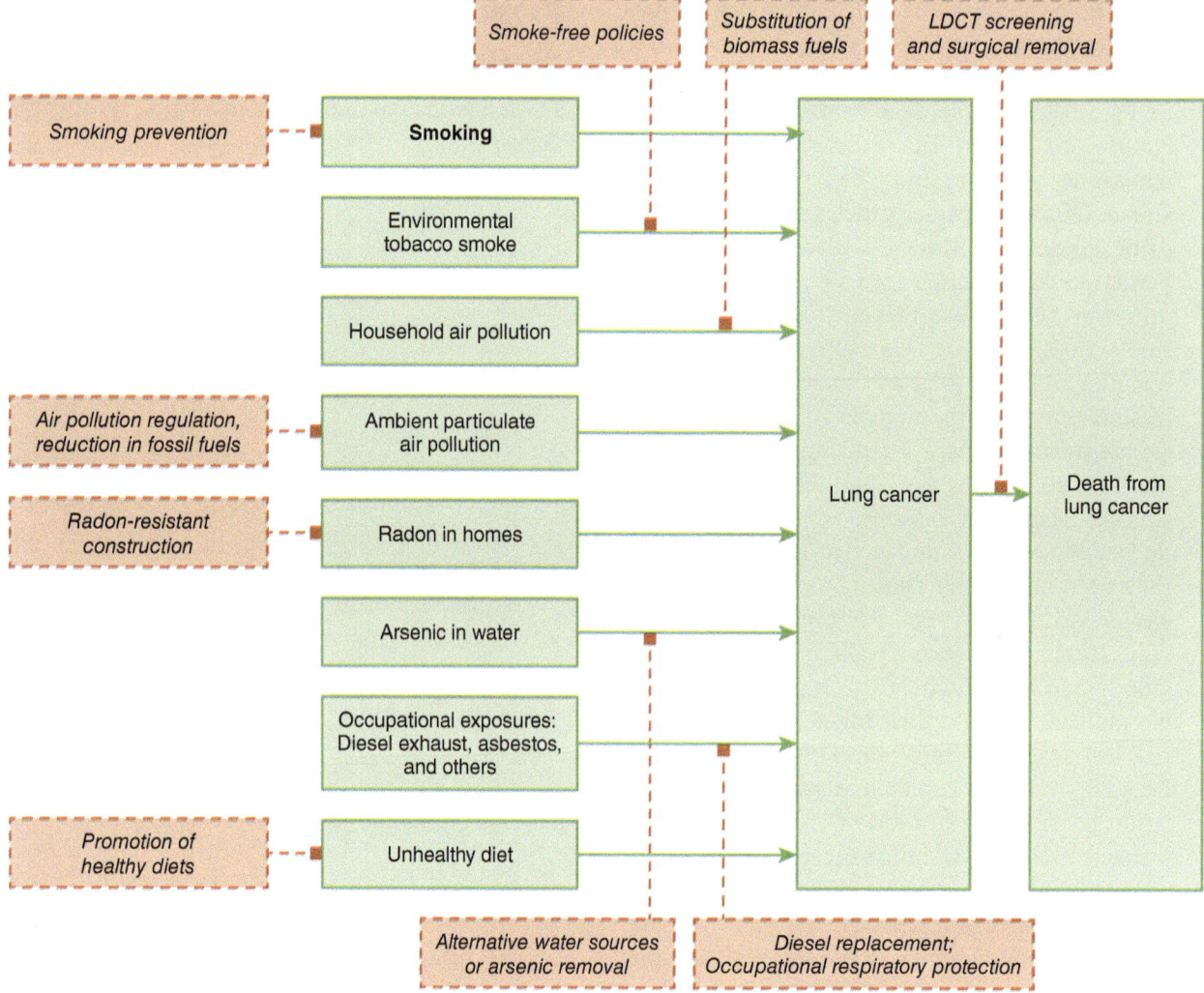

Figure 3.9 Cause-and-Effect Diagram for Lung Cancer, with Preventive Interventions.

breathing chemicals and particles in the air. In the United States, these standards are enforced by the Occupational Health and Safety Administration (OSHA).[8,21] Asbestos is especially dangerous. Its use is currently banned in 71 countries (not including the United States) and should be banned worldwide.[12,22] The EPA and OSHA have regulations to protect people from exposure to asbestos when buildings are renovated.[23]

- *Promotion of healthy diets.* Promotion of healthy diets is discussed in Chapter 14. Nutrition.

Secondary Prevention

A type of x-ray imaging called **low-dose computed tomography** (LDCT) can now identify early lung cancers that surgeons can remove. However, LDCT also finds false positives, that is, changes in the lung that are not cancer, which often results in people undergoing unnecessary and

Box 3.2 Summary–Prevention of Lung Cancer

- Primary prevention
  - Smoking prevention
  - Smoke-free policies
  - Substitution of biomass fuels
  - Air pollution regulation and reduction in fossil fuel use
  - Radon-resistant construction
  - Alternative water sources or arsenic removal systems
  - Replacement of diesel engines
  - Occupational respiratory protection standards
  - Promotion of healthy diets
- Secondary prevention
  - LDCT screening of people who have smoked heavily and surgical removal of early cancers

risky surgery. [7] For that reason, this test should be reserved for people at very high risk of lung cancer. The U.S. Preventive Services Task Force recommends that people ages 50 to 80 who have smoked for 20 or more "pack-years" (packs of cigarettes per day multiplied by years) be screened by LDCT once a year.[12,24] This reduces their mortality from lung cancer by about 20%.[12] However, the testing is expensive and not widely available, and most eligible people are not being tested. [12]

Box 3.3 **Key Words–Lung Cancer**

Alveolus (of the lung), plural alveoli
Ambient air pollution
Biomass
Bronchiole
Bronchus, bronchi
Capillary
Low-dose computed tomography (LDCT)
N-nitrosamines
Particulate matter
Polycyclic aromatic hydrocarbons
Radon
Respirator

Resources–Lung Cancer

- Leiter A, Veluswamy RR, Wisnivesky JP. The global burden of lung cancer: current status and future trends. *Nat Rev Clin Oncol.* 2023;20(9):624-639. doi:10.1038/s41571-023-00798-3
- Bade BC, Dela Cruz CS. Lung Cancer 2020: Epidemiology, Etiology, and Prevention. *Clin Chest Med.* 2020;41(1):1-24. doi:10.1016/j.ccm.2019.10.001

Cancer of the Breast

Introduction

Breast cancer is the most common and the deadliest type of cancer for women worldwide. Today this disease is much more common in high-income countries, but rates are rising quickly in low- and middle-income countries. Central to the development of breast cancer is the female hormone **estrogen**. Also important are several risk factors for multiple types of cancer, particularly alcohol use and overweight. Most of the attention on breast cancer prevention has focused on mammography but many cases can be prevented by addressing these risk factors.

Physiology of the Breast

The primary biologic function of the female breast is to produce milk for babies. The breast is composed of 15–20 sections called **lobes**, with each lobe composed of many more tiny **lobules**. When a mother is nursing a baby, the bulbs in these lobules (called **alveoli**) produce milk. The milk then travels through a network of tiny channels called **ducts** to the nipple (**Figure 3.10**).[25]

The lining of the ducts and the alveoli is a layer of epithelial cells. These cells respond to estrogen, which is produced by the ovaries and by fat tissue. In each month's menstrual cycle, a woman's level of estrogen rises and falls, peaking in the middle of the cycle just before ovulation. That rise in estrogen stimulates the epithelial cells to proliferate so that they can be ready to produce milk if pregnancy were to occur. If it does not, in the second half of the cycle, many of these newly-formed epithelial cells die, to be replaced by proliferating cells in the next cycle.[26]

Pathophysiology of Breast Cancer

Almost all breast cancers arise from the breast's epithelial cells, typically those in the smallest branches of the ducts.[3] The more often these epithelial cells are stimulated by estrogen, the more often they divide, and the greater the risk that one cell line will be transformed into cancer cells.[3] The central role that estrogen plays in the development of breast cancer explains some of the key risk factors for the disease, such as having no pregnancies (leading to more menstrual cycles), taking medications containing estrogen, and perhaps obesity.[27]

Breast cancers are classified based on whether the cancer cells have three key hormone **receptors**. Hormone receptors are molecules present in cells that change the operations of cells when a hormone is present. These receptors involved in breast cancer are the **estrogen receptor (ER)**, the **progesterone receptor (PR)**, and the **human epidermal growth factor receptor (HER2)**.[3]

- Cancers that have ER but not HER2 are called **luminal cancers**. (These cancers usually also have PR.) This is the most common form of breast cancer. Luminal cancers tend to occur in older women and Caucasian women and tend to grow slowly, so they are typically discovered by a mammogram.[3]

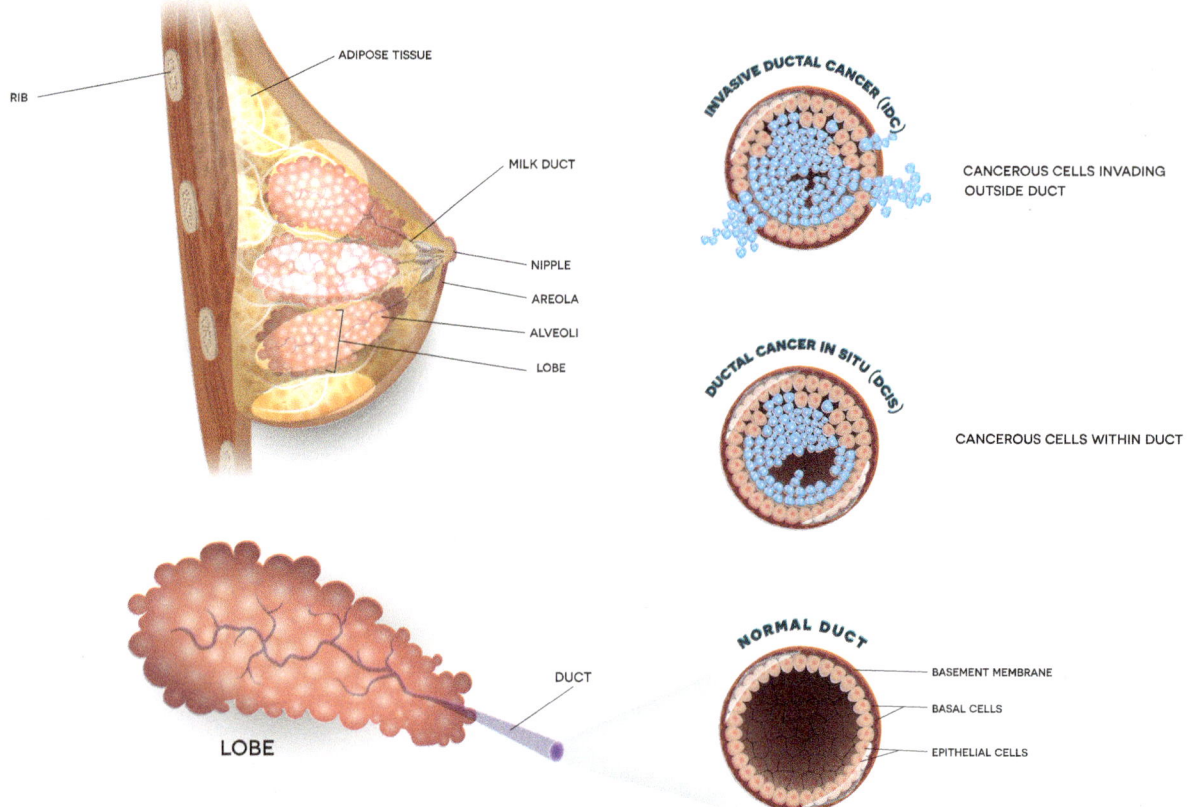

Figure 3.10 The Breast, Breast Ducts, and Breast Cancer. The breast is composed of 15–20 lobes, each of which has many small lobules. The bulbs in these lobules are called alveoli. In a parent who is nursing, the alveoli make milk, which flows through the milk ducts to the nipple. Breast cancer arises from the cells that line the smallest branches of these ducts.

© TimeLineArtist/Shutterstoc

- Cancers that have HER2, regardless of whether they have ER or PR, are called **HER2 cancers**. About 20% of breast cancers are of this type. These cancers are found more often in younger women.[3]
- Cancers that do not have ER, HER2, or PR are called **triple-negative cancers**. About 15% of breast cancers are of this type. These cancers are more common in younger women and women of African descent. They tend to be more aggressive and are more likely to noticed by the affected person as a lump in the breast.[3]

Breast cancers develop slowly, over years, and go through **stages** of development. In the earliest stage, the proliferating epithelial cells stay inside the breast ducts (Figure 3.10). This stage is called **ductal carcinoma in situ or DCIS** ("in situ" in Latin means "in place"). Because it has not spread, DCIS can almost always be fully cured by surgery and medical treatment.[28]

When cancer cells invade past the epithelium into the rest of the breast or beyond, the cancer is called an **invasive carcinoma**. For invasive carcinomas, the stage is classified by the size of the primary cancer, whether cancer cells have spread to nearby **lymph nodes** (clusters of immune cells), and whether cells have invaded distant tissues. Those without any spread beyond the breast are called **localized**, those with spread only to lymph nodes are called **regional**, and those with metastases are called **distant** or **metastatic**.[3]

The larger the primary cancer is and the more it has spread, the more difficult it is to cure. Only about one-third of women in the United States with metastases survive 5 years after their diagnosis, but 98% of those with no metastases or spread to lymph nodes do.[5] With more screening and improvements in treatments, the survival rate for breast cancer is far better than it once was: the 5-year survival rate in the United States overall for women diagnosed in 2016 was about 91%, but for those diagnosed in 1973 it was 61%.[27,29]

Epidemiology: Patterns and Trends

Thanks to early identification and better treatments, there is a big difference between the incidence and mortality rates from breast cancer. In the United

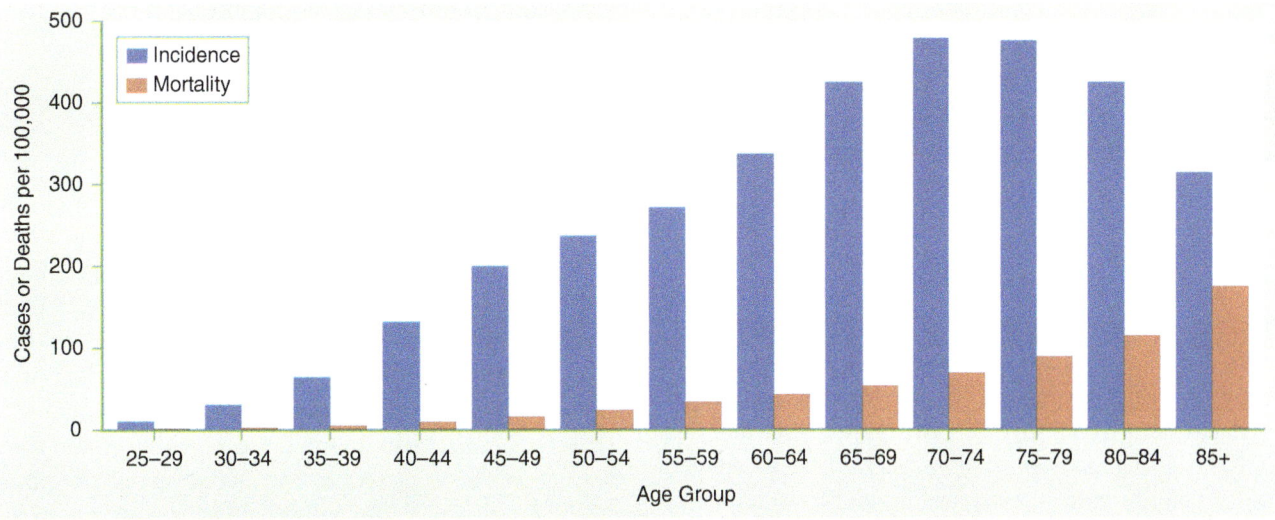

Figure 3.11 **Breast Cancer Incidence and Mortality in the United States by Age Group.** The incidence of breast cancer starts at about age 30 and peaks in the 70–79 year age group. Mortality rates peaks in the 80s. (In this graph, incidence data is from 2017–2021 and mortality data is from 2018–2022.)

Data from U.S. Cancer Statistics Working Group. U.S. Cancer Statistics Data Visualizations Tool. U.S. Department of Health and Human Services, Centers for Disease Control and Prevention and National Cancer Institute, released in June 2024. https://www.cdc.gov/cancer/dataviz

States, about 250,000 women are diagnosed with breast cancer every year, and more than 40,000 die from it.[5] The disease is so common that about one in eight women living to 90 will develop breast cancer at some point.[29]

Breast cancer incidence rates rise with age, starting in the early 30s and peaking in the 70s (**Figure 3.11**). Rates vary by race and ethnicity (**Figure 3.12**). Although White women are more likely to be diagnosed with breast cancer, Black women are more likely to die from it.[5] That racial difference may result from both differences in access to timely medical treatment and the fact that Black women are more likely to have aggressive tumors, such as triple-negative cancer.[3] Breast cancer incidence rates in all racial groups are higher in women of higher socioeconomic status, which may be explained in part by their having fewer pregnancies and using more medications containing estrogen.[30,31]

The incidence of breast cancer in the United States has not changed much in the past 20 years.[5] Fortunately, for most women, breast cancer is detected early; for about two-thirds the initial cancer is localized, for about one-fourth it is regional, and for about 5% it is distant.[5]

Mortality rates from breast cancer in the United States have been falling about 1–2% per year over the past 20 years.[5]

Globally, some 2.3 million women develop breast cancer every year and nearly 700,000 die from it.[11]

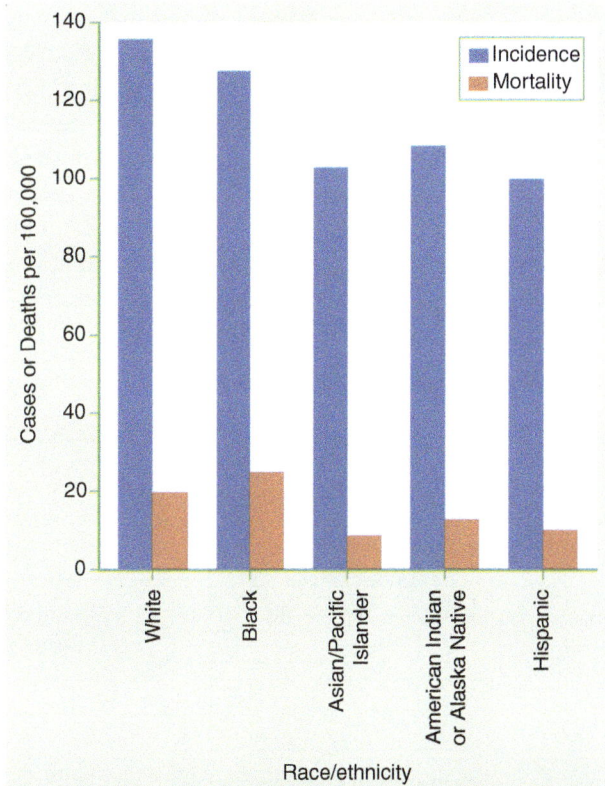

Figure 3.12 **Breast Cancer Incidence and Mortality in the United States by Race/Ethnicity.** The incidence of breast cancer is highest in White women but the mortality rate is highest in Black women. (Note that incidence data is from 2017–2021 and mortality data is from 2018–2022.)

Data from U.S. Cancer Statistics Working Group. U.S. Cancer Statistics Data Visualizations Tool. U.S. Department of Health and Human Services, Centers for Disease Control and Prevention and National Cancer Institute, released in June 2024. https://www.cdc.gov/cancer/dataviz

Disease rates vary greatly from one country to another. The incidence of breast cancer is highest in high-income countries in North America and Europe, with rates about twice those of sub-Saharan Africa and four times those of South Asia.[11] The difference is probably because women in high-income countries have more estrogen-related risk (such as fewer pregnancies and more use of estrogen-containing medications) and because they have other risks, such as use of alcohol, being overweight, and physical inactivity.[11] However, rates are rising quickly in low-income countries. For example, in sub-Saharan Africa, breast cancer incidence rates have more than tripled between the 1960s and the 2010s.[32] And already, mortality rates from breast cancer are actually highest in low- and middle-income countries,[11] probably because people in these countries do not have full access to screening and treatments.

Risk Factors

There is a strong element of genetic risk to breast cancer.[3] If a woman has a first-degree relative with breast cancer, she is about three times as likely to develop the disease.[27] Two genes have been identified that strongly predict breast cancer risk—the **BRCA1** and **BRCA2** genes. Ordinarily, these genes are responsible for repairing damaged DNA. This DNA repair must be needed often, because women with defective versions of these genes have a 70% chance of developing breast cancer by age 80.[33] Fortunately, BRCA1 and BRCA2 mutations are not common, so women with these mutations account for only 3–6% of the cases of breast cancer.[3]

Modifiable risk factors for breast cancer include (**Figure 3.13**):

- *Estrogen exposure.* It seems that any exposure or condition that leads to high levels of estrogen, temporarily or permanently, increases the risk of breast cancer.[3] Because each menstrual cycle brings with it a temporary surge in estrogen levels, women are more likely to develop breast cancer if they have more menstrual cycles over the course of their lives—for example, if they go through puberty early (before age 12) or if they go through menopause late (after age 55).[27] This is also why women are at higher risk if they never become pregnant, have fewer pregnancies, or are older when they have a first pregnancy.[27] For women who do become pregnant and have children, breastfeeding reduces breast cancer risk because it slows or stops their menstrual cycles.[3,27] And women are slightly more likely to develop breast cancer if they take birth control pills containing estrogen, or later if they take pills containing estrogen for symptoms after menopause.[27,34,35]

- *Alcohol consumption.* Alcohol is classified by the U.S. Department of Health and Human Services as a carcinogen,[36] and it has been linked specifically to breast cancer.[37] The risk of breast cancer in women increases with the amount of alcohol they drink. Women drinking on average less than one drink per day have a 4% increase in risk, those averaging 1–3 drinks per day have

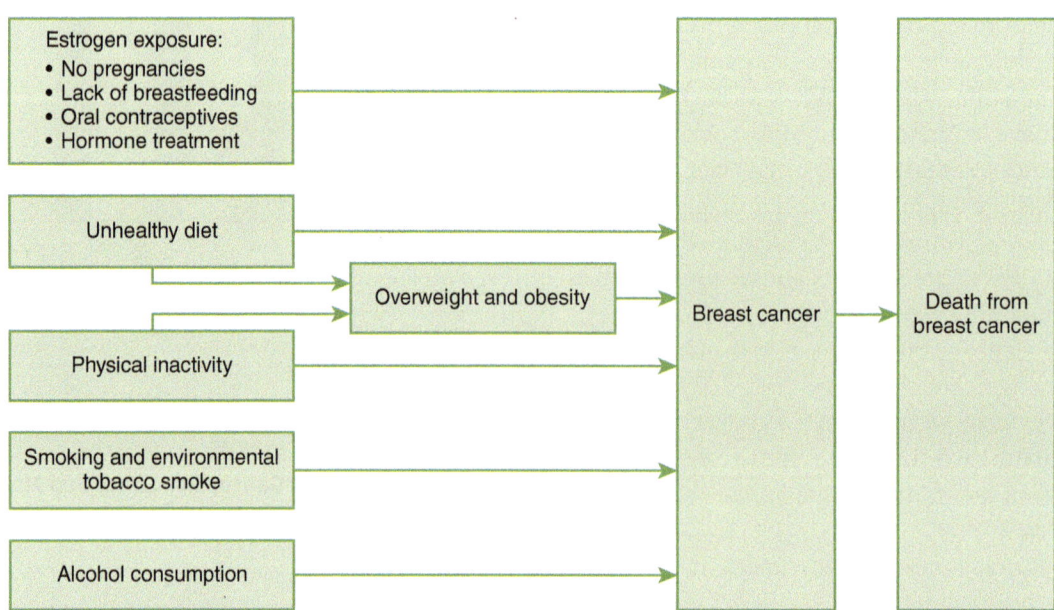

Figure 3.13 **Cause-and-Effect Diagram for Breast Cancer.**

about a 25% increase, and those drinking more than 3 drinks per day about a 60% increase in risk.[38]

- *Overweight and obesity.* Women who are overweight are more likely to develop breast cancer after menopause (but not before menopause).[3,27,37] The more overweight they are, the greater the risk. On average, for each 5 kg/m² increase in the **body mass index**, the risk of breast cancer rises 11%.[39,40] The reasons are not clear, but after menopause, fat tissue is the main producer of estrogens in the body.[40] Also, women who are overweight have higher circulating levels of the hormone **insulin** and a similar hormone called **insulin-like growth factor (ILGF)**, both of which increase mitosis and reduce apoptosis (programmed death) of cells.[27]

- *Physical inactivity.* Women who are physically active are less likely to develop breast cancer, with the most active having about a 14% lower risk.[27,37] This may be because exercise reduces the amount of body fat, which reduces estrogen levels as well as reducing insulin and ILGF.

- *Unhealthy diet.* Expert groups reviewing studies on the connection between diet and breast cancer concluded that there was "moderate evidence" that diets high in red meat, processed meat, sugar-sweetened beverages and foods, and refined grains increase the risk, while diets rich in whole grains, fruit, and vegetables reduce risk.[37,41,42]

- *Smoking* and *exposure to environmental tobacco smoke* appear to increase the risk of breast cancer, although the relationship is much weaker than it is for lung cancer.[37,43] While the mechanisms are not clear, the carcinogens in tobacco smoke do reach the breast epithelial cells.

Of all the modifiable risk factors, the ones that studies attribute the greatest fraction of breast cancer to in the United States are alcohol use (15% of cases) and being overweight (11% of cases).[14]

Preventive Interventions

Primary Prevention

While primary prevention efforts are likely to be less successful for breast cancer than for cancer of the lung or colon, many cases could be prevented by addressing modifiable risk factors.[14,44] Specific interventions include (**Figure 3.14**):

- *Avoidance of estrogen-containing medications.* After menopause, women's bodies produce less estrogen, and some experience hot flashes and other

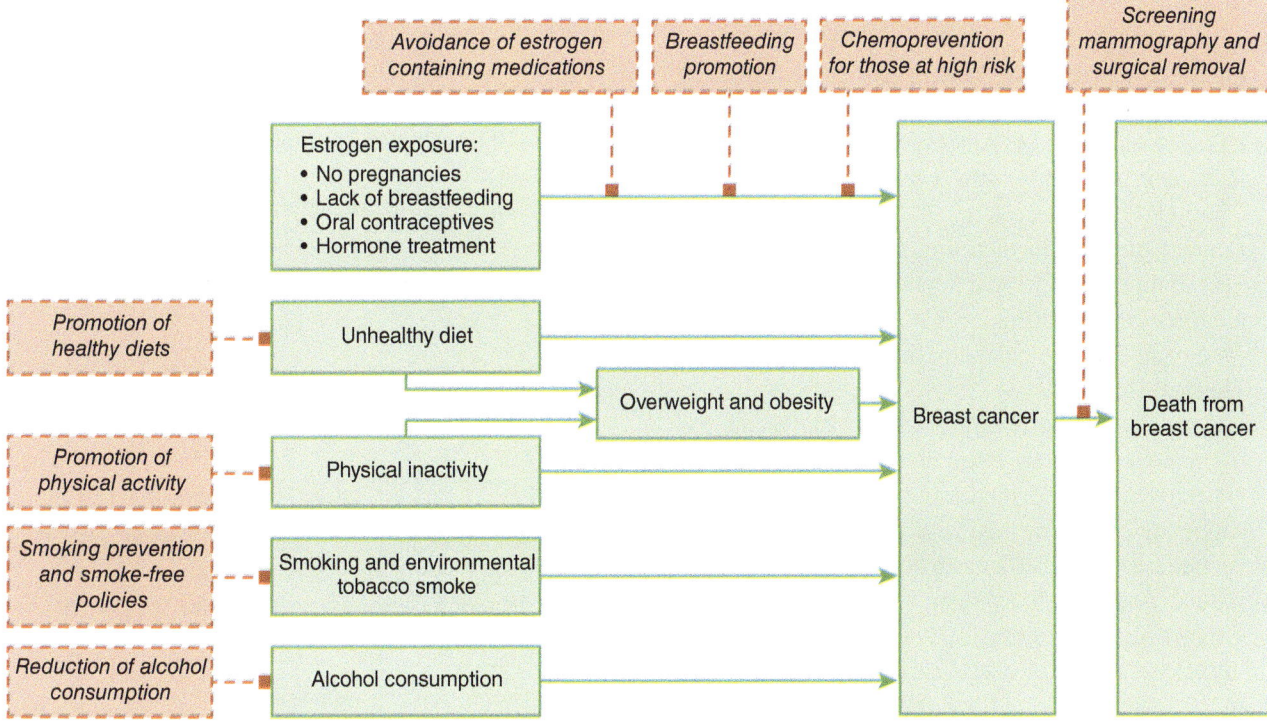

Figure 3.14 **Cause-and-Effect Diagram for Breast Cancer, with Preventive Interventions.**

symptoms from this sudden loss of estrogen. These symptoms improve by taking medications containing estrogen and progesterone, which is known as **hormone replacement therapy**. Many took these medications in the 1990s and some take them today. However, because of the risk of breast cancer and other diseases, experts now recommend against taking hormone replacement therapy.[45] Also, many women today take birth control pills that contain estrogen. The connection of these oral contraceptives to a small increase in breast cancer risk suggests it is safer to choose other reliable contraceptives, such as those that contain only **progesterone** or intrauterine devices (IUDs).

- *Breastfeeding promotion.* Breastfeeding clearly has important health benefits for both infants and mothers in high-income countries like the United States and across the world. A reduction in breast cancer risk is one of those benefits. The Dietary Guidelines for Americans recommend that mothers breastfeed their infants for 12 months, and the World Health Organization recommends that mothers breastfeed their infants for 24 months. Programs that educate and support breastfeeding can increase the number of mothers who start nursing their babies and the duration that they continue.[46]

- *Reduction of alcohol consumption.* A later chapter discusses many policies that can reduce alcohol consumption, such as warning labels, communications campaigns, raising the price through taxes, and limiting the number of alcohol outlets. See Chapter 14. Alcohol Use.

- *Reduction of smoking* and *smoke-free policies.* See Chapter 11. Tobacco Use.

- *Promotion of healthy diets* and *prevention of obesity.* See Chapter 7. Chronic Metabolic Diseases and Chapter 14. Nutrition.

- *Promotion of physical activity.* See Chapter 15. Physical Inactivity.

- *Chemoprevention* for women at high risk. Recognizing that estrogen can cause breast cancer, researchers have developed medications to prevent breast cancer by counteracting this hormone. Some drugs (including two called anastrozole and exemestane) reduce how much estrogen the body produces. Other drugs (including two called tamoxifen and raloxifene) block the effect that estrogen has on cells in the breast.[3,47] Using these medications to prevent breast cancer is called **chemoprevention**. Chemoprevention is recommended for women at high risk of developing breast cancer, which experts

define as having an estimated 5-year risk of 3% of more. (Risk can be estimated by using a risk assessment calculator on the National Cancer Institute website at https://bcrisktool.cancer.gov/calculator.html.)[47] Examples of those with risks above 3% are 65-year-old women who have had no children and have a single first-degree relative with breast cancer, and those above age 45 who have more than one first-degree relative with breast cancer.[47] Experts recommend that those with risks above 3% take one of these drugs for 5 years. The drugs have their own risks and side effects, though, and today few eligible women are choosing to take these drugs.[47]

Some women at extremely high risk, such as those with BRCA1 or BRCA2 mutations, choose to have their breasts removed to prevent cancer.[3] This is a major decision that only they can make, but for this small number of people, it almost eliminates the risk of breast cancer.[47]

Secondary Prevention

Some breast cancers can be identified early by *screening mammography* and then being surgically removed.[3] The U.S. Preventive Services Task Force recommends that women age 40–74 years who are at average risk have screening mammograms every two years.[48] The World Health Organization recommends this screening every 2 years for women ages 50–69 "in well-resourced settings."[11] In the United States, three-fourths of women age 50–74 are meeting this recommendation.[5]

While screening mammography has helped many, there are many cancers that it does not detect early enough. Studies show screening mammography reduces breast cancer mortality by 15–20%. And that benefit comes at a cost of identifying many false positives, which can lead to anxiety, additional tests, and sometimes unnecessary treatment.[49]

Box 3.4 **Summary–Prevention of Breast Cancer**

- Primary prevention
  - Avoidance of estrogen-containing medications
  - Breastfeeding promotion
  - Reduction of alcohol consumption
  - Smoking prevention and smoke-free policies
  - Promotion of healthy diets and prevention of obesity
  - Promotion of physical activity
  - Chemoprevention (for women at high risk)
- Secondary prevention
  - Promotion of screening mammography

Resources–Breast Cancer

- Farkas AH, Nattinger AB. Breast Cancer Screening and Prevention. *Ann Intern Med.* 2023;176(11):ITC161-ITC176. doi:10.7326/AITC202311210. This summarizes information relevant to prevention of breast cancer in a primary care setting.
- Terry MB, Colditz GA. Epidemiology and Risk Factors for Breast Cancer: 21st Century Advances, Gaps to Address through Interdisciplinary Science. *Cold Spring Harb Perspect Med.* 2023;13(9). doi:10.1101/cshperspect.a041317. This is an update on population-based risk factors for breast cancer and unresolved questions.

Cancer of the Colon and Rectum

Introduction

Cancer of the **colon** or **rectum**, called **colorectal cancer** and often just referred to as colon cancer, is the third leading type of cancer and the second leading cause of cancer deaths in the world.[11] The epithelial cells lining the colon and rectum are susceptible to acquiring cancer mutations because they turn over very quickly and are heavily exposed to carcinogens in food. Unhealthy diets, a lack of exercise, smoking, and drinking alcohol make colon cancer common in high-income countries and increasingly common in low-income countries. Fortunately, abnormal growths in the colon can be identified and removed, preventing not just cancer deaths but also cancer itself.

Physiology of the Colon and Rectum

The colon and the rectum are the final segments of the gastrointestinal tract, just after the small intestine (**Figure 3.15**). The small intestine absorbs nutrients from food into the blood. The undigested parts of food then pass into the colon, which absorbs fluids and stores the remaining feces until defecation.

The colon and rectum are lined with epithelial cells (**Figure 3.16**). Inside the colon there are a very large number of bacteria, which make up the **gut microbiome**. These bacteria ferment unabsorbed compounds from digested food. The bacteria also interact with the epithelial cells in complex ways that researchers are just beginning to understand.

The epithelial cells have a very high turnover, lasting just a few days before they are shed into the feces. As they are shed, these epithelial cells are replaced by **stem cells** that also live in the lining of the colon. To replace the epithelial cells, the stem cells divide repeatedly, and as they do, they gradually take on epithelial cells' appearance and function.

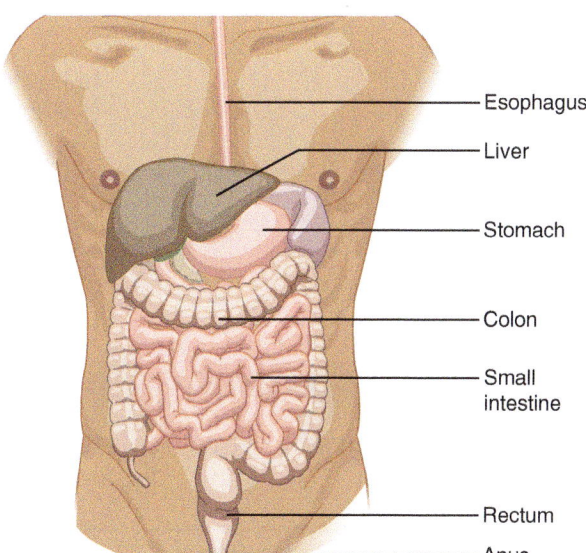

Esophagus
Liver
Stomach
Colon
Small intestine
Rectum
Anus

Figure 3.15 **The Gastrointestinal Tract.** The colon and rectum are the final segment of the gastrointestinal tract, just after the small intestine.

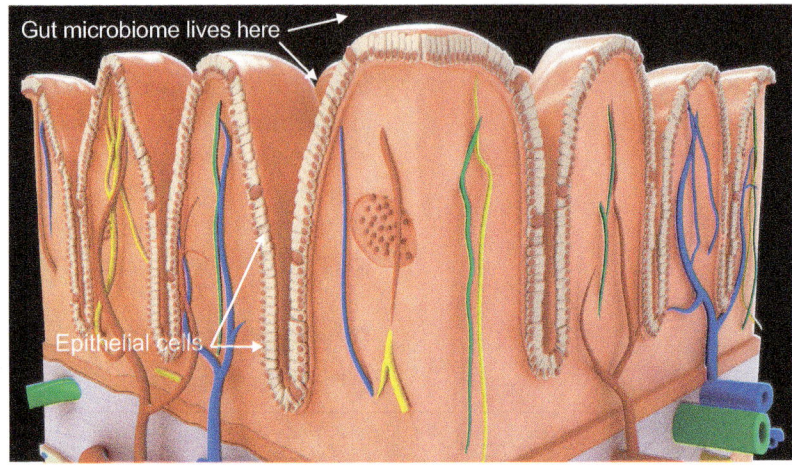

Figure 3.16 **The Epithelium of the Colon and the Microbiome.** The colon and rectum are lined with epithelial cells. Inside the colon there are a very large number of bacteria, which make up the gut microbiome.

Pathophysiology of Colon Cancer

The stem cells and epithelial cells, like all human cells, have genetic mechanisms to keep their growth under control. But each time they divide, the copying of their DNA creates a chance that a mutation will occur in these control genes and cell lines will begin to grow uncontrollably. Some sequences of mutations are particularly common and dangerous. About 80% of colon cancers involve mutations of a specific control gene called the adenomatous polyposis coli (APC) gene.[50] The transformation into cancer is the result of mutations that accumulate over many years.

As colon epithelial cells begin to proliferate abnormally, they form growths called **adenomas**.

Adenomas can then grow into the interior space of the colon or rectum, forming **polyps**. About 30% of American adults have these polyps by the time they turn 60.[50] Polyps themselves are considered benign tumors, and many people live with them for years without problems. However, if the cells in polyps become aggressive and invade the tissue underneath the epithelium or other parts of the body, these tumors are labeled **adenocarcinomas**, i.e., colorectal cancer (**Figure 3.17**).

It should not be surprising that the type of food ingested influences the risk that the colon's epithelial cells will become cancerous. Some foods contain carcinogens that directly induce mutations in the cells that they touch. Other foods contain compounds that are metabolized by bacteria in the gut microbiome into carcinogens. And yet other foods

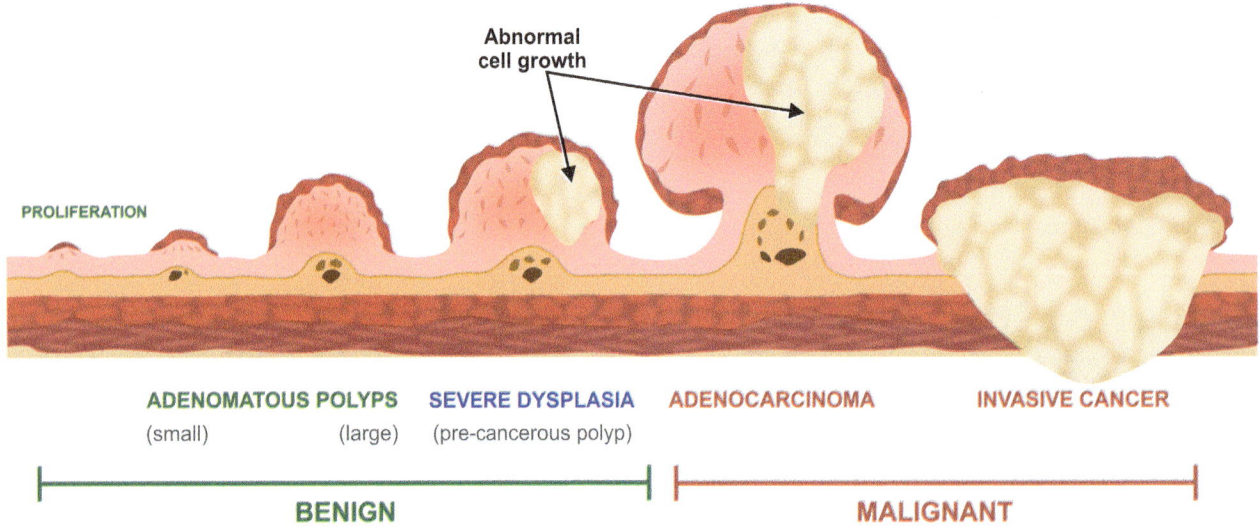

Figure 3.17 **Development of Polyps and Colorectal Cancer.** Colorectal cancer develops over many years, progressing from proliferation of epithelial cells to adenomas, polyps, and adenocarcinomas, which then invade the underlying tissue.

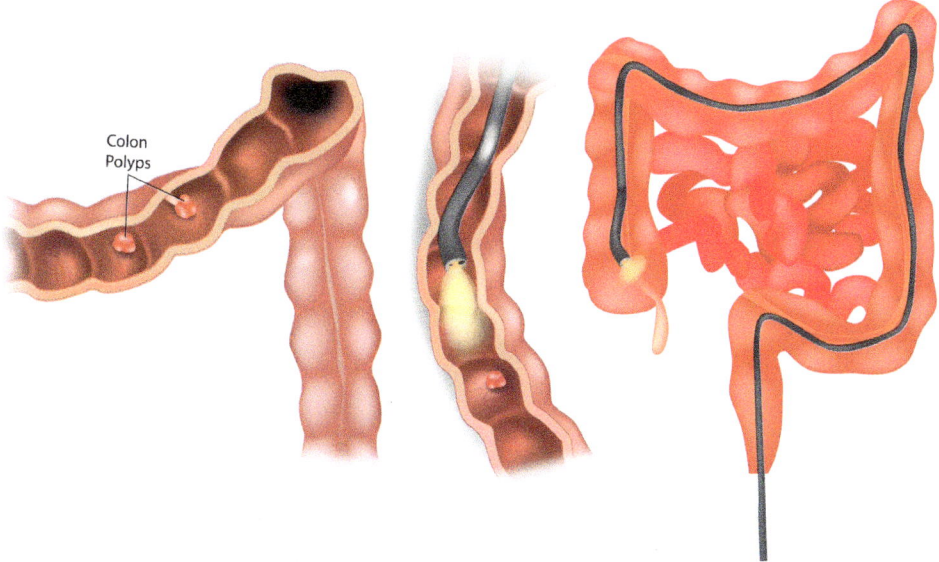

Colon
Polyps

Figure 3.18 **Identification and Removal of Polyps.** During a colonoscopy, a flexible tube called a colonoscope is inserted into the colon. Polyps in the lining of the colon can be seen and removed with this colonoscope.

may have an indirect effect by altering the type of bacteria that are in the microbiome. While many of the mechanisms involved are not understood, studies have shown that diets high in red and processed meats, saturated fats, refined grains, and added sugars increase the risk of colon cancer. Diets high in whole grains, fruits, vegetables, and legumes reduce this risk.[42]

Once colon epithelial cells have mutated to become cancer cells, those cancer cells invade the tissue on the wall of the colon, travel to **lymph nodes** in the abdomen, and spread through the blood to the liver and other parts of the body. As with breast cancer, colon cancers are classified into stages: **localized** (confined to the colon), **regional** (spread to lymph nodes), and **distant** (metastases to other organs).[50]

During the years that it takes for normal epithelium to develop into adenomas, polyps, and then cancer, the abnormal tissue often breaks down, leaving trace amounts of blood in the feces. The blood is so scant that it is usually not noticed ("occult"), but tests of feces can identify it. If tests of feces show blood, the source of the bleeding can be found with a **sigmoidoscope** or **colonoscope**, which are flexible tubes inserted into the colon that transmit images using fiber optics. Even better, these scopes include tiny tools that allow physicians to immediately snip off any polyps that they find (**Figure 3.18**). Because nearly all colorectal cancers start as polyps, removing polyps during a **colonoscopy** or **sigmoidoscopy** can often prevent the development of cancer.[50]

Epidemiology: Patterns and Trends

In the United States, about 153,000 people develop colorectal cancer and 52,500 die from it each year.[51] Because colorectal cancer takes many years to develop, disease rates rise sharply with age (**Figure 3.19**). The incidence in the 70–74 year age group is 17 times that in the 35–39 year age group.[51] The incidence varies by race and ethnicity (**Figure 3.20**). Compared to rates in non-Hispanic Whites, colorectal cancer incidence is about 15% higher in non-Hispanic Blacks, 30% higher in American Indians, and more than twice as high in Alaskan Natives, who have the highest known case rates in the world, for unknown reasons.[51]

Studies have shown that people with lower income or education have a 25–50% higher incidence of colorectal cancer, even after taking race and ethnicity into account.[52] Between one-third and one-half of these socioeconomic differences can be explained by differences in risk factors, such as smoking and obesity.[53]

The overall incidence and mortality of colorectal cancer in the United States, while still very high by global standards, have been falling since about 1980. This could be because fewer Americans smoke and because many are undergoing colon cancer screening tests and having polyps removed. However, for unknown reasons, colorectal cancer rates have been increasing in adults ages 20–39 years since the mid-1980s and in adults ages 40–54 years since the mid-1990s (**Figure 3.21**).[51]

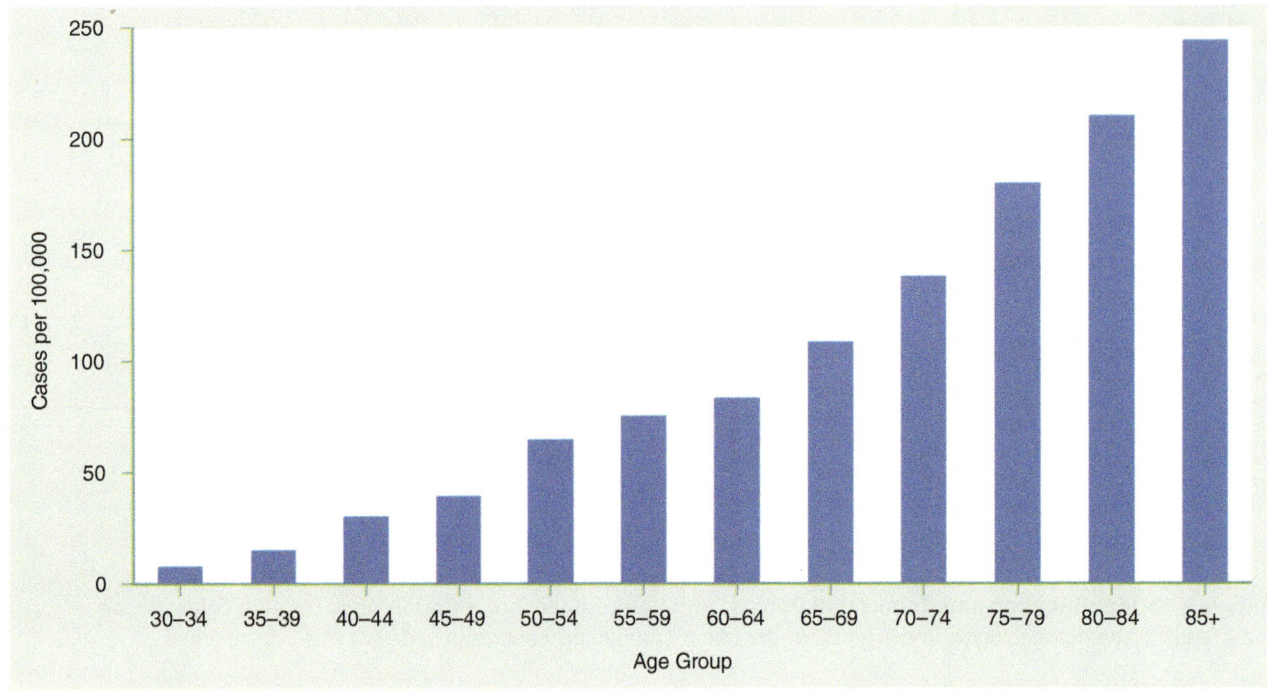

Figure 3.19 **Incidence of Colorectal Cancer in the United States by Age Group, 2015–2019.**

Data from Siegel RL, Wagle NS, Cercek A, Smith RA, Jemal A. Colorectal cancer statistics. CA Cancer J Clin. 2023;73:233-254.

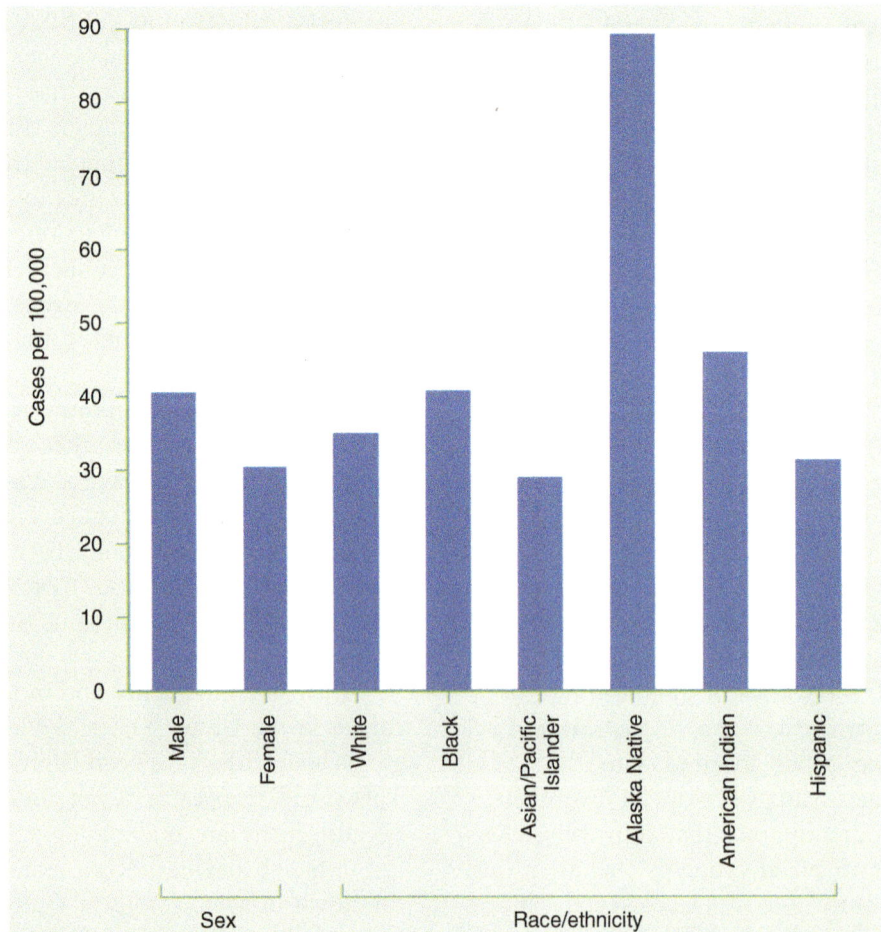

Figure 3.20 **Incidence of Colorectal Cancer in the United States by Sex and Race/Ethnicity, 2015–2019.**

Data from Siegel RL, Wagle NS, Cercek A, Smith RA, Jemal A. Colorectal cancer statistics. CA Cancer J Clin. 2023;73:233-254.

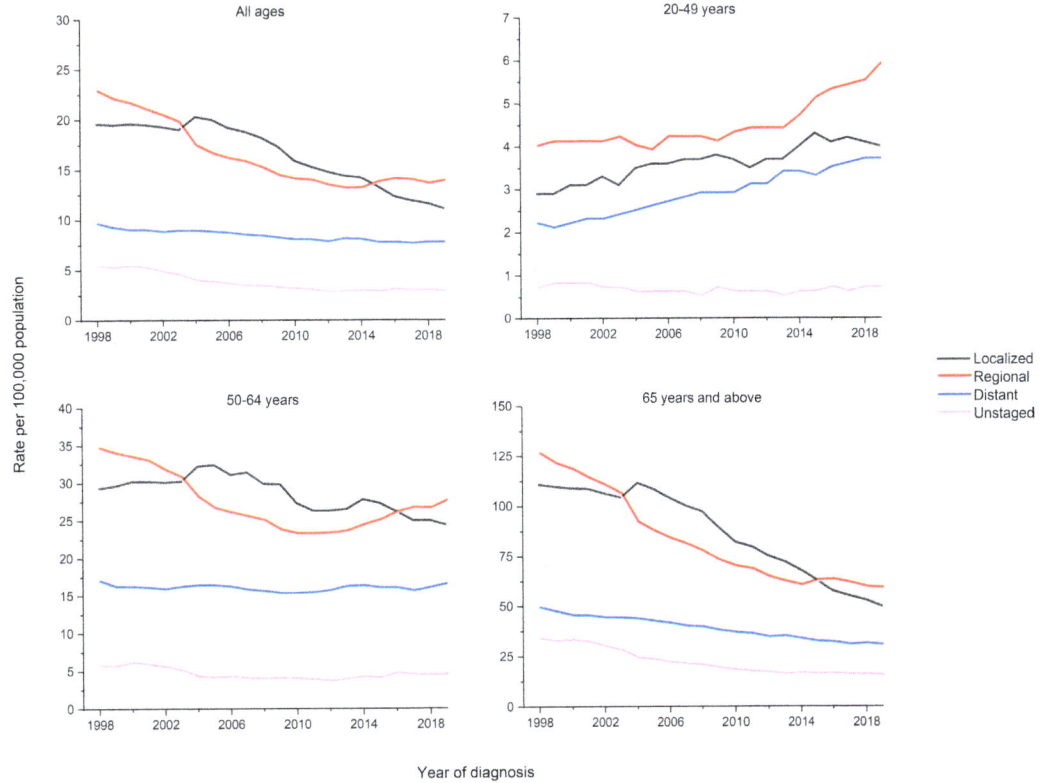

Figure 3.21 **Trends in Colorectal Cancer Incidence in the United States by Age Group, 1998–2019.** The overall incidence of colon cancer has been falling since the 1980s, but the incidence in adults ages 20–49 is rising.

Reproduced from Siegel RL, Wagle NS, Cercek A, Smith RA, Jemal A. Colorectal cancer statistics. CA Cancer J Clin. 2023;73:233-254.

Globally, nearly 1.9 million people are diagnosed with cancer of the colon or rectum each year, and more than 900,000 people die from this cancer.[11] The incidence of colorectal cancer is lowest in Africa and South-Central Asia, where people eat more traditional plant-based diets and are less likely to smoke. It is highest in Europe, Australia, New Zealand, and North America. The differences are very large: Colorectal cancer rates are about six times higher in Europe than in sub-Saharan Africa.[11]

Risk Factors

An *unhealthy diet* is the largest known modifiable risk factor for colorectal cancer (**Figure 3.22**). Foods that increase the risk of colorectal cancer are:

- *Red meat.* The link to colon cancer is likely through a compound called **heme**, which is used by red blood cells to carry iron and is present in high levels in red meat (but not poultry). Heme stimulates bacteria in the gut microbiome

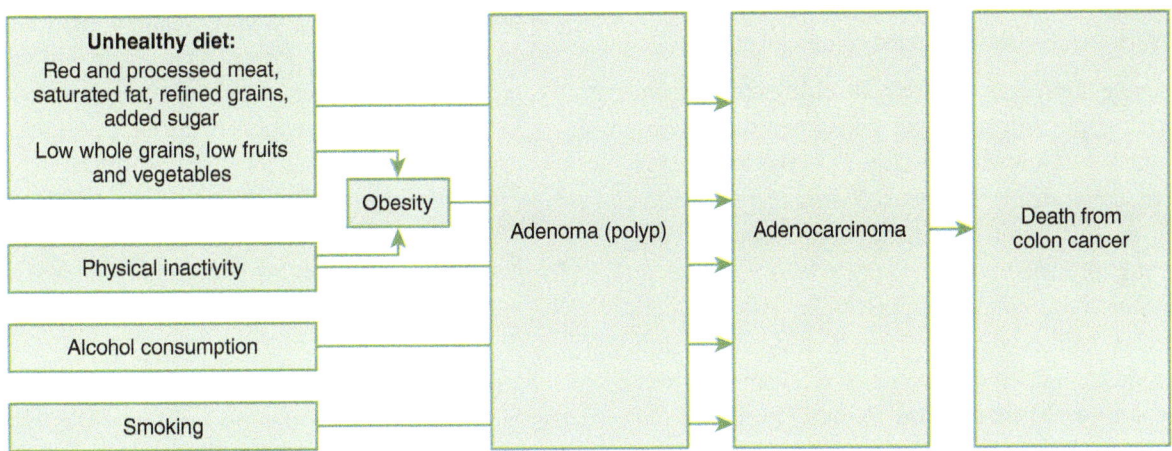

Figure 3.22 **Cause-and-Effect Diagram for Colorectal Cancer.**

of the colon to produce **N-nitrosamines**, the same class of cancer-causing chemicals found in tobacco smoke.[54] In addition, cooking red meats at high temperatures produces chemicals called heterocyclic amines and polycyclic aromatic hydrocarbons, which likewise are carcinogenic.[54,55]

- *Processed meat,* such as ham, bacon, sausage, and hot dogs. Besides containing heme, some processed meat contains chemical preservatives called **nitrites**. Under the right conditions within the intestines, these nitrites can lead to production of N-nitrosamines.[56,57] Other possible mechanisms also exist.[56]
- *Saturated fat.* Fat in the diet prompts the liver to produce **bile acids** to help digest this fat. These bile acids appear to support the growth of certain bacteria in the microbiome that cause epithelial cells to proliferate.[42,58]
- *Sugar-sweetened beverages and refined grains.* The mechanism by which these foods increase colon cancer risk are not clear but may involve the insulin resistance caused by sugar intake (see Chapter 7. Chronic metabolic diseases) or to the effect of sugar on the gut microbiome.[42,59]

Foods that reduce the risk of colorectal cancer are the following:

- *Whole grains and fiber.* Dietary fiber in the intestines is metabolized to **short-chain fatty acids**, at least one of which reduces epithelial cell proliferation. Whole grains are a rich source of dietary fiber as well as a source of other compounds that may protect against cancer cell formation.[55]
- *Fruits and vegetables.* The mechanism is not clear, but chemicals in these may suppress the transformation of normal epithelial cells into cancer cells.[60]

Four non-dietary behaviors are also important (and often overlooked) risk factors for colorectal cancer:

- *Smoking* increases the risk of colorectal cancer, with people smoking two packs per day having about a 40% increased risk.[61] This risk may come from carcinogens in tobacco smoke that circulate in the blood, affecting high-turnover cells throughout the body.
- *Alcohol consumption* increases the risk for colorectal cancer by about 10% for each drink per day.[55] The mechanism is unclear but may involve **acetaldehyde**, which is produced from alcohol by the liver and can be carcinogenic to epithelial cells.[55]

- *Physical inactivity.* People who are physically active have about a 20% lower risk of developing colorectal cancer.[55] This protective effect may be due to exercise increasing the body's sensitivity to **insulin**, which leads the body to produce less insulin.[62] Insulin promotes epithelial cell proliferation. Another theory is that exercise reduces the "transit time" for feces in the colon, which reduces the exposure of epithelial cells to carcinogens in foods.
- *Obesity.* Many studies have shown an increase in colorectal cancer risk in persons with higher levels of body fat. Persons with a body mass index of 30 have about a 30% increased risk of developing colorectal cancer, even after taking into account many other factors.[55] People with more body fat have higher circulating levels of insulin.[63] Also, a higher level of body fat is accompanied by more inflammation throughout the body, and inflammation can promote colon cancer development.[64]

Estimates by different experts are that more than half of colorectal cancer deaths could be avoided by people having healthier diets and eliminating these other four risk factors.[6,65] Consistent with that estimate, one study showed that health professionals who never smoked, were not obese, consumed low or moderate amounts of alcohol, and exercised regularly were about 60% less likely than the general U.S. population to have or die from colorectal cancer.[66]

Preventive Interventions
Primary Prevention

Primary prevention of colon cancer involves addressing these risk factors (**Figure 3.23**), which includes the following:

- *Promotion of healthy diets* by reducing the promotion of red meat, processed meat, and high-fat foods, and increasing the availability, accessibility, and promotion of whole grains, foods containing natural fiber, and dairy products. *Prevention of obesity* would also reduce colon cancer risk, and the greatest potential for obesity prevention is through promotion of healthier diets. See Chapter 14. Nutrition.
- *Promotion of physical activity.* See Chapter 15. Physical Inactivity.
- *Reduction of smoking.* See Chapter 11. Tobacco Use.
- *Reduction of alcohol consumption.* See Chapter 12. Alcohol Use.

Many studies have shown that taking *aspirin* regularly can prevent the occurrence of polyps or cause existing polyps to shrink, reducing the risk of colorectal cancer.[67,68] This may be because aspirin

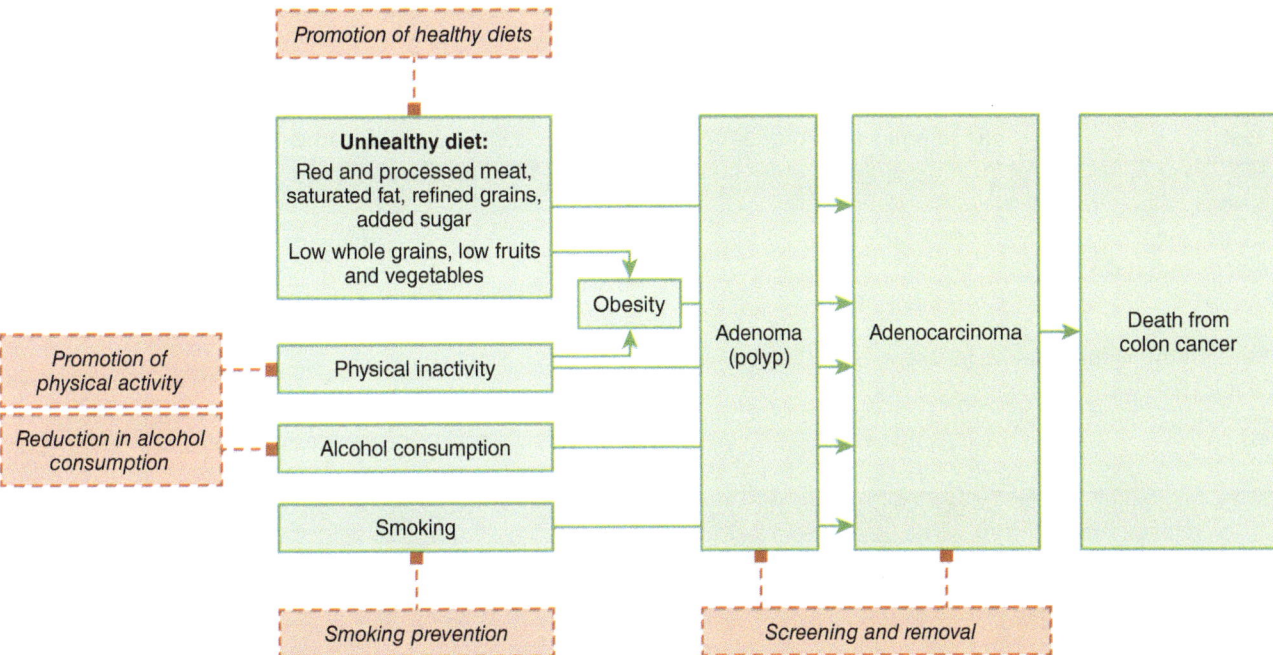

Figure 3.23 **Cause-and-Effect Diagram for Colorectal Cancer, with Preventive Interventions.**

slows the production of a compound that prompts epithelial cells to proliferate.[50] These studies have led some experts to recommend that people take daily aspirin for primary prevention.[68] However, taking aspirin every day leads to an increased risk of bleeding, and most experts have concluded that for most people, this risk of bleeding from daily aspirin use is greater than the benefits in colorectal cancer prevention.[68,69]

Secondary Prevention

In theory, a large majority of colorectal cancer cases could be prevented through regular screening to identify polyps and then removing them. A study of health professionals found that those who had had colonoscopy screening were about 50% less likely to develop colorectal cancer and 70% less likely to die from it.[70]

Experts recommend regular screening for people 45–75 years old.[71] If colorectal cancer rates continue to rise in younger adults, experts may lower the recommended age to begin screening.

Several tests are available for colorectal cancer screening (**Table 3.2**):[71]

- *Screening tests for blood in stool* are fairly simple to perform and can be done at home. These include the high-sensitivity **guaiac fecal occult blood test (gFOBT)**, the **fecal immunochemical test (FIT)**, and a newer test that combines FIT with detection of DNA often present in cancer cells (**sDNA-FIT**).[71] The gFOBT is less sensitive than the other two tests, so it requires three separate stool samples, while the others require

one sample only. The gFOBT and the FIT should be conducted once a year. The sDNA-FIT, which is the most sensitive test, can be conducted every one to three years. The FIT is the test used most because of its accuracy and low cost.

- *Direct visualization tests* are complicated to do, must be done in a medical facility, and require preparation beforehand to empty the colon of feces. These tests include colonoscopy, flexible sigmoidoscopy, and **CT colonography**. A colonoscopy views the entire colon and can be performed only once every 10 years, but it carries a very small risk (about 3 per 10,000 procedures) of perforating the colon.[71] Flexible sigmoidoscopy views only the final section of the colon and rectum, but it is safer and it does not require the extensive preparation or anesthesia needed for colonoscopy. A major advantage of these tests is that if polyps are seen, they can be removed immediately. Flexible sigmoidoscopy should be combined with annual stool blood tests to detect cancers beyond the range of sigmoidoscope. CT colonography (sometimes called "virtual colonoscopy") is a relatively new x-ray test of the large intestine to detect polyps and cancers. It does not require anesthesia and does not carry a risk of perforation, but if polys are found, a colonoscopy is then needed to remove them.[71]

Screening for colorectal cancer is a partial success story in the United States. The CDC estimates that in 2020, more than 70% of American adults ages 50–75 have had at least one screening test at the recommended

Table 3.2 Recommended Colorectal Cancer Screening Tests

Several different tests for colon cancer are available. Each has its advantages and disadvantages.

Test	Recommended Frequency	Advantages	Disadvantages
Stool-Based Tests			
Guaiac fecal occult blood test (gFOBT)	Every year	Low cost	Requires 3 stool samples Dietary restrictions needed when testing
Fecal immunochemical test (FIT)	Every year	Requires only 1 stool sample	
sDNA-FIT	Every 1-3 years	Requires only 1 stool sample	Involves collecting entire bowel movement
Direct Visualization Tests			
Colonoscopy	Every 10 years	Views entire colon Polyps can be removed during procedure	Uncomfortable bowel preparation before procedure Requires sedation or anesthesia Small risk of perforation
CT colonography	Every 5 years	Views entire colon Does not require sedation or anesthesia	Uncomfortable bowel preparation before procedure If polyps found, colonoscopy needed to remove them
Flexible sigmoidoscopy	Every 5 years, or every 10 years with FIT every year	Safer than colonoscopy Polyps can be removed during procedure	Requires bowel preparation before procedure Views only final section of the colon and rectum; to detect cancers in other regions, must be combined with stool-based tests

Data from U.S. Preventive Services Task Force. Screening for Colorectal Cancer: U.S. Preventive Services Task Force Recommendation Statement. JAMA 2021;325:1965-1977.

Box 3.6 Summary–Prevention of Colorectal Cancer

- Primary prevention
  - Smoking prevention
  - Reduction of alcohol consumption
  - Promotion of healthy diets
    - Reducing red meat, processed meat, and high-fat foods; increasing whole grains, high-fiber foods, and dairy products
  - Prevention of obesity
  - Promotion of physical activity
- Secondary prevention
  - Screening for and removal of polyps and noninvasive adenocarcinomas

Box 3.7 Key Words–Colorectal Cancer

Acetaldehyde
Adenocarcinoma
Adenoma
Bile acids
Colon
Colonoscope, colonoscopy
Colorectal
CT colonography
Distant cancer stage
Fecal immunochemical test (FIT)
Guaiac fecal occult blood test (gFOBT)
Gut microbiome
Heme
Insulin
Localized cancer stage

interval, an increase from less than 40% in 2000.[72,73] About half of the reduction in colon cancer mortality in the United States since 1975 has been attributed to this screening.[72] While other high-income countries in Europe and Asia have similar colorectal cancer screening programs, most lower-income countries—with lower rates of colorectal cancer and less funding for medical care—do not.[74]

Resources–Colorectal Cancer

- Brenner H, Kloor M, Pox CP. Colorectal cancer. *Lancet*. 2014;383:1490-1502. doi:10.1016/S0140-6736(13)61649-9
- Davidson KW, Barry MJ, Mangione CM, et al. Screening for Colorectal Cancer: US Preventive Services Task Force Recommendation Statement. *JAMA - Journal of the American Medical Association*. 2021;325(19):1965-1977. doi:10.1001/jama.2021.6238

Cancer of the Pancreas

Introduction

It is easy to be pessimistic about cancer of the pancreas. Because it spreads before people notice it, pancreatic cancer has a very low survival rate after diagnosis. Unlike lung cancer, pancreatic cancer has no single driving risk factor. And unlike deaths from breast cancer and colon cancer, deaths from pancreatic cancer cannot be prevented by screening and removal of early cancers or pre-cancers.

But there are proven, modifiable (and familiar) risk factors for pancreatic cancer: smoking, excessive weight, and alcohol use. And the disease is so deadly that many lives could be saved if the incidence of the disease were to be reduced by only 5–10%. In fact, rates of pancreatic cancer in the United States are rising steadily, so even preventing further increases would be a meaningful success.

Physiology: Normal Biology of the Pancreas

The pancreas is two very different glands combined in one organ. One gland—the **exocrine pancreas**—produces enzymes to digest food in the small intestine. Most of what we eat could not be fully digested without these enzymes. The other gland—the **endocrine pancreas**—produces **insulin** and other hormones to regulate levels of glucose in the blood (see Chapter 7. Chronic Metabolic Diseases). The most common type of cancer involves the exocrine pancreas—specifically, the cells responsible for producing and transporting the digestive enzymes.

The cells that produce these enzymes are grouped in tiny hollow bulbs called **acini** (singular acinus). The enzymes travel down through a branched network of ducts to reach the small intestine (**Figure 3.24**). When they are first produced and are in transit, these enzymes are in inactive forms called **proenzymes**; the proenzymes become activated when they arrive in the small intestine by a second set of enzymes. It is important that the proenzymes remain inactive until they reach the intestine, because when they are in their active form, they can be toxic. In fact, in some abnormal conditions, the activated forms of the enzymes come in direct contact with the pancreatic tissue, and when they do, they can "digest" the entire organ in a matter of hours.

Pathophysiology of Pancreatic Cancer

Cancer of the pancreas arises from either the cells in the acini or the cells lining the ducts.[75] It is unclear why these cells are at risk, but the cells in the acini have a remarkable ability to divide and transform themselves into other types of cells in the pancreas.[76] That stem cell-like potential may make them vulnerable to losing control over their growth. Most cancers begin as growths inside the ducts called **pancreatic intraepithelial neoplasia (PaIN)**.[75-77] These PaIN growths are very common and usually benign (about ¾ of older adults have them without problems) but occasionally they are transformed into cancer, called **pancreatic ductal adenocarcinoma**.[75,78]

The transformation into cancer cells is like the development of cancer everywhere else: a stepwise series of mutations, each increasing the chances that additional mutations will happen, resulting in a cell line that proliferates uncontrollably and evades the immune system.[77,78] On average, pancreatic cancer

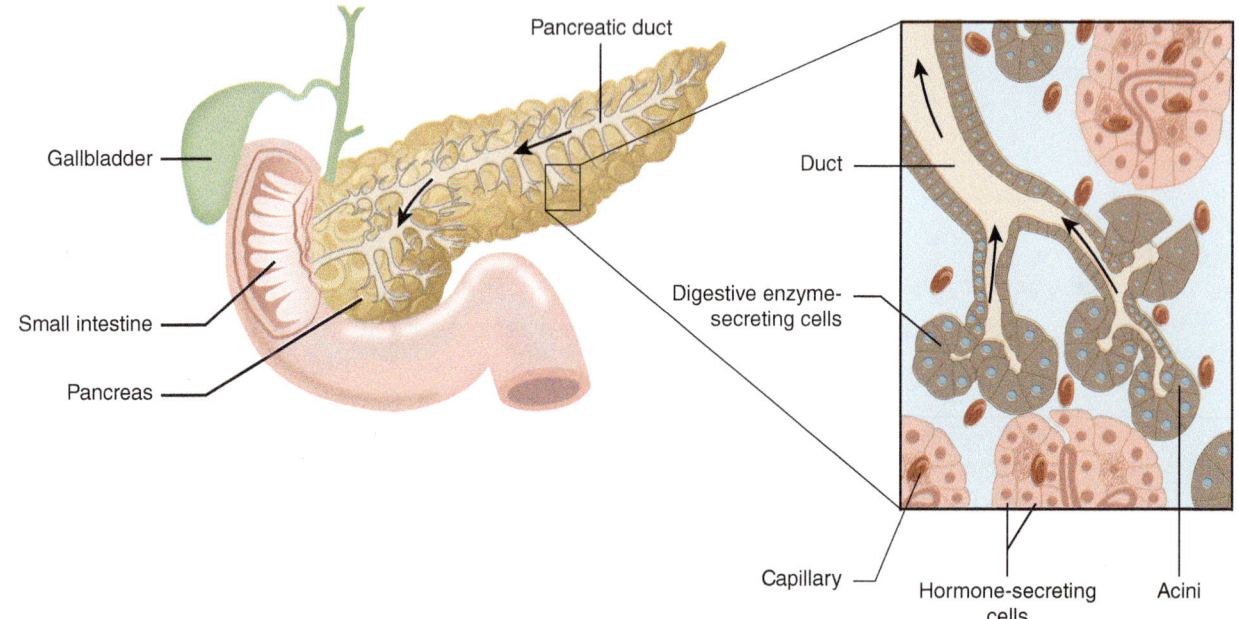

Figure 3.24 The Pancreas. The pancreas is two different glands combined in one organ. One gland produces enzymes to digest food in the small intestine, and the other produces insulin and other hormones. The cells that produce enzymes are grouped in tiny bulbs called acini. The enzymes travel from the acini through a network of ducts into the small intestine. Cancer of the pancreas arises from cells in the acini or the ducts.

cells have 60–70 mutations that distinguish them from normal cells.[76]

One factor that seems to influence that transformation in the pancreas is the immune system in the immediate area. When the immune system is activated, some cells suppress the activity of others. Cells in the pancreas that become cancerous seem to appear in areas where there is more suppression taking place.[75] Perhaps that suppression allows cancerous cells that would otherwise be killed by the immune system instead to survive and proliferate.

As with breast cancer, people carrying certain genes are more likely to develop pancreatic cancer. In fact, some of the same genes are involved. For example, people with the BRCA1 or BRCA2 genes that predispose them to breast cancer are also several times more likely to develop pancreatic cancer.[77] But, as with breast cancer, a large majority of people who have pancreatic cancer do not have these genetic defects.[77]

By the time the symptoms of a pancreatic cancer are noticed, there is an 85% chance it has already spread to lymph nodes in the region or metastasized to distant organs, so surgically removing the cancer is not possible.[79] Even when the pancreatic cancers removed by surgery seem localized, the cancers tend to recur and are usually deadly.[78] Only 14% of people with pancreatic cancer in the United States survive five years after their diagnosis, which is the lowest survival rate of all cancer types.[5]

Epidemiology: Patterns and Trends

In the United States, about 64,000 people are diagnosed with pancreatic cancer and 50,000 die from the disease each year.[51] Those numbers have been rising by about 1% per year since 2000, perhaps driven by the nation's epidemic of obesity. Like most cancers that grow over many years, pancreatic cancer is mainly a disease of older adults (**Figure 3.25**). For unknown reasons, disease rates are higher in men than in women and higher in African Americans than other racial or ethnic groups (**Figure 3.26**).[5]

Globally, nearly 500,000 people are diagnosed with pancreatic cancer and more than 450,000 die from it each year.[11] Rates (adjusted for age) are four to five times higher in high-income countries than in low- and middle-income countries.[11] Part of that difference may be that some people in low-income countries die from pancreatic cancer without getting a diagnosis. However, the differences are also likely due in part to higher rates of smoking and obesity in high-income countries.

Risk Factors

Modifiable risk factors for pancreatic cancer include (**Figure 3.27**):

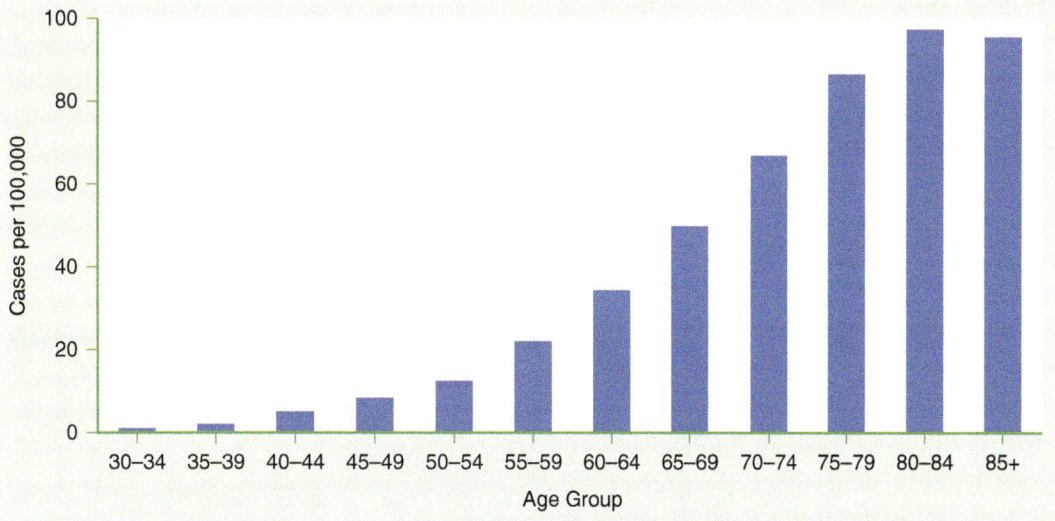

Figure 3.25 Incidence of Pancreatic Cancer in the United States by Age Group, 2017–2021.

Data from U.S. Cancer Statistics Working Group. U.S. Cancer Statistics Data Visualizations Tool. U.S. Department of Health and Human Services, Centers for Disease Control and Prevention and National Cancer Institute, released in June 2024. https://www.cdc.gov/cancer/dataviz

- *Cigarette smoking.* People who smoke are about 75% more likely to develop pancreatic cancer.[80] The longer people smoke, the greater the risk. Of the carcinogenic chemicals in tobacco smoke, one specific **N-nitrosamine** called **NNK** has been shown to cause not only lung cancer but also pancreatic cancer when given to laboratory rats.[81] While the lungs get the heaviest dose of N-nitrosamines, these chemicals also enter the bloodstream and circulate throughout the body, reaching the pancreas.

- *Overweight and obesity.* The risk of pancreatic cancer rises with increasing body mass index.[77,78,80] People who are obese are about 35% more likely

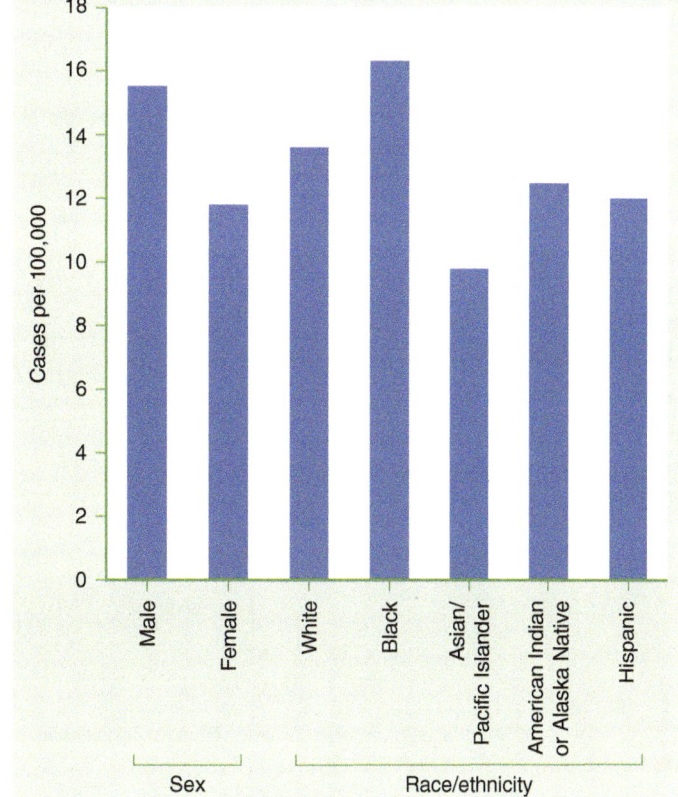

Figure 3.26 Incidence of Pancreatic Cancer in the United States by Race and Sex, 2017–2021.

Data from U.S. Cancer Statistics Working Group. U.S. Cancer Statistics Data Visualizations Tool. U.S. Department of Health and Human Services, Centers for Disease Control and Prevention and National Cancer Institute, released in June 2024. https://www.cdc.gov/cancer/dataviz

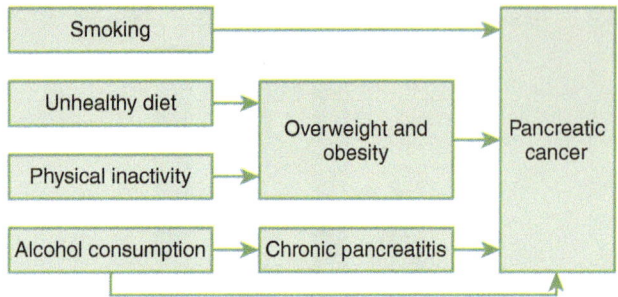

Figure 3.27 Cause-and-Effect Diagram for Pancreatic Cancer.

to develop the disease, and the more years that people are overweight or obese, the greater the risk.[82,83] The mechanism is not clear, but insulin may provide the link: people with obesity show more resistance to the effects of insulin and have higher blood levels of insulin. These insulin patterns have been shown to promote pancreatic cancer in laboratory animals.[82] Related to this, people with Type 2 Diabetes Mellitus, who also have insulin resistance and may have high levels of insulin in the blood, are about 50% more likely to develop pancreatic cancer.[78]

- *Alcohol consumption.* People who drink more than two alcoholic beverages per day are about 20% more likely to develop pancreatic cancer.[80] Alcohol has been shown in laboratory studies to transform normal pancreatic epithelial cells into cancer cells.[84] Also, some very heavy drinkers develop a condition called **chronic pancreatitis**, a condition in which there is a high level of inflammation of the pancreas.[78] This condition has a very strong link to pancreatic cancer, with a 13-fold increase in risk.[80,85]

The most recent estimates are that 16% of cases of pancreatic cancer in the United States are attributable to overweight and obesity and 10% are attributable to cigarette smoking.[14] As obesity rates rise and smoking rates fall in the United States, the importance of obesity to the development of pancreatic cancer is likely to rise. Globally, the rank of these two risk factors is the reverse: an estimated 21% of cases are attributable to smoking and 6% to excessive weight and obesity.[86] Regardless, these estimates suggest that at least one quarter of the cases of pancreatic cancer are preventable.

Preventive Interventions

Primary Prevention

While there are virtually no initiatives specifically designed to prevent pancreatic cancer, addressing these risk factors should have that effect (**Figure 3.28**):

- *Smoking prevention.* See Chapter 11. Tobacco Use.
- *Obesity prevention through promotion of a healthy diet and physical activity.* Obesity and diabetes are discussed in Chapter. Chronic Metabolic Diseases, and the prevention of unhealthy diets and physical activity are discussed in Chapter 14. Nutrition and Chapter 15. Physical Inactivity.
- *Reduction in alcohol consumption.* There are two potential benefits here: prevention of the small increase in cancer risk for moderate drinkers, and prevention of chronic pancreatitis by reducing the number of long-term heavy drinkers. See Chapter 12. Alcohol Use

Secondary Prevention

Researchers have developed tests to detect pancreatic cancer early. These tests involve ultrasound imaging with a scope inserted into the upper intestinal tract or computed tomography (CT) imaging. Unfortunately, these tests do not distinguish cancer from normal pancreatic tissue very well, and except for people with a very high genetic risk, the tests are not recommended.[78]

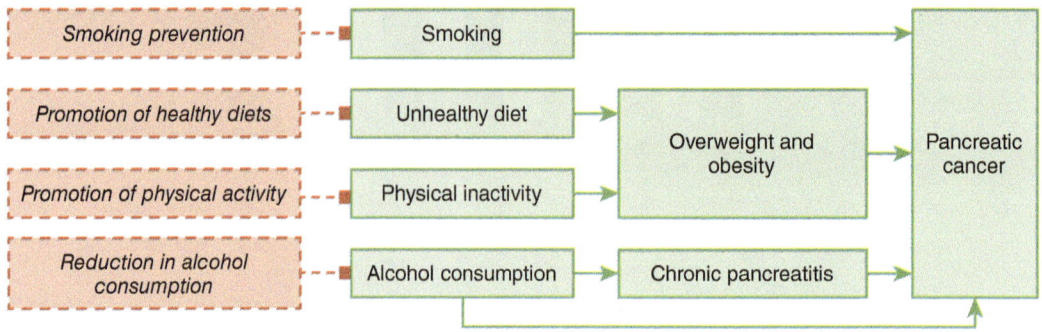

Figure 3.28 Cause-and-Effect Diagram for Pancreatic Cancer, with Preventive Interventions.

Box 3.8 Summary–Prevention of Pancreatic Cancer

- Smoking prevention
- Obesity prevention through promotion of a healthy diet and physical activity
- Reduction in alcohol use

Box 3.9 Key Words–Pancreatic Cancer

Acinus, acini (of the pancreas)
Chronic pancreatitis
Endocrine pancreas
Exocrine pancreas
Insulin
Microbiome, gut
N-nitrosamines
NNK
Pancreatic ductal adenocarcinoma
Pancreatic intraepithelial neoplasia (PaIN)
Proenzymes

Resources–Pancreatic Cancer

- Mizrahi JD, Surana R, Valle JW, Shroff RT. Pancreatic Cancer. *Lancet* 2020;395:2008-2020. doi:10.1016/S0140-6736(20)30974-0. This is a detailed review of the biological and medical aspects of pancreatic cancer.
- Pourshams A, Sepanlou SG, Ikuta KS, et al. The global, regional, and national burden of pancreatic cancer and its attributable risk factors in 195 countries and territories, 1990–2017: A systematic analysis for the Global Burden of Disease Study 2017. *Lancet Gastroenterol Hepatol.* 2019;4(12):934-947. doi:10.1016/S2468-1253(19)30347-4

References

1. Kumar V. Neoplasia. In: Kumar V, Abbas AK, Aster JC, Turner JR, eds. *Robbins & Cotran Pathologic Basis of Disease.* 10th ed. Elsevier; 2021:267-336.

2. Martincorena I, Campbell PJ. Somatic mutation in cancer and normal cells. *Science (1979).* 2015;349(6255):1483-1489. doi:10.1126/science.aab4082

3. Lester SC. Carcinoma of the Breast. In: Kumar V, Abbas AK, Aster JC, Turner JR, eds. *Robbins & Cotran Pathologic Basis of Disease.* 10th ed. Elsevier; 2021:1046-1061.

4. Gallagher EJ, LeRoith D. Hyperinsulinaemia in cancer. *Nat Rev Cancer.* 2020;20(11):629-644. doi:10.1038/s41568-020-0295-5

5. Centers for Disease Control and Prevention. United States Cancer Statistics. Published 2023. Accessed December 10, 2023. Available at: https://www.cdc.gov/cancer/uscs/index.htm

6. Global Burden of Disease Collaboration, Institute for Health Metrics and Evaluation. GBD Results Tool. Published July 12, 2023. Accessed July 11, 2023. Available at: https://vizhub.healthdata.org/gbd-results/

7. Husain AN. Tumors of the Lung. In: Kumar V, Abbas A, Aster JC, Turner JR, eds. *Robbins & Cotran Pathologic Basis of Disease.* 10th ed. Elsevier; 2021:715-725.

8. Bade BC, Dela Cruz CS. Lung Cancer 2020: Epidemiology, Etiology, and Prevention. *Clin Chest Med.* 2020;41(1):1-24. doi:10.1016/j.ccm.2019.10.001

9. Clegg LX, Reichman ME, Miller BA, et al. Impact of socioeconomic status on cancer incidence and stage at diagnosis: Selected findings from the surveillance, epidemiology, and end results: National Longitudinal Mortality Study. *Cancer Causes and Control.* 2009;20(4):417-435. doi:10.1007/s10552-008-9256-0

10. Sidorchuk A, Agardh EE, Aremu O, Hallqvist J, Allebeck P, Moradi T. Socioeconomic differences in lung cancer incidence: A systematic review and meta-analysis. *Cancer Causes and Control.* 2009;20(4):459-471. doi:10.1007/s10552-009-9300-8

11. Sung H, Ferlay J, Siegel RL, et al. Global Cancer Statistics 2020: GLOBOCAN Estimates of Incidence and Mortality Worldwide for 36 Cancers in 185 Countries. *CA Cancer J Clin.* 2021;71(3):209-249. doi:10.3322/caac.21660

12. Leiter A, Veluswamy RR, Wisnivesky JP. The global burden of lung cancer: current status and future trends. *Nat Rev Clin Oncol.* 2023;20(9):624-639. doi:10.1038/s41571-023-00798-3

13. Li Y, Hecht SS. Carcinogenic components of tobacco and tobacco smoke: A 2022 update. *Food Chem Toxicol.* 2022;165:113179. doi:10.1016/j.fct.2022.113179

14. Islami F, Goding Sauer A, Miller KD, et al. Proportion and number of cancer cases and deaths attributable to potentially modifiable risk factors in the United States. *CA Cancer J Clin.* 2018;68:31-54. doi:10.3322/caac.21440

15. Ajrouche R, Ielsch G, Cléro E, et al. Quantitative health risk assessment of indoor aadon: A systematic review. *Radiat Prot Dosimetry.* 2017;177(1-2):69-77. doi:10.1093/rpd/ncx152

16. Pope D, Bruce N, Dherani M, Jagoe K, Rehfuess E. Real-life effectiveness of 'improved' stoves and clean fuels in reducing PM 2.5 and CO: Systematic review and meta-analysis. *Environ Int.* 2017;101:7-18. doi:10.1016/j.envint.2017.01.012

17. World Health Organization. *Ambient (Outdoor) Air Pollution.* Published December 19, 2022. Accessed June 10, 2024. Available at: https://www.who.int/news-room/fact-sheets/detail/ambient-(outdoor)-air-quality-and-health

18. Cohen AJ, Brauer M, Burnett R, et al. Estimates and 25-year trends of the global burden of disease attributable to ambient air pollution: an analysis of data from the Global Burden of Diseases Study 2015. *Lancet*. 2017;389(10082):1907-1918. doi:10.1016/S0140-6736(17)30505-6

19. United States Environmental Protection Agency. *The National Radon Action Plan—A Strategy for Saving Lives*. Published March 29, 2024. Accessed June 10, 2024. Available at: https://www.epa.gov/radon/national-radon-action-plan -strategy-saving-lives#2021-2025

20. UNICEF. *Arsenic Primer. Guidance on the Investigation and Mitigation of Arsenic Contamination*. Published 2018. Accessed June 10, 2024. Available at: https://www.unicef.org/documents /arsenic-primer-guidance-investigation-mitigation-arsenic -contamination

21. Occupational Health and Safety Administration. Respiratory Protection. Published 2023. Accessed December 11, 2023. Available at: https://www.osha.gov/respiratory-protection /standards

22. Furuya S, Chimed-Ochir O, Takahashi K, David A, Takala J. Global asbestos disaster. *Int J Environ Res Public Health*. 2018;15:1000. doi:10.3390/ijerph15051000

23. Environmental Protection Agency. Asbestos Laws and Regulations. Published 2023. Accessed December 11, 2023. Available at: https://www.epa.gov/asbestos/asbestos -laws-and-regulations

24. U.S. Preventive Services Task Force. Lung Cancer: Screening. Published 2021. Accessed December 11, 2023. Available at: https://www.uspreventiveservicestaskforce .org/uspstf/recommendation/lung-cancer-screening

25. Alex A, Bhandary E, McGuire KP. Anatomy and physiology of the breast during pregnancy and lactation. *Adv Exp Med Biol*. 2020;1252:3-7. doi:10.1007/978-3-030-41596-9_1

26. Arendt LM, Kuperwasser C. Form and function: How estrogen and progesterone regulate the mammary epithelial hierarchy. *J Mammary Gland Biol Neoplasia*. 2015;20(1-2): 9-25. doi:10.1007/s10911-015-9337-0

27. Rojas K, Stuckey A. Breast cancer epidemiology and risk factors. *Clin Obstet Gynecol*. 2016;59(4):651-672.

28. Delaloge S, Khan SA, Wesseling J, Whelan T. Ductal carcinoma in situ of the breast: finding the balance between overtreatment and undertreatment. *Lancet*. 2024;403(10445):2734 –2746. doi:10.1016/S0140-6736(24)00425-2

29. Surveillance Research Program, National Cancer Institute. SEER*Explorer: An interactive website for SEER cancer statistics. Published June 27, 2024. Accessed October 9, 2024. Available at: https://seer.cancer.gov/statistics-network /explorer/

30. Yin D, Morris C, Allen M, Cress R, Bates J, Liu L. Does socioeconomic disparity in cancer incidence vary across racial /ethnic groups? *Cancer Causes and Control*. 2010;21(10):1721-1730. doi:10.1007/s10552-010-9601-y

31. Lundqvist A, Andersson E, Ahlberg I, Nilbert M, Gerdtham U. Socioeconomic inequalities in breast cancer incidence and mortality in Europe: A systematic review and meta-analysis. *Eur J Public Health*. 2016;26(5):804-813. doi:10.1093/eurpub /ckw070

32. Joko-Fru WY, Jedy-Agba E, Korir A, et al. The evolving epidemic of breast cancer in sub-Saharan Africa: Results from the African Cancer Registry Network. *Int J Cancer*. 2020;147(8):2131-2141. doi:10.1002/ijc.33014

33. Kuchenbaecker KB, Hopper JL, Barnes DR, et al. Risks of breast, ovarian, and contralateral breast cancer for BRCA1 and BRCA2 mutation carriers. *JAMA*. 2017;317(23): 2402-2416. doi:10.1001/jama.2017.7112

34. Collaborative Group. Type and timing of menopausal hormone therapy and breast cancer risk: individual participant meta-analysis of the worldwide epidemiological evidence. *Lancet*. 2019;394(10204):1159-1168. doi:10.1016 /S0140-6736(19)31709-X

35. National Cancer Institute. Oral Contraceptives and Cancer Risk. Published 2018. Accessed December 13, 2023. Available at: https://www.cancer.gov/about-cancer/causes -prevention/risk/hormones/oral-contraceptives-fact-sheet

36. National Toxicology Program, U.S. Department of Health and Human Services. *15th Report on Carcinogens*. Published December 21, 2921. Accessed October 9, 2024. Available at: https://ntp.niehs.nih.gov/whatwestudy/assessments/cancer /roc

37. Terry MB, Colditz GA. Epidemiology and risk factors for breast cancer: 21st century advances, gaps to address through interdisciplinary science. *Cold Spring Harb Perspect Med*. 2023;13:a041317. doi:10.1101/cshperspect.a041317

38. Bagnardi V, Rota M, Botteri E, et al. Alcohol consumption and site-specific cancer risk: A comprehensive dose-response meta-analysis. *Br J Cancer*. 2015;112(3):580-593. doi:10.1038/bjc.2014.579

39. Kyrgiou M, Kalliala I, Markozannes G, et al. Adiposity and cancer at major anatomical sites: Umbrella review of the literature. *BMJ (Online)*. 2017;356:j477. doi:10.1136/bmj.j477

40. American Institute for Cancer Research, World Cancer Research Fund. *Diet, Nutrition, Physical Activity and Breast Cancer*. Published 2018. Accessed December 11, 2024. Available at: https://www.wcrf.org/wp-content/uploads /2024/10/Breast-cancer-report.pdf

41. Dietary Guidelines Advisory Committee. *Scientific Report of the 2020 Dietary Guidelines Advisory Committee Advisory Report to the Secretary of Agriculture and Secretary of Health and Human Services*. Published 2020. Accessed June 12, 2024. Available at: https://www.dietaryguidelines.gov/2020 -advisory-committee-report

42. U.S. Department of Agriculture. *USDA Nutrition Evidence Systematic Review*. Published 2024. Accessed July 14, 2024. Available at: https://nesr.usda.gov/

43. Luo J, Margolis KL, Wactawski-Wende J, et al. Association of active and passive smoking with risk of breast cancer among postmenopausal women: A prospective cohort study. *BMJ*. 2011;342(7796):536. doi:10.1136/bmj.d1016

44. Song M, Giovannucci E. Preventable incidence and mortality of carcinoma associated with lifestyle factors among white adults in the United States. *JAMA Oncol*. 2016;2(9):1154-1161. doi:10.1001/jamaoncol.2016.0843

45. U.S. Preventive Services Task Force. *Hormone Therapy in Postmenopausal Persons: Primary Prevention of Chronic Conditions*. Published November 1, 2022. Accessed December 14, 2023. Available at: https://www.uspreventiveservicestaskforce .org/uspstf/recommendation/menopausal-hormone-therapy -preventive-medication

46. Keats EC, Das JK, Salam RA, et al. Effective interventions to address maternal and child malnutrition: an update of the evidence. *Lancet Child Adolesc Health*. 2021;5(5): 367-384. doi:10.1016/S2352-4642(20)30274-1

47. Shieh Y, Tice JA. Medications for primary prevention of breast cancer. *JAMA*. 2020;324(3):291. doi:10.1001/jama.2020.9246

48. Nicholson WK, Silverstein M, Wong JB, et al. Screening for breast cancer: US Preventive Services Task Force

recommendation statement. *JAMA.* 2024;331(22):1918-1930. doi:10.1001/jama.2024.5534

49. Farkas AH, Nattinger AB. Breast cancer screening and prevention. *Ann Intern Med.* 2023;176(11):ITC161–ITC176. doi:10.7326/AITC202311210

50. Kumar V, Abbas AK, Aster JC, Turner JR. Adenocarcinoma. In: Kumar V, Abbas AK, Aster JC, Turner JR, eds. *Robbins & Cotran Pathologic Basis of Disease.* 10th ed. Elsevier; 2021: 813-818.

51. Siegel RL, Wagle NS, Cercek A, Smith RA, Jemal A. Colorectal cancer statistics, 2023. *CA Cancer J Clin.* 2023;73:233-254. doi:10.3322/caac.21772

52. Doubeni CA, Laiyemo AO, Major JM, et al. Socioeconomic status and the risk of colorectal cancer: An analysis of more than a half million adults in the National Institutes of Health–AARP Diet and Health Study. *Cancer.* 2012;118(14):3636-3644. doi:10.1002/cncr.26677

53. Doubeni CA, Major JM, Laiyemo AO, et al. Contribution of behavioral risk factors and obesity to socioeconomic differences in colorectal cancer incidence. *J Natl Cancer Inst.* 2012;104(18):1353-1362. doi:10.1093/jnci/djs346

54. Sasso A, Latella G. Role of heme iron in the association between red meat consumption and colorectal cancer. *Nutr Cancer.* 2018;70(8):1173-1183. doi:10.1080/01635581.2018.1521441

55. American Institute of Cancer Research, World Cancer Research Fund. *Diet, Nutrition, Physical Activity and Colorectal Cancer.* Published 2018. Accessed July 2, 2023. Available at: https://dietandcancerreport.org

56. Santarelli RL, Pierre F, Corpet DE. Processed meat and colorectal cancer: A review of epidemiologic and experimental evidence. *Nutr Cancer.* 2008;60(2). doi:10.1080/01635580701684872

57. Vernia F, Longo S, Stefanelli G, Viscido A, Latella G. Dietary factors modulating colorectal carcinogenesis. *Nutrients.* 2021;13:143. doi:10.3390/nu13010143

58. Yang J, Wei H, Zhou Y, et al. High-fat diet promotes colorectal tumorigenesis through modulating gut microbiota and metabolites. *Gastroenterology.* 2022;162(1):135-149. doi:10.1053/j.gastro.2021.08.041

59. Hur J, Otegbeye E, Joh HK, et al. Sugar-sweetened beverage intake in adulthood and adolescence and risk of early-onset colorectal cancer among women. *Gut.* 2021;70(12):2330-2336. doi:10.1136/gutjnl-2020-323450

60. Song M, Garrett WS, Chan AT. Nutrients, foods, and colorectal cancer prevention. *Gastroenterology.* 2015;148(6):1244-1260.e16. doi:10.1053/j.gastro.2014.12.035

61. Liang PS, Chen TY, Giovannucci E. Cigarette smoking and colorectal cancer incidence and mortality: Systematic review and meta-analysis. *Int J Cancer.* 2009;124(10):2406-2415. doi:10.1002/ijc.24191

62. Bird SR, Hawley JA. Update on the effects of physical activity on insulin sensitivity in humans. *BMJ Open Sport Exerc Med.* 2017;2:e000143. doi:10.1136/bmjsem-2016-000143

63. Tran TT, Naigamwalla D, Oprescu AI, et al. Hyperinsulinemia, but not other factors associated with insulin resistance, acutely enhances colorectal epithelial proliferation in vivo. *Endocrinology.* 2006;147(4):1830-1837. doi:10.1210/en.2005-1012

64. Zhou B, Shu B, Yang J, Liu J, Xi T, Xing Y. C-reactive protein, interleukin-6 and the risk of colorectal cancer: A meta-analysis. *Cancer Causes and Control.* 2014;25(10). doi:10.1007/s10552-014-0445-8

65. Islami F, Goding Sauer A, Gapstur SM, Jemal A. Proportion of cancer cases attributable to excess body weight by US state, 2011-2015. *JAMA Oncol.* 2019;5(3):384-392. doi:10.1001/jamaoncol.2018.5639

66. Song M, Giovannucci E. Preventable incidence and mortality of carcinoma associated with lifestyle factors among white adults in the United States. *JAMA Oncol.* 2016;2(9):1154-1161. doi:10.1001/jamaoncol.2016.0843

67. Rothwell PM, Fowkes FGR, Belch JF, Ogawa H, Warlow CP, Meade TW. Effect of daily aspirin on long-term risk of death due to cancer: Analysis of individual patient data from randomised trials. *Lancet.* 2011;377(9759):31-41. doi:10.1016/S0140-6736(10)62110-1

68. Guirguis-Blake J, Evans C, Perdue L, Bean S, Senger C. *Aspirin Use to Prevent Cardiovascular Disease and Colorectal Cancer: An Evidence Update for the U.S. Preventive Services Task Force Evidence Synthesis No. 211. AHRQ Publication No. 21-05283-EF-1.* Agency for Healthcare Research and Quality; 2022.

69. Rodríguez LAG, Martín-Pérez M, Hennekens CH, Rothwell PM, Lanas A. Bleeding risk with long-term low-dose aspirin: A systematic review of observational studies. *PLoS One.* 2016;11(8):e0160046. doi:10.1371/journal.pone.0160046

70. Lin JS, Perdue LA, Henrikson NB, Bean SI, Blasi PR. *Evidence Synthesis Number 202 Screening for Colorectal Cancer: An Evidence Update for the U.S. Preventive Services Task Force.* Published. 2021. Available at: https://www.ahrq.gov

71. Davidson KW, Barry MJ, Mangione CM, et al. Screening for colorectal cancer: US Preventive Services Task Force Recommendation Statement. *JAMA.* 2021;325(19):1965-1977. doi:10.1001/jama.2021.6238

72. Zauber AG. The impact of screening on colorectal cancer mortality and incidence: Has it really made a difference? *Dig Dis Sci.* 2015;60(3):681-691. doi:10.1007/s10620-015-3600-5

73. U.S. Cancer Statistics Working Group. *Colorectal Cancer Screening. United States Cancer Statistics: Data Visualizations.* Published June 2023. Accessed July 20, 2023. Available at: https://gis.cdc.gov/Cancer/USCS/#/CancerScreening/

74. Klabunde C, Blom J, Bulliard JL, et al. Participation rates for organized colorectal cancer screening programmes: An international comparison. *J Med Screen.* 2015;22(3):119-126. doi:10.1177/0969141315584694

75. Wood LD, Canto MI, Jaffee EM, Simeone DM. Pancreatic cancer: pathogenesis, screening, diagnosis, and treatment. *Gastroenterology.* 2022;163(2):386-402.e1. doi:10.1053/j.gastro.2022.03.056

76. Grimont A, Leach SD, Chandwani R. Uncertain beginnings: Acinar and ductal cell plasticity in the development of pancreatic cancer. *Cell Mol Gastroenterol Hepatol.* 2022;13(2):369-382. doi:10.1016/j.jcmgh.2021.07.014

77. Maitra A. Pancreatic carcinoma. In: Kumar V, Abbas AK, Aster JC, Turner JR, eds. *Robbins & Cotran Pathologic Basis of Disease.* 10th ed. Elsevier; 2021:890-893.

78. Mizrahi JD, Surana R, Valle JW, Shroff RT. Pancreatic cancer. *Lancet.* 2020;395:2008-2020.

79. Siegel RL, Miller KD, Wagle NS, Jemal A. Cancer statistics, 2023. *CA Cancer J Clin.* 2023;73(1):17-48. doi:10.3322/caac.21763

80. Park W, Chawla A, O'Reilly EM. Pancreatic cancer: A review. *JAMA.* 2021;326(9):851-862. doi:10.1001/jama.2021.13027

81. Schuller HM. Mechanisms of smoking-related lung and pancreatic adenocarcinoma development. *Nat Rev Cancer.* 2002;2(6):455-463. doi:10.1038/nrc824

82. Stolzenberg-Solomon RZ, Schairer C, Moore S, Hollenbeck A, Silverman DT. Lifetime adiposity and risk of pancreatic cancer in the NIH-AARP Diet and Health Study cohort. *American Journal of Clinical Nutrition.* 2013;98(4):1057-1065. doi:10.3945/ajcn.113.058123

83. Dobbins M, Decorby K, Choi BCK. The association between obesity and cancer risk: A meta-analysis of observational studies from 1985 to 2011. *ISRN Prev Med.* 2013;2013:1-16. doi:10.5402/2013/680536

84. Yu W, Ma Y, Roy SK, Srivastava R, Shankar S, Srivastava RK. Ethanol exposure of human pancreatic normal ductal epithelial cells induces EMT phenotype and enhances pancreatic cancer development in KC (Pdx1-Cre and LSL-KrasG12D) mice. *J Cell Mol Med.* 2022;26(2):399-409. doi:10.1111/jcmm.17092

85. Raimondi S, Lowenfels AB, Morselli-Labate AM, Maisonneuve P, Pezzilli R. Pancreatic cancer in chronic pancreatitis: Aetiology, incidence, and early detection. *Best Pract Res Clin Gastroenterol.* 2010;24(3):349-358. doi:10.1016/j.bpg.2010.02.007

86. Pourshams A, Sepanlou SG, Ikuta KS, et al. The global, regional, and national burden of pancreatic cancer and its attributable risk factors in 195 countries and territories, 1990–2017: A systematic analysis for the Global Burden of Disease Study 2017. *Lancet Gastroenterol Hepatol.* 2019;4(12):934-947. doi:10.1016/S2468-1253(19)30347-4

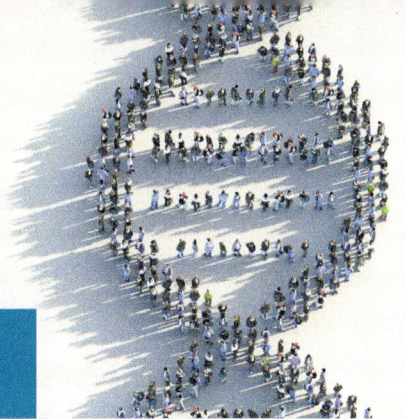

CHAPTER 4

Musculoskeletal Disorders

Most of the body's weight is in the musculoskeletal system. This system includes muscles, bones, the **tendons** that connect muscles to bones, the joints that connect the bones, and the **ligaments** that hold bones together at the joints.

When an external force is applied to musculoskeletal tissues, it causes them to stretch, compress, or otherwise change shape. A measure of the force applied per unit of cross-sectional area of the tissue is called **stress**. (In this chapter, the term *stress* is used to refer to physical stress, not psychological stress.) Stress on tissues that occurs repeatedly over years can damage these tissues and cause pain, leading to **musculoskeletal disorders**. These disorders do not kill people—not directly, at least—so they are not often viewed as public health problems. But they can be disabling and cause much unnecessary suffering.

As people age, their musculoskeletal tissues become less resilient, and the damage from repeated stress accumulates. To some degree, musculoskeletal problems are inevitable if we live long enough, but these problems can be delayed.

Interestingly, the right amount and timing of stress on musculoskeletal tissues can *prevent* musculoskeletal disorder. Muscles, bones, and other tissues weaken when they are not used and respond to the right kind of stress by becoming stronger. Prevention is based on promoting the kind of graded stress needed to strengthen tissues, giving those tissues appropriate rest, and avoiding the sudden, high-force stress that can tear tissues.

Across entire populations, there are risk factors other than stress that also play important and often overlooked roles in the development of musculoskeletal disorders. Obesity, smoking, and psychosocial problems can increase not only rates of heart disease, cancer, and mental illnesses, but also of aches and pains.

This chapter covers the two musculoskeletal problems causing the greatest public health burden in the United States, as measured by disability-adjusted life years (DALYs) lost (see Figure 1.8 in Chapter 1. Disease Prevention and Populations)[1]: osteoarthritis and low back pain.

Osteoarthritis

Introduction

Arthritis is a general term for **inflammation** of one or more joints. Inflammation is a condition in which the body's immune system is activated, prompting immune cells and antibodies to attack a tissue that has been damaged. While the main purpose of the immune system is to kill invading organisms, inflammation is triggered by damaged tissues even when there are no invaders.

Arthritis can be a feature of many diseases. The disease that most often causes arthritis is called **osteoarthritis**, which is also called **degenerative joint disease**.[2] Osteoarthritis is a chronic disease in which the cartilage lining in one or more joints gradually breaks down, causing people to have pain, stiffness in their joints, deformities, and ultimately, difficulty walking, standing, or using their hands.

It is only recently that health experts have begun to think of osteoarthritis as a public health problem.

Their responses so far have focused mainly on helping people who already have the disease manage their symptoms.[3] However, there are interventions that should delay the onset or slow the development of osteoarthritis population-wide.

For many years, doctors thought osteoarthritis was simply the result of "wear and tear" on joints. They were partly right; repeated stress on joints is the primary determinant of osteoarthritis. But in recent years, research has shown that the immune system's response to that stress also plays a big role. And the concept of "wear and tear" does not adequately describe the physical stress that causes osteoarthritis. The invention of labor-saving devices—from tractors to washing machines to industrial robots—has reduced humans' need to push, pull, bend, and lift things. One might predict that these devices would prevent osteoarthritis. Instead, as the world modernizes, rates of osteoarthritis are rising, even after taking aging into account. Preventing osteoarthritis will require engineering the right kind and amount of physical activity back into people's daily lives, as well as better management of the immune response.

Physiology of Synovial Joints

Joints are the meeting of two or more bones. The joints that are most vulnerable to osteoarthritis are called **synovial joints**. In synovial joints, the ends of the bones are wrapped in tough fibrous tissue called the **joint capsule** and are separated from each other by a **joint space** that is filled with **synovial fluid** (**Figure 4.1**). The inside lining of the joint capsule is a thin layer of tissue called **synovium**, and the ends of the bones are covered by **articular cartilage**. Ligaments that are outside of the joint capsule stabilize the joint, holding the bones together even as they move.

Cartilage is a spongy tissue composed mostly of water, held together by fibers made of a protein called **collagen** and cells called **chondrocytes**. Cartilage acts as a shock absorber for the joint, and the smooth surface of the cartilage and the synovial fluid lubricate the joint.[2] The chondrocytes keep the cartilage healthy,[4] but if the cartilage is damaged or torn, they cannot replace it with a new cartilage.[2] In a healthy person, cartilage does not contain either blood vessels or nerve fibers, so pain does not originate from it. But vessels and

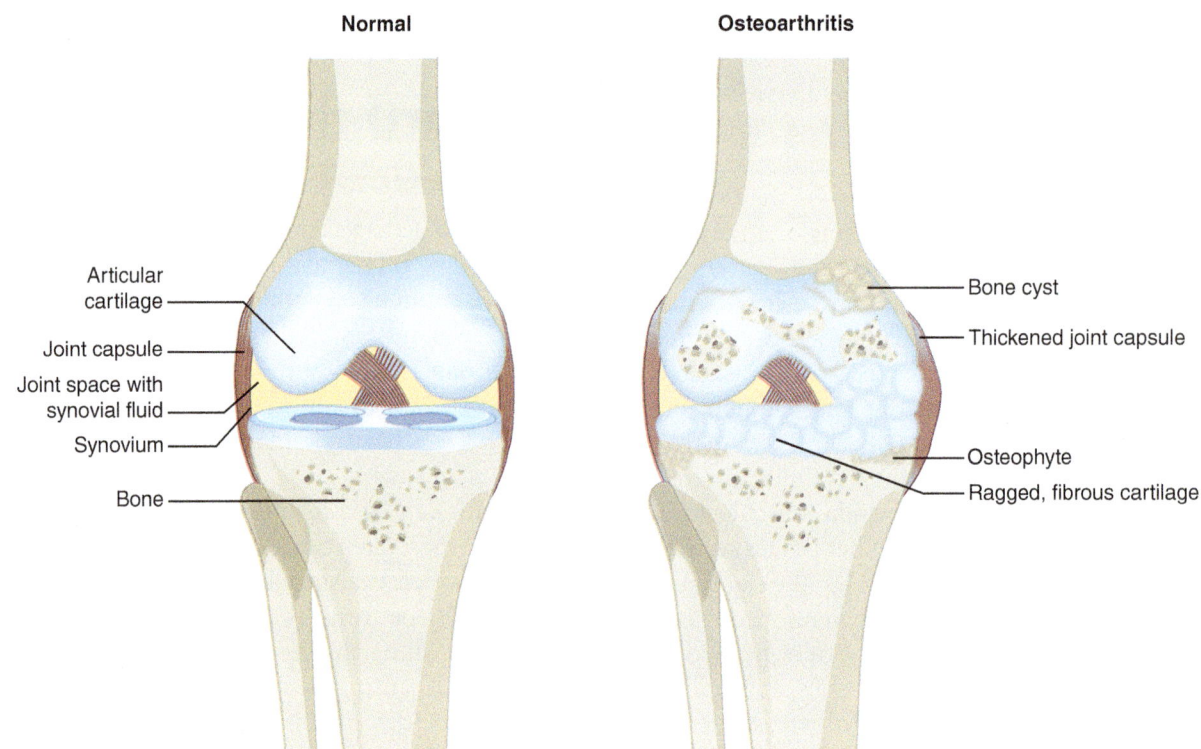

Normal   **Osteoarthritis**

Articular cartilage
Joint capsule
Joint space with synovial fluid
Synovium
Bone

Bone cyst
Thickened joint capsule
Osteophyte
Ragged, fibrous cartilage

Figure 4.1 Normal Synovial Joint and Joint with Osteoarthritis. In a synovial joint, the ends of the bones are covered by a joint capsule and separated from each other by a space that is filled with fluid. The ends of the bones are covered by cartilage. If the joint has osteoarthritis, the cartilage is thinner and ragged, and the bones develop fluid-filled spaces called bone cysts and areas of new growth called bone spurs or osteophytes.

Modified from Robinson WH et al. Low-grade inflammation as a key mediator of the pathogenesis of osteoarthritis. Nat Rev Rheumatol 2016 Oct;12(10):580–92. doi: 10.1038/nrrheum.2016.136

nerves are present in the ends of bones, so joint damage that extends beneath the cartilage can be very painful.

Pathophysiology of Osteoarthritis

If a person sprains an ankle, the next day the ankle is swollen, red, and painful. This is a demonstration of how stress can damage tissue and how that damaged tissue provokes a response of inflammation from the body's immune system. It is the inflammation, not the ankle sprain itself, that causes swelling, redness, and pain. In osteoarthritis, a lesser stress on joints stimulates a lesser amount of inflammation in the cartilage and the synovium, but this stress is ultimately more damaging because it is repeated thousands of times.[2,5]

Inflammation is a complex response by the immune system that has many components. Some aspects of the inflammatory response help restore tissues, but some are destructive to tissues. If the stress and inflammatory response from an injury were to happen only once, as with a sprained ankle, in time the joint would heal itself and maybe become even stronger. But tissues need time to heal and to become stronger after physical stress. When stress on a knee or a hip is repeated throughout the day, hundreds of days a year for many years (as it is for someone carrying excess weight from obesity), there is no time for healing, and the unrelenting inflammation causes permanent damage to the articular cartilage.[6] Furthermore, damaged cartilage is more susceptible than healthy cartilage to injury from physical stress, setting up a vicious circle that partly explains why osteoarthritis gets worse over time.[5]

Conditions that activate the immune system in other ways may accelerate this process. In particular, obesity is a biologic condition that activates the body's immune system (see Chapter 7. Chronic Metabolic Diseases); people with obesity have constant low-level inflammation throughout the body, and for them, osteoarthritis progresses more quickly.

As osteoarthritis does its damage, the cartilage gradually becomes thinner and ragged (Figure 4.1).[2,5] With less shock absorption, the ends of the bones also become damaged, developing small fluid-filled spaces called **bone cysts**.[6] Unlike cartilage, bones that are damaged regrow, and in the later stages of osteoarthritis, the ends of the bones grow inappropriately into the sides of joints with **osteophytes**, also called **bone spurs**.[2,6] An x-ray of a joint with osteoarthritis will show a narrower-than-normal joint space, bone cysts, and osteophytes.

One demonstration of the feedback that underlies osteoarthritis is its link to acute knee injuries. A teenager and young adult who tears a ligament in the knee playing soccer or basketball usually recovers with or without surgery, only to develop osteoarthritis in that knee many years later. The inflammation from that single injury apparently initiates a process that gradually damages the joint over decades.

Some joints are much more susceptible than others. The joints most commonly affected are the knee and hip, probably because they carry most of the body's weight, and the small joints of the fingers, probably because they get the most use. By far the most troublesome joints are the knees,[2] affecting some 85% of people with osteoarthritis (**Figure 4.2**).[5,7]

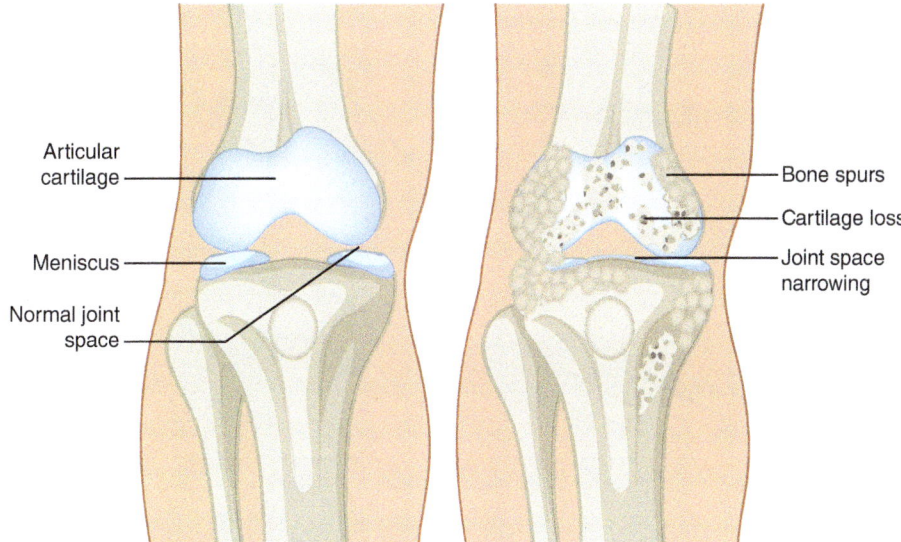

Figure 4.2 **Normal Knee and Knee with Osteoarthritis.** When the knee develops osteoarthritis, the cartilage breaks down, the joint space becomes narrower, and bone spurs grow.

Many people have signs of osteoarthritis on x-rays without experiencing any symptoms at all.[5] That may be because there are no nerve fibers in the cartilage, which is where the damage begins. But as the disease progresses and the cartilage disintegrates, blood vessels and nerve endings grow into the joint surface, making them painful.[5,6,8]

Osteoarthritis can be disabling. People with osteoarthritis may give up on walking or being physically active (taking on the health risks of inactivity), can have difficulty sleeping, and become depressed.[9] No medical treatments today can prevent or stop the disease's progress. Physicians can only treat people with medications for pain, encourage them to keep active, and when the disability is bad enough, replace their hips or knees with artificial joints.[2]

The difference between x-ray images and people's symptoms has led doctors to make a distinction between osteoarthritis *disease* (changes to the biology of the joint) and osteoarthritis *illness* (symptoms caused by those biologic changes).[4] The distinction is necessary to interpret statistics; the prevalence of osteoarthritis based on x-rays is many times higher than the prevalence based on symptoms or on a physician's diagnosis. And the distinction may also be important to prevention. The public health goal is to prevent the *illness* of osteoarthritis so that people remain active and do not suffer from pain. In theory there may be interventions that prevent one but not the other.[4]

Epidemiology: Patterns and Trends

The prevalence of osteoarthritis increases with age and varies by sex, body weight, and the joints involved. About 10–20% of Americans over age 60 have symptoms from osteoarthritis of the knee.[5] The estimates of the percentage with osteoarthritis of the knee diagnosed by physicians are shown in **Figure 4.3**.[10] Women are about 30% more likely than men to have knee osteoarthritis, with larger gaps among those who are obese.[5,6,11] While there are many theories about why women are at higher risk, this difference is not yet explained.[12]

Osteoarthritis of the hip is about half as common as osteoarthritis of the knee.[5] The prevalence of osteoarthritis of the hand varies enormously by the definition used and the population studied, and there is an especially large difference between x-ray signs and symptoms because most older adults have x-ray signs of the disease, with women affected more than men, but few of them have symptoms.[5,13]

There is an inconsistent pattern of osteoarthritis and race. People of African descent are more likely than Whites to have osteoarthritis of the knee but are less likely to have osteoarthritis of the hip or hand.[13-15] People with lower incomes or less education who live in rural areas have a higher prevalence of osteoarthritis of the knee and hip.[14] These demographic differences are also not explained.

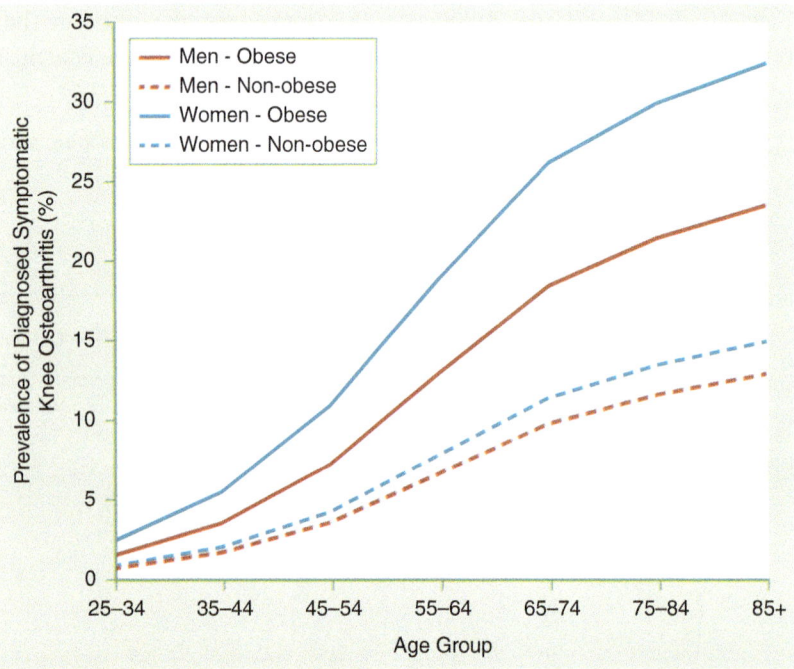

Figure 4.3 **Estimated Prevalence of Knee Osteoarthritis in the United States, by Age Group.** Osteoarthritis is more common in older adults, in women, and in persons who are obese.

Data from Losina E et al. Lifetime risk and age at diagnosis of symptomatic knee osteoarthritis in the U.S. Arthr Care Res 2013;64(5):7023-711 doi 10.1002/acr.21898

Globally, the prevalence of osteoarthritis is higher in countries with higher incomes, the highest in North America, Australia and New Zealand, and the Middle East. The prevalence is about half as high in sub-Saharan Africa.[16] But in all regions of the world, osteoarthritis is increasing, rising about 10% from 1990 to 2017. North America, which is the region that already had the highest prevalence, is also experiencing the biggest increase (22%), most likely driven by the obesity epidemic.[16]

Risk Factors

Researchers have found several risk factors for osteoarthritis that unfortunately cannot be modified. People are at greater risk if they naturally do not have straight *alignment* of the bones connected by the joints — for example, if their knees angle inwards or bow outwards.[4-6] Similarly, babies born with **dislocated hips** are more likely to develop hip osteoarthritis as adults.[4] And there are *genetic* risk factors, which are stronger for hip than knee disease and are particularly strong for osteoarthritis of the hand.[4]

Three risk factors that are modifiable have been clearly and strongly linked to the development and progression of osteoarthritis (**Figure 4.4**):

- *Overweight and obesity.* The risk of developing osteoarthritis of the knee rises sharply with increasing **body mass index** (BMI). People with BMI of 25-30 (overweight) are at about twice the risk, those with BMI between 30 and 35 (obese Class 1) are at about three times the risk, and those with BMI above 35 (obese Class 2 or 3) are nearly five times the risk.[17] The strength of this association, combined with obesity's high (and rising) prevalence, means that obesity is a driving force for knee osteoarthritis globally. In developed countries around the world, about 25% of knee osteoarthritis is attributable to overweight and obesity.[11]

In the United States, with nearly the highest obesity rates in the world, approximately 50% of knee osteoarthritis is attributable to obesity.[18] Obesity is linked to osteoarthritis of other joints too, but less strongly. Interestingly, obesity even increases the risk of osteoarthritis of the hand, which shows that the increase in risk is not just due to the physical stress of excess body weight but also may involve body-wide inflammation.[13,17]

- *Joint injury.*[11] People who have a torn knee ligament or torn meniscus from an injury (such as from sports) are about five times as likely to develop osteoarthritis years later.[4,14] High-risk sports include football, soccer, basketball, hockey, and rugby. By one estimate, about 5% of osteoarthritis of the knee can be attributed to previous acute injuries.[5]

- *Occupational repetitive joint stress.* Certain occupations involve people putting frequent stress on specific joints, for example, by squatting, climbing, lifting, or kneeling.[19] People in these occupations are more likely to develop osteoarthritis in the joints that are stressed. Workers who frequently kneel or squat—such as floor layers, brick layers, carpenters, and house cleaners—are more likely to develop osteoarthritis of the knee.[5,19] Construction workers and farmers, who frequently lift objects, are more likely to develop osteoarthritis of the hip.[5] Professional athletes in high-impact sports like football, hockey, and weightlifting are more likely to develop osteoarthritis of both the knee and the hip.[14] People who constantly use their hands at work, such as clothing workers, and food workers, have higher rates of osteoarthritis of the hand.[13]

There is one other risk factor, which is less well understood but also probably very important:

- *Physical inactivity and muscle weakness.* This may seem contradictory, but physical *inactivity* also

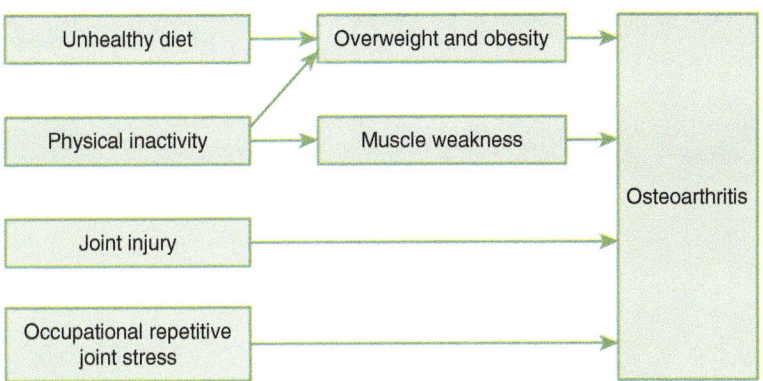

Figure 4.4 **Cause-and-Effect Diagram for Osteoarthritis.**

appears to increase the risk of osteoarthritis—at least involving the knee. To put it another way, studies suggest that people who engage in low-impact exercise or recreational running are less likely to develop osteoarthritis of the knee than those who do not exercise.[9,14,20-22] (Professional runners, though, who frequently put high levels of stress on their knees, are at higher risk.[20]) In what may be related to this, people who have weak knee extensor muscles (like the quadriceps) are also more likely to develop knee osteoarthritis.[4-6] And a core medical recommendation for people who already have osteoarthritis is exercise—both **aerobic** and **muscle-strengthening**.[9] More research is needed on the relationship of different types and amounts of physical activity to the development of osteoarthritis, but at this point, it seems that while frequent *movement* of joints and *strengthening* of muscles that span joints is needed to maintain the health and resilience of joint tissues, heavy or frequent *impact* on joints, especially with inadequate rest or healing, does more damage than good.

These risk factors do not fully explain the increasing trend in osteoarthritis. In a fascinating study, a group of anthropologists examining skeletons found that osteoarthritis of the knee was roughly twice as common in people living in the 1900s as in either people living in the 1800s or pre-historic farmers and hunter-gatherers, even after taking body weight into account.[23] The study hints at unrecognized or underestimated risk factors for knee osteoarthritis in our modern environment.

Preventive Interventions

There has been little attention given to osteoarthritis as a public health problem and very little hard proof of interventions to prevent it. But the risk factors listed above are strong and clear enough that preventing them ought to reduce the incidence and prevalence of this disease (**Figure 4.5**).

The following are primary preventive measures to reduce the prevalence of osteoarthritis:

Primary Prevention

- *Promotion of healthier diets* to prevent overweight and obesity. The highest priority for prevention of osteoarthritis lies in halting or reversing the obesity epidemic. See Chapter 7. Chronic Metabolic Diseases and Chapter 14. Nutrition.

- *Promotion of low-impact aerobic and muscle-strengthening physical activity.* Interventions to promote the right kind of physical activity in populations should reduce osteoarthritis of the knee and maybe of other joints. Exercises that should help are those that improve the strength of knee extensor muscles, such as weightlifting and jumping, as well as those that maintain the mobility and flexibility of joints, such as walking and recreational running.[4] This sort of activity may help people who have had a previous knee joint injury like a cartilage tear as well as everyone else. See Chapter 15. Physical Inactivity.

- *Muscle-strengthening exercise programs to prevent knee injuries.* Preventing tears of the knee ligaments or cartilage in children and young adults playing sports can prevent some from developing osteoarthritis as they age.[4] Since there are many health benefits to sports and exercise, we should encourage, rather than limit, these activities. Fortunately, targeted exercise programs have been proven to reduce knee injuries in sports.[4,5,24-26] These programs have many components, but it seems that the most important ones are strengthening and **plyometric exercises** (involving jumping), which strengthen

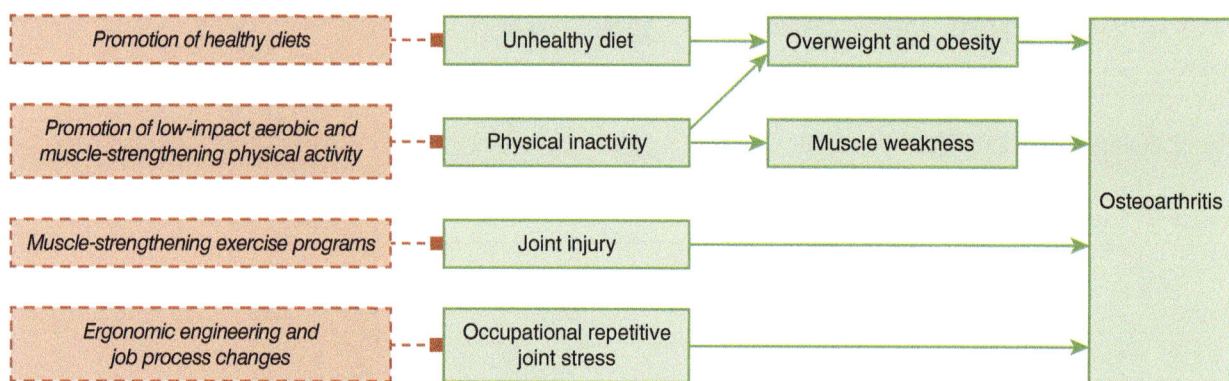

Figure 4.5 Cause-and-Effect Diagram for Osteoarthritis, with Preventive Interventions.

muscles and maybe other tissues that stabilize the knee joint.[25]

- *Ergonomic engineering and job process changes* to prevent repetitive joint stress by reducing squatting, lifting, kneeling, and climbing. For example, machines have been developed that reduce the need for people who lay flooring to kneel.[27] Each task requires a somewhat different solution, but ergonomic solutions can be found for every occupation.

Secondary Prevention

Because osteoarthritis develops slowly over years, the line between primary and secondary prevention is blurry. But interventions that should prevent osteoarthritis from occurring at all should also help slow its progression in people who have started experiencing joint pain and stiffness. For people who are overweight or obese, *weight loss* reduces the pain from knee osteoarthritis.[4,5,9] People who tear a knee ligament or cartilage should *avoid surgery* unless the knee is unstable, and continue *low-impact aerobic and strengthening exercises.*[4,5]

It is also important to avoid using treatments that are ineffective and dangerous. Doctors should especially avoid prescribing opioids for osteoarthritis because they are no better at reducing pain than over-the-counter pain medicines and they are addictive and potentially fatal.[28]

Box 4.1 Summary–Prevention of Osteoarthritis

- Promotion of healthier diets to prevent overweight and obesity
- Promotion of low-impact aerobic and muscle-strengthening physical activity
- Muscle-strengthening exercise programs to prevent knee joint injuries
- Ergonomic engineering and job process changes to prevent repetitive joint stress

---

Box 4.2 Key Words–Osteoarthritis

Aerobic exercise or physical activity
Arthritis
Articular cartilage
Body mass index
Bone cysts
Bone spurs
Cartilage
Chondrocytes
Collagen
Degenerative joint disease
Dislocated hip
Inflammation
Joint
Joint capsule
Joint space
Ligament
Muscle-strengthening exercise or physical activity
Musculoskeletal disorders
Osteoarthritis
Osteophytes
Plyometric exercises
Stress (physical)
Synovial fluid
Synovial joint
Synovium
Tendon

Resources–Osteoarthritis

- Hunter DJ, Bierma-Zeinstra S. Osteoarthritis. *The Lancet.* 2019;393(10182). doi:10.1016/S0140-6736(19)30417-9. This includes a comprehensive review of the epidemiology, pathogenesis, and treatment of osteoarthritis.
- Whittaker JL, Runhaar J, Bierma-Zeinstra S, Roos EM. A lifespan approach to osteoarthritis prevention. *Osteoarthritis Cartilage.* 2021;29(12):1638-1653. doi:10.1016/j.joca.2021.06.015. This is a thoughtful discussion of primary prevention of osteoarthritis.
- The Centers for Disease Control and Prevention has many resources on osteoarthritis available at www.cdc.gov/arthritis, including *A National Public Health Agenda for Osteoarthritis: 2020 Update.*
- *Remain in the Game: A Joint Effort* is one of several training programs to prevent knee and hip joint injuries in sports. Videos and print materials are available at https://oaaction.unc.edu/remain-in-the-game-a-joint-effort/

Low Back Pain

Introduction

Pain in the lower back is so common that it is tempting to view it as a normal part of being a two-legged, upright human. For some people, though, low back pain is severe and persistent, making this condition the leading cause of disability in the United States and globally.[29]

Low back pain often causes people to miss days of work or stop working entirely. And low back pain is often caused *by* work. This makes it a condition that employers and workers' compensation programs care very much about.[29]

It is natural to assume that low back pain results from bending and lifting objects that are too heavy, and that it can be prevented by simply avoiding these activities. But the causes and approaches to prevention are a little more complicated. Certainly, bending and lifting at work can be dangerous for the lower back, but exercise programs that strengthen spine muscles, which involve some amount of bending and lifting, can help prevent the problem. And low back pain has strong psychosocial determinants that may be as important as—or more important than—bending and lifting.[30] In addition, low back pain is a condition for which medical care often makes the problem worse. A key preventive step is avoiding treatments that are unnecessary and risky.

Anatomy of the Spine

The **spine** is a column of bones called **vertebrae** that are stacked like poker chips and that support the abdomen, chest, upper body, and skull. The **cervical** (neck) section has seven vertebrae, the **thoracic** (chest) section has 12 vertebrae that connect to ribs, and the **lumbar** section has five vertebrae (**Figure 4.6**).[31] These vertebrae sit on top of the **coccyx** and **sacrum** at the lower end of the spine.

Each **vertebra** has a round- or oval-shaped **vertebral body** at the front, an oval-shaped hole behind the body, and spikes that stick out on the back and the sides, like points on a star (**Figures 4.7** and **4.8**).[32] The holes in the vertebrae line up to form a tube called the **spinal canal** that surrounds and protects the **spinal cord**.

The spinal cord is a central part of the body's **nervous system**. (The nervous system is the organ system that controls other organ systems; it includes the brain, spinal cord, and a very large number of nerves.) The spinal cord contains **neurons** (brain cells) and **axons**, which are very long extensions of neurons that interface with muscles or other neurons.

The spinal cord is like a bundle of electric wires (axons) that connect the brain to the rest of the body. These axons transmit electrical signals down *from* the brain to control the body's muscles. The axons also transmit electrical signals up *to* the brain from the skin, muscles, and other tissues for sensations like pain.

In each of the gaps between the vertebrae, two bundles of axons called **nerve roots** leave the spinal canal to connect the spinal cord to muscles and other tissues on the two sides of the body (Figure 4.7

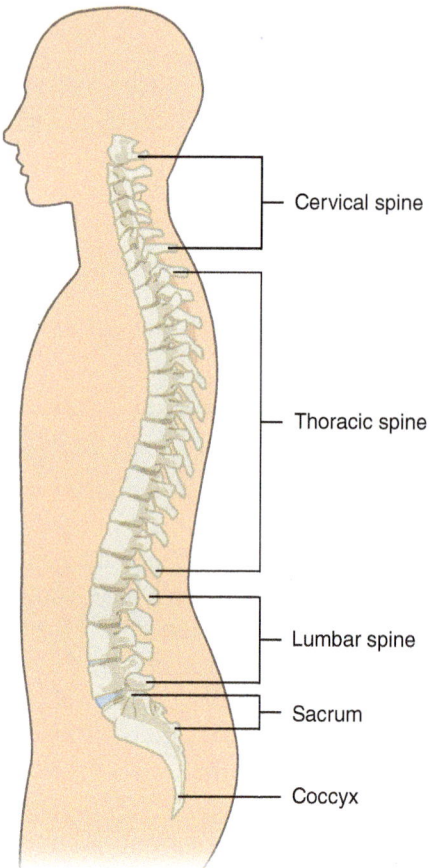

Figure 4.6 The Spine. The spine is a column of bones called vertebrae that are stacked like poker chips. These vertebrae sit on top of the sacrum and coccyx.

Modified from Park DK. Spine Basics. OrthoInfo - American Academy of Orthopaedic Surgeons. Published June 2020. Accessed July 24, 2024. https://orthoinfo.aaos.org/en/diseases–conditions/spine-basics/

and 4.8). If these nerve roots are stretched, squeezed, or chemically irritated, the damage interferes with the electrical signals, which can cause muscles to become weak or even paralyzed and sensations of pain to be sent to the brain.

The vertebrae do not sit directly on top of each other. They are separated by specialized **cartilage** called **intervertebral discs**. Each disk has a soft gel-like center called the **nucleus pulposus**, surrounded by a tough, fibrous ring called the **annulus fibrosus** (**Figure 4.8**).[30] These discs act as shock absorbers for the spine and are squeezed when a person lifts heavy objects.[30] The discs are flexible enough to allow for the spine to bend and twist.

Each vertebra also connects to the one below it with two spikes called **facets** (Figure 4.8). The **facet joints** between each vertebra and the one below it can also stretch and wiggle, but like all joints, they can be a source of pain if they become damaged.

The vertebrae are also connected to each other by muscles and **ligaments** (bands of dense fibrous tissue) attached to the spikes (Figure 4.7). It is the

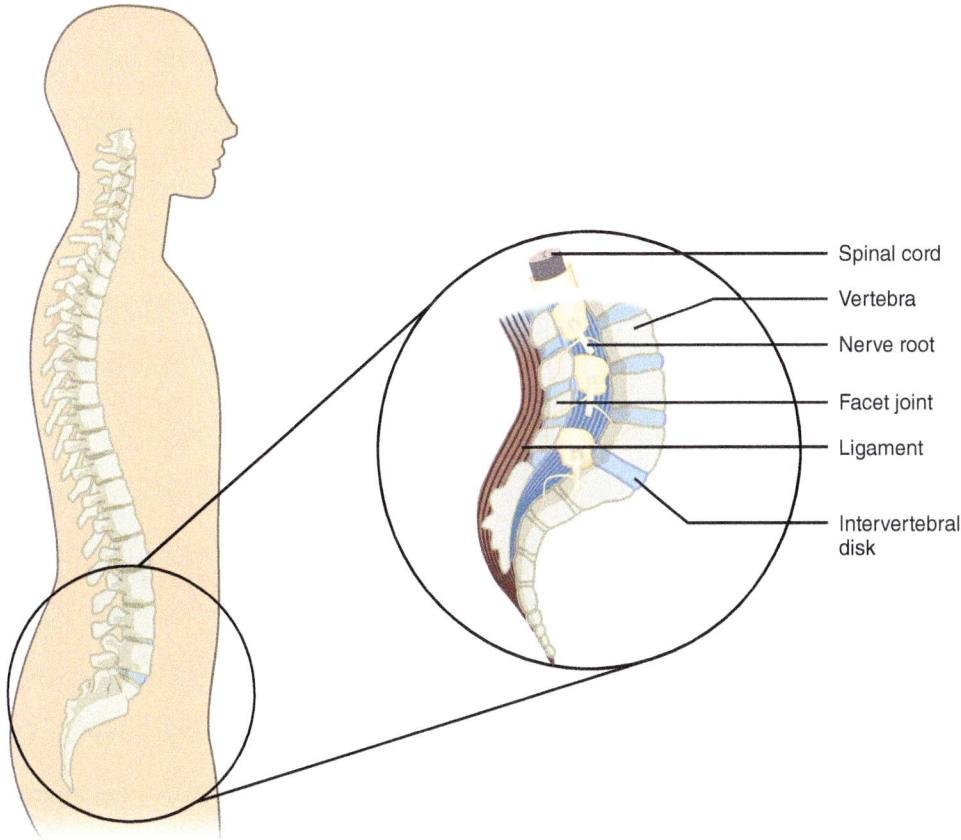

Figure 4.7 **Anatomy of Healthy Lumbar Spine.** Vertebrae are separated from each other by intervertebral disks. The vertebrae have holes in them that align to form the spinal canal. The spinal cord fills the spinal canal, and nerve roots extend from the spinal cord into the gaps between vertebrae.

Modified from Park DK. Herniated Disk in the Lower Back. OrthoInfo - American Academy of Orthopaedic Surgeons. Published January 2022. Accessed July 24, 2024. https://orthoinfo.aaos.org/en/diseases--conditions/herniated-disk-in-the-lower-back/

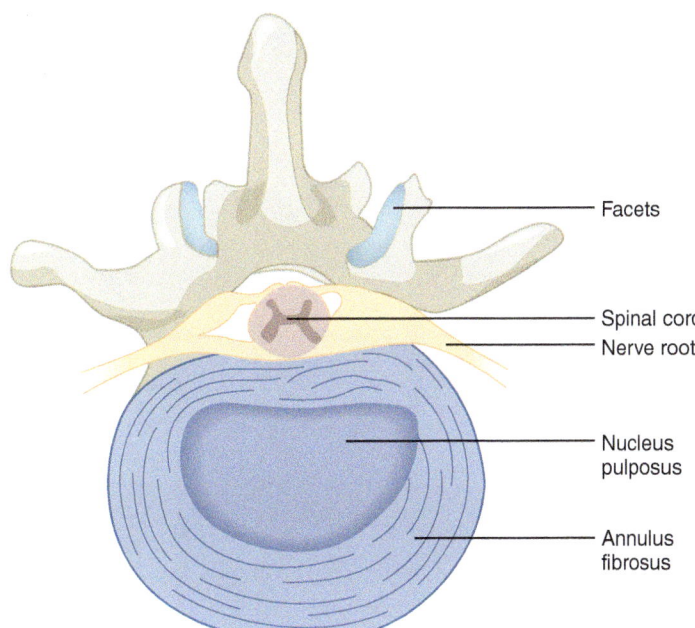

Figure 4.8 **Lumbar Vertebra with Healthy Intervertebral Disk.** This is a view of a healthy vertebra from above, showing also the spinal cord and the two nerve roots. The intervertebral disk has a soft gel-like center called the nucleus pulposus, surrounded by a tough, fibrous ring called the annulus fibrosus.

Modified from Park DK. Herniated Disk in the Lower Back. OrthoInfo - American Academy of Orthopaedic Surgeons. Published January 2022. Accessed July 24, 2024. https://orthoinfo.aaos.org/en/diseases--conditions/herniated-disk-in-the-lower-back/

muscles that, by contracting and relaxing, make the spine bend and twist. The ligaments support the spine so that it does not bend or twist too far.

Pathophysiology of Low Back Pain

The human spine is shaped like an S, with the thoracic section convex and the lumbar and cervical sections concave (Figure 4.6). It is the concave lumbar spine that allows humans to walk on only two legs, freeing up humans' hands for making tools and throwing spears. This shape is very different from that of four-legged animals. As important as the concave shape is to our evolution as a species, it also unfortunately makes the lower back very vulnerable to injury.

With all the different structures crowded together in the lumbar spine, much can go wrong. Low back pain can originate from muscles, ligaments, joints, or from pressure on axons in the spinal cord or nerve roots. The most commonly recognized causes are:

- *Herniated disk.*[30] If a person lifts a heavy object or if the vertebrae otherwise take on a very heavy load, the pressure can squeeze the intervertebral disc so much that the gel-like nucleus pulposus bulges or squirts out, tearing into (or through) the annulus fibrosus (**Figure 4.9**).[32,33] This abnormal bulging is called a **herniation** or a **herniated** disc. The disc itself (like cartilage in other joints) does not

have pain nerve fibers in it, so the herniation does not itself cause pain; in fact, studies show that a large fraction of adults without back pain have discs that have herniated in the past.[30] But if the herniated disc presses on or irritates a nerve root, it can produce pain that can be severe—including pain that is felt down an entire leg—and can cause weakness and loss of sensation in the legs.[30,34] Herniations are more likely to occur in a person whose intervertebral discs have degenerated (became weaker), which occurs with aging and may be accelerated by smoking.[35,36] But, interestingly, herniated discs tend to occur in younger or middle-aged adults (age 30–50), maybe because they are more likely to do strenuous activities. It may seem that surgery would be needed to relieve pressure from a herniated disc on a nerve root, but most herniated discs heal on their own, and people who avoid surgery do as well as or better than those who have an operation.[30,37]

- *Spinal stenosis.* In older adults the spinal canal can become narrower, which is called **stenosis**. This can be caused by collapsed intervertebral discs, thickened ligaments, or osteoarthritis of the vertebral joints causing **osteophytes** (bone spurs), all of which tend to get worse with aging.[30,38,39] Although for many people this condition causes no symptoms, for some it can press on the spinal cord or nerve roots, causing pain in the lower

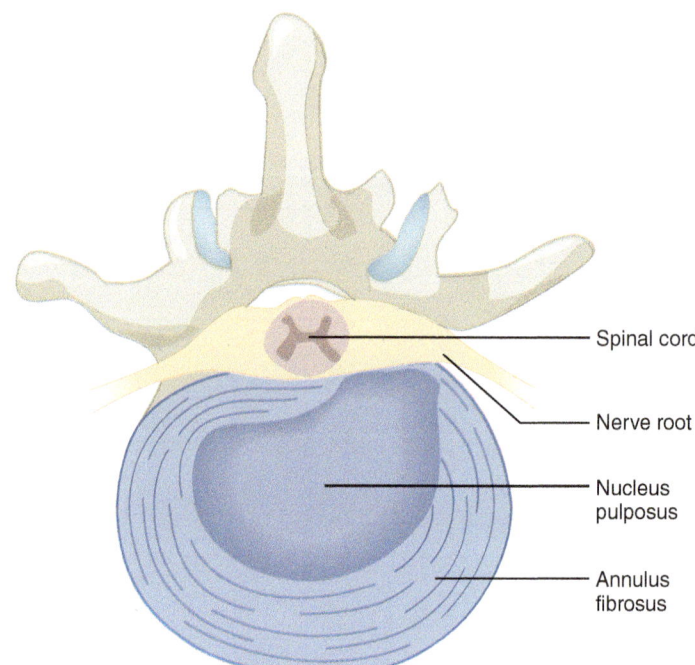

Spinal cord

Nerve root

Nucleus pulposus

Annulus fibrosus

Figure 4.9 Herniated Lumbar Disc. When a disk is herniated, the nucleus pulposus bulges into or through the annulus fibrosus. It then presses on a nerve root and can cause pain, weakness, and loss of sensation in the leg.

Modified from Park DK. Herniated Disk in the Lower Back. OrthoInfo - American Academy of Orthopaedic Surgeons. Published January 2022. Accessed July 24, 2024. https://orthoinfo.aaos.org/en/diseases--conditions/herniated-disk-in-the-lower-back/

back and legs, which is sometimes accompanied accompanied by weakness in the legs.[30]

- *Muscle strain or ligament sprain.* If the spine's muscles and ligaments are stretched with a force greater than they are accustomed to, they can tear, partially or completely.[30] A tear in a muscle is called a **strain** and a tear in a ligament is called a **sprain**. This can happen when a person lifts a heavy object. For example, the normal concave shape of the lumbar spine changes to a convex shape when a person bends over to lift an object and reverts to the concave shape returning to an upright position; if that shape change happens suddenly, while the person is holding a heavy load, it can stretch the spine's muscles and ligaments with a sudden force (**Figure 4.10**). But strains and sprains can also occur when a person just bends or twists the spine quickly, such as during exercise, especially when in an awkward or unfamiliar posture.[40] These injuries are less likely to occur in people who have stronger spinal muscles, which is why exercise that strengthens core muscles helps prevent them. Muscle strains can also result from frequently-repeated stretching or contraction of the spinal muscles, for example, in a worker using machines that cause vibrations to the entire body.[30] Like herniated discs, tears in muscles and ligaments heal by themselves over time. But if a person responds

to the injury by avoiding activity or exercise, it can lead to weaker muscles, which increases the chances of another injury. Or if the cause of the damage is a repeated motion at work, the back pain can become persistent.

- *Osteoarthritis of joints in spine.* The joints between the vertebral bodies and the joints between the facets can develop **osteoarthritis**, just like any other joint in the body (see earlier section in this chapter).[30] As with osteoarthritis in other joints, in the early years, osteoarthritis of the spine does not usually cause pain.[30] But over time, as joint cartilage deteriorates, bone spurs grow, bones begin to rub against each other, and the joint become painful.

For most people, the exact source of low back pain is not clear, so they are labeled as having **nonspecific low back pain**. MRI images in these people do not show herniated discs or spinal stenosis, which hints that the most common cause of nonspecific low back pain may be muscle strain or ligament sprain.[34]

Pain in the low back often starts as a sudden injury, from which most people recover within six weeks (**acute low back pain**).[34] But for a small percentage of people the pain persists, that is, it becomes **chronic low back pain** and a cause of long-term disability.[41] Even within chronic pain there

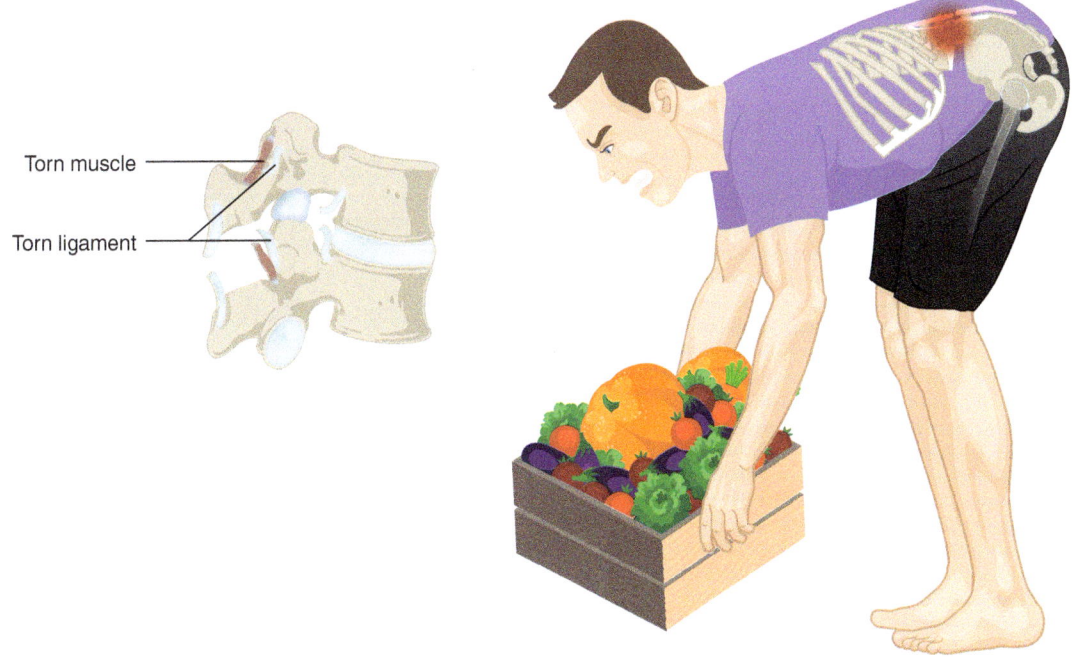

Torn muscle

Torn ligament

Figure 4.10 Stress on the Lower Back Causing Tears in Muscle and Ligament. When the lower spine is suddenly stressed, for example, when a person is lifting, the muscles or ligaments at the back of the vertebrae can tear.

are differences, with some people having severe, constant pain and others having pain that comes and goes in episodes over months or years.[41] It is not clear why pain persists in some people but not in others. However, there is an important psychosocial element to back pain. For example, people who are anxious or depressed may be more afraid to be physically active after a back injury, so they avoid it, even to the point of staying in bed for long periods of time. And avoiding activity can set up a vicious circle of muscle weakness and repeated injury.[30]

Some people develop chronic neck pain instead of (or in addition to) chronic low back pain. Much less is known about the causes of chronic neck pain than low back pain. People who have neck pain are less likely than those with low back pain to have a herniated disk, muscle sprain, or ligament strain, but working in sustained or awkward postures is a common risk factor.[42] Psychosocial factors seem to be particularly important in chronic neck pain.[42]

Epidemiology: Patterns and Trends

The best estimates are that, on any given day, 12% of people have low back pain, and that over the course of a year, 38% of people have an episode of low back pain lasting a least one day.[43] Low back pain affects a younger group of people than osteoarthritis, beginning in teenage years and rising with age but peaking in people in their 60s.[43] Women are about 80% more likely to have the problem than men for unknown reasons.[29,30]

Low back pain is more common in people with lower socioeconomic status,[34] and the information available suggests that it may be more common in Whites, Blacks, and Native Americans than Hispanics or Asians.[44]

Because of varying definitions and lack of data in much of the world, it is very difficult to assess the differences in low back pain between countries, but according to estimates by the Global Burden of Disease project, the highest prevalence of low back pain is in higher-income countries, including the United States, Europe, Russia, Australia, and New Zealand, with lower rates it the low-income countries of sub-Saharan Africa.[29] This suggests that the lifestyle changes involved in moving from a farming- or factory-based economy to an information- and services-based economy do not necessarily prevent low back pain and may even promote it.

Risk Factors

About 40% of chronic low back pain can be attributed to three risk factors (**Figure 4.11**):[1]

- *Overweight and obesity.*[29,30,34,45,46] People who are overweight (body mass index 25–29 kg/m²) are about 15% more likely and those who are obese (body mass index more than 30 kg/m²) are about 60% more likely to develop low back pain. It is not clear why. Perhaps it is simply because the additional weight puts a constant stress on spinal joints and muscles, or perhaps the inflammation that occurs in obesity makes injured tissues more painful.[46-48] Estimates by the Global Burden of Disease project are that 12% of the disability of low back pain globally and in the United States is attributable to overweight and obesity.[29]

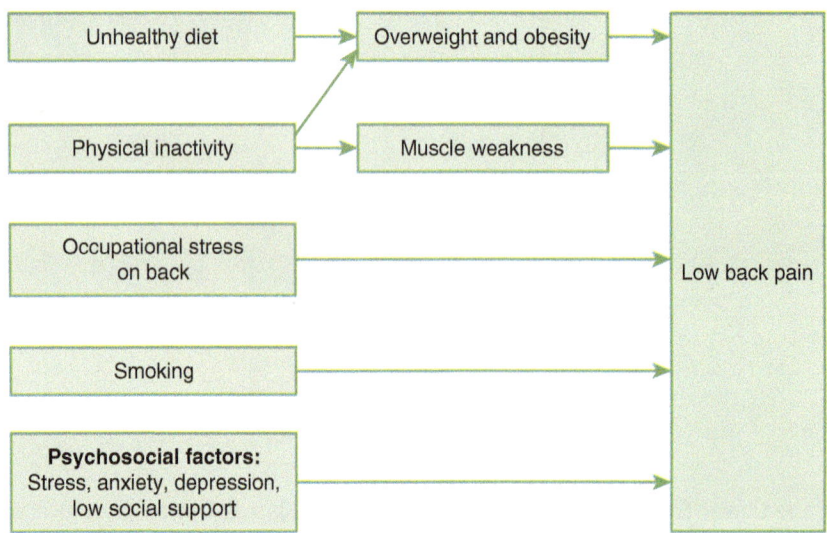

Figure 4.11 Cause-and-Effect Diagram for Low Back Pain.

- *Smoking.*[30,46] The link between smoking and low back pain is not nearly as strong as the link between smoking and heart disease or cancer, but it is nonetheless important. People who smoke are about 60% more likely to have low back pain.[46] Globally, an estimated 13% of low back pain is attributable to smoking;[29] in the United States, where smoking rates are higher, it is closer to 20%.[1] The mechanism for this link is not clear, but it may be tobacco smoke causing the cartilage in intervertebral discs to deteriorate.[35,36] Former smokers have a prevalence of low back pain that is between that of smokers and non-smokers, suggesting that if a smoker quits, the smoker reduces but does not eliminate the risk.[49]

- *Occupational stress on the back.*[30,34] Even in our modern world of industrial robots, many people's jobs require them to put physical stress on their backs by lifting and carrying things. Jobs that involve repeatedly lifting heavy objects and jobs that involve bending or twisting are associated with about a 50% increase in the risk of back pain.[46,50] Unlike people exercising voluntarily, people who stress their back muscles on the job often must do so repeatedly, without taking breaks, even when they are tired or are already experiencing pain. Also, people are more likely to get low back pain if they are subjected at work to frequent whole-body vibrations—like truck drivers and some machine operators.[45] On the other hand, people who sit or stand in the same position at work, such as computer workers or security guards, do not appear to be at higher risk.[50] The Global Burden of Disease project estimates that 22% of low back pain globally can be attributed to this occupational stress.[29]

Two other risk factors are important, but less well quantified:

- *Muscle weakness and physical inactivity.* Muscle weakness is difficult to measure at a population level, but exercise programs in which people strengthen their core muscles reliably reduce rates of low back pain (see section below), so weakness of core muscles must increase people's risk. The relationship between general physical inactivity and chronic low back pain is less clear,[30] with some studies showing no difference and some showing that the most physically active people are 10–15% less likely to have the problem.[51]

- *Psychosocial factors.* No one has pinpointed the precise psychosocial factors that increase the risk of low back pain or fully explained the connection, but these factors make a big difference. Researchers have used varying labels to describe this contributor, like psychological stress, anxiety, depression, and low levels of social support.[30,34,45] Together they describe people who are facing social, psychological, or psychiatric problems that make it difficult for them to manage their low back pain.

Preventive Interventions

Primary Prevention

Interventions to reduce these risk factors include (**Figure 4.12**):

- *Prevention of smoking.* There are dozens of excellent health reasons to avoid or quit smoking. Reducing low back pain is one of them. See Chapter 11. Tobacco Use.

- *Prevention of overweight and obesity* through promotion of healthier diets and physical activity. People who are overweight suffer many different musculoskeletal problems, including osteoarthritis (see earlier in this chapter), low back pain, and other aches and pains. Prevention of overweight and obesity would have the reliable effect of improving the quality of life for many people. The changes required to prevent obesity are mostly in promoting healthier diets, but physical activity has a dual benefit in preventing low back pain by helping reduce obesity and strengthening core muscles. See Chapter 14. Nutrition for a discussion of promotion of healthy diets and Chapter 15. Physical Inactivity for a discussion of physical activity.

- *Exercise* programs to prevent back pain are proven to work, reducing the incidence by about one third.[52,53] The successful programs contain many components, but most include exercises to strengthen core muscles. Although more general physical fitness programs may also work, they have not been proven.[45]

- *Ergonomic changes* in job tasks to reduce heavy lifting, bending, twisting, and vibration. Most experts today recommend that if people must lift objects, they stand as close to the object as possible, keep their back straight rather than flexed, avoid twisting their backs, and bend at the knees to lift with the legs.[54] While this squatting technique does not reduce the load on the

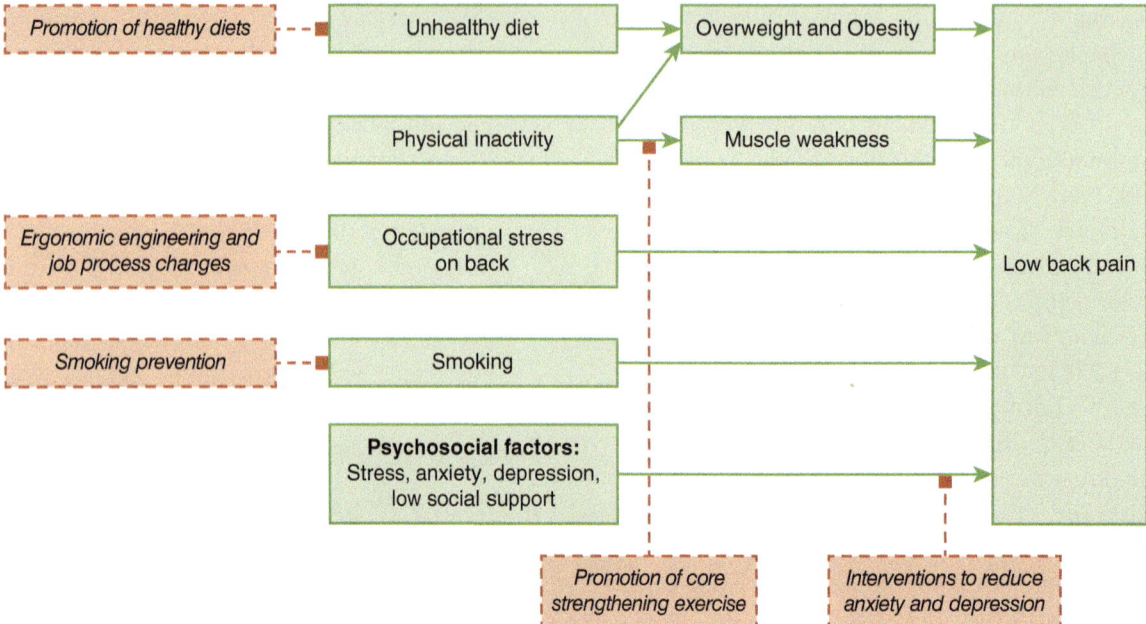

Figure 4.12 **Cause-and-Effect Diagram for Low Back Pain, with Preventive Interventions.**

intervertebral discs (it may actually increase it), it may reduce the forceful stretching of the spine's muscles and ligaments.[55] The National Institute of Occupational Safety and Health (NIOSH) has published guidelines for employers on how to design tasks that involve lifting and carrying objects. The core of the guidelines is the **Revised NIOSH Lifting Equation**, which sets a maximum weight for an object that a worker can lift safely, based on factors like how close the object is to the employee and how far and how often it must be lifted.[56,57]

- *Interventions to reduce anxiety and depression.* Although studies have not proven this, psychosocial factors like anxiety and depression play such an important role that any actions that reduce them should reduce low back pain. Chapter 5. Mental Illnesses discusses what is known about the causes of anxiety and depression and suggests interventions to reduce them. While some interventions have such a long lag time that they seem impractical as methods to prevent back pain, others like improving social connections and reducing loneliness may make a difference relatively quickly.

Some interventions that may seem logical have been proven to *not* prevent low back pain. Specifically, back braces and back support belts do not work.[45] Shoe insoles also have no benefit.[52] And education programs or advice on safer lifting techniques by themselves have been shown to be ineffective.[45,52]

Secondary Prevention

Many studies have been done on ways to help people who already have back pain get better or avoid recurrences. The effective approaches are like those for primary prevention. *Exercise programs* definitely help.[53] All exercise programs that have been studied work better than no exercise, but the ones that seem the most effective are those that strengthen core muscles (such as Pilates), often paired with psychological support and individualized help with managing pain.[58] Various *behavioral therapy programs* seem to help with the psychosocial aspect of back pain, in particular a type of treatment called **cognitive behavioral therapy** and mindfulness-based stress-reduction programs.[34,45]

Maybe more important is what studies show should *not* be done for people with low back pain. Several popular treatments have been found not just ineffective, but also capable of making back pain worse or causing other serious health problems. In particular, *bed rest* after an acute back injury can increase pain and delay recovery.[45] *Opioids* are no more effective for relieving pain than over-the-counter pain medications like ibuprofen (Advil, Motrin), and are addictive and potentially fatal.[45] Unless a herniated disk is causing a full or partial paralysis, experts recommend avoiding *surgery* because it generally does not help and it carries its own risks.[37] And *steroid injections in the spine* do not help over the long term and sometimes cause severe neurologic damage.[37]

These unnecessary and risky treatments are so widely used that they have become public health problems of their own, large enough to warrant interventions to prevent them.[29] In Australia, Scotland, Norway, and Canada, organizations have paid for mass media campaigns recommending that people with back pain stay active and avoid unnecessary treatment.[59] In Australia, the campaign not only changed people's attitudes about back pain, but it also changed physician's beliefs and reduced the number of days people had to claim worker's compensation insurance for back pain.[60]

Box 4.3 Summary–Prevention of Low Back Pain.

- Prevention of smoking
- Promotion of healthier diets to prevent overweight and obesity
- Exercise programs that include core strengthening
- Ergonomic changes in job tasks to reduce heavy lifting, bending, twisting, and vibration.
- Interventions to reduce anxiety and depression
- Avoidance of bed rest and unnecessary surgery, injections, and medications for back pain

---

Box 4.4 Key Words–Low Back Pain

Acute low back pain
Annulus fibrosus
Axon
Bone spurs
Cartilage
Cervical
Chronic low back pain
Coccyx
Cognitive behavioral therapy
Facet joint
Facets
Herniate (v), herniation (n)
Intervertebral disk
Ligament
Lumbar
Nerve root
Nervous system
Neuron
Nonspecific low back pain
Nucleus pulposus
Osteoarthritis
Osteophytes
Revised NIOSH Lifting Equation
Sacrum
Spinal canal
Spinal cord
Spine
Sprain
Stenosis
Strain
Thoracic
Vertebra, pl. vertebrae
Vertebral body

Resources–Low Back Pain

- Knezevic NN, Candido KD, Vlaeyen JWS, Van Zundert J, Cohen SP. Low back pain. *Lancet*. 2021;398(10294):78-92. doi:10.1016/S0140-6736(21)00733-9. This is a detailed review of the problem, its prevention, and its treatment.
- Ferreira ML, De Luca K, Haile LM, et al. Global, regional, and national burden of low back pain, 1990–2020, its attributable risk factors, and projections to 2050: A systematic analysis of the Global Burden of Disease Study 2021. *Lancet Rheumatol*. 2023;5(6):e316-e329. doi:10.1016/S2665-9913(23)00098-X
- MedlinePlus. Lifting and bending the right way. National Library of Medicine. https://medlineplus.gov/ency/patientinstructions/000414.htm. This is an example of standard advice today about how to lift objects safely.
- The American Academy of Orthopaedic Surgeons has excellent plain-language summaries of back injuries and back pain, at https://orthoinfo.aaos.org/en/diseases--conditions/
- The Revised NIOSH Lifting Equation can be applied to workplace safety using an app and manual available at https://www.cdc.gov/niosh/topics/ergonomics/nlecalc.html

References

1. Global Burden of Disease Collaboration, Institute for Health Metrics and Evaluation. *GBD Results Tool*. Published July 12, 2023. Accessed July 11, 2023. Available at: https://vizhub.healthdata.org/gbd-results/
2. Horvai A. Joints. In: Kumar V, Abbas AK, Aster JC, Turner JR, eds. *Robbins & Cotran Pathologic Basis of Disease*. 10th ed. Elsevier; 2021:1197-1208.
3. Centers for Disease Control and Prevention. *A National Public Health Agenda for Osteoarthritis: 2020 Update*. Published 2020. Accessed June 13, 2024. Available at: https://www.cdc.gov/arthritis/docs/oaagenda2020.pdf
4. Whittaker JL, Runhaar J, Bierma-Zeinstra S, Roos EM. A lifespan approach to osteoarthritis prevention. *Osteoarthritis Cartilage*. 2021;29(12):1638-1653. doi:10.1016/j.joca.2021.06.015

5. Hunter DJ, Bierma-Zeinstra S. Osteoarthritis. *Lancet.* 2019;393(10182). doi:10.1016/S0140-6736(19)30417-9

6. Coaccioli S, Sarzi-Puttini P, Zis P, Rinonapoli G, Varrassi G. Osteoarthritis: New insight on its pathophysiology. *J Clin Med.* 2022;11(20). doi:10.3390/jcm11206013

7. Sheth NP, Foran JRH. Arthritis of the Knee. OrthoInfo— *American Academy of Orthopaedic Surgeons.* Published February 2023. Accessed July 24, 2024. Available at: https:// orthoinfo.aaos.org/en/diseases--conditions/arthritis-of-the -knee/

8. Dimitroulas T, Duarte R V., Behura A, Kitas GD, Raphael JH. Neuropathic pain in osteoarthritis: A review of pathophysiological mechanisms and implications for treatment. *Semin Arthritis Rheum.* 2014;44(2):145-154. doi:10.1016/j.semarthrit.2014 .05.011

9. Sharma L. Osteoarthritis of the Knee. Solomon CG, ed. *N Engl J Med.* 2021;384(1):51-59. doi:10.1056/NEJMcp1903768

10. Losina E, Weinstein AM, Reichmann WM, et al. Lifetime risk and age at diagnosis of symptomatic knee osteoarthritis in the US. *Arthritis Care Res (Hoboken).* 2013;65(5):703-711. doi:10.1002/acr.21898

11. Silverwood V, Blagojevic-Bucknall M, Jinks C, Jordan JL, Protheroe J, Jordan KP. Current evidence on risk factors for knee osteoarthritis in older adults: A systematic review and meta-analysis. *Osteoarthritis Cartilage.* 2015;23(4):507-515. doi:10.1016/j.joca.2014.11.019

12. Hernandez PA, Bradford JC, Brahmachary P, et al. Unraveling sex-specific risks of knee osteoarthritis before menopause: Do sex differences start early in life? *Osteoarthritis Cartilage.* 2024;32(9):1032-1044. doi:10.1016/j.joca.2024.04.015

13. Plotz B, Bomfim F, Sohail MA, Samuels J. Current epidemiology and risk factors for the development of hand osteoarthritis. *Arth Rheum Rep.* 2021. doi:10.1007/s11926 -021-01025-7/Published

14. Allen KD, Thoma LM, Golightly YM. Epidemiology of osteoarthritis. *Osteoarthritis Cartilage.* 2022;30(2):184-195. doi:10.1016/j.joca.2021.04.020

15. Callahan LF, Cleveland RJ, Allen KD, Golightly Y. Racial/ ethnic, socioeconomic, and geographic disparities in the epidemiology of knee and hip osteoarthritis. *Rheumatic Disease Clinics of North America.* 2021;47(1):1-20. doi:10 .1016/j.rdc.2020.09.001

16. Safiri S, Kolahi AA, Smith E, et al. Global, regional and national burden of osteoarthritis 1990-2017: A systematic analysis of the Global Burden of Disease Study 2017. *Ann Rheum Dis.* 2020. doi:10.1136/annrheumdis-2019-216515

17. Reyes C, Leyland KM, Peat G, Cooper C, Arden NK, Prieto-Alhambra D. Association between overweight and obesity and risk of clinically diagnosed knee, hip, and hand osteoarthritis: A population-based cohort study. *Arthritis Rheumatol.* 2016;68(8):1869-1875. doi:10.1002/art.39707

18. Muthuri SG, Hui M, Doherty M, Zhang W. What if we prevent obesity? Risk reduction in knee osteoarthritis estimated through a meta-analysis of observational studies. *Arthritis Care Res (Hoboken).* 2011;63(7):982-990. doi:10.1002 /acr.20464

19. Wang X, Perry TA, Arden N, et al. Occupational risk in knee osteoarthritis: A systematic review and meta-analysis of observational studies. *Arthritis Care Res (Hoboken).* 2020;72(9):1213-1223. doi:10.1002/acr.24333

20. Alentorn-Geli E, Samuelsson K, Musahl V, Green CL, Bhandari M, Karlsson J. The association of recreational and competitive running with hip and knee osteoarthritis: A systematic review and meta-analysis. *J Orthop and Sports Phys Ther.* 2017;47(6):373-390. doi:10.2519/jospt.2017.7137

21. Lo GH, Driban JB, Kriska AM, et al. Is there an association between a history of running and symptomatic knee osteoarthritis? A cross-sectional study from the osteoarthritis initiative. *Arthritis Care Res (Hoboken).* 2017;69(2):183-191. doi:10.1002/acr.22939

22. Timmins KA, Leech RD, Batt ME, Edwards KL. Running and knee osteoarthritis: A systematic review and meta-analysis. *Am J Sports Med.* 2017;45(6):1447-1457. doi:10 .1177/0363546516657531

23. Wallace IJ, Worthington S, Felson DT, et al. Knee osteoarthritis has doubled in prevalence since the mid-20th century. *Proc Natl Acad Sci U S A.* 2017;114(35):9332-9336. doi:10.1073/pnas.1703856114

24. Crossley KM, Patterson BE, Culvenor AG, Bruder AM, Mosler AB, Mentiplay BF. Making football safer for women: A systematic review and meta-analysis of injury prevention programmes in 11,773 female football (soccer) players. *Br J Sports Med.* 2020;54(18):1089-1098. doi:10.1136 /bjsports-2019-101587

25. Lauersen JB, Bertelsen DM, Andersen LB. The effectiveness of exercise interventions to prevent sports injuries: A systematic review and meta-analysis of randomised controlled trials. *Br J Sports Med.* 2014;48(11):871-877. doi:10.1136/bjsports-2013-092538

26. Emery CA, Roy TO, Whittaker JL, Nettel-Aguirre A, Van Mechelen W. Neuromuscular training injury prevention strategies in youth sport: A systematic review and meta-analysis. *Br J Sports Med.* 2015;49(13):865-870. doi:10.1136/bjsports-2015-094639

27. Visser S, van der Molen HF, Kuijer PPFM, Sluiter JK, Frings-Dresen MHW. Stand up: comparison of two electrical screed levelling machines to reduce the work demands for the knees and low back among floor layers. *Ergonomics.* 2016;59(9): 1224-1231. doi:10.1080/00140139.2015.1122233

28. Thorlund JB, Simic M, Pihl K, et al. Similar effects of exercise therapy, nonsteroidal anti-inflammatory drugs, and opioids for knee osteoarthritis pain: A systematic review with network meta-analysis. *J Orthop Sports Phys Ther.* 2022;52(4):207-216. doi:10.2519/jospt.2022.10490

29. Ferreira ML, De Luca K, Haile LM, et al. Global, regional, and national burden of low back pain, 1990–2020, its attributable risk factors, and projections to 2050: A systematic analysis of the Global Burden of Disease Study 2021. *Lancet Rheumatol.* 2023;5(6):e316-e329. doi:10.1016 /S2665-9913(23)00098-X

30. Knezevic NN, Candido KD, Vlaeyen JWS, Van Zundert J, Cohen SP. Low back pain. *Lancet.* 2021;398(10294):78-92. doi:10.1016/S0140-6736(21)00733-9

31. Park DK. *Spine Basics. OrthoInfo—American Academy of Orthopaedic Surgeons.* Published June 2020. Accessed July 24, 2024. Available at: 9781284297164_CH01_Farley1e_CE .docx

32. Park DK. *Herniated Disk in the Lower Back. OrthoInfo— American Academy of Orthopaedic Surgeons.* Published January 2022. Accessed July 24, 2024. Available at: https:// orthoinfo.aaos.org/en/diseases--conditions/herniated -disk-in-the-lower-back/

33. American Academy of Orthopaedic Surgeons. *Herniated Disk in the Lower Back. OrthoInfo.* Published August 2021. Accessed January 4, 2024. Available at: https://orthoinfo.aaos.org/en /diseases--conditions/herniated-disk-in-the-lower-back/

34. Chiarotto A, Koes BW. Nonspecific low back pain. *N Engl J Med.* 2022;386(18):1732-1740. doi:10.1056/nejmcp2032396

35. Nasto LA, Ngo K, Leme AS, et al. Investigating the role of DNA damage in tobacco smoking-induced spine degeneration. *Spine J.* 2014;14(3):416-423. doi:10.1016/j.spinee.2013.08.034

36. Battié MC, Videman T, Kaprio J, et al. The Twin Spine Study: Contributions to a changing view of disc degeneration. *Spine Jl.* 2009;9(1):47-59. doi:10.1016/j.spinee.2008.11.011

37. Foster NE, Anema JR, Cherkin D, et al. Prevention and treatment of low back pain: Evidence, challenges, and promising directions. *Lancet.* 2018;391(10137):2368-2383. doi:10.1016/S0140-6736(18)30489-6

38. American Academy of Orthopaedic Surgeons. *Low Back Pain. OrthoInfo.* Published August 2021. Accessed January 4, 2024. Available at: https://orthoinfo.aaos.org/en/diseases--conditions/low-back-pain/

39. American Academy of Orthopaedic Surgeons. *Lumbar Spinal Stenosis. OrthoInfo.* Published August 2021. Accessed January 4, 2024. Available at: https://orthoinfo.aaos.org/en/diseases--conditions/lumbar-spinal-stenosis/

40. Steffens D, Ferreira ML, Latimer J, et al. What triggers an episode of acute low back pain? A case-crossover study. *Arthritis Care Res (Hoboken).* 2015;67(3):403-410. doi:10.1002/acr.22533

41. Kongsted A, Kent P, Axen I, Downie AS, Dunn KM. What have we learned from ten years of trajectory research in low back pain? *BMC Musculoskelet Disord.* 2016;17(1). doi:10.1186/s12891-016-1071-2

42. Kim R, Wiest C, Clark K, Cook C, Horn M. Identifying risk factors for first-episode neck pain: A systematic review. *Musculoskelet Sci Pract.* 2018;33:77-83. doi:10.1016/j.msksp.2017.11.007

43. Hoy D, Bain C, Williams G, et al. A systematic review of the global prevalence of low back pain. *Arthritis Rheum.* 2012;64(6):2028-2037. doi:10.1002/art.34347

44. Waterman BR, Belmont PJ, Schoenfeld AJ. Low back pain in the United States: Incidence and risk factors for presentation in the emergency setting. *Spine J.* 2012;12(1):63-70. doi:10.1016/j.spinee.2011.09.002

45. Chou R. Low back pain. *Ann Intern Med.* 2021;174(8):ITC113-ITC128. doi:10.7326/AITC202108170

46. Shiri R, Falah-Hassani K, Heliövaara M, et al. Risk factors for low back pain: A population-based longitudinal study. *Arthritis Care Res (Hoboken).* 2019;71(2):290-299. doi:10.1002/acr.23710

47. Zhang TT, Liu Z, Liu YL, et al. Obesity as a risk factor for low back pain: A meta-analysis. *Clin Spine Surg.* 2018;31(1):22-27.

48. Elgaeva EE, Tsepilov Y, Freidin MB, Williams FMK, Aulchenko Y, Suri P. ISSLS Prize in Clinical Science 2020. Examining causal effects of body mass index on back pain: A Mendelian randomization study. *Eur Spine Jl.* 2020;29(4):686-691. doi:10.1007/s00586-019-06224-6

49. Shiri R, Falah-Hassani K. The effect of smoking on the risk of sciatica: A meta-analysis. *Am J Med.* 2016;129(1):64-73.e20. doi:10.1016/j.amjmed.2015.07.041

50. Jahn A, Andersen JH, Christiansen DH, Seidler A, Dalbøge A. Occupational mechanical exposures as risk factor for chronic low-back pain: A systematic review and meta-analysis. *Scand J Work Environ Health.* 2023;49(7):453-465. doi:10.5271/sjweh.4114

51. Shiri R, Falah-Hassani K. Does leisure time physical activity protect against low back pain? Systematic review and meta-analysis of 36 prospective cohort studies. *Br J Sports Med.* 2017;51(19):1410-1418. doi:10.1136/bjsports-2016-097352

52. Steffens D, Maher CG, Pereira LSM, et al. Prevention of lowback pain a systematic review and meta-Analysis. *JAMA Intern Med.* 2016;176(2):199-208. doi:10.1001/jamainternmed.2015.7431

53. Roren A, Daste C, Coleman M, et al. Physical activity and low back pain: A critical narrative review. *Ann Phys Rehabil Med.* 2023;66(2). doi:10.1016/j.rehab.2022.101650

54. MedlinePlus. Lifting and bending the right way. National Library of Medicine. Published August 12, 2023. Accessed January 6, 2024. Available at: https://medlineplus.gov/ency/patientinstructions/000414.htm

55. von Arx M, Liechti M, Connolly L, Bangerter C, Meier ML, Schmid S. From stoop to squat: A comprehensive analysis of lumbar loading among different lifting styles. *Front Bioeng Biotechnol.* 2021;9:769117. doi:10.3389/fbioe.2021.769117

56. National Institute for Occupational Safety and Health. *Applications Manual for the Revised NIOSH Lifting Equation.* Published 2021. Accessed June 13, 2024. https://doi.org/10.26616/NIOSHPUB94110revised092021

57. Waters TR, Putz-Anderson V, Garg A, Fine LJ. Revised NIOSH equation for the design and evaluation of manual lifting tasks. *Ergonomics.* 1993;36(7):749-776. doi:10.1080/00140139308967940

58. Hayden JA, Cartwright J, van Tulder MW, Malmivaara A. Exercise therapy for chronic low back pain. *Cochrane Database of Syst Rev.* 2012;CD009790. doi:10.1002/14651858.cd009790

59. Gross DP, Russell AS, Ferrari R, et al. Evaluation of a Canadian back pain mass media campaign. *Spine (Phila Pa 1976).* 2010;35(8):906-913.

60. Buchbinder R, Jolley D, Wyatt M. Population based intervention to change back pain beliefs and disability: Three part evaluation. *BMJ.* 2001;322(7301):1516-1520. doi:10.1136/bmj.322.7301.1516

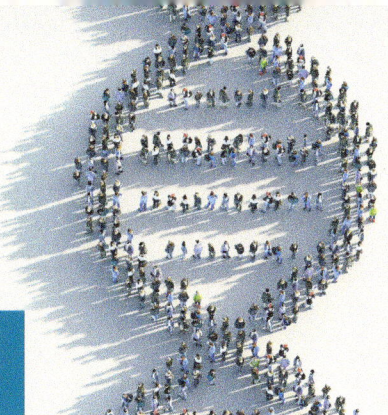

CHAPTER 5

Mental Illnesses

As communicable diseases become less common and people live longer, illnesses involving the brain are becoming more important to society's health. Unlike illnesses of other organs, mental illnesses rarely kill directly. But they can cause death indirectly from complications like smoking, drug overdose, and suicide. And even when they do not kill, mental illnesses cause suffering and disability that can last many years, making them important public health problems. For example, depression now ranks within the top 10 causes of disability-adjusted life years (DALYs) lost in the United States (see Chapter 1. Disease Prevention and Population).

The brain is by far the most complicated organ in the body and the least understood. This command-and-control organ is a network of some 86 billion brain cells sending signals to each other,[1] like transistors in a computer chip. The heart, as important as it is, has only one main function—to pump blood. But the brain does thousands of things, many of which are so complex that we have trouble finding words to describe them. We are left using terms like "memory," "thought," and "mood" that we struggle to define. Likewise, the disorders and diseases of the brain are poorly understood. It is much harder to define depression and explain its causes than to define and explain heart disease.

Advocates for mental health tend to focus on increasing the availability of treatment for people suffering from mental illnesses.[2] There is certainly a pressing need for more and better treatment. But unlike, for example, heart disease, for which there are national prevention programs promoting exercise and healthy eating, there are few organized efforts to *prevent* mental illnesses. Nonetheless, modifiable risk factors for mental illness have been identified, which

suggests that primary prevention is possible. This chapter will discuss ways that the most important mental illnesses might be prevented in populations.

The Brain

The **nervous system** is an organ system that senses the environment, interprets that input, and gives direction to other organs. It is composed of the **central nervous system** (the brain and the **spinal cord**) and the **peripheral nervous system** (**nerves** that connect the brain and spinal cord to other organs and tissues). The brain sits on top of the spinal cord and includes the **brain stem**, the **cerebral cortex**, the **cerebellum**, and other brain centers (**Figure 5.1**).

The key cells of the nervous system are called **neurons**. These cells are responsible for sending signals to each other and to other organs and tissues. Neurons are clustered in different brain centers, each of which is responsible for leading specific brain functions. For example, the neurons in the spinal cord send signals to muscles to contract, and the neurons in the cerebellum help groups of muscles move in a smooth, coordinated way.

The largest and most advanced area of the brain is the cerebral cortex, which carries out many high-level functions, including planning and directing complex movements, interpreting the images sent by the eyes and ears, speaking and interpreting the speech of others, learning, and "thinking." Between the spinal cord and the cerebral cortex are several centers that are involved in mental illnesses, including the **thalamus**, **hypothalamus**, and **hippocampus**. These centers play key roles in emotions, mood, and memory, as well as the regulation of body temperature,

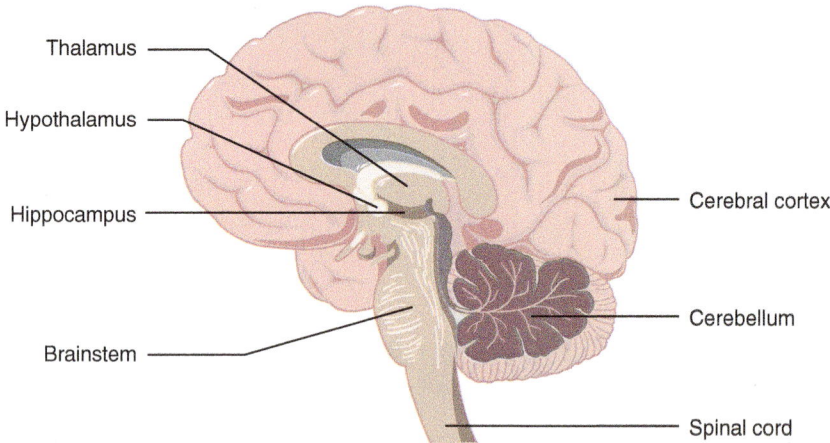

Figure 5.1 The Human Brain and Regions Important to Mental Illness. The brain sits on top of the spinal cord. Between the cerebral cortex and the brainstem are several brain centers that are involved in mental illness, including the thalamus, the hypothalamus, and the hippocampus.

hunger, thirst, and sleep. As this chapter will show, some mental disorders primarily involve problems with thought and others with emotions and mood.

The neurons that make up the brain are strange-looking cells, not oval-shaped, but instead shaped more like a bush, with a central root and many tiny branches called **dendrites** (**Figure 5.2**). A neuron may also have one extremely long branch called an **axon**, which connects it to other neurons in the brain, spinal cord, muscles, or other organs.

The dendrites and axons are like wires through which neurons send electrical signals to each other. At the interface between a dendrite or axon of one neuron and a dendrite of another neuron is a tiny gap called a **synapse**. Electrical signals that run down dendrites or axons do not cross these synapses. Instead, the neurons pass on the message using small chemicals called **neurotransmitters**. The neuron that is sending a message releases small packets of these neurotransmitters into the synapse; when the

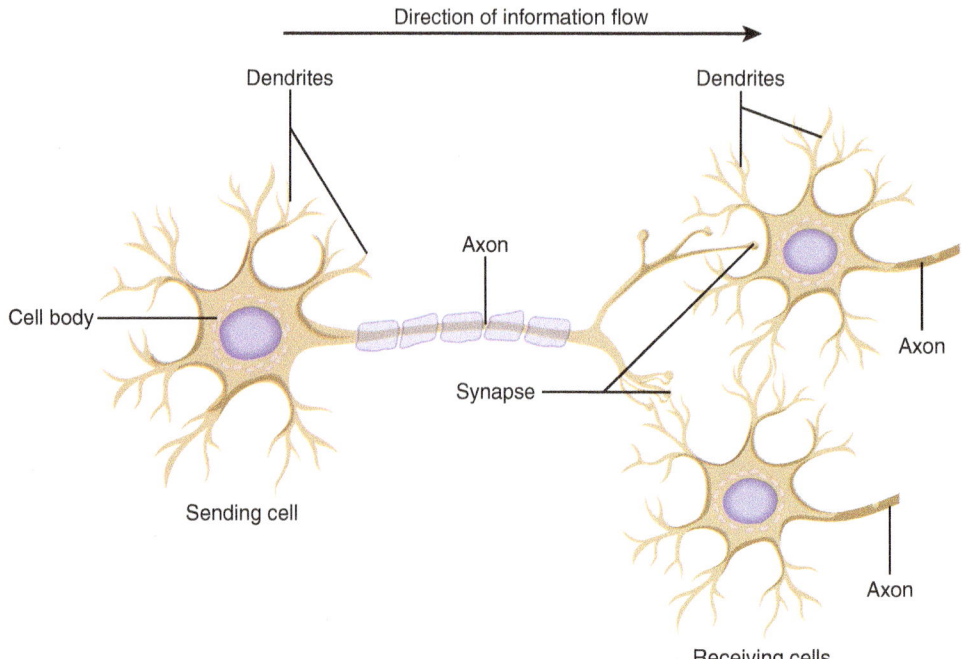

Figure 5.2 Neurons, Axons, and Dendrites. The brain operates by neurons sending electrical signals to each other through their axons and dendrites. The interfaces between the axon of one neuron and a dendrite or cell body of another neuron is called a synapse. The neurons communicate across the synapses by sending and receiving chemicals called neurotransmitters. These neurotransmitters play key roles in both mental illness and drug addiction.

receiving neuron picks these neurotransmitters, that receiving neuron changes its function.

There are many different neurotransmitter chemicals that play key roles in different centers of the brain. Most medications to treat mental illness seem to have their effect by increasing or decreasing the activity of specific neurotransmitters. Likewise, drugs that people use recreationally—like alcohol, amphetamine and cocaine—work by mimicking, stimulating, or blocking neurotransmitters (see Chapter 13. Use of Addictive Drugs).

Overview of Mental Illnesses (Disorders)

When a person has thoughts, emotions, or behaviors that cause that person severe distress or difficulty carrying out daily activities, the condition is labeled a mental illness. Mental illnesses differ from illnesses involving other organ systems in many ways, but especially by being much more difficult to define and distinguish. Doctors have no laboratory tests with which to make a diagnosis of schizophrenia, depression, or anxiety. They are left defining mental illnesses based on combinations of behaviors and symptoms that often occur together. Common combinations of behavior and symptoms are called **syndromes**. These syndromes are somewhat subjective, and the behaviors and symptoms (and thus, the syndromes) may change over time.

That means it is often difficult for psychiatrists to consistently distinguish one mental illness from another. Psychiatrists have tried to create consistency in how mental illnesses are diagnosed, named, and grouped with a guidebook called the **Diagnostic and Statistical Manual of Mental Disorders**, or DSM.[3] The fifth edition of this guidebook was published in 2013 and updated in 2022. As experts learn more about how the brain operates, the criteria for diagnosis, labels, and classifications of mental illness syndromes are likely to change.[3]

Another complication is that symptoms of mental illness are much worse in some people than in others. On one end of the spectrum, psychiatrists may assign a label of "serious mental illness" when the illness is disabling, for example, interfering with a person's ability to go to school, hold a job, or live independently.[4] On the other end of the spectrum, it can be very difficult to make a clear distinction between having a mental illness and being "normal" when everyone's thoughts are somewhat illogical and when everyone experiences periods of sadness, elation, and fear. In part because of these gray areas, psychiatry as a field

is moving away from the words "illness" and "disease" and instead using the term mental "disorders."

This chapter will discuss three mental disorders responsible for the most DALYs lost in the United States. **Schizophrenia** is often called a "thought disorder" because it affects a person's thinking—that is, their higher-level interpretation of experiences. **Depression** is called a "mood disorder" because it alters how positively or negatively a person feels about their situation. **Anxiety** is a group of disorders involving persistent fear or a sense of threat. This chapter will also discuss **dementia**, which is usually called a "neurologic illness" instead of a "mental illness" but which, like the other disorders in this chapter, interferes with how the brain works. These four disorders overlap with each other, influence each other, and share some risk factors.

Box 5.1 Key Words—Mental Illness

Anxiety
Axon
Brain stem
Central nervous system
Cerebellum
Cerebral cortex
Dementia
Dendrite
Depression
Diagnostic and Statistical Manual of Mental
    Disorders (DSM)
Hippocampus
Hypothalamus
Nerves
Nervous system
Neuron
Neurotransmitter
Peripheral nervous system
Schizophrenia
Spinal cord
Synapse
Syndrome
Thalamus

Resources—Mental Illness

- The Substance Abuse and Mental Health Services Administration (SAMHSA) conducts the National Survey on Drug Use and Health every year. This project surveys a large representative sample of Americans 12 years of age or older about their use of drugs, mental health symptoms, and treatment. Each year SAMHSA publishes a readable, high-level national summary report, as well as detailed tables, available at https://www.samhsa .gov/data/data-we-collect/nsduh-national-survey -drug-use-and-health

- World Health Organization. *Mental Health Atlas 2020*. Geneva; 2021. This summarizes mental health services in countries around the world.

Schizophrenia

Introduction

Schizophrenia is a serious, long-term mental disorder. The term schizophrenia, which means "splitting of the mind" in ancient Greek, was invented in the early 1900s by a German psychiatrist to emphasize people's differing reactions to their experiences.[5,6] Unlike the story told in the movies, people with schizophrenia do not have split or multiple "personalities." Instead, those with schizophrenia have unusual interpretations of their experiences—to the point that many seem out of touch with the reality perceived by those around them—and disorganized thought processes that can leave them severely disabled.

Over the years, dozens of theories have been proposed to explain the biologic causes of schizophrenia. The pathophysiology of the disease is still not understood very well. But experts increasingly agree about how schizophrenia develops and some factors and experiences that are risk factors.

Definition and Description of the Disease

Schizophrenia is a syndrome with three key features:[7]

- *Hallucinations and delusions.* **Hallucinations** are perceptions—things that people see, hear, smell, taste, or feel—that do not come from objective sources. Often, hallucinations in schizophrenia involve hearing "voices" that no one else hears. **Delusions** are false beliefs that persist despite clear evidence that they are not true. For example, the affected persons may believe they have magical powers or are Jesus Christ. Often, the delusions are **paranoid**, for example, believing that others are plotting to hurt them. Hallucinations and delusions are referred to as the **positive symptoms of schizophrenia**. **Psychosis** is term for any mental disorder that causes hallucinations and delusions (which are also called **psychotic symptoms**); schizophrenia is one type of psychosis.
- *Reduced drive and interest.* People with schizophrenia tend to show little motivation and withdraw from others. They may not talk much without prompting, and their faces tend to display little emotion. These are called the **negative symptoms of schizophrenia**.
- *Impaired cognition.* **Cognition** is what most people call "thought." A more precise definition would be mental processes involved in gaining knowledge and understanding, including attention, perception, learning, memory, and language. People with schizophrenia have various problems with cognition. Among them, while most people have trains of thought in which one idea is linked to the next, people with schizophrenia often string together thoughts that are not logically connected, in what some psychiatrists call "loose associations."

While young children who later develop schizophrenia are often withdrawn and have difficulties in school, the disease usually appears only when those children become teenagers or young adults. In those years, persons with schizophrenia typically have a "first break" episode that includes hallucinations and delusions.[8] Afterwards, their hallucinations and delusions may come and go,[8] but the "negative symptoms" and the impaired cognition usually persist.[9]

Schizophrenia is more severe for some people than others. After their first break, about one-third of people with the disorder recover to the point that they can function fairly well, about one-third have constant psychotic symptoms, and about one-third have intermittent psychotic symptoms.[10,11]

Medications and supportive mental health workers can help people with schizophrenia. The drugs used most are called **antipsychotic medications** because they reduce the hallucinations and delusions. Unfortunately, these drugs do not help the impaired cognition.[10] For that reason, people with schizophrenia, even on treatment, are usually unemployed,[9] so they need financial and other forms of support.[10] Their need for help often puts a heavy burden on their families.

The antipsychotic drugs also have unhealthy side effects, causing people taking them to gain weight and have high blood cholesterol.[10] People with schizophrenia tend to die early, either from suicide or from heart disease linked to their weight gain, high blood cholesterol, and smoking.[9,10,12]

Pathophysiology of Schizophrenia

Most experts now believe schizophrenia involves a faulty development of the brain, resulting from a combination of a genetic vulnerability and harmful exposures during childhood or before a child is born.[8,10,13]

Genes are particularly important. People with close family members with schizophrenia are several times more likely to develop the disease themselves.[10] But genes are not destiny; even when one of two identical twins has schizophrenia, there is only a 50% chance that the other will.[14]

As the brain develops in a fetus, it grows billions of neurons and builds trillions of synapses that connect them. This growth of synapses continues into a child's pre-school years. In a healthy child, during late childhood and adolescence, the brain "prunes" away synapses that are not needed, like pruning an unruly bush, eliminating about half of the synapses by adulthood.

According to a current theory, in people who develop schizophrenia, the synapses are "over-pruned" in the teenage years, as if an overly enthusiastic gardener were to chop off too many branches of a bush, leaving behind a scraggly, unhealthy plant.[14,15] With fewer synapses in the cerebral cortex, the brain cannot handle higher-level tasks, so this may explain the impaired cognition in people with schizophrenia.

The over-pruning of synapses happens in genetically susceptible people who have some kind of harmful exposures. Many different exposures can do this, including infections, violence, psychological stress, or drugs. And these harmful exposures can occur at any time that the brain is still building or pruning synapses, from before birth through the teenage years (**Figure 5.3**).

At the same time, the neurons in some areas of the brain in persons with schizophrenia seem to produce too much of a neurotransmitter called **dopamine**.[10] Dopamine has specialized roles in different areas of the brain, and it is particularly involved in drug addiction. People abusing amphetamines ("crystal meth") have abnormally high levels of dopamine activity in their brains, and they have hallucinations and delusions like those caused by schizophrenia, in what is called "drug-induced psychosis".[16] In people with schizophrenia, the antipsychotic medications lessen the hallucinations and delusions by blocking the effect of dopamine.[10]

While dopamine levels in the brains of people with schizophrenia appear to be too high, some studies suggest that levels of another neurotransmitter called **glutamate** may be too low.[17] Glutamate is used by neurons throughout the brain and tends to stimulate other neurons.

A simplified but useful way to think of the biology of schizophrenia is that dopamine excess causes the positive symptoms (hallucinations and delusions), glutamate deficiency causes the negative symptoms (reduced drive and interest), and a deficiency of synapses causes the impaired cognition.

Today, schizophrenia and recreational drug use form an unfortunate negative feedback loop. People with schizophrenia are about three times as likely as those without the disease to use drugs, particularly tobacco, alcohol, cannabis, and cocaine.[18] These drugs—especially cannabis—tend to make their positive and negative symptoms worse, which may lead them to use the drugs more.[10,18]

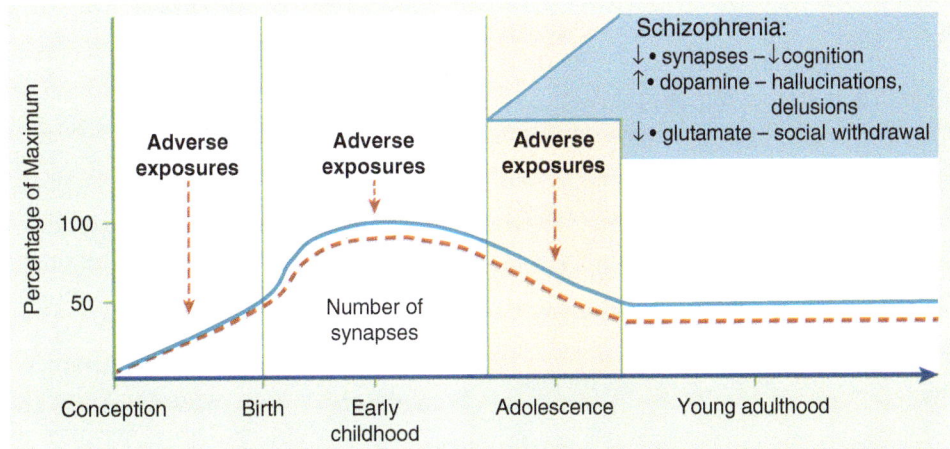

Figure 5.3 **Model of Relationships of Adverse Exposures During Development and Schizophrenia Among Vulnerable Persons.** Illustration of the possible causes of schizophrenia. Ordinarily, the number of synapses between neurons grows in the brain from before birth into a child's pre-school years, but these synapses are "pruned" during adolescence and the young adult years. One theory is that adverse exposures prenatally or during childhood, adolescence, or early adulthood cause "over-pruning" of synapses, leaving fewer synapses and the brain less capable. This overpruning may also lead to abnormal levels of the neurotransmitters dopamine and glutamate.

Data from Owen MJ, Sawa A, Mortensen PB. Schizophrenia. The Lancet. 2016;388(10039):86-97. doi:10.1016/S0140-6736(15)01121-6

While schizophrenia can be a very severe disease, it may be that the disease is only the tip of a much larger iceberg of people with less severe symptoms.[19] As many as 5% of people without diagnosed mental illness—or more than 10 times the number with schizophrenia—admit to having some hallucinations and delusions.[9,19] Perhaps a genetic vulnerability to schizophrenia is fairly common, and exposures before birth or throughout childhood simply push people who would otherwise have mild "normal" positive symptoms toward more severe symptoms and a psychiatrist's diagnosis.

Epidemiology: Patterns and Trends

Schizophrenia is a relatively uncommon mental illness, affecting about 3 persons per 1,000.[20,21] It occurs throughout the world, but it is as much as five times more common in some countries and regions than in others.[8,20,21]

Within the United States, rates of schizophrenia are about twice as high in African Americans as in White Americans, and in between those groups are Hispanics.[22,23] Similarly, in the United Kingdom, rates of schizophrenia are higher in non-White immigrants from Africa and the Caribbean.[8] These differences are thought to be caused by the harmful effects of racial discrimination and adverse childhood experiences.[8,24]

Risk Factors

The wide range in the prevalence of schizophrenia among countries suggests that the environments in which people live can have a large impact on the disease's development. That in turn implies that schizophrenia may be preventable through changes to the environment.

Children whose biologic fathers are older are more likely to develop schizophrenia. The risk increases steadily from father's age in the early 20s to above age 55, with children of the oldest fathers about three times as likely to have the illness.[8,10]

Other risk factors for schizophrenia include (**Figure 5.4**):

- *Adverse exposures during pregnancy.* Children are more likely to develop schizophrenia if, when they were in the womb, their mothers had *infections, diabetes, pre-eclampsia,* or *severe malnutrition.*[8,14,25-27] (**Pre-eclampsia** is an abnormal condition of pregnancy in which the mother has high blood pressure and kidney problems.

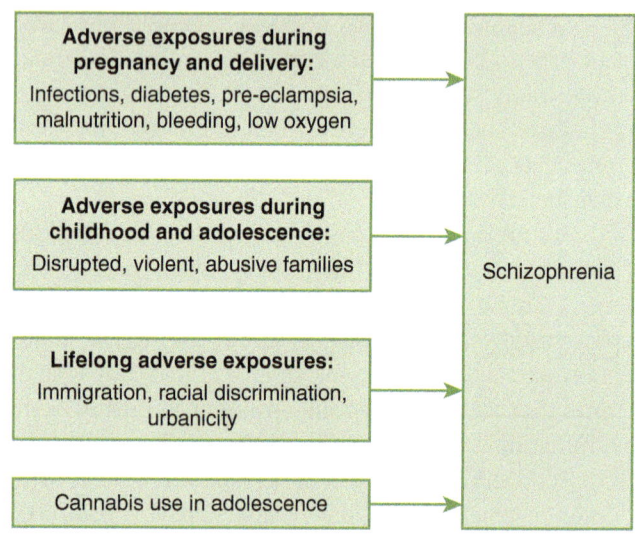

Figure 5.4 **Cause-and-Effect Diagram for Schizophrenia.**

It is discussed in Chapter 10. Diseases of the Newborn.) And children who go on to develop schizophrenia are more likely to have abnormally small heads, a possible sign that during the pregnancy their brains were not getting enough blood, oxygen, or nutrients.[8]

- *Adverse exposures during delivery.* Schizophrenia is more common in children who were born after a difficult delivery with problems such as *bleeding,* a brief *period without oxygen,* or an emergency caesarean section.[8]

- *Adverse experiences during childhood and adolescence.* Children growing up in families that are disrupted, violent, or abusive are more likely to develop schizophrenia.[28-30] By one estimate, about one-third of schizophrenia cases can be attributed to these adverse experiences in childhood.[28]

- *Lifelong exposures.* People are about three times more likely to develop schizophrenia if they are first- or second-generation *immigrants,* particularly if they are immigrants from Africa or the Caribbean, to high-income countries with predominantly White populations.[31] Experts speculate that this is a biologic consequence of *racial discrimination.*[8-10] Another risk is *living in an urban area,* which increases the risk twofold to fourfold, possibly because people in urban areas live with the psychological stress of being both socially isolated and surrounded by strangers.[32] If the "tip of the iceberg" theory is correct, immigration and urban residence may not cause schizophrenia so much as they make the symptoms worse, but the result is the same: more people with overt psychosis.[10]

- *Cannabis use* among young people has been strongly associated with the subsequent development of schizophrenia, with the heaviest users having about four times the risk.[33] This association may be partly explained by people who are destined to develop schizophrenia using more drugs, but that does not fully explain the connection. Even young adults who are evaluated psychologically and found to be free of mental illness are about three times more likely to later develop schizophrenia if they use cannabis, suggesting that cannabis use is causing or contributing to the disease.[34] The higher the potency of cannabis used, the higher the risk.[35] One group of experts estimated that 12% of people with first episodes of psychosis in Europe could be attributed to high-potency marijuana.[35] It is not understood how cannabis use could cause or trigger psychosis, but cannabis activates some neurotransmitters that have wide-ranging effects on the brain.[36]

Preventive Interventions

While genes cannot be changed, it may be possible to reduce the incidence of schizophrenia by reducing adverse exposures to pregnant women, children, and adolescents. In fact, many people are already working to reduce these harmful exposures. Interventions that might prevent schizophrenia include (**Figure 5.5**):

- *Promotion of healthy pregnancies and prevention of birth trauma* to protect the fetus and infant while the brain is developing. This includes helping women have healthy diets and avoiding alcohol, tobacco, and other drugs during pregnancy. Prevention of adverse outcomes of pregnancy is discussed more in Chapter 10. Diseases of the Newborn.

- *Prevention of adverse childhood experiences.* Mental health advocates have appropriately focused attention on the severe lifelong consequences of family violence, child abuse, and child neglect. Often though, their emphasis has been on providing mental health services to children who have already had damaging experiences. A better approach, if possible, is to support families with young children in ways that reduce the number who have these adverse experiences. This includes *treating mental illness or substance use in parents*, *providing financial support to low-income families*, and working with families in other ways to *prevent child abuse*. While there are already government programs to do this, child welfare agencies are often overwhelmed by the need, so they may require more resources for this.

- *Prevention of cannabis use by adolescents.* Reducing cannabis use by adolescents should reduce schizophrenia rates. In the United States, cannabis use is becoming not just legalized but also actively promoted, resulting in a sharp rise in both its use by young adults and the potency of the drug. In 2019, 7% of American teens ages 12–17 and 23% of American young adults ages 18–25 were using marijuana (increasing from 16% in 2006).[37] Shockingly, the marijuana sold in 2023 is more than 10 times as potent as the marijuana sold in 1975.[38] Even with use of the drug legal, there are many ways society could

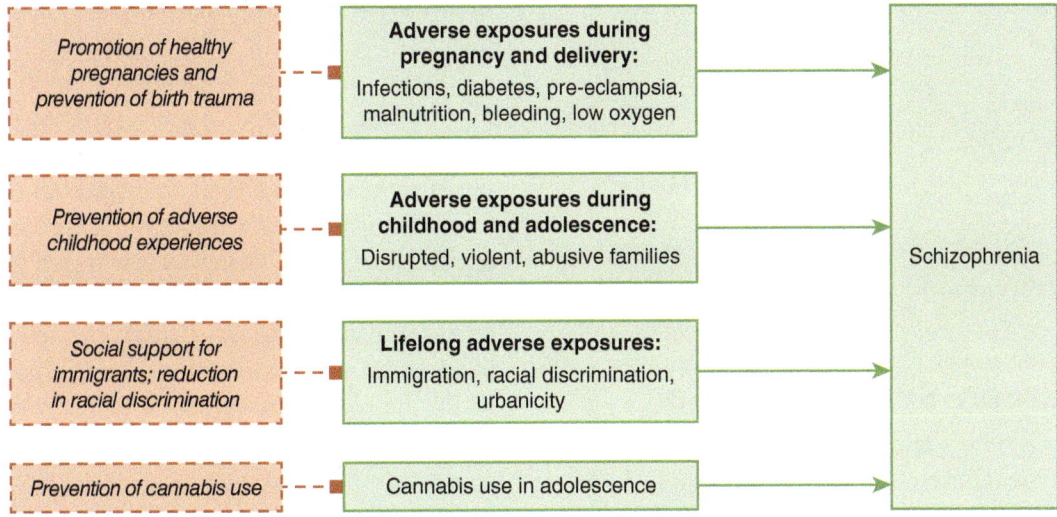

Figure 5.5 Cause-and-Effect Diagram for Schizophrenia, with Preventive Interventions.

discourage its use and protect adolescents from drug promotion—for example, prohibiting advertising of the drug, requiring lower potency, and restricting sales outlets. Prevention of recreational drug use is discussed in Chapter 13. Use of Addictive Drugs.

- *Social support for immigrants* and *reduction in racial discrimination.* Millions of immigrants from low-income countries live in the United States and other high-income countries. Their children may be less likely to develop schizophrenia if they have greater support in learning the language and integrating into the social and economic life of their new countries. At the same time, reduction in racial discrimination should reduce schizophrenia rates in longstanding minority racial populations.

Box 5.2 Summary–Prevention of Schizophrenia

- Promotion of healthy pregnancies and prevention of birth trauma
- Prevention of adverse childhood experiences
  - Treatment of mental illness and substance use in parents
  - Financial support for low-income families
  - Prevention of child abuse
- Prevention of cannabis use by adolescents
- Social support for immigrants and reduction in racial discrimination

Box 5.3 Key Words–Schizophrenia

Antipsychotic medications
Cognition
Delusions
Dopamine
Glutamate
Hallucinations
Negative symptoms of schizophrenia
Paranoid
Positive symptoms of schizophrenia
Pre-eclampsia
Psychosis
Psychotic symptoms

Resources–Schizophrenia

- Jauhar S, Johnstone M, McKenna PJ. Schizophrenia. *The Lancet*. 2022;399(10323):473-486. doi:10.1016/S0140-6736(21)01730-X. This is a medical description of schizophrenia,

along with up-to-date thinking on the disease's causes, treatment, prevention, and current controversies.

- The National Institute of Mental Health maintains a website with information about schizophrenia for non-experts at https://www.nimh.nih.gov/health/topics/schizophrenia

Depression

Introduction

Depression is a large and frustrating public health problem—large because it affects many people for long stretches of time in a profound way, and frustrating because it is both difficult to prevent and to treat. It is known that genetics influence a person's susceptibility to depression and that depression can be initiated by psychologically stressful events. These stressful events can induce depression at any age, but those that happen in childhood seem particularly hazardous, with harms that can last a lifetime.

Definition and Description of the Disease

The word **mood** is difficult to define, but everyone knows the difference between being in a good mood and being in a bad mood. It is normal for mood to rise and fall during a day, or to drop very low after a painful event like the death of a loved one. But people with **mood disorders** experience moods that are intensely high or low—enough to seriously impact their daily lives—and that can last weeks or months. **Major depressive disorder** (or **major depression**) is the most common type of mood disorder.

Major depression goes far beyond sadness. People who are depressed may experience no pleasure in anything, wonder if they will ever be able to feel pleasure again, and tend to blame themselves. To meet medical criteria for major depression, a person must have a persistently low mood nearly every day for at least two weeks, together with other psychological and physical symptoms severe enough to interfere with the ability to work, go to school, or do the routine activities of daily living.[39] People with **persistent depressive disorder** (formerly called **dysthymia**) may have less severe symptoms but the depression is present most of the time for at least two years.

Major depression and persistent depressive disorder differ from **bipolar disorder**, another mood disorder in which a person has some periods of depression and other periods of **mania**, an abnormally positive mood that leaves them excited, impulsive, and dangerously optimistic.

Most people with major depression experience a first episode in their late teens or early adult years.[39] For those who are treated by mental health professionals, the episode lasts a few months to a year. Most will recover, only to have more bouts of depression over their lifetime.[39]

Depression is more severe in some people than in others, and many people with it never visit mental health professionals. In one community survey, only about 30% who were depressed were classified as having "serious" illness, meaning that they were not able to work, were depressed for at least 30 days, or had attempted suicide.[40]

People with major depression are more likely to experience:

- *Anxiety.* More often than not, people with major depression have a second diagnosis termed an **anxiety disorder**.[41]
- *Alcohol and drug problems.* About one in four have a diagnosed **substance use disorder**.[41]
- *Marital, family, and job problems.* They are less likely to marry, more likely to get divorced, and more likely to lose their jobs.[42]
- *Suicide.* Major depression increases the risk of suicide at least tenfold.[43] Experts estimate that as many as 15% of people who have been hospitalized for major depression ultimately die by suicide.[43]
- *Chronic diseases,* such as ischemic heart disease, stroke, diabetes, and certain cancers.[42] These diseases may stem from depression itself, from the unhealthy habits of people who are depressed (particularly alcohol use, drug use, physical inactivity, unhealthy diets), or from a combination.

Physiology: The Brain and Mood

Depression involves a group of structures deep in the brain called the **limbic system**. The limbic system includes the **hypothalamus**, the **hippocampus**, and the **amygdala**, among other structures (**Figure 5.6**). These brain centers work together to control mood, memory, and the response to psychologically stressful events.[44]

- The hypothalamus controls the release of many of the body's **hormones**, which are chemicals that circulate in the blood and regulate other organs in many ways. In a stressful event, the hypothalamus is activated, and when activated, it directs the body to release hormones that cause the heart to beat quickly and the person to breathe faster.[45]
- The hippocampus plays an important role in memory.[44]
- The amygdala is where memories of stressful events are stored.[46] It is discussed more in the section on anxiety disorders later in this chapter.

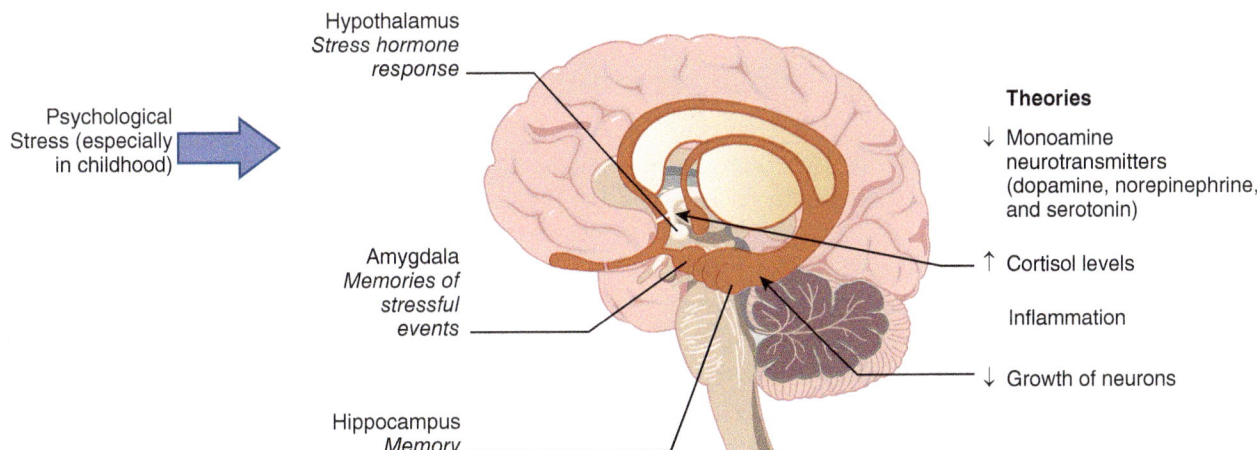

Figure 5.6 Theories of the Limbic System's Role in Depression. An illustration of four theories of the causes of depression. In susceptible people, psychological stress produces changes to the brain that cause depression. Stress in childhood seems particularly influential. These theories propose that depression may result from: 1) reduced levels of monoamine transmitters, 2) stress-induced cortisol, 3) inflammation in the brain, and/or 4) a reduced growth of neurons in parts of the hippocampus.

Pathophysiology of Depression

Unfortunately, there is no single theory of the biologic cause of depression that can explain all of the illness' patterns.[39,47-49]

It is known that depression is more likely to occur in people who are genetically susceptible and who then go through psychologically stressful experiences, particularly when they are children.[50-53] **Psychological stress** is a response by the body to a threat that the person feels they cannot overcome or handle.[53] (Psychological stress differs from physical stress discussed in Chapter 4. Musculoskeletal Disorders. In this chapter, for simplicity, the term **stress** will be used to mean psychological stress.) For children, stress could be caused by violence (for example, child abuse), the threat of violence (for example, bullying), witnessing violence (for example, domestic violence or a neighborhood shooting), separation from parents, or deprivation from food, shelter, or love.[53] For adults, stress can likewise be caused by violence, but it can also be provoked by longer-term threats like the loss of a job or a romantic partner.[39,48]

It is also known that parts of the limbic system, beyond responding to stress, are somehow involved in depression.[48]

Putting those facts together, there are four theories that each partly explain the biologic causes of major depression (Figure 5.6):

- *Increased cortisol levels caused by stress.*[39] In this theory, in response to stressful life events, the hypothalamus directs the body to release large amounts of **cortisol** (often called a "stress hormone") as well as other neurotransmitters and hormones.[48] Cortisol helps the body manage brief stressful situations, but when the cortisol level is too high for too long, it can lead to depression.[48] It may be that experiencing too many stressful events in childhood makes the hypothalamus permanently more likely to stimulate the release of cortisol.

- *Inflammation in the brain.* A more recent theory is that some elements of the **immune system** become abnormally active in someone who has experienced stress, causing **inflammation** in the brain.[39] The immune system is a group of cells that the body maintains to recognize and fight off invading organisms like bacteria or viruses. Inflammation is the process that the immune system uses to fight those invaders, and it involves the migration of immune cells to the site of the infection and the release of compounds like antibodies. According to this theory, some of these compounds released by immune cells cause depression by interfering with the functioning of neurons.

- *Less growth of neurons.* For many years, scientists believed that no new neurons were formed after birth. However, more recent studies show that in healthy people, new neurons are constantly growing in parts of the hippocampus.[48,54] According to this theory, in people with depression, stress somehow slows the growth of these neurons.[39]

- *Low levels of monoamine neurotransmitters.* For many years, the dominant theory was that depression was caused by abnormally low levels of the neurotransmitters **serotonin**, **norepinephrine**, and **dopamine** in the limbic system.[49] These neurotransmitters are all chemicals called **monoamines**.[48] The drugs used most to treat depression are thought to work because they raise the levels of these neurotransmitters. It is not clear in this theory why these neurotransmitter levels would become low, though.

Epidemiology: Patterns and Trends

Depending on the definition used, about 6-10% of adults in the United States have at least one episode of depression over a year, and about twice that many have had at least one episode over their lifetimes.[55,56] That means that depression is about 20 times as common as schizophrenia.

In the National Survey of Drug Use and Health, about 6% of adults reported having an episode of depression that severely impaired their ability to function, such as working or going to school, in the past year that lasted at least two weeks.[55] Depression with severe impairment is more common in women than men and more common in Whites than people in other racial groups (**Figure 5.7**).[55] The reasons for these demographic differences are not known. Depression peaks in young adults and is less common in older age groups (**Figure 5.8**).[55]

Depression is linked to social disadvantage, but the relationship is not a simple one. In the United States, people in poverty are about twice as likely to have an episode of major depression.[41,56] But in low- and middle-income countries, poverty does not seem to be related to risk of major depression at all.[42]

Waves of major depression tend to follow social disruptions, from war to financial crises, that create stress in people's lives.[57] The most striking and well-documented example of this is that during the

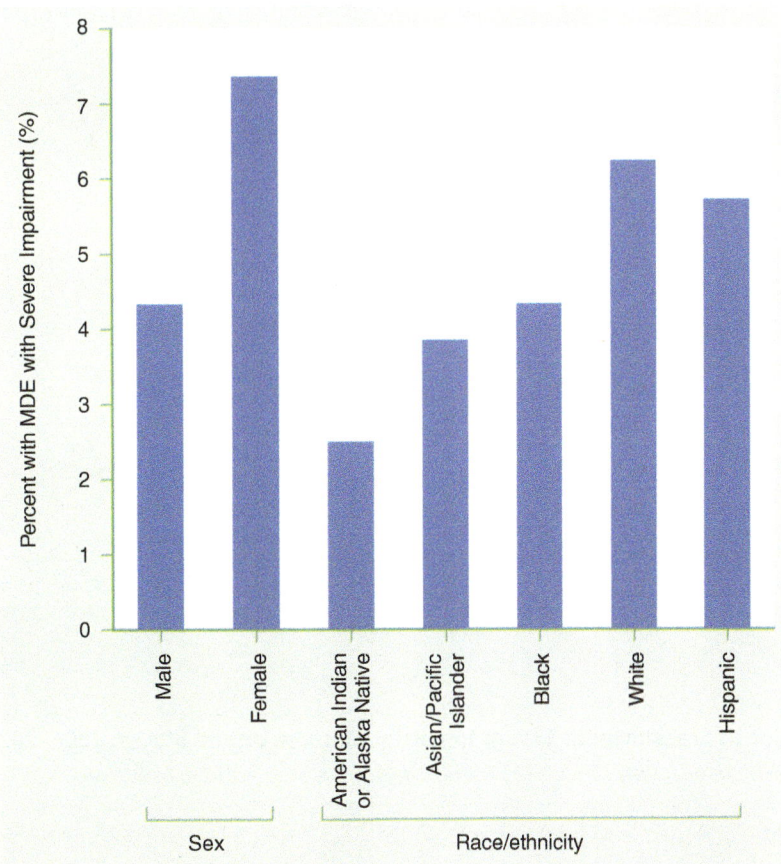

Figure 5.7 **Major Depressive Episode with Severe Impairment in Past Year in Adults Age 18 and Older, 2023.** The graph shows the percent of adults who had an episode of depression that severely impaired their ability to function, such as being unable to work or attend school, and that lasted for at least two weeks in the past year,. Depression is more common in women and in White people.

Data from Substance Use and Mental Health Services Administration. National Survey of Drug Use and Health: National Releases for 2023. Accessed July 26, 2024. https://www.samhsa.gov/data/nsduh/national-releases

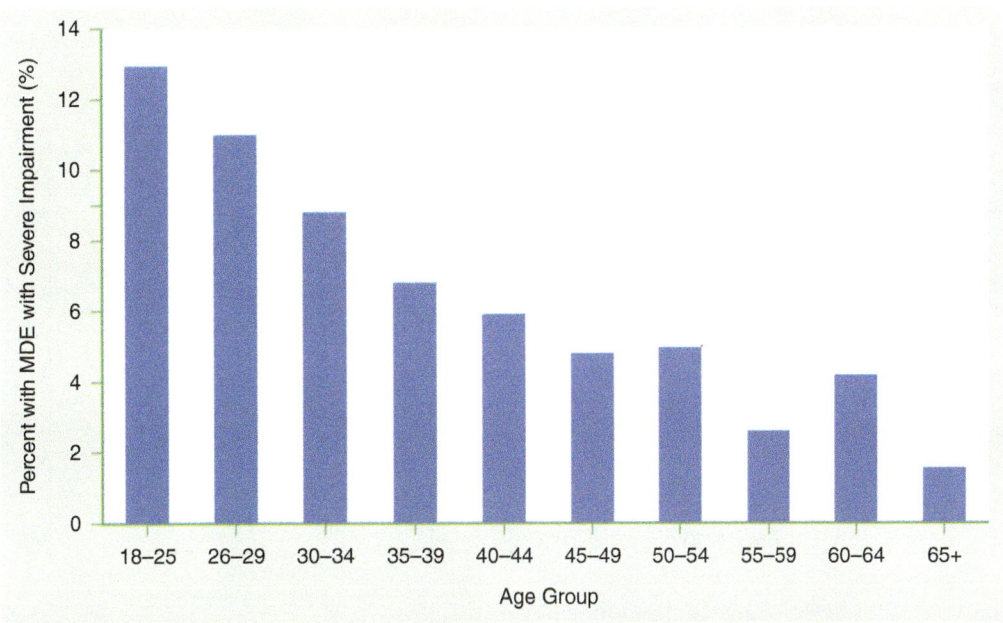

Figure 5.8 **Major Depression with Severe Impairment in the Past Year by Age Group, 2023.** Younger adults are more likely than older adults to have an episode of depression with impairment.

Data from Substance Use and Mental Health Services Administration. National Survey of Drug Use and Health: National Releases for 2023. Accessed July 26, 2024. https://www.samhsa.gov/data/nsduh/national-releases

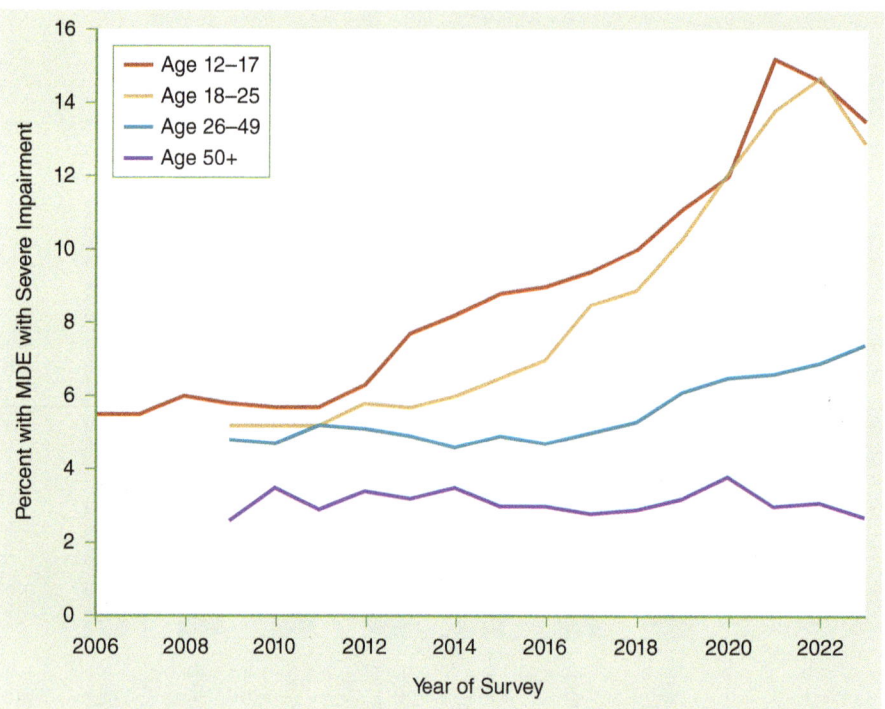

Figure 5.9 Trend in Major Depression with Severe Impairment in the United States, 2006–2023. The percent of teenagers and younger adults with depression rose sharply in the 2010s and early 2020s.

Data from Substance Use and Mental Health Services Administration. National Survey of Drug Use and Health: National Releases for 2023. Accessed July 26, 2024. https://www.samhsa.gov/data/nsduh/national-releases

first year of the COVID-19 pandemic, the rates of major depression increased by about 25%, with the increase larger in women than in men.[57]

Annual surveys are showing a very worrisome trend in depression that cannot be explained by the COVID-19 pandemic. The percentage of adolescents and young adults in the United States with major depression and severe impairment began to rise in about 2012, nearly tripling by 2022 (**Figure 5.9**).[55,58-60] This surge in depression occurred at about the same time in other countries, too.[61,62] Most worrisome, it was paralleled by increases in suicide attempts and completed suicides in both teens and younger adults.[60,63]

Risk Factors

Major depression has a strong genetic aspect to it, although it is less strong than the genetic risk of schizophrenia. People with a parent or sibling with major depression are about three times as likely to develop depression themselves.[64]

After genetics, there are several clearly established risk factors for depression (**Figure 5.10**). Some risk factors sit in negative feedback loops—that is, they increase the likelihood of developing depression, and depressed people are more likely to take on these risks. For example, physical inactivity increases the risk for depression, and people who are depressed are

likely to become less physically active. Nonetheless, most of these risk factors show that there are opportunities for prevention:

- *Adverse childhood experiences.* Adults are about twice as likely to have depression if as children they were raised by parents who were violent, abusive, neglectful, or had their own problems with mental illness or drug use.[65] Adults raised by

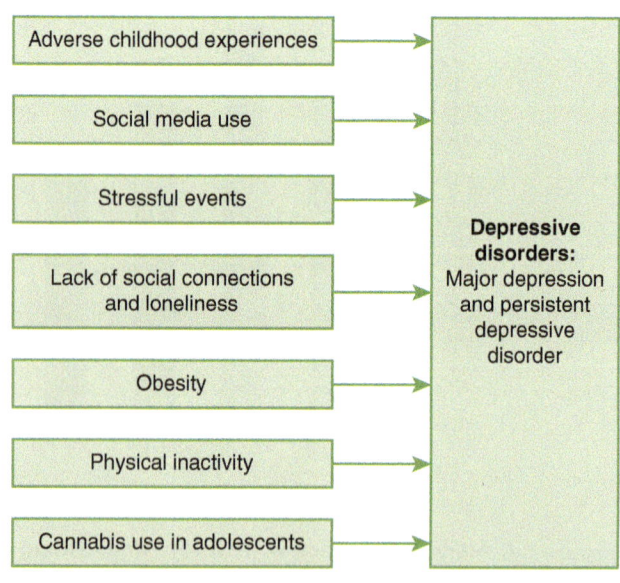

Figure 5.10 Cause-and-Effect Diagram for Depression.

families experiencing divorce, loss of a parent, or poverty but that were not abusive are also at an increased risk, but less so.[65] Stress in childhood seems to make episodes of depression not only more likely to occur, but also longer and more severe.[39] By one estimate, nearly one-fourth of depression in adults is attributable to these damaging experiences of children.[65]

- *Stressful events in adult years.* Experts have long recognized that a bout of depression often follows severe or life-threatening events, such as the death of spouse, divorce, an unwanted pregnancy, rape, a major accident, being a victim of violence, or losing a job.[39,48] And depression is less likely to occur after positive life events, such as marriage, the birth of a baby, career success, or financial success.[48]

- *Social media use.* Apparently, using social media is, or can be, extremely stressful. Adolescents who spend more time on social media, such as Facebook, Snapchat, Instagram, and YouTube, are about 60% more likely to have symptoms of depression. The harm is greater in females than males.[66] Adolescents who spend more time on social media are also more likely to have symptoms of anxiety and to deliberately hurt themselves, for example, by cutting the skin on their thighs or arms.[67-69] It is likely that surges in depression, anxiety, attempted suicides, and completed suicides in recent years are linked and are related to increases in social media use.[58,59,61,63,70-73]

- *Lack of social connections and loneliness.* People are more likely to have symptoms of depression if they do not have others they can turn to for help or to confide in, that is, **social connections**.[74-76] Older adults are more likely to have an episode of major depression if they have fewer social connections. Similarly, people are more likely to become depressed if they are lonely—that is, they do not have as much contact with others as they would like.[74,77,78] And people who live alone or are lonely are more likely to die by suicide or hurt themselves.[79] It is not known biologically how social connections might prevent depression, but social support is known to reduce inflammation and to help people handle stressful experiences.[80] The link between social connections and depression may explain why depression is far more common in adults who are separated or divorced than those who are married.[42] This risk factor is particularly important at the population level because it is so common—about half of Americans report on surveys that they experience loneliness. Unfortunately, social isolation is increasing.[80] The sharp

increase in major depression from the COVID-19 pandemic could have been caused by the stress of this event in people's lives, the loss of social connections caused by the lockdowns, the increase in social media use during the lockdowns, or a combination.[57,81]

- *Obesity.* People who are obese are more likely to have symptoms of depression or an episode of major depression.[82-84] The connection of depression to obesity is not understood, but it may be because obesity tends to cause inflammation, and inflammation acts on the brain to cause depression.[82]

- *Physical inactivity.* People who do not get exercise or spend more time watching television or using computers are about 20% more likely to experience depression, unrelated to the effect of physical activity on obesity.[76,85,86] When people who are sedentary become more active, their symptoms of depression improve.[86] The biologic mechanism behind this benefit is not clear, but exercise has effects on stress hormones, the growth of neurons, and the immune system.[87]

- *Cannabis use.* Teens who use cannabis are about 40% more likely to become depressed when they become young adults.[88] It is not clear how cannabis use might cause depression, but cannabis use in adolescents alters neurotransmitters and the growth of the brain. The effect of cannabis on depression is not as strong as its effect on schizophrenia, but this drug is so pervasive that it makes a meaningful difference population-wide.[88]

Finally, the higher rates of depression found in people with lower incomes suggests that social disadvantage is a key risk factor for depression. The downstream impact of this is significant, because depression harms physical health in many ways. It may be that depression (and anxiety, as discussed in the next section) are key bridges between social disadvantage and poor physical health. The relationship of social disadvantage to illness is discussed in Chapter 16. Social Disadvantage.

Preventive Interventions
Primary Prevention

There are many risks for major depression that cannot be changed in populations. Human genes will remain as they are, and people will continue to experience stressful life events. But the list of risk factors points to some opportunities for primary prevention of depression (**Figure 5.11**):

- *Prevention of adverse childhood experiences.* The work is not easy, but protecting children from

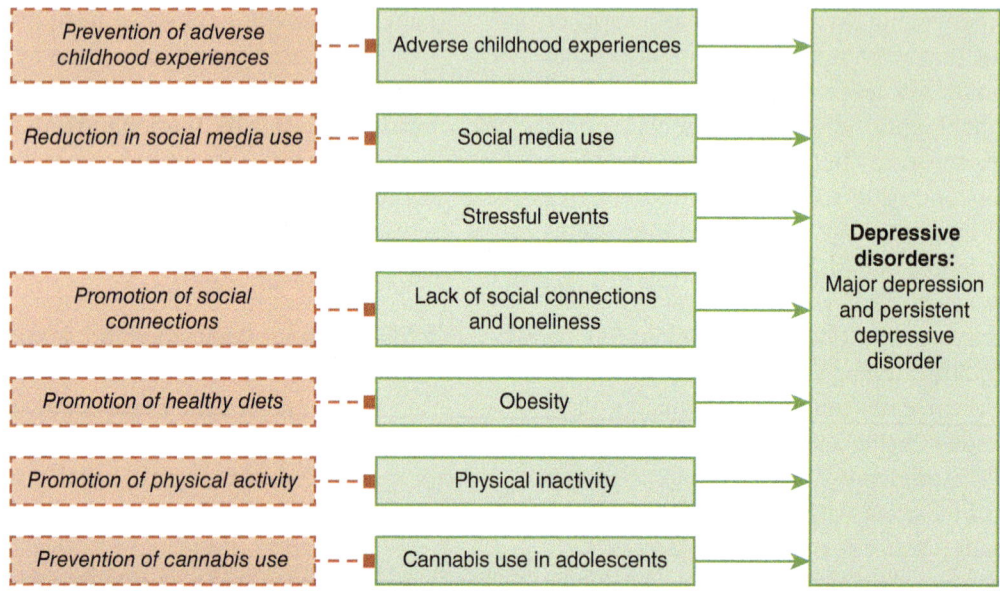

Figure 5.11 Cause-and-Effect Diagram for Depression, with Preventive Interventions.

violence, abuse, or neglect within families should reduce rates of depression in future adults. Protecting children involves both supporting families who are themselves stressed and, at times, intervening to shield them from abusive parents.

- *Reduction in social media use.* The connection between social media use and depression suggests that cutting back on social media would reduce the number of teenagers and young adults who develop depression, and might also reduce rates of suicide. In 2022, teenagers on average spent 3.5 hours per day on social media, and one in four spent five or more hours per day.[89] In 2023, the U.S. Surgeon General warned about the dangers of social media in his *Advisory on Social Media and Youth Mental Health*. He recommended that technology companies remove features in their platforms designed to grab users' attention and keep them glued to their phones, and that policy-makers set rules that limit these features.[89] And in 2024, the Surgeon General took the additional step of asking Congress to require warning labels on social media platforms.[90]
- *Promotion of social connections.* While lack of social connections and loneliness is subjective—measuring not people's situations but instead their responses to those situations—they are nonetheless risk factors that can be changed at the population level. In 2023, the U.S. Surgeon General addressed this problem with his report *Our Epidemic of Loneliness and Isolation*. This report makes recommendations on how to strengthen social connections, including redesigning the built environment with common places like libraries and parks, supporting

programs that bring people together, and revamping information technology so that it builds rather than breaks down connections among people.[80]
- *Promotion of healthy eating* to prevent obesity. Chapter 14 Nutrition discusses the promotion of healthy eating.
- *Promotion of physical activity.* Physical activity has an immediate benefit by reducing depression directly and a longer-term benefit by helping combat obesity. See Chapter 15. Physical Inactivity.
- *Prevention of cannabis use in adolescents.* Cannabis use is actively promoted in the United States today. Even with use of the drug legal in many states, there are many ways society could discourage its use and protect adolescents from drug promotion—for example, prohibiting advertising of the drug, requiring lower potency, and restricting sales outlets.

Secondary Prevention

The U.S. Preventive Services Task Force recommends that primary care providers screen all their patients for depression. There are several simple questionnaires providers can use for this screening, but the most popular are the **PHQ-2** and the **PHQ-9** (using two and nine questions, respectively). People who are found to be depressed can be treated with psychotherapy, antidepressant medications, or both.[91] Neither form of treatment cures the disease or makes the symptoms disappear, but both forms help people somewhat, and the two are about equally effective.[91]

While many people are undoubtedly helped by this treatment, there are limitations to this approach for entire populations. Many people who are depressed do not go to primary providers. Those primary providers are often overwhelmed with other problems, leaving little time to spend evaluating or helping those who are depressed. Often, the most that they can do is refer patients to mental health professionals, who may not be easy for patients to access. And both psychotherapy and treatment with medication involve many steps over weeks or months, which many people (especially those who are depressed) may have difficulty completing. Overall, only about 40% of people with major depression receive any treatment for it, with treatment less common in men, racial and ethnic minority populations, and those who are unemployed.[92]

Box 5.4 Summary–Prevention of Depression

- Prevention of adverse childhood experiences
- Reduction in social media use
- Promotion of social connections
- Promotion of healthy eating to reduce or prevent obesity
- Promotion of physical activity
- Prevention of cannabis use in adolescents

Box 5.5 Key Words–Depression

Amygdala
Anxiety disorder
Bipolar disorder
Cortisol
Dopamine
Dysthymia
Hippocampus
Hormone
Hypothalamus
Immune system
Inflammation
Limbic system
Major depression, Major depressive disorder
Mania
Monoamines
Mood
Mood disorder
Norepinephrine
Persistent depressive disorder
PHQ-2 and PHQ-9
Psychological stress
Serotonin
Social connection
Stress
Substance use disorder

Resources–Depression

- Kessler RC, McLaughlin KA, Green JG, et al. Childhood adversities and adult psychopathology in the WHO world mental health surveys. *British Journal of Psychiatry*. 2010;197(5):378-385. doi:10.1192/bjp.bp.110.080499. This summarizes the research from a consistent set of surveys in many countries on the connection between adverse childhood experiences and mental illness in adults.

- *Social Media and Youth Mental Health: The U.S. Surgeon General's Advisory* (Health and Human Services, 2023, available at SurgeonGeneral.gov) summarizes the evidence of the link between social media use and mental health problems and provides recommendations to technology companies, policy-makers, and parents about how to reduce the harm of social media.

- *Our Epidemic of Loneliness and Isolation: The U.S. Surgeon General's Advisory on the Healing Effects of Social Connection and Community* (Health and Human Services, 2023, available at SurgeonGeneral.gov) provides an excellent review of the links between social connections and mental illness as well as a summary of steps that individuals and organizations of all types can take to strengthen social connections.

- Nemeroff CB. The state of our understanding of the pathophysiology and optimal treatment of depression: Glass half full or half empty? *American Journal of Psychiatry*. 2020;177(8):671-685. doi:10.1176/appi.ajp.2020.20060845. This is a technical paper that explains current thinking about the biologic causes of depression.

- The National Institute of Mental Health maintains a webpage on depression at https://www.nimh.nih.gov/health/topics/depression that explains the illness and its treatment in simple terms and has links to other resources.

Anxiety

Introduction

Anxiety is a very common problem in which worries and fears are amplified to the point that they can be paralyzing.[93] Anxiety is so closely tied to depression that for many years mental health experts considered it to be just another symptom of depression. About 60% of people with depression meet criteria for anxiety disorder[39,41] and roughly the same proportion of people with anxiety disorders also have major depression.[93] The recommended medical treatments for anxiety and depression are similar, and the risk factors for the two disorders are much the same, as are the interventions to prevent them.

Definition and Description of the Disease

It is normal and healthy for a person to feel afraid when threatened. If a person is afraid of a threatening situation that *might* happen in the future, that person has **anxiety**. Like fear, anxiety is a helpful, protective response to genuine threats. Anxiety becomes unhealthy enough to earn the label of an **anxiety disorder** if the symptoms last at least a few months and are: 1) out of proportion to the threat, 2) severe and persistent, or 3) disruptive of a person's ability to function.[93,94] People with anxiety disorders not only feel worried, nervous, or fearful, but they also have physical symptoms, like tense muscles, dizziness, a racing heart rate, and breathlessness.[95] Having these symptoms—or worrying that they might—makes people with anxiety disorders avoid certain situations, which interferes with their ability to work, go to school, or manage their daily lives.[93]

There are many different types of anxiety disorders, each with their own labels, and they often occur in combinations.[93] The most common are:

- **Generalized anxiety disorder**, in which people are anxious about their routine activities, such as their performance at work or school.
- **Social anxiety disorder**, in which people are afraid of and avoid interacting with others, often feeling that they are being scrutinized, judged, or the focus of attention.
- **Panic disorder**, in which people have recurring, unexpected attacks of panic, with physical symptoms.
- **Agoraphobia**, in which people are afraid to be in crowded public settings, or even just out of the home.
- **Specific phobias**, in which people have marked fear of (and avoid) specific objects or situations, such as insects, thunderstorms, heights, or enclosed spaces.[94]

In the past, **post-traumatic stress disorder (PTSD)** and **obsessive-compulsive disorder** were considered anxiety disorders, but they are now classified separately by the Diagnostic and Statistical Manual for Mental Disorders.

Anxiety disorders often first appear in the teenage or young adult years.[93,94] But younger children can also have anxiety disorders, such as **separation anxiety disorder**, in which they are abnormally afraid of separating from a parent, and **selective mutism**, in which they do not speak when people other than family members are present.

Grouping and classifying mental illnesses is always difficult, as is drawing lines between what is normal and what is a disorder. But classifying and labeling are especially difficult in anxiety. Probably most people are hampered by anxiety at one time or another. Even people who meet strict criteria for anxiety disorders may have symptoms that are not very severe or long-lasting. In one survey that identified people with anxiety in the community, only one in four were labeled as having "serious" problems, meaning that they had symptoms that severely limited their ability to function or lasted more than 30 days.[40]

The symptoms of people with anxiety disorders wax and wane over their lifetimes but generally are at their worst in young adult years and then ease with age.[94] Nonetheless, people with anxiety disorders are more likely to develop other health problems, including drug or alcohol addiction and heart disease.[93,95]

Pathophysiology of Anxiety Disorders

Humans, like all animals, are more likely to survive if they can learn from dangerous situations. When animals are injured or threatened, they remember the details of what happened. If they later recognize a similar set of details, they have a **fear response**, in which they snap to attention and become suspicious and afraid.

The limbic system is involved in managing both the brain's response to stressful events and memory, so it makes sense that it would handle memories of stressful events. The center most involved is the **amygdala**.[46] When a human is in a situation that reminds that person of a painful or threatening experience, the amygdala generates a fear response in the rest of the brain, setting the heart racing, the palms sweating, and the brain on high alert. Most people experiencing a fear response quickly leave that situation; afterwards, many people anticipating that response avoid getting into that situation.

For example, if a person riding a bicycle is hit by a car and breaks an arm, that person will have a memory that links bicycle riding with danger and pain. If that person later straddles a bicycle, it may trigger panic, chasing that person off the bike. For a long time afterward, that person may avoid getting on any bicycle. Over time, though, memories fade and mounting a bicycle triggers a lesser fear response or no fear response at all. To put it in words of psychology, over time there has been **extinction** of a **conditioned fear response**.

In people with anxiety disorders, it seems that the amygdala becomes hyperactive, doing its job too well. When it does, the fear response may be prompted by situations that are much less related to a painful memory, such as just seeing a bicycle, or the fear response may occur with no prompts at all. That free-floating anxiety undergirds general anxiety disorder and social anxiety disorder. Or the fear-provoking memory may never fade—that is, there is failure of extinction of the conditioned fear response—which may lead to a specific phobia.[94]

It seems that the amygdala becomes hyperactive in people with a genetic predisposition who then experience stressful events and situations, especially in childhood, while the brain is still developing (**Figure 5.12**). It has been shown that the amygdala grows in size in children who have experienced psychological stress, and that it stays large after the period of stress ends.[96] Related to this, some experts believe that anxiety can be traced to altered levels of neurotransmitters in the amygdala.

Epidemiology: Patterns and Trends

In the United States and in the world as a whole, about 12% of adults meet criteria for an anxiety disorder over a 12-month period, making anxiety the most common mental disorder. Women are twice as likely to be affected as men.[92-94]

In the United States, the prevalence of anxiety disorders is higher in those with lower incomes,[94,97] but the disorder is slightly more common in Whites than African Americans or Hispanics.[40,98]

Interestingly, globally there is a large variation in prevalence of anxiety across countries, with higher prevalence in high-income countries.[99] One study found that anxiety was most prevalent in English-speaking countries, about half as prevalent in Asian and African countries, and in between elsewhere.[99] The prevalence was also higher in regions with recent war or other conflicts.[100]

Like depression, anxiety began to rise in prevalence in the United States in about 2012, especially in teens and younger adults. From 2011 to 2018, annual surveys showed an increase in anxiety symptoms in every age group below 50, with the most rapid rise (a 50% increase) in adults age 18–25.[71] Over about the same time period, anxiety symptoms also surged among children ages 3–17.[68]

Risk Factors

As with all the mental illnesses covered in this chapter, genetics contributes to the risk of anxiety disorders, although less so than it does for schizophrenia. The genetic risk for anxiety overlaps with that for depression—that is, having a parent or close relative with either an anxiety disorder or major depression increases a person's risk of developing an anxiety disorder.[93,94]

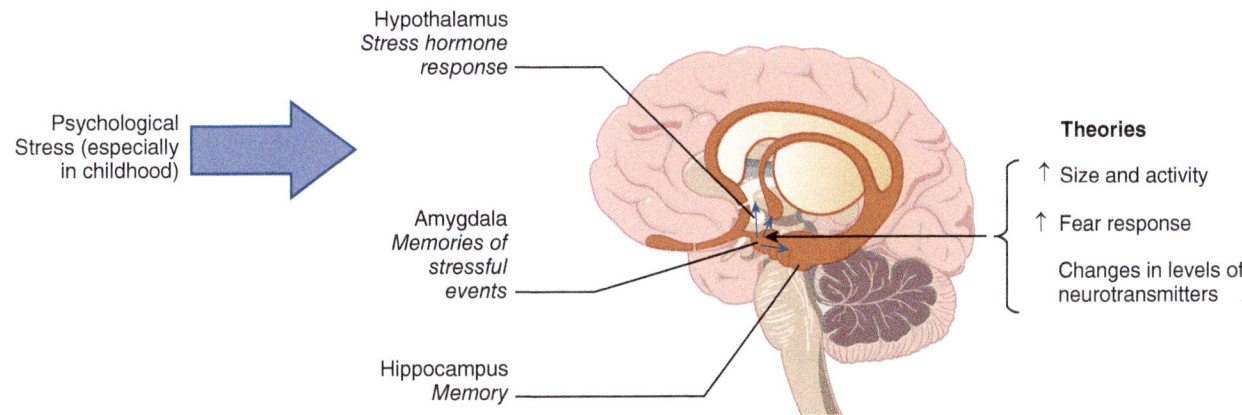

Figure 5.12 Theories of the Amygdala's Role in Anxiety Disorders. Illustration of a theory of the causes of anxiety disorders. The amygdala is the brain center responsible for storing memories of stressful events and generating a fear response to similar situations. In susceptible people exposed to stress, especially during childhood, the amygdala becomes hyperactive, producing a fear response to situations that are not even threatening.

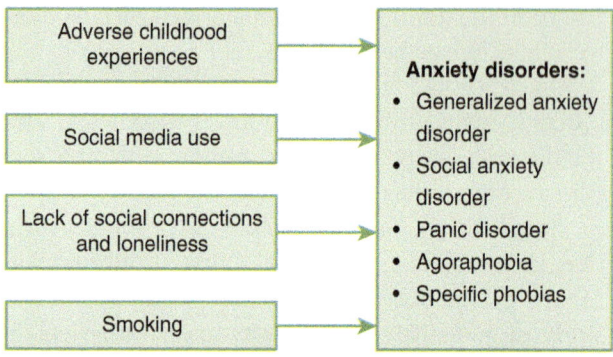

Figure 5.13 Cause-and-Effect Diagram for Anxiety Disorders.

Modifiable known risk factors for anxiety disorders are (**Figure 5.13**):

- *Adverse childhood experiences*, such as child abuse or neglect, or parents with mental illness or substance use.[65,101,102] These adverse experiences may be the stressful situations that cause the amygdala to become hyperactive. One study estimated that about 30% of anxiety disorders in adults were attributable to adverse childhood experiences.[65]
- *Social media use*. It is not difficult to understand how social media use—with the constant flow of judgmental and threatening comments—might provoke stress and anxiety. Adolescents who spend more time on social media are more likely to have symptoms of anxiety.[68,69] The surge in anxiety beginning in the early 2010s, like the surge in depression, is likely driven by an increase in social media use.[58,70,71]
- *Lack of social connections and loneliness*. Both adolescents and older adults who have no one they can confide in or who are lonely are more likely to develop anxiety (and depression).[80,103]
- *Smoking* has been identified as a risk factor for agoraphobia, panic disorder, generalized anxiety disorder, and social anxiety disorder.[97,104] While

this may be in part because anxiety induces people to smoke, some studies have found that when people quit, their symptoms of anxiety lessen.[105]

Preventive Interventions

Primary Prevention

Based on the risk factors above, these interventions should ultimately reduce the prevalence of anxiety disorders (**Figure 5.14**):

- *Prevention of adverse childhood experiences*. As with depression, prevention of adverse experiences for children, such as violent, abusive, or neglectful home environments, should reduce anxiety in those children as they become adults.
- *Reduction in social media use*. The previous section on depression discusses how reduction in social media use may prevent depression, and it should similarly reduce anxiety disorders. The 2023 U.S. Surgeon General's *Advisory on Social Media and Youth Mental Health* makes recommendations for how to protect adolescents from the harmful effects of social media.[89]
- *Promotion of social connections*. The report of the U.S. Surgeon General makes recommendations on how to strengthen social connections.[80]
- *Prevention of smoking*. See Chapter 11. Tobacco Use.

Secondary Prevention

As with depression, the U.S. Preventive Services Task Force recommends that primary care providers screen their patients for anxiety, although it is less clear that the screening and treatment is helpful for anxiety.[95] The screening tool used most is called the General Anxiety Disorder questionnaire, which comes in a 2-item and a 7-item version (the **GAD-2** and **GAD-7**).[94,95] Anxiety is so common that about one in five patients in primary care practices will show up on

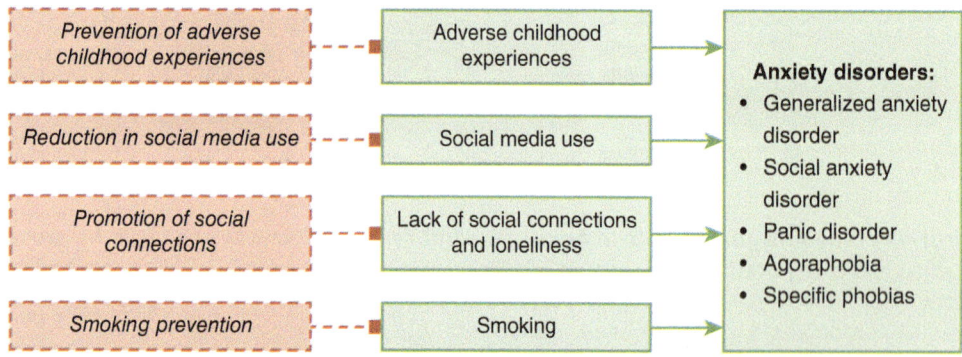

Figure 5.14 Cause-and-Effect Diagram for Anxiety Disorders, with Preventive Interventions.

screening as having an anxiety disorder.[95] Those who do can be treated with psychotherapy—giving people ways to manage their anxiety and the situations that provoke it—or with medications used to treat depression.[93] These treatments have some benefit, but they are far from cures.[106] Both psychotherapy and medications take weeks to have an effect. Also, people taking medications may have difficulty stopping because their symptoms can return, causing panic attacks.[106] Only about one in four adults in the United States who meet criteria for anxiety disorder in the past 12 months receives treatment for it.[92]

Box 5.6 Summary–Prevention of Anxiety Disorders.

- Prevention of adverse childhood experiences
- Reduction in social media use
- Promotion of social connections
- Prevention of smoking

Box 5.7 Key Words–Anxiety

Agoraphobia
Amygdala
Anxiety
Anxiety disorder
Conditioned fear response
Extinction (of a conditioned responses)
Fear response
GAD-2 and GAD-7
Generalized anxiety disorder
Obsessive-compulsive disorder
Panic disorder
Post-traumatic stress disorder
Selective mutism
Separation anxiety disorder
Social anxiety disorder
Specific phobias

Resources–Anxiety

- Kessler RC, McLaughlin KA, Green JG, et al. Childhood adversities and adult psychopathology in the WHO world mental health surveys. *British Journal of Psychiatry*. 2010;197(5):378-385. doi:10.1192/bjp.bp.110.080499. This summarizes the research from a consistent set of surveys in many countries on the connection between adverse childhood experiences and mental illness in adults.
- *Social Media and Youth Mental Health: The U.S. Surgeon General's Advisory* (Health and Human Services, 2023, available at SurgeonGeneral.gov) summarizes the evidence of the link between social media use and mental health problems and provides recommendations to technology companies, policy-makers, and parents about how to reduce the harm of social media.
- *Our Epidemic of Loneliness and Isolation: The U.S. Surgeon General's Advisory on the Healing Effects of Social Connection and Community* (Health and Human Services, 2023, available at SurgeonGeneral.gov) provides an excellent review of the links between social connections and mental illness as well as a summary of steps that individuals and organizations of all types can take to strengthen social connections.
- Penninx BW, Pine DS, Holmes EA, Reif A. Anxiety disorders. *Lancet*. 2021;397(10277):914-927. doi:10.1016/S0140-6736(21)00359-7. This is a detailed technical summary of current thinking on the types of anxiety disorders, their biologic causes, and treatment of them.
- The National Institute of Mental Health maintains a webpage on anxiety disorders at https://www.nimh.nih.gov/health/topics/anxiety-disorders that explains the illnesses and their treatment in simple terms and has links to other resources.

Dementia

Introduction

Dementia is a condition tied to aging in which the brain gradually loses neurons and shrinks, causing a person to lose mental abilities like memory and language. As people live longer, dementia is rising in the rankings as a cause of death and disability. There is no cure for dementia, but reducing its risk factors—many of which are also risks for heart disease and stroke—can greatly delay it.[107]

Definition and Description of the Disease

Dementia can be caused by several different diseases. The most common is **Alzheimer's disease**, named for the early 20th century German psychiatrist who first described it.[108] For many years, the Alzheimer's label was reserved for people who developed dementia before age 65, but now experts recognize it as the same condition that affects older people. A second cause is **vascular dementia**, which is caused by insufficient blood flow to the brain. These two diseases overlap; the symptoms are very similar, most people with dementia show evidence of both diseases,[108] and the diseases share risk factors.

People with dementia gradually lose their **cognitive** abilities—that is, their ability to remember, learn, understand, speak, and think clearly. They may become forgetful and lose their car keys. They may have difficulty finding words, planning for events, using a cell phone, or following a plot in a movie. In the beginning, these problems are called **mild cognitive impairment**.[109] The problems earn the label of dementia when they interfere with people's ability to care for themselves.[110]

The specific difficulties that people have depend somewhat on which disease is primarily causing dementia. People with Alzheimer's disease typically first have difficulty forming new short-term memories.[109] They may not remember a conversation that took place earlier in the day, despite clearly remembering events that happened years earlier. Often, they next have difficulty speaking, such as finding words, remembering people's names, or explaining themselves.[111] As the disease worsens, they have trouble planning and achieving even simple goals, in what is called a loss of **executive function**.[111] Later, they have difficulty finding objects or become lost, even in familiar places.[109]

At some point, most people with Alzheimer's disease also develop symptoms seen in psychiatric illnesses. They may become suspicious or fearful. Or they can develop depression, anxiety, and sometimes even hallucinations and delusions.[109,111]

Alzheimer's disease and vascular dementia unfold very slowly. The entire process—from when symptoms are so mild that no one notices them to a person's death—may last 20 years.[112]

Pathophysiology of Dementia

In dementia, the brain gradually loses its capabilities because it loses **neurons** (brain cells) and **synapses** (the interfaces between neurons). As the brain loses neurons, it shrinks. This loss of neurons happens in both the cerebral cortex, which explains the loss of cognitive capabilities, and in parts of the limbic system (especially the hippocampus and amygdala), which explains the memory loss and the psychiatric symptoms.[113]

Two biologic processes cause the brain to lose neurons and synapses in Alzheimer's disease and in vascular dementia.[111,114] Remember, though, that these two diseases greatly overlap, so both processes may contribute to either disease.

- *Accumulation of protein fragments in amyloid plaques.* Neurons produce a protein that, after leaving the cell, is chopped into small pieces called **amyloid beta fragments**.[109,111] These fragments are probably just waste products, but in people with Alzheimer's disease, instead of being recycled or washed away, they accumulate, clumping together to form **amyloid plaques** (**Figure 5.15**). Over time, these amyloid plaques grow large enough to be seen under a microscope. These plaques damage neurons and synapses. It is as if the brain were a chemical factory that, instead of hauling away its toxic wastes, continues to store them in piles of leaky barrels, even as the spills kill the factory's workers. Over years, as the amyloid plaques pile up and neurons die, the brain shrinks in size (**Figure 5.16**).

  The amyloid plaques also interfere with how neurons handle other proteins called **tau proteins**.[111,112] The tau proteins then form their

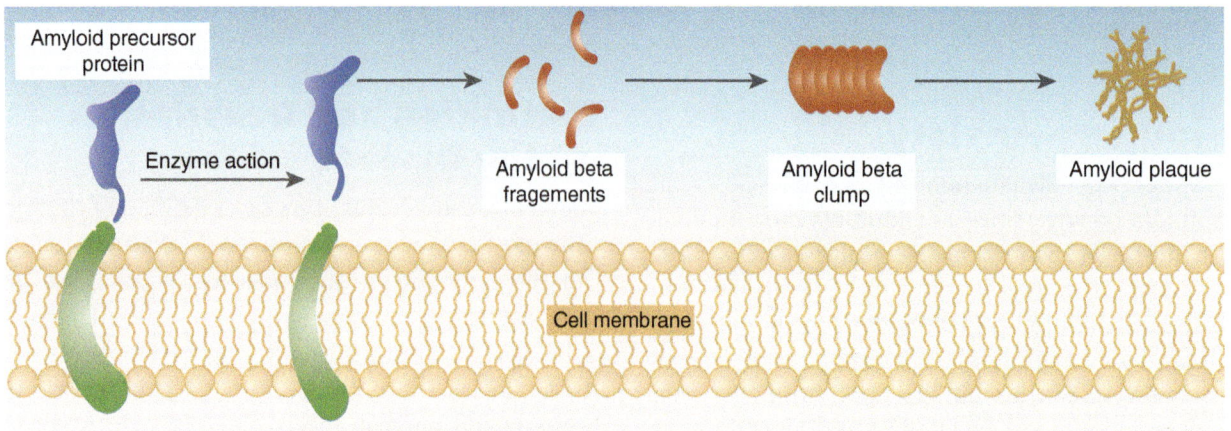

Figure 5.15 Development of Amyloid Plaques. Neurons produce a protein called amyloid precursor protein. After enzymes act on this protein, they leave amyloid beta fragments outside of cells. In Alzheimer's disease, these amyloid beta fragments clump together to form amyloid plaques. Amyloid plaques damage neurons and synapses.

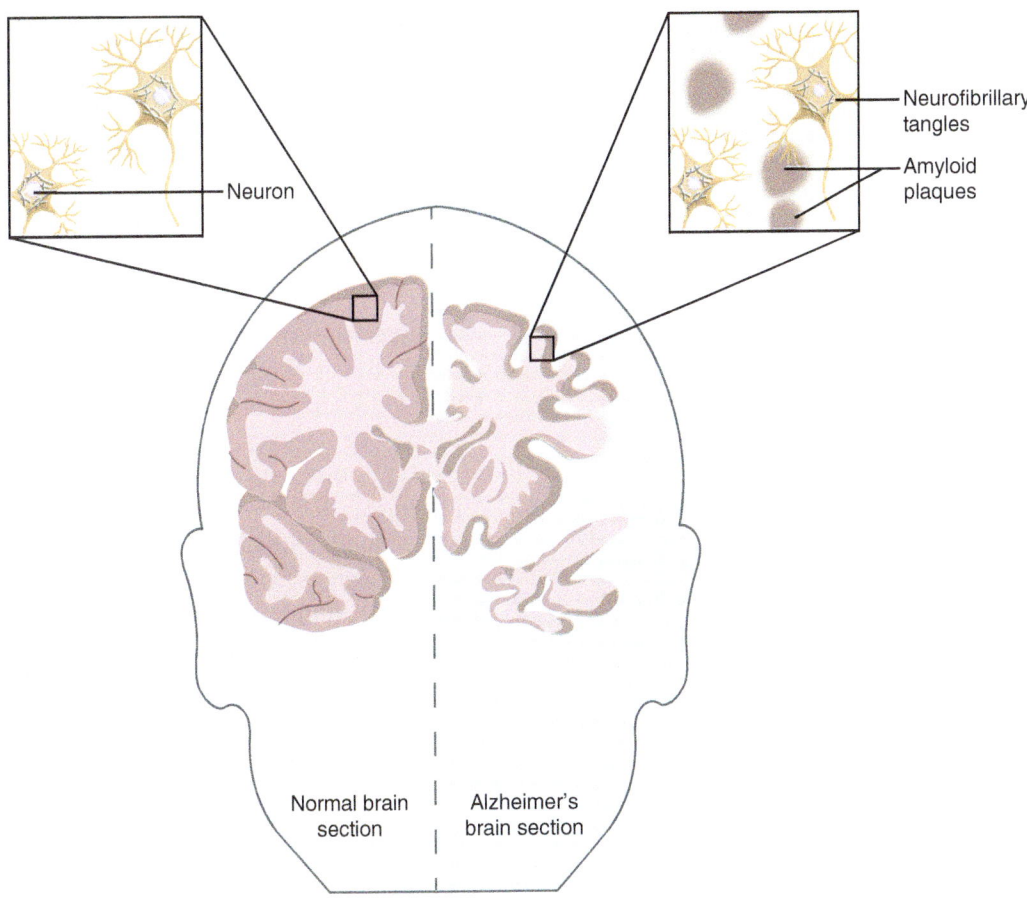

Neurofibrillary tangles

Amyloid plaques

Neuron

Normal brain section

Alzheimer's brain section

Figure 5.16 Changes to the Brain in Alzheimer's Disease. The brain in Alzheimer's disease is shrunken in size. Viewed with a microscope, it shows accumulation of amyloid plaques outside of neurons and neurofibrillary tangles inside of neurons.

own clumps, called **neurofibrillary tangles** (or just **tangles**). These tangles also grow big enough to be seen under a microscope and are likewise toxic to neurons.[111]

People who have a head injury causing a **concussion** (a disruption in brain function) are nearly twice as likely to develop Alzheimer's disease, even years later.[107] That may be because severe head injuries induce the brain to produce clumps of these tau proteins.[115]

Neurons do not generally regrow after they die, so a loss of one neuron means a permanent loss of its contribution to the brain's capabilities. Fortunately, the brain seems to have excess capacity, like a computer packed with spare RAM chips. This extra capacity has been called **cognitive reserve**. At first, this spare capacity picks up the slack when the brain loses neurons, so the appearance of amyloid plaques and tangles goes on for years before anyone notices a loss of mental ability.[109] But eventually that cognitive reserve is depleted and people show signs of dementia.

The brain seems to behave like a muscle, growing in strength when used and weakening if left inactive. People who have had more education or who regularly do more difficult mental tasks are able to handle more of these amyloid plaques and tangles without showing signs of dementia. One theory is that these people can delay dementia because, over a lifetime, they have built up more cognitive reserve that they draw on when they lose neurons.[111]

- *Reduction in blood flow to the brain from damaged arteries.*

The brain is a metabolically active organ that needs a constant and rich supply of blood to survive. When the vessels carrying blood to the brain are narrowed, neurons die from lack of oxygen or nutrients, causing vascular dementia.[111,116,117] This starving of neurons can happen when: 1) large or medium-sized arteries become narrowed from **atherosclerosis** (**Figure 5.17**), causing repeated strokes, including small **silent strokes** that no one notices, or 2) the tiny arteries called **arterioles** are damaged and narrowed from longstanding high

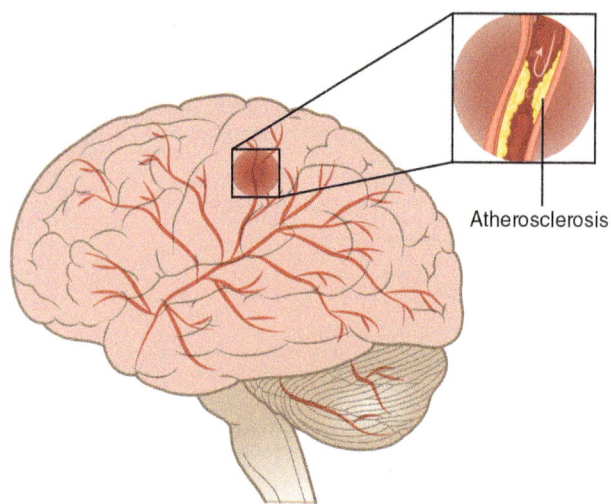

Figure 5.17 Vascular Dementia. In vascular dementia, plaques of atherosclerosis cause narrowing of arteries supplying blood to the brain. This reduces blood flow to neurons.

blood pressure or diabetes.[116] For more on atherosclerosis and high blood pressure, see Chapter 2. Heart Disease and Stroke.

Epidemiology: Patterns and Trends

The prevalence of dementia rises sharply with age (**Figure 5.18**). About one person per 1000 in their late 40s has dementia, and the prevalence roughly doubles every five years of age after that.[118] Although not everyone fortunate enough to reach age 95 has dementia, most do. For unknown reasons, women tend to develop dementia somewhat sooner than men.[112,119]

Alzheimer's disease rates vary by race, with the highest rates in African Americans, Native Americans and Hispanics, the lowest in Asians, and Whites falling between them.[111] These racial differences are probably related to income. People with lower levels of income are more likely to develop dementia for reasons that are not known but may be related to their having less education and more exposure to factors that promote atherosclerosis.[120–122]

Worldwide, the age-specific prevalence of dementia is rising slowly, but the number of people with dementia is rising quickly because people are living longer and the world's population is growing so rapidly.[123] Dementia is more prevalent in high-income countries like the United States than in low-income countries, even after taking age into account.[118] But in those high-income countries, age-adjusted rates of dementia have been slowly falling over the past few decades.[107,112,114] It is not known why dementia rates are falling, but rates of ischemic heart disease are also falling (see Chapter 2. Heart Disease and Stroke), and the two diseases share many risk factors.

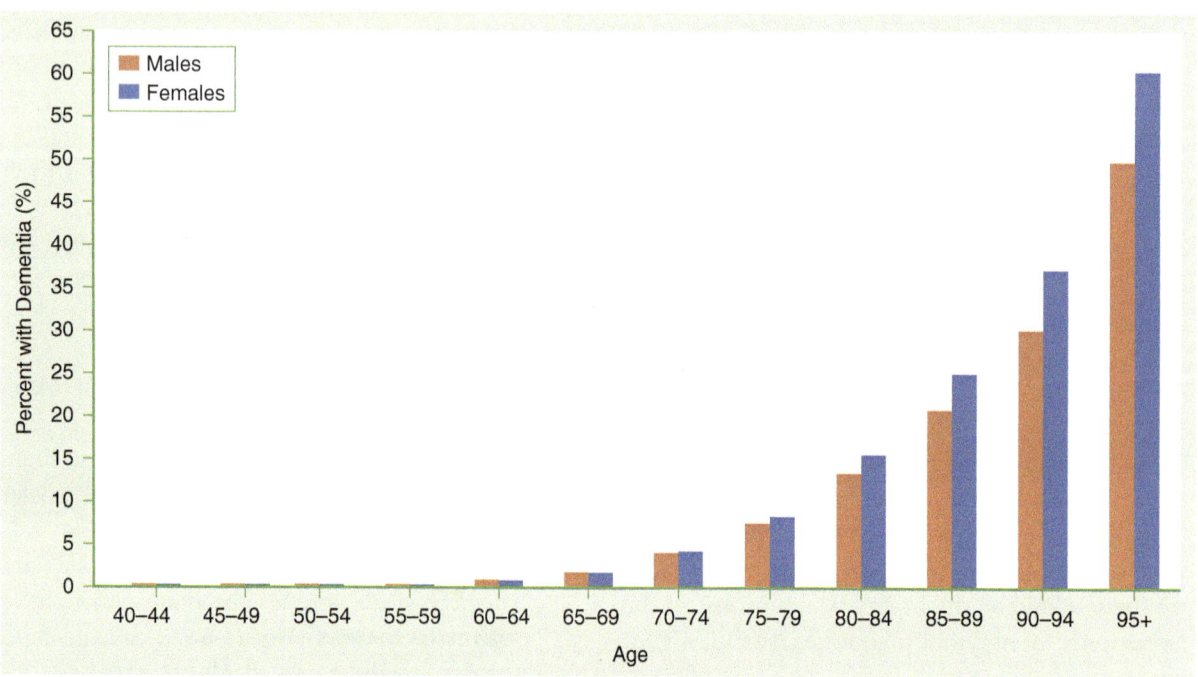

Figure 5.18 Estimated Prevalence of Dementia by Age and Sex in the United States.

Data from Global Burden of Disease Collaboration, Institute for Health Metrics and Evaluation. GBD Results Tool. Published July 12, 2023. Accessed July 11, 2023. https://vizhub.healthdata.org/gbd-results/

Risk Factors

As for most other diseases, there are genetic risks for dementia. People carrying a gene called **ApoE4** develop amyloid plaques earlier in life and are about three times as likely to develop Alzheimer's disease as others.[124] About 25% of Americans, but 60% of those with Alzheimer's disease, carry this gene.[125,126] Many other genes pose a smaller increase in risk.

Nonetheless, there are many risk factors for dementia that can be modified to delay the disease. By one estimate, addressing these risk factors could prevent up to 40% of cases of dementia globally.[107] Most of these risk factors fall in three groups: those that hurt the brain directly, those that limit cognitive reserve, and those that damage and narrow the arteries supplying the brain. The risk factors are (**Figure 5.19**):

- *Traumatic brain injury.* Head injuries that cause concussions and increase the risk of Alzheimer's disease are not uncommon. People get concussions in contact sports (not just football and boxing but also soccer, baseball, and basketball), military actions, falls, and crashes involving cars, motorcycles, and bicycles.[107] And it may be that lesser blows to the head, if they are frequent,

cause similar damage. Alzheimer's disease has parallels with a brain disease called **chronic traumatic encephalopathy (CTE)** that has recently been recognized in athletes in contact sports, and the reason may be these repeated smaller head injuries.[107,115]

- *Excessive alcohol use.* People who have more than about 1–2 alcoholic drinks per day are more likely to develop dementia.[107] That may be because alcohol is toxic to neurons or that people who drink heavily develop a deficiency of the B vitamin thiamine, which is essential to neurons.[127] (In some studies, people who drink small amounts of alcohol seem to have a *lower* risk of dementia than those who abstain, but because of its toxicity overall, no experts recommend drinking alcohol to prevent dementia.)[107,114]

- *Less active use of the brain.* People who have used their brains less actively over a lifetime are more likely to develop dementia. Specifically, *people with less education, especially in childhood,* are at higher risk, as are those who spend *less time engaged in activities* like social events, playing music, creating art, reading, or speaking a second language.[107] Likewise, people who are

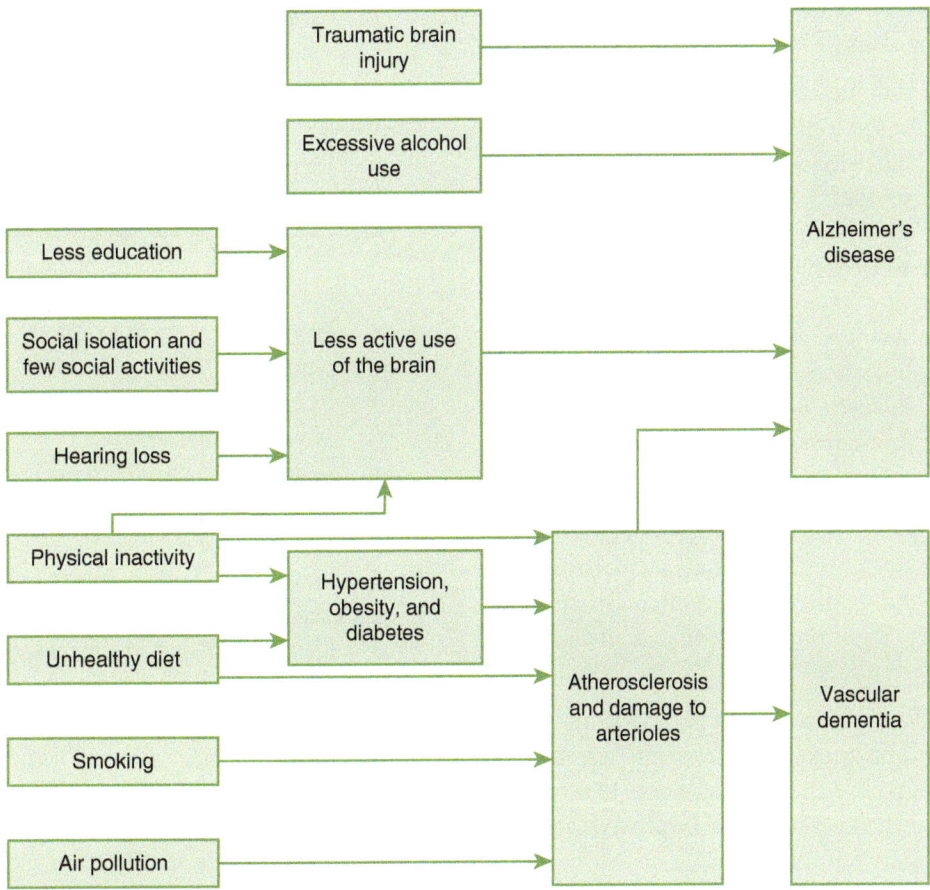

Figure 5.19 Cause-and-Effect Diagram for Dementia.

socially isolated or have low social contact are at greater risk, perhaps because talking and listening stimulate the brain and build cognitive reserve.[107,114] And people who have *hearing loss in mid-life* are also at much higher risk, because losing the ability to listen to language leaves the brain less active.

- *Atherosclerosis and damage to arterioles.* Behaviors or exposures that increase the risk for heart disease and stroke (see Chapter 2 Heart Disease and Stroke) also damage and narrow the arteries supplying the brain, so they increase the risk of dementia. They include:
  - *Unhealthy diet,* which raises **cholesterol** levels in the blood, causing atherosclerosis.[111]
  - *Physical inactivity,* which has both indirect and direct harmful effects on the brain.[107,114] It damages and narrows arteries by increasing the risk of atherosclerosis, **hypertension** (high blood pressure), and diabetes. In addition, physical inactivity leaves the brain less active.
  - *Smoking,* because the chemicals in tobacco smoke damage the lining of arteries and lead to atherosclerosis.[107]
  - *Air pollution* (including second-hand tobacco smoke), probably because breathing polluted air damages arteries in the same way that smoking does.[107]

And people with metabolic conditions that cause or are caused by damage to tiny arteries are also at much greater risk. Those risky conditions include *hypertension* (high blood pressure), *obesity,* and *diabetes.*[107,111,114]

Two other factors have been consistently and strongly linked to dementia. People are more likely to develop dementia if they have *depression* that began late in life or if they have *disturbed sleep patterns*—that is, sleeping too little, too much, or at odd or irregular times.[107,114] However, it is unclear if these actually cause dementia or are just early signs of dementia.

Preventive Interventions

Preventing dementia involves taking steps to reduce the behaviors and exposures that increase risk, as well as treating the conditions that increase risk (**Figure 5.20**):[107,114]

- *Prevention of traumatic brain injuries.* Many brain injuries can be prevented or made less severe through changes to the rules of sports that reduce blows to the head, as well as improved helmets and other safety equipment.
- *Reduction in alcohol use.* See Chapter 14. Alcohol Use.

- *Promotion of brain activity.* Interventions that may increase brain activity for groups and populations:
  - *Strengthening and broadening education,* both for children and adults.
  - *Cognitive training.* To help people build cognitive reserve, the World Health Organization has recommended cognitive training programs in which people at risk for dementia are given regular "brain exercises," such as puzzles to solve.[128,129] Activities like music lessons may have a similar effect. While it is not easy to see how these can be brought to scale in an entire population, they may be valuable for higher-risk groups, such as people living in retirement homes.
  - *Promotion of social connections* and social activities. The U.S. Surgeon General's Advisory *Our Epidemic of Loneliness and Isolation* provides practical recommendations to build social connections, which include social activities that likely build cognitive reserve.[80]
  - *Prevention of hearing loss* and *provision of hearing aids to people with hearing loss.* Hearing loss is a public health problem of its own, caused by a variety of factors, including exposure to noise. It can be prevented by reducing exposure to excessive noise, particularly at workplaces and when using personal audio devices, or it can be managed by use of hearing aids.
- *Reduction of heart disease and stroke.* Chapter 2 discusses strategies to prevent heart disease and stroke. Primary prevention elements of these strategies that should also prevent dementia are:
  - *Reduction of smoking.* See Chapter 11. Tobacco Use.
  - *Promotion of healthy diets.* See Chapter 14. Nutrition.
  - *Promotion of physical activity.* See Chapter 15. Physical Inactivity.
  - *Reduction in air pollution.* Air pollution is discussed more in Chapter 8. Chronic Respiratory Diseases.
- Secondary prevention interventions that should also reduce dementia are:
  - *Identification and treatment of persons with hypertension* (high blood pressure). See Chapter 2. Heart Disease and Stroke.
  - *Identification of persons with high blood cholesterol and treatment with statins.* See Chapter 2. Heart Disease and Stroke.
  - *Identification and treatment of diabetes* to reduce hemoglobin A1c levels. See Chapter 7. Chronic Metabolic Diseases.

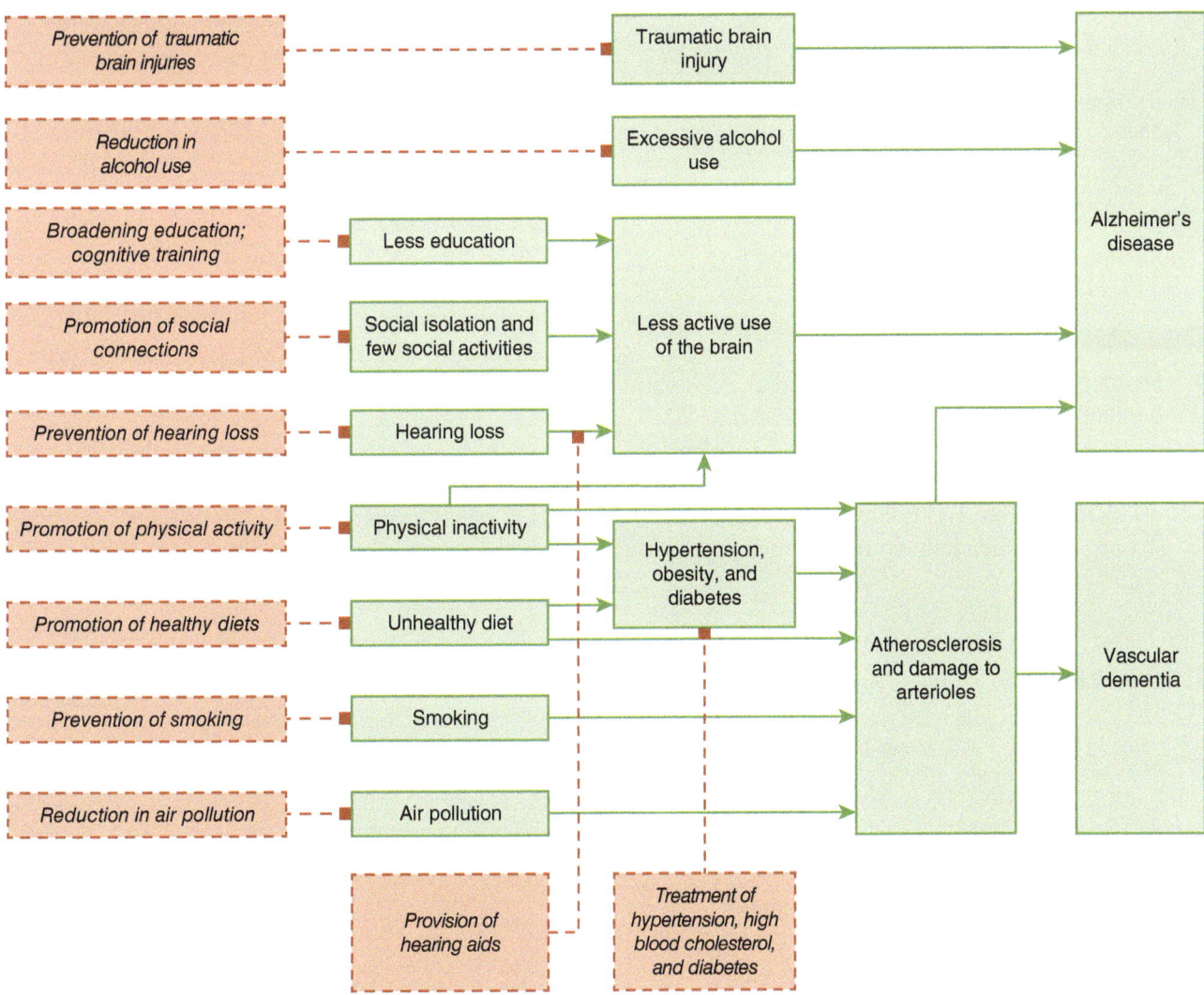

Figure 5.20 Cause-and-Effect Diagram for Dementia, with Preventive Interventions.

Box 5.8 Summary–Prevention of Dementia

- Prevention of traumatic brain injuries
- Reduction in alcohol use
- Strengthening and broadening education
- Cognitive training
- Promotion of social connections and social activities
- Prevention of hearing loss and provision of hearing aids to people with hearing loss
- Prevention of smoking
- Promotion of healthy diets
- Promotion of physical activity
- Reduction in air pollution
- Identification and treatment of hypertension
- Identification of persons with high blood cholesterol and treatment with statins
- Identification and treatment of diabetes

Box 5.9 Key Words–Dementia

Alzheimer's disease
Amyloid beta fragments
Amyloid plaques
ApoE4
Arterioles
Atherosclerosis
Cholesterol
Chronic traumatic encephalopathy (CTE)
Cognitive
Cognitive reserve
Concussion
Executive function
Hypertension
Mild cognitive impairment
Neurofibrillary tangles
Neuron

(continues)

Box 5.9 Key Words–Dementia *(continued)*

Silent stroke
Synapse
Tangles
Tau proteins
Vascular dementia

Resources–Dementia

- Livingston G, Huntley J, Sommerlad A, et al. Dementia prevention, intervention, and care: 2020 report of the Lancet Commission. *The Lancet.* 2020;396(10248):413-446. doi:10.1016/S0140-6736(20)30367-6. This Commission makes evidence-based recommendations for population-based prevention of dementia, and this report summarizes both the recommendations and the evidence.

- *Risk Reduction of Cognitive Decline and Dementia: WHO Guidelines.* Geneva: World Health Organization; 2019. This report also summarizes evidence-based recommendations to prevent dementia.

- *National Plan to Address Alzheimer's Disease: 2022 Update,* available at https://aspe.hhs.gov/topics/aging-disability/alzheimers-dementia. This summarizes the U.S. national plan for dementia, focusing more on services for people with dementia than on prevention.

- CDC's National Brain Health Initiative, at https://www.cdc.gov/aging/nationalinitiatives/national-healthy-nhbi.html provides plain-language resources for policy-makers, health professionals, persons with dementia, and their caregivers.

References

1. Azevedo FAC, Carvalho LRB, Grinberg LT, et al. Equal numbers of neuronal and nonneuronal cells make the human brain an isometrically scaled-up primate brain. *J Comp Neurol.* 2009;513(5):532-541. doi:10.1002/cne.21974

2. World Health Organization. *Mental Health Atlas 2020.* Geneva; 2021.

3. American Psychiatric Association. *Diagnostic and Statistical Manual of Mental Disorders, Fifth Edition, Text Revision.* 5th ed. American Psychiatric Association; 2022. doi:10.1176/appi.books.9780890425596

4. Gonzales L, Kanani A, Pereyra A. Policy definitions for "serious mental Illness" across 56 United States, districts and territories. *Community Ment Health J.* 2023;59(3):595-599. doi:10.1007/s10597-022-01026-5

5. Jablensky A. The diagnostic concept of schizophrenia: Its history, evolution, and future prospects. *Dialogues Clin Neurosci.* 2010;12(3):271-287.

6. Kuhn R, Cahn CH. Eugen Bleuler's concepts of psychopathology. *Hist Psychiatry.* 2004;15(3):361-366. doi:10.1177/0957154X04044603

7. Jauhar S, Johnstone M, McKenna PJ. Schizophrenia. *Lancet.* 2022;399(10323):473-486. doi:10.1016/S0140-6736(21)01730-X

8. Messias EL, Chen CY, Eaton WW. Epidemiology of schizophrenia: Review of findings and myths. *Psychiatric Clinics of North America.* 2007;30(3):323-338. doi:10.1016/j.psc.2007.04.007

9. Owen MJ, Sawa A, Mortensen PB. Schizophrenia. *Lancet.* 2016;388(10039):86-97. doi:10.1016/S0140-6736(15)01121-6

10. van Os J, Kapur S. Schizophrenia. *Lancet.* 2009;374(9690):635-645. doi:10.1016/S0140-6736(09)60995-8

11. Wiersma D, Nienhuis FJ, Slooff CJ, Giel R. Natural course of schizophrenic disorders: A 15-year follow-up of a Dutch incidence cohort. *Schizophr Bull.* 1998;24(1):75-85. doi:10.1093/oxfordjournals.schbul.a033315

12. Hjorthøj C, Stürup AE, McGrath JJ, Nordentoft M. Years of potential life lost and life expectancy in schizophrenia: A systematic review and meta-analysis. *Lancet Psychiatry.* 2017;4(4):295-301. doi:10.1016/S2215-0366(17)30078-0

13. Murray RM, Bhavsar V, Tripoli G, Howes O. Thirty years on: How the neurodevelopmental hypothesis of schizophrenia morphed into the developmental risk factor model of psychosis. *Schizophr Bull.* 2017;43(6):1190-1196. doi:10.1093/schbul/sbx121

14. McCutcheon RA, Reis Marques T, Howes OD. Schizophrenia: An overview. *JAMA Psychiatry.* 2020;77(2):201-210. doi:10.1001/jamapsychiatry.2019.3360

15. Feinberg I. Schizophrenia: caused by a fault in programmed synaptic elimination during adolesence? *J Psychiatr Res.* 1982;17:319-334.

16. Mullen J, Richards J, Crawford A. Amphetamine-related psychiatric disorders. *StatPearls.* 2023.

17. McCutcheon RA, Reis Marques T, Howes OD. Schizophrenia: An overview. *JAMA Psychiatry.* 2020;77(2):201-210. doi:10.1001/jamapsychiatry.2019.3360

18. Khokhar JY, Dwiel LL, Henricks AM, Doucette WT, Green AI. The link between schizophrenia and substance use disorder: A unifying hypothesis. *Schizophr Res.* 2018;194:78-85. doi:10.1016/j.schres.2017.04.016

19. Van Os J, Linscott RJ, Myin-Germeys I, Delespaul P, Krabbendam L. A systematic review and meta-analysis of the psychosis continuum: Evidence for a psychosis proneness-persistence-impairment model of psychotic disorder. *Psychol Med.* 2009;39(2):179-195. doi:10.1017/S0033291708003814

20. McGrath J, Saha S, Chant D, Welham J. Schizophrenia: A concise overview of incidence, prevalence, and mortality. *Epidemiol Rev.* 2008;30(1):67-76. doi:10.1093/epirev/mxn001

21. Charlson FJ, Ferrari AJ, Santomauro DF, et al. Global epidemiology and burden of schizophrenia: Findings from the global burden of disease study 2016. *Schizophr Bull.* 2018;44(6):1195-1203. doi:10.1093/schbul/sby058

22. Bresnahan M, Begg MD, Brown A, et al. Race and risk of schizophrenia in a US birth cohort: Another example of

health disparity? *Int J Epidemiol.* 2007;36(4):751-758. doi:10.1093/ije/dym041

23. Kendler KS, Gallagher TJ, Abelson JM, Kessler RC. Lifetime prevalence, demographic risk factors, and diagnostic validity of nonaffective psychosis as assessed in a US community sample: The National Comorbidity Survey. *Arch Gen Psychiatry.* 1996;53:1022-1031.

24. Devylder J, Anglin D, Munson MR, et al. Ethnoracial variation in risk for psychotic experiences. *Schizophr Bull.* 2023;49(2):385-396. doi:10.1093/schbul/sbac171

25. Davies C, Segre G, Estradé A, et al. Prenatal and perinatal risk and protective factors for psychosis: A systematic review and meta-analysis. *Lancet Psychiatry.* 2020;7(5):399-410. doi:10.1016/S2215-0366(20)30057-2

26. Fuglewicz AJ, Piotrowski P, Stodolak A. Relationship between toxoplasmosis and schizophrenia: A review. *Adv Clin Exp Med.* 2017;26(6):1033-1038. doi:10.17219/acem/61435

27. Brown AS, Derkits EJ. Prenatal infection and schizophrenia: A review of epidemiologic and translational studies. *Am J Psychiatry.* 2010;167:261-280.

28. Rosenfield PJ, Jiang D, Pauselli L. Childhood adversity and psychotic disorders: Epidemiological evidence, theoretical models and clinical considerations. *Schizophr Res.* 2022;247:55-66. doi:10.1016/j.schres.2021.06.005

29. Matheson SL, Shepherd AM, Pinchbeck RM, Laurens KR, Carr VJ. Childhood adversity in schizophrenia: A systematic meta-analysis. *Psychol Med.* 2013;43(2):225-238. doi:10.1017/S0033291712000785

30. Varese F, Smeets F, Drukker M, et al. Childhood adversities increase the risk of psychosis: A meta-analysis of patient-control, prospective-and cross-sectional cohort studies. *Schizophr Bull.* 2012;38(4):661-671. doi:10.1093/schbul/sbs050

31. Cantor-Graae E, Selten JP. Schizophrenia and migration: A meta-analysis and review. *Am J Psychiatry.* 2005;162:12-24.

32. Vassos E, Pedersen CB, Murray RM, Collier DA, Lewis CM. Meta-analysis of the association of urbanicity with schizophrenia. *Schizophr Bull.* 2012;38(6):1118-1123. doi:10.1093/schbul/sbs096

33. Marconi A, Di Forti M, Lewis CM, Murray RM, Vassos E. Meta-analysis of the association between the level of cannabis use and risk of psychosis. *Schizophr Bull.* 2016;42(5):1262-1269. doi:10.1093/schbul/sbw003

34. Zammit S, Allebeck P, Andreasson S, Lundberg I, Lewis G. Self-reported cannabis use as a risk factor for schizophrenia in Swedish conscripts of 1969: Historical cohort study. *BMJ.* 2002;325:1199-1204.

35. Di Forti M, Quattrone D, Freeman TP, et al. The contribution of cannabis use to variation in the incidence of psychotic disorder across Europe (EU-GEI): A multicentre case-control study. *Lancet Psychiatry.* 2019;6(5):427-436. doi:10.1016/S2215-0366(19)30048-3

36. Little R, D'Mello D. Theories on cannabis and schizophrenia. *Innov Clin Neurosci.* 2022;19(7-9):38-43.

37. SAMHSA. National survey of drug use and health 2019 detailed tables. *2019 National Survey of Drug Use and Health Releases.* Published 2020. Accessed September 25, 2023. Available at: https://www.samhsa.gov/data/report/2019-nsduh-detailed-tables

38. Freeman TP, Craft S, Wilson J, et al. Changes in delta-9-tetrahydrocannabinol (THC) and cannabidiol (CBD) concentrations in cannabis over time: Systematic review and meta-analysis. *Addiction.* 2021;116(5):1000-1010. doi:10.1111/add.15253

39. Malhi GS, Mann JJ. Depression. *Lancet.* 2018;392(10161):2299-2312. doi:10.1016/S0140-6736(18)31948-2

40. Kessler RC, Tat Chiu W, Demler O, Walters EE. Prevalence, severity, and comorbidity of 12-month DSM-IV disorders in the National Comorbidity Survey Replication. *Arch Gen Psychiatry.* 2005;62:617-627.

41. Kessler RC, Berglund P, Demler O, et al. The epidemiology of major depressive disorder. *JAMA.* 2003;289(23):3095. doi:10.1001/jama.289.23.3095

42. Kessler RC, Bromet EJ. The epidemiology of depression across cultures. *Annu Rev Public Health.* 2013;34:119-138. doi:10.1146/annurev-publhealth-031912-114409

43. Angst J, Angst F, Stassen HH. Suicide risk in patients with major depressive disorder. *J Clin Psych.* 1999;60(suppl 2):57-62.

44. Hall JE, Hall ME. The limbic system and the hypothalamus: behavioral and motivational mechanisms in the brain. In: *Guyton and Hall Textbook of Medical Physiology.* 14th ed. Elsevier; 2021:741-752.

45. Harvard Health Publishing. Understanding the stress response. Published July 6, 2020. Accessed October 15, 2023. Available at: https://www.health.harvard.edu/staying-healthy/understanding-the-stress-response

46. Möhler H. The GABA system in anxiety and depression and its therapeutic potential. *Neuropharmacology.* 2012;62:42-53. doi:10.1016/j.neuropharm.2011.08.040

47. Krishnan V, Nestler EJ. The molecular neurobiology of depression. *Nature.* 2008;455(7215):894-902. doi:10.1038/nature07455

48. Jesulola E, Micalos P, Baguley IJ. Understanding the pathophysiology of depression: From monoamines to the neurogenesis hypothesis model—are we there yet? *Behav Brain Res.* 2018;341:79-90. doi:10.1016/j.bbr.2017.12.025

49. Nemeroff CB. The state of our understanding of the pathophysiology and optimal treatment of depression: Glass half full or half empty? *Am J Psychiatry.* 2020;177(8):671-685. doi:10.1176/appi.ajp.2020.20060845

50. Cohen S, Janicki-Deverts D, Miller GE. Psychological stress and disease. *JAMA.* 2007;298(14):1685-1678.

51. Lo CC, Gerling HM, Ash-Houchen W, Cheng TC. Violent victimization, stressful events, and depression: A longitudinal study of young adults in the U.S. *Community Ment Health J.* 2021;57(3):502-511. doi:10.1007/s10597-020-00673-w

52. Yang L, Zhao Y, Wang Y, et al. The effects of psychological stress on depression. *Curr Neuropharmacol.* 2015;13:494-504.

53. Juruena MF. Early-life stress and HPA axis trigger recurrent adulthood depression. *Epilepsy & Behav.* 2014;38:148-159. doi:10.1016/j.yebeh.2013.10.020

54. Cameron HA, Glover LR. Adult neurogenesis: Beyond learning and memory. *Annu Rev Psychol.* 2015;66:53-81. doi:10.1146/annurev-psych-010814-015006

55. Substance Use and Mental Health Services Administration. Key substance use and mental health indicators in the United States: Results from the 2022 National Survey on Drug Use and Health. Published 2023. Accessed June 17, 2024. Available at: https://www.samhsa.gov/data/sites/default/files/reports/rpt42731/2022-nsduh-nnr.pdf

56. Hasin DS, Sarvet AL, Meyers JL, et al. Epidemiology of adult DSM-5 major depressive disorder and its specifiers in the United States. *JAMA Psychiatry.* 2018;75(4):336-346. doi:10.1001/jamapsychiatry.2017.4602

57. Santomauro DF, Mantilla Herrera AM, Shadid J, et al. Global prevalence and burden of depressive and anxiety disorders in 204 countries and territories in 2020 due to the COVID-19 pandemic. *Lancet*. 2021;398(10312):1700-1712. doi:10.1016/S0140-6736(21)02143-7

58. Twenge JM, Martin GN, Campbell WK. Decreases in psychological well-being among American adolescents after 2012 and links to screen time during the rise of smartphone technology. *Emotion*. 2018;18(6):765-780. doi:10.1037/emo0000403

59. Twenge JM, Cooper AB, Joiner TE, Duffy ME, Binau SG. Age, period, and cohort trends in mood disorder indicators and suicide-related outcomes in a nationally representative dataset, 2005-2017. *J Abnorm Psychol*. 2019;128(3):185-199. doi:10.1037/abn0000410

60. Substance Use and Mental Health Services Administration. Key substance use and mental health indicators in the United States: Results from the 2020 National Survey on Drug Use and Health. Published 2021. Accessed June 17, 2024. Available at: https://www.samhsa.gov/data/sites/default/files/reports/rpt42731/2022-nsduh-nnr.pdf

61. Krokstad S, Weiss DA, Krokstad MA, et al. Divergent decennial trends in mental health according to age reveal poorer mental health for young people: Repeated cross-sectional population-based surveys from the HUNT Study, Norway. *BMJ Open*. 2022;12(5). doi:10.1136/bmjopen-2021-057654

62. Thapar A, Eyre O, Patel V, Brent D. Depression in young people. *Lancet*. 2022;400(10352):617-631. doi:10.1016/S0140-6736(22)01012-1

63. Centers for Disease Control and Prevention. WISQARS: Web-based injury statistics query and reporting system. Published 2023. Accessed June 17, 2024. Available at: https://wisqars.cdc.gov/

64. Sullivan PF, Michael Neale FC, Kendler KS. Reviews and overviews genetic epidemiology of major depression: Review and meta-analysis. *Am J Psychiatry*. 2000;157:1552-1562.

65. Kessler RC, McLaughlin KA, Green JG, et al. Childhood adversities and adult psychopathology in the WHO world mental health surveys. *Br J Psychiatry*. 2010;197(5):378-385. doi:10.1192/bjp.bp.110.080499

66. Liu M, Kamper-DeMarco KE, Zhang J, Xiao J, Dong D, Xue P. Time spent on social media and risk of depression in adolescents: A dose–response meta-analysis. *Int J Environ Res Public Health*. 2022;19:5164. doi:10.3390/ijerph19095164

67. McAllister C, Hisler GC, Blake AB, Twenge JM, Farley E, Hamilton JL. Associations between adolescent depression and self-harm behaviors and screen media use in a nationally representative time-diary study. *Res Child Adolesc Psychopathol*. 2021;49(12):1623-1634. doi:10.1007/s10802-021-00832-x

68. Chochol MD, Gandhi K, Croarkin PE. Social media and anxiety in youth: A narrative review and clinical update. *Child Adolesc Psychiatr Clin N Am*. 2023;32(3):613-630. doi:10.1016/j.chc.2023.02.004

69. Riehm KE, Feder KA, Tormohlen KN, et al. Associations between time spent using social media and internalizing and externalizing problems among US youth. *JAMA Psychiatry*. 2019;76(12):1266-1273. doi:10.1001/jamapsychiatry.2019.2325

70. Twenge JM. Why increases in adolescent depression may be linked to the technological environment. *Curr Opin Psychol*. 2020;32:89-94. doi:10.1016/j.copsyc.2019.06.036

71. Goodwin RD, Weinberger AH, Kim JH, Wu M, Galea S. Trends in anxiety among adults in the United States, 2008-2018: Rapid increases among young adults. *J Psychiatr Res*. 2020;130:441-446. doi:10.1016/j.jpsychires.2020.08.014

72. Burstein B, Agostino H, Greenfield B. Suicidal attempts and ideation among children and adolescents in US Emergency Departments, 2007-2015. *JAMA Pediatr*. 2019;173(6):598. doi:10.1001/jamapediatrics.2019.0464

73. Hedegaard H, Curtin SC, Warner M. Suicide Mortality in the United States, 1999-2019. *NCHS Data Brief*. 2021;(398):1-7.

74. Wickramaratne PJ, Yangchen T, Lepow L, et al. Social connectedness as a determinant of mental health: A scoping review. *PLoS One*. 2022;17(10):e0275004. doi:10.1371/journal.pone.0275004

75. Gariépy G, Honkaniemi H, Quesnel-Vallée A. Social support and protection from depression: Systematic review of current findings in Western countries. *British Journal of Psychiatry*. 2016;209(4):284-293. doi:10.1192/bjp.bp.115.169094

76. Choi KW, Stein MB, Nishimi KM, et al. An exposure-wide and Mendelian randomization approach to identifying modifiable factors for the prevention of depression. *American Journal of Psychiatry*. 2020;177(10):944-954. doi:10.1176/appi.ajp.2020.19111158

77. Domènech-Abella J, Mundó J, Haro JM, Rubio-Valera M. Anxiety, depression, loneliness and social network in the elderly: Longitudinal associations from The Irish Longitudinal Study on Ageing (TILDA). *J Affect Disord*. 2019;246:82-88. doi:10.1016/j.jad.2018.12.043

78. Mann F, Wang J, Pearce E, et al. Loneliness and the onset of new mental health problems in the general population. *Soc Psychiatry Psychiatr Epidemiol*. 2022;57(11):2161-2178. doi:10.1007/s00127-022-02261-7

79. Shaw RJ, Cullen B, Graham N, et al. Living alone, loneliness and lack of emotional support as predictors of suicide and self-harm: A nine-year follow up of the UK Biobank cohort. *J Affect Disord*. 2021;279:316-323. doi:10.1016/j.jad.2020.10.026

80. Department of Health and Human Services, Office of Assistant Secretary for Health. *Our Epidemic of Loneliness and Isolation: The U.S. Surgeon General's Advisory on the Healing Effects of Social Connection and Community*. Published 2023. Accessed June 17, 2024. Available at: https://www.hhs.gov/sites/default/files/surgeon-general-social-connection-advisory.pdf

81. Gabarrell-Pascuet A, García-Mieres H, Giné-Vázquez I, et al. The association of social support and loneliness with symptoms of depression, anxiety, and posttraumatic stress During the COVID-19 pandemic: A meta-analysis. *Int J Environ Res Public Health*. 2023;20(4). doi:10.3390/ijerph20042765

82. Frank P, Jokela M, Batty GD, Lassale C, Steptoe A, Kivimäki M. Overweight, obesity, and individual symptoms of depression: A multicohort study with replication in UK Biobank. *Brain Behav Immun*. 2022;105:192-200. doi:10.1016/j.bbi.2022.07.009

83. Luppino FS, De Wit LM, Bouvy PF, et al. Overweight, obesity, and depression: A systematic review and meta-analysis of longitudinal studies. *Arch Gen Psychatriry*. 2010;67(3).

84. Jokela M, Laakasuo M. Obesity as a causal risk factor for depression: Systematic review and meta-analysis of Mendelian randomization studies and implications for

population mental health. *J Psychiatr Res.* 2023;163:86-92. doi:10.1016/j.jpsychires.2023.05.034

85. Schuch FB, Vancampfort D, Firth J, et al. Physical activity and incident depression: A meta-analysis of prospective cohort studies. *Am J Psychiatry.* 2018;175(7):631-648. doi:10.1176/appi.ajp.2018.17111194

86. Kandola AA, del Pozo Cruz B, Osborn DPJ, Stubbs B, Choi KW, Hayes JF. Impact of replacing sedentary behaviour with other movement behaviours on depression and anxiety symptoms: A prospective cohort study in the UK Biobank. *BMC Med.* 2021;19(1). doi:10.1186/s12916-021-02007-3

87. Kandola A, Ashdown-Franks G, Hendrikse J, Sabiston CM, Stubbs B. Physical activity and depression: Towards understanding the antidepressant mechanisms of physical activity. *Neurosci Biobehav Rev.* 2019;107. doi:10.1016/j.neubiorev.2019.09.040

88. Gobbi G, Atkin T, Zytynski T, et al. Association of cannabis use in adolescence and risk of depression, anxiety, and suicidality in young adulthood: A systematic review and meta-analysis. *JAMA Psychiatry.* 2019. doi:10.1001/jamapsychiatry.2018.4500

89. Department of Health and Human Services, Office of the Assistant Secretary for Health. *Social Media and Youth Mental Health; Advisory of the US Surgeon General.* Published 2023. Accessed June 17, 2024. Available at: https://www.hhs.gov/sites/default/files/sg-youth-mental-health-social-media-advisory.pdf

90. Murthy VH. Surgeon General: Why I'm calling for a warning label on social media platforms. *The New York Times.* Published June 17, 2024. Accessed June 16, 2024. Available at: https://www.nytimes.com/2024/06/17/opinion/social-media-health-warning.html

91. O'Connor EA, Perdue LA, Coppola EL, Henninger ML, Thomas RG, Gaynes BN. Depression and suicide risk screening: Updated evidence report and systematic review for the US Preventive Services Task Force. *JAMA.* 2023;329(23):2068-2085. doi:10.1001/jama.2023.7787

92. Olfson M, Blanco C, Wall MM, Liu SM, Grant BF. Treatment of common mental disorders in the United States: Results from the national epidemiologic survey on alcohol and related conditions-III. *J Clin Psychiatry.* 2019;80(3). doi:10.4088/JCP.18m12532

93. Penninx BW, Pine DS, Holmes EA, Reif A. Anxiety disorders. *Lancet.* 2021;397(10277):914-927. doi:10.1016/S0140-6736(21)00359-7

94. Craske MG, Stein MB. Anxiety. *Lancet.* 2016;388(10063): 3048-3059. doi:10.1016/S0140-6736(16)30381-6

95. Szuhany KL, Simon NM. Anxiety disorders: A review. *JAMA.* 2022;328(24):2431-2445. doi:10.1001/jama.2022.22744

96. Teicher MH, Samson JA. Annual research review: Enduring neurobiological effects of childhood abuse and neglect. *J Child Psychol Psychiatry.* 2016;57(3):241-266. doi:10.1111/jcpp.12507

97. Moreno-Peral P, Conejo-Cerón S, Motrico E, et al. Risk factors for the onset of panic and generalised anxiety disorders in the general adult population: A systematic review of cohort studies. *J Affect Disord.* 2014;168:337-348. doi:10.1016/j.jad.2014.06.021

98. Kessler RC, Berglund P, Demler O, et al. Lifetime prevalence and age-of-onset distributions of DSM-IV disorders in the National Comorbidity Survey Replication. *Arch Gen Psychiatry.* 2005;62:593-602.

99. Baxter AJ, Scott KM, Vos T, Whiteford HA. Global prevalence of anxiety disorders: A systematic review and meta-regression. *Psychol Med.* 2013;43(5):897-910. doi:10.1017/S003329171200147X

100. Baxter AJ, Vos T, Scott KM, et al. The regional distribution of anxiety disorders: Implications for the Global Burden of Disease Study, 2010. *Int J Methods Psychiatr Res.* 2014;23(4):422-438. doi:10.1002/mpr.1444

101. Gardner MJ, Thomas HJ, Erskine HE. The association between five forms of child maltreatment and depressive and anxiety disorders: A systematic review and meta-analysis. *Child Abuse Negl.* 2019;96. doi:10.1016/j.chiabu.2019.104082

102. Whitaker RC, Dearth-Wesley T, Herman AN, et al. The interaction of adverse childhood experiences and gender as risk factors for depression and anxiety disorders in US adults: A cross-sectional study. *BMC Public Health.* 2021;21(1). doi:10.1186/s12889-021-12058-z

103. Loades M, Chatburn E, Higson-Sweeney N, et al. Rapid systematic review: The impact of social isolation and loneliness on the mental health of children and adolescents in the context of COVID-19. *J Am Acad Child Adolesc Psychiatry.* 2020;59(11):1218-1239. www.jaacap.org.

104. Zimmermann M, Chong AK, Vechiu C, Papa A. Modifiable risk and protective factors for anxiety disorders among adults: A systematic review. *Psychiatry Res.* 2020;285:112705. doi:10.1016/j.psychres.2019.112705

105. Taylor GMJ, Lindson N, Farley A, et al. Smoking cessation for improving mental health. *Cochrane Database of Systematic Reviews.* 2021;2021(3):CD013522. doi:10.1002/14651858.CD013522.pub2

106. Nasir M, Trujillo D, Levine J, Dwyer JB, Rupp ZW, Bloch MH. Glutamate systems in DSM-5 anxiety disorders: Their role and a review of glutamate and GABA psychopharmacology. *Front Psychiatry.* 2020;11. doi:10.3389/fpsyt.2020.548505

107. Livingston G, Huntley J, Sommerlad A, et al. Dementia prevention, intervention, and care: 2020 report of the Lancet Commission. *Lancet.* 2020;396(10248):413-446. doi:10.1016/S0140-6736(20)30367-6

108. Knopman DS, Gottesman RF, Sharrett AR, et al. Mild cognitive impairment and dementia prevalence: The Atherosclerosis Risk in Communities Neurocognitive Study. *Alzheimer's and Dementia: Diagnosis, Assessment and Disease Monitoring.* 2016;2:1-11. doi:10.1016/j.dadm.2015.12.002

109. Soria Lopez JA, González HM, Léger GC. Alzheimer's disease. In: *Handbook of Clinical Neurology.* Vol 167. Elsevier B.V.; 2019:231-255. doi:10.1016/B978-0-12-804766-8.00013-3

110. Oh ES, Rabins PV. Dementia. *Ann Intern Med.* 2019;171(5):ITC33–ITC46. doi:10.7326/AITC201909030

111. Yarns BC, Holiday KA, Carlson DM, Cosgrove CK, Melrose RJ. Pathophysiology of Alzheimer's disease. *Psychiatr Clin North Am.* 2022;45(4):663-676. doi:10.1016/j.psc.2022.07.003

112. Scheltens P, De Strooper B, Kivipelto M, et al. Alzheimer's disease. *Lancet.* 2021;397(10284):1577-1590. doi:10.1016/S0140-6736(20)32205-4

113. Margeta M, Perry A. Alzheimer Disease. In: Kumar V, Abbas AK, Aster JC, Turner JR, eds. *Robbins and Cotran Pathologic Basis of Disease.* 10th ed. Elsevier; 2021:1275-1279.

114. Dintica CS, Yaffe K. Epidemiology and risk factors for dementia. *Psychiatr Clin North Am.* 2022;45(4):677-689. doi:10.1016/j.psc.2022.07.011

115. Hay J, Johnson VE, Smith DH, Stewart W. Chronic traumatic encephalopathy: The neuropathological legacy of traumatic brain injury. *Annual Review of Pathology: Mechanisms of Disease*. 2016;11:21-45. doi:10.1146/annurev-pathol-012615-044116

116. Wong EC, Chui HC Chui C. Vascular cognitive impairment and dementia. *Continuum (NY)*. 2022;28(3):750-780.

117. Kalaria RN. The pathology and pathophysiology of vascular dementia. *Neuropharmacology*. 2018;134:226-239. doi:10.1016/j.neuropharm.2017.12.030

118. Global Burden of Disease Collaboration, Institute for Health Metrics and Evaluation. GBD Results. Published July 12, 2023. Accessed July 11, 2023. Available at: https://vizhub.healthdata.org/gbd-results/

119. Cao Q, Tan CC, Xu W, et al. The prevalence of dementia: A systematic review and meta-analysis. *J Alzheimer's Dis*. 2020;73(3):1157-1166. doi:10.3233/JAD-191092

120. Wang X, Bakulski KM, Paulson HL, Albin RL, Park SK. Associations of healthy lifestyle and socioeconomic status with cognitive function in U.S. older adults. *Sci Rep*. 2023;13:7513. doi:10.1038/s41598-023-34648-0

121. Koster A, Penninx BWJH, Bosma H, et al. Socioeconomic differences in cognitive decline and the role of biomedical factors. *Ann Epidemiol*. 2005;15(8):564-571. doi:10.1016/j.annepidem.2005.02.008

122. Yaffe K, Falvey C, Harris TB, et al. Effect of socioeconomic disparities on incidence of dementia among biracial older adults: Prospective study. *BMJ (Online)*. 2013;347:f7051. doi:10.1136/bmj.f7051

123. Nichols E, Steinmetz JD, Vollset SE, et al. Estimation of the global prevalence of dementia in 2019 and forecasted prevalence in 2050: An analysis for the Global Burden of Disease Study 2019. *Lancet Public Health*. 2022;7(2):e105–e125. doi:10.1016/S2468-2667(21)00249-8

124. Farrer LA, Cupples LA, Haines JL, et al. Effects of age, sex, and ethnicity on the association between apolipoprotein E genotype and Alzheimer disease: A meta-analysis. *JAMA*. 1997;278(16):1349-1356.

125. Ward A, Crean S, Mercaldi CJ, et al. Prevalence of apolipoprotein E4 genotype and homozygotes (APOE e4/4) among patients diagnosed with Alzheimer's disease: A systematic review and meta-analysis. *Neuroepidemiology*. 2012;38(1):1-17. doi:10.1159/000334607

126. Gharbi-Meliani A, Dugravot A, Sabia S, et al. The association of APOE ε4 with cognitive function over the adult life course and incidence of dementia: 20 years follow-up of the Whitehall II study. *Alzheimers Res Ther*. 2021;13(1). doi:10.1186/s13195-020-00740-0

127. Ridley NJ, Draper B, Withall A. Alcohol-related dementia: An update of the evidence. *Alzheimers Res Ther*. 2013;5:3. doi:10.1186/alzrt157

128. World Health Organization. *Risk Reduction of Cognitive Decline and Dementia: WHO Guidelines*. Published 2019. Accessed June 17, 2024. Available at: https://www.who.int/publications/i/item/9789241550543

129. Strout KA, David DJ, Dyer EJ, Gray RC, Robnett RH, Howard EP. Behavioral interventions in six dimensions of wellness that protect the cognitive health of community-dwelling older adults: A systematic review. *J Am Geriatr Soc*. 2016;64(5):944-958. doi:10.1111/jgs.14129

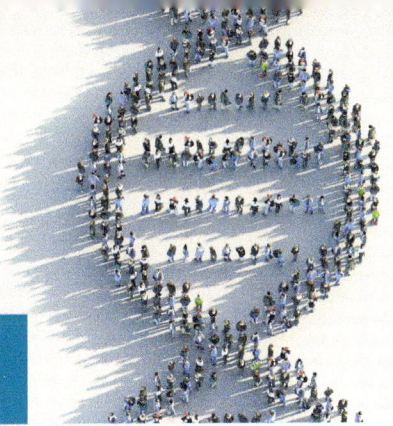

CHAPTER 6

Injuries

Taken as a group, injuries kill more than 250,000 Americans per year, ranking them just below heart disease and cancer among leading causes of death.[1] And unlike heart disease or cancer, injuries tend to kill people when they are young, so they are even more important causes of years of life lost (YLL).[1] Injuries can be prevented, though, by applying some of the same public health principles that have been used to reduce rates of heart disease and cancer.

Overview of Injuries

Injuries are classified in two ways: by the **intent** of the person(s) involved—also known as the **manner** of injury—and by the **mechanism**. The intent or manner of an injury is grouped into:

- **Unintentional**, which are often called accidents.
- **Intentional**:
  - **Self-harm** or **suicide** if the injury resulted from a person attempting to harm themselves.
  - **Assault** or **homicide** if the injury resulted from one person attempting to harm another.
- **Legal intervention**, in which law enforcement officers injure a person while acting in the line of duty. These injuries might be considered assaults or homicides, but the CDC maintains this distinction in national data.
- **Undetermined**, if the intent of the person(s) involved is not known.

All injuries involve an external object or substance coming into contact with a person and causing tissue damage. There are hundreds of different mechanisms by which this can happen, including motor vehicle crashes, firearm shootings, and falls. And poisonings (for example, opioid overdoses) are classified as injuries also because they involve damage from an external substance.

Any intent can be paired with any injury mechanism. For example, fatal firearm injuries can be unintentional, suicides, homicides, or the result of legal intervention. Likewise, fatal falls can be unintentional, suicides (that is, jumps), homicides (for example, one person pushing another off a balcony), or legal intervention. By tradition, all injuries from motor vehicle crashes for which the manner is unknown are classified on death certificates as unintentional, even though some of those crashes are probably suicidal and a few may be homicidal.

Figure 6.1 shows injury deaths in the United States by intent and mechanism.[2] The most common manner is unintentional. The most common mechanisms are poisonings, firearms, falls, and motor vehicle crashes. Most poisoning deaths are unintentional, but some are suicidal. In contrast, most firearm injuries are intentional, with suicide a more common intent than homicide.

This chapter covers motor vehicle crash injuries, firearm injuries, and falls and has a small section on suicides regardless of mechanism. Poisonings are discussed in Chapter 13. Use of Addictive Drugs.

Injury Prevention Strategy and the Haddon Matrix

Much of the progress in injuries in the past century has come from finding opportunities for prevention that had been overlooked. Figure 6.1 illustrates a key concept that helps identify these opportunities. It is natural to consider injuries grouped by their intent—that is, how can we prevent homicides, suicides, and accidents? When the questions are framed this way,

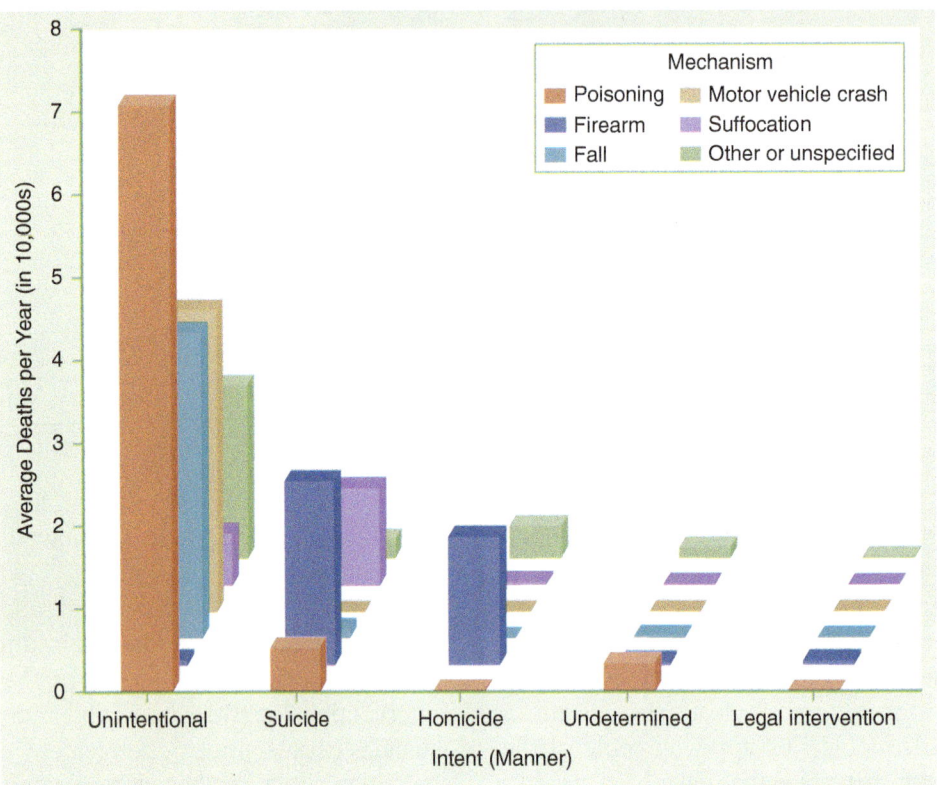

Figure 6.1 Injury Deaths in the United State by Intent and Mechanism, 2018–2021. Injuries are classified by both the intent (also known as the manner) and the mechanism involved. The most common manner of injury death is unintentional, and the most common mechanisms are poisonings, firearms, falls, and motor vehicle crashes. Most firearm deaths are intentional (suicide or homicide) but most deaths from other mechanisms are unintentional.

Data from National Center for Health Statistics, Centers for Disease Control and Prevention. Underlying Cause of Death Data on CDC WONDER. Published 2023. Accessed June 12, 2024. https://wonder.cdc.gov/Deaths-by-Underlying-Cause.html

the answers often are police, mental health treatment, and safety education. But when injuries are instead grouped by mechanism, the questions change. How can we prevent motor vehicle crashes? How can we prevent firearm injuries? The reframed questions prompt different answers, such as designing safer cars or safer guns.

The person who first applied public health concepts like these to injury prevention was the physician and epidemiologist William Haddon. He described all injuries as interactions among three actors: a human, a "vehicle" (such as a car or gun), and the "environment" in which the injury takes place.[3] Factors of any of those three can affect the likelihood and severity of an injury. For example, a motor vehicle rollover crash injury is more likely if the human who is driving is drunk, the car has a high center of gravity, or the roadway is poorly lit.

Haddon took the model one step further with what is now called the Haddon Matrix. Factors relating to humans, vehicles, and the environment can influence the risk of injury in any of three phases: *pre-event*, *event*, and *post-event*, in which the "event" is the motor vehicle crash, shooting, fall, etc.[3]

Table 6.1 shows how the matrix can be applied to motor vehicle crash injuries. Pre-event factors affect the likelihood that a crash will take place, and they include alcohol use by the human or speed limits in the environment. Event factors affect the likelihood that an injury will take place if a crash were to occur, and they include energy-absorbing steering columns and use of seat belts. Post-event factors influence the outcome of an injury after it occurs, such as systems of emergency medical care and the ease of access to a crashed vehicle.

The Haddon Matrix shows that preventing injuries is complicated. The matrix has nine cells, and within each cell there are several actions that could be taken. As the section below on motor vehicle crashes shows, this leads to a long list of very diverse preventive interventions, such as roadway roundabouts, electronic stability control, motorcycle helmet laws, and alcohol taxes. Individually these interventions may prevent only a small fraction of injuries, but together they can prevent many. The section after that on firearm injuries shows how this kind of multifaceted approach might be applied to a persistent problem that needs public health solutions.

Table 6.1 The Haddon Matrix Describing Factors Influencing Motor Vehicle Crash Injuries

Factors that influence the risk of injury include human factors, vehicle factors, and environment factors, and these factors can exert their influence in any of three phases: pre-event, event, or post-event. The table shows examples of factors of each type for each phase involved in motor vehicle crash injuries.

Phase	Human Factors	Vehicle Factors	Environment Factors
Pre-event	Alcohol use	Rollover potential	Road design
	Distracted driving	Video screens on car consoles	Traffic-calming devices
	Driver education	Automatic emergency braking	Speed limits
		Electronic stability control	Sidewalks and bicycle lanes
Event	Use of seat belts	Airbags	Guardrails
	Use of motorcycle helmets	Seat belts	Breakaway light poles
		Energy-absorbing steering column	
Post-event	First-aid skills	Ease of access to crashed vehicles	EMS system
		Fire risk	

Box 6.1 Key Words–Injuries

Assault
Homicide
Intent (of an injury)
Intentional injury
Legal intervention
Manner (of an injury)
Mechanism (of an injury)
Self-harm
Suicide
Unintentional injury

Motor Vehicle Crash Injuries

Introduction

The story of motor vehicle crash (MVC) injuries in the United States was once considered a major public health achievement.[4]

In the first half of the 20th century, as more people owned and drove cars, the mortality rate from MVCs rose sharply.[5] During this time, safety experts viewed car crashes to be "accidents" caused by careless drivers.[6] That view pointed to one solution—driver education—which was never very effective.[7,8]

But in the 1960s, health and safety experts underwent a crucial shift in how they thought about car crashes. In 1966, Congress passed the Highway Safety Act, which established what is now the National Highway Traffic Safety Administration (NHTSA). The person chosen to lead the new agency was William Haddon. Haddon introduced the idea that MVC injuries do not have one cause, like driver error, but instead have multiple **component causes**, including the designs of cars and roads. (For more on component causes of disease, see Chapter 1. Disease Prevention and Populations.) Haddon used his matrix to clarify those component causes for MVC injuries.[3] After identifying many different prevention opportunities, his agency established standards for safer roads and safer cars that protected drivers even when they made errors. Haddon's rules saved tens of thousands of lives within a decade and led to a plummeting of MVC deaths into the 2000s.[9]

Unfortunately, as discussed below, in recent years that public health victory has been partly reversed. The concepts of prevention that Haddon used in the 1960s are still valuable, but they need to keep up with changes in technology and society.

Mechanisms of MVC Injuries

Designing safer roads and vehicles requires understanding exactly how roads and vehicles injure people. Among NHTSA's contributions to prevention are detailed systems to collect standardized data on vehicle crashes to improve that understanding. Countless different interactions of roadways, vehicles, and people can end in injuries, but the data show that a few mechanisms are especially common. It helps to think of them separately as mechanisms for crashes (pre-event phase, using the Haddon Matrix) and mechanisms for injuries resulting from crashes (event phase).

Common Mechanisms for Crashes

Most fatal crashes in the United States are one of four types, in this order of frequency (**Figure 6.2**):

- *Multiple vehicle crashes.* About 40% of fatal crashes involve one motor vehicle (car, truck, or motorcycle) colliding with another. Most fatal multiple-vehicle crashes occur not on limited-access highways and not on local roads, but instead on **arterial** or **collector roads** between them.[10] These roads typically have traffic flowing in opposite directions, often without **median barriers** separating them. That design poses a risk of vehicles colliding with others going in the opposite direction by straying across the center line or when making left turns. Also, these roads often have many **driveway access points**, that is, places where cars can enter the roadway between intersections (for example, from strip malls), risking collisions with those on the road.[11,12]
- *Single vehicle crashes* (often called run-off-road crashes). Nearly 30% of fatal crashes involve a single vehicle running off the road and hitting a fixed object, like a ditch, tree, or pole.[10] These are more likely to occur on roads in rural areas with tight turns, narrow lanes, narrow shoulders, fixed objects close to roadways, or road designs that change abruptly.[13,14]
- *Vehicle-on-pedestrian or -bicyclist crashes.* Just under one-fourth of fatal crashes involve a vehicle hitting a pedestrian or bicyclist. Most crashes involving pedestrians occur in urban areas, during dark hours, with the pedestrian on the road between intersections.[10,15] Most bicyclists fatally hit by vehicles are also on roads, usually between intersections.[10,16] Designs that favor these types of crashes are roads that do not have sidewalks or crosswalks for pedestrians and that do not have separate protected lanes or traffic signals for bicyclists.
- *Rollover crashes.* When a vehicle is driving through a curve, the driver can steer too much ("oversteer"), causing the rear of the car to "spin out" and the vehicle to turn sideways and then roll over. Rollover crashes are more common on roads that have curves and hills, and during wet or snowy weather.[17] They usually involve pickup trucks or sports-utility vehicles that have high centers of gravity.[10]

All types of crashes are more likely to occur if the vehicle is moving at a high speed and if any person involved is under the influence of alcohol or other drugs, or distracted by a smart phone or other device.

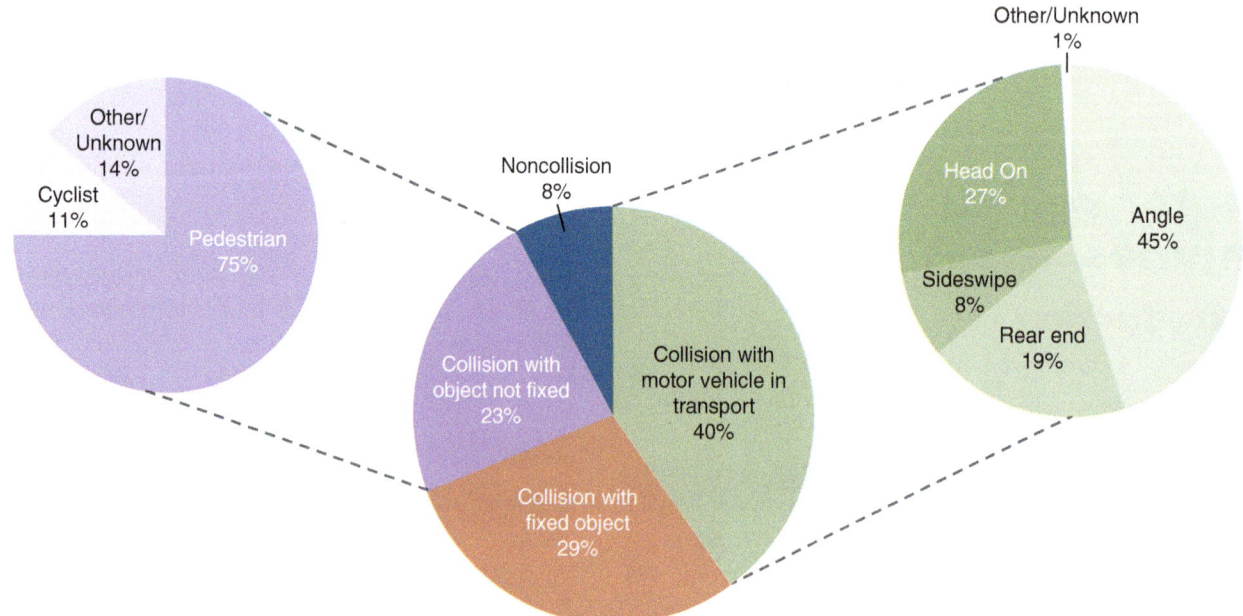

Figure 6.2 First Harmful Event for Fatal Crashes in the United States, 2021. Mechanisms of crashes in which a death occurred. Of these, 40% are multiple vehicle crashes ("collision with a motor vehicle in transport"), 29% are single vehicle crashes ("collision with a fixed object"), 23% involve a vehicle hitting a pedestrian, bicyclist, or other moving object ("collision with an object not fixed"), and 8% are non-collision (mostly rollover) crashes.

Data from National Highway Traffic Safety Administration. Traffic Safety Facts 2021: A Compilation of Motor Vehicle Traffic Crash Data (Table 29). Washington; 2022. https://crashstats.nhtsa.dot.gov/

Common Mechanisms for Injuries in a Crash

Cars are much better designed than they once were to protect drivers and passengers in crashes, but they still allow many serious injuries.

- *Vehicle occupant injuries.* In a head-on crash, drivers and passengers are thrown forward, risking injuries to the head (hitting the windshield) or chest (hitting the steering wheel or dashboard).[18-22] Side crashes are much less common but more deadly because a car door absorbs less impact than an engine compartment.[18,23] Intrusion of the door can cause injuries to the chest, abdomen, and pelvis.[18-20] When the crash impact is from the rear, vehicle occupants are thrown backward and can have neck (whiplash) injuries.[19] Vehicle rollovers are especially dangerous. If passengers are not wearing seatbelts, they are tossed around within the vehicle or thrown from it (ejected). Even if they are wearing seat belts, they can be crushed by a collapse of the vehicle's roof.[19]
- *Motorcyclists* who crash do not have steel cages protecting them, so they are about five times as likely to be injured and about ten times as likely to die as people who crash in cars.[10] Those who

do not wear helmets are most likely to get head injuries, which are particularly lethal. These crashes are especially common in low-and middle-income countries, where motorcycles are used much more than they are in the United States.[24]
- *Pedestrians* involved in crashes are typically not run over but instead are "run under" by the front of the vehicle. That causes head injuries as they hit the car's hood or windshield.[25]
- *Bicyclists* struck by vehicles can have injuries to many body parts, but injuries to the head are particularly likely to be fatal.[26]

Epidemiology: Patterns and Trends

Figure 6.3 shows 50-year trends in MVC deaths in the United States. Between 1966 and 2010, deaths per vehicle mile traveled dropped by an astonishing 80%.[10] Unfortunately, that benefit was blunted by Americans driving more; during those years, the average number of vehicle miles traveled per person more than doubled.[10] Then, since 2011, except for an interruption during the COVID-19 pandemic, MVC death rates have been rising, measured either as deaths per 100,000 persons or deaths per vehicle-mile traveled.

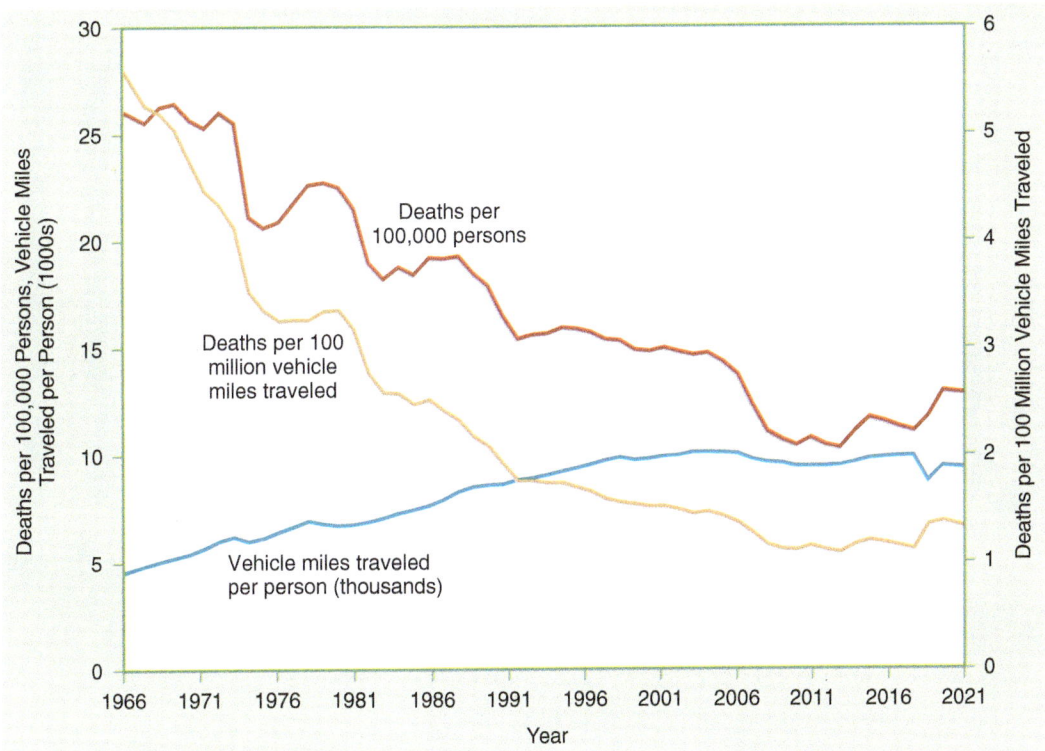

Figure 6.3 Trends in Motor Vehicle Crash Deaths in the United States, 1966–2022. Deaths per capita or per vehicle-mile traveled fell from 1966 to 2011, even as the average vehicle miles traveled more than doubled. However, these two measures of mortality from motor vehicle crashes have been rising since about 2011.

Data from National Highway Traffic Safety Administration. Traffic Safety Facts 2021: A Compilation of Motor Vehicle Traffic Crash Data. Washington; 2022. https://crashstats.nhtsa.dot.gov/

The number and pedestrians and bicyclists killed is increasing even faster than the number of drivers and passengers.[10]

In the early 2020s, more than 40,000 Americans died in MVCs each year.[10] Of those, about half were drivers and about 15% each were passengers, motorcyclists, and pedestrians (**Figure 6.4**).

Figure 6.5 shows MVC mortality rates in the United States by age, race, and sex.[2] Unlike for most diseases, mortality rates for MVC crashes are high in young adults. Men are far more likely than women to die from MVCs. Mortality rates are higher in African American and American Indian/Alaska Native populations than in White populations, and are much lower in Asian populations.[2]

Deaths from MVCs are a major public health problem across the globe, too. Worldwide, MVCs kill more people than malaria, tuberculosis, HIV/AIDS, and most forms of cancer and are the sixth leading cause of years of life lost.[27] Among high-income countries, the United States has one of the highest MVC mortality

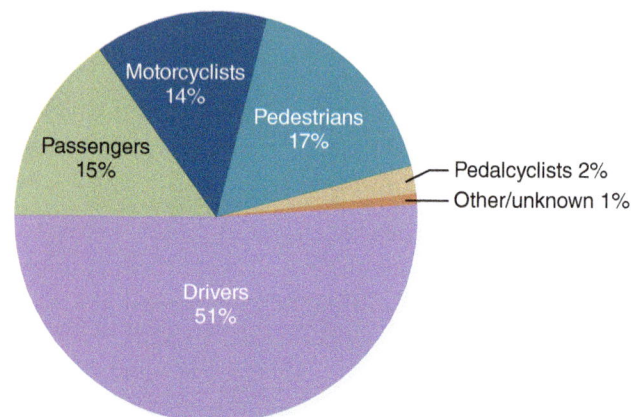

Figure 6.4 Victims in Fatal Motor Vehicle Crashes, United States, 2021.

Data from National Highway Traffic Safety Administration. Traffic Safety Facts 2021: A Compilation of Motor Vehicle Traffic Crash Data. Washington; 2022. https://crashstats.nhtsa.dot.gov/

rates in the world, with a rate about five times that of Norway and Sweden.[28] But MVC mortality rates are even higher in low-income countries, especially those in Southeast Asia (**Figure 6.6**).[29]

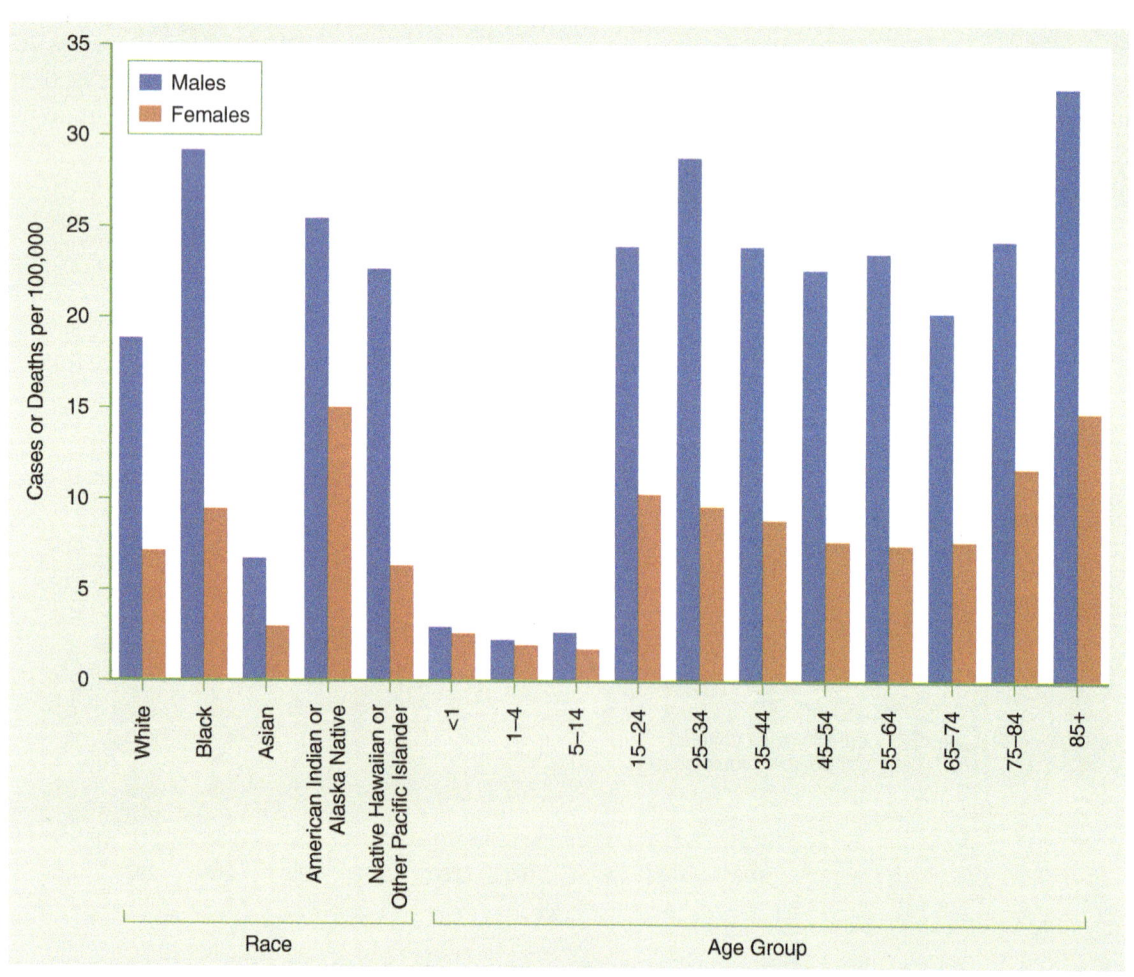

Figure 6.5 Motor Vehicle Traffic Mortality Rates in the United States by Age, Race, and Sex, 2021. Deaths from motor vehicle crashes are more common in men, in Black populations, and in both younger adults and the oldest adults.

Data from National Center for Health Statistics, Centers for Disease Control and Prevention. Underlying Cause of Death Data on CDC WONDER. Published 2023. Accessed June 12, 2024. https://wonder.cdc.gov/Deaths-by-Underlying-Cause.html

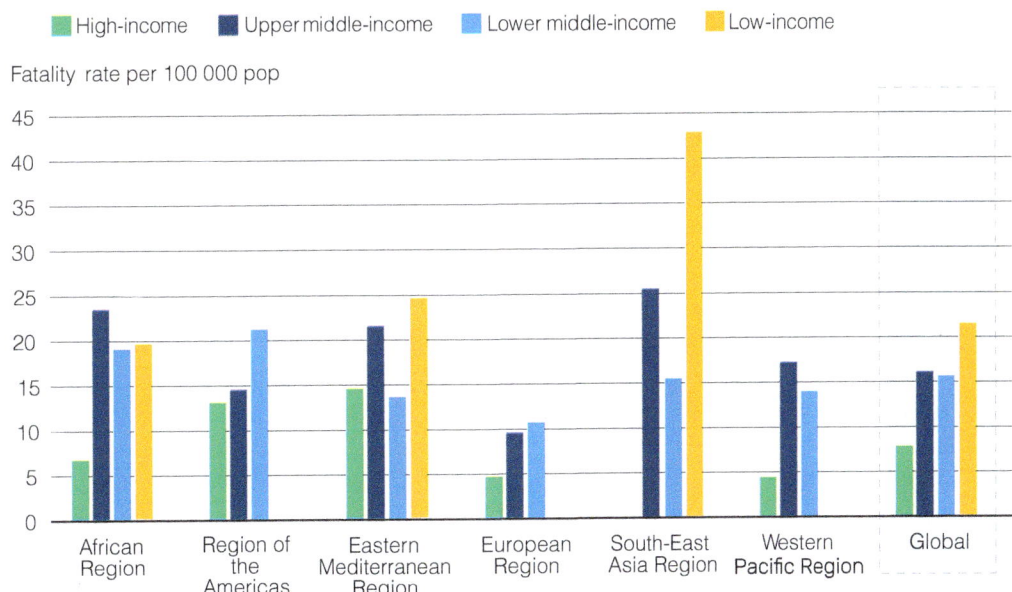

Figure 6.6 **Motor Vehicle Crash Mortality Rates Worldwide, by Region and Country Income, 2021.** While the United States has among the highest motor vehicle crash mortality rates among high-income countries, rates are higher in low-and middle-income countries, especially those in Southeast Asia.

Reproduced from World Health Organization. Global Status Report on Road Safety 2023. Geneva; 2023. Accessed July 27, 2024. https://www.who.int/publications/i/item/9789240086517

Risk Factors

The most important risk factors for MVC injuries are (**Figure 6.7**):

- *Land use-created dependence on motor vehicles.* When people drive more, more are likely to crash and become injured. A risk factor for MVC injuries that is often overlooked is people's

dependence on vehicles for transportation, which stems from how communities assign uses for land. Where land is segregated into separate residential, commercial, and industrial zones, people must travel long distances to buy groceries, go to school, or go to work, leaving little choice other than to drive. The dependence on cars is greater if the streets do not have sidewalks, crosswalks,

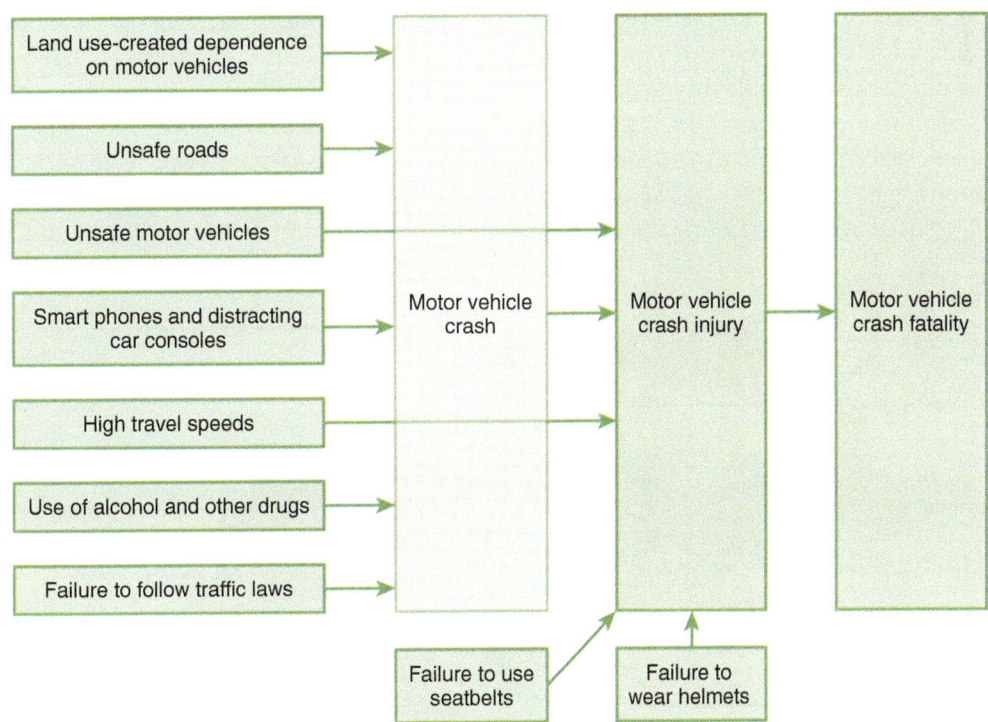

Figure 6.7 **Cause-and-Effect Diagram for Motor Vehicle Crash Injuries.**

or bicycle lanes, and if public transit systems are inconvenient.

- *Unsafe roads.* While communities are continuously working to improve road safety, there are still too many road segments with dangerous features, such as having *multiple driveway access points*, and the *absence of median barriers, turn lanes, or, traffic signals at intersections*, or the *absence of streetlights*.[11,30] Pedestrians are often at risk because of the the *absence of sidewalks, crosswalks at intersections, or pedestrian phases at traffic lights.* Bicyclists are often at risk because of a *lack of protected bike lanes.*

- *Unsafe motor vehicles.* Safety features now built into cars include crumple zones in the front and rear, high-strength steel "cages" surrounding occupants, head restraints, energy-absorbing steering columns, seat belts, and airbags (**Figure 6.8**).[31] Still, cars and trucks could be even safer. For example, they do not protect drivers enough in side-impact crashes, have blind spots for drivers, and cause head injuries to pedestrians and bicyclists. And children are not effectively protected in a crash by safety belts that are designed for adults.

- *Smart phones and distracting car consoles.* Distracted driving is a large and growing problem because people and cars carry technology that is designed to grab and hold people's attention.[32] If a driver takes his eyes off the road for 5 seconds while looking at a text, at a speed of 60 mph, that driver has effectively driven the length of 1½ football fields with his eyes closed.[33] Texting or talking on a mobile phone while driving increases the crash risk threefold to fourfold.[34] In a very disturbing national survey, more than one-fifth of drivers admitted that they watched videos, made video calls, or used social media on most or all of

their driving trips.[35] Increasingly, drivers are also distracted by car consoles. These consoles have not only many confusing controls, but also digital screens that allow people to watch videos or play video games while driving.[36]

- *High travel speeds.* When people drive faster, they are both more likely to get into a crash (with shorter reaction times and longer stopping distances), and more likely to cause an injury if they do crash. The risk of injury from a crash rises not in proportion to the speed of vehicles, but instead exponentially.[37] Those who face the greatest risk are pedestrians and bicyclists hit by cars. About 90% of pedestrians will survive a collision with a car traveling at 25 mph (40 kph), but only about 50% will survive if the car is traveling at 50 mph (80 kph).[38]

- *Unsafe behaviors by drivers, riders, and pedestrians.* Errors by drivers contribute to nearly all MVCs.[32] Unsafe behavior by cyclists and pedestrians also contributes to the problem. The behaviors (other than distracted driving) that are most important are:
  - *Use of alcohol and other drugs.* People under the influence of alcohol are more aggressive, less perceptive of risks, more likely to take risks that they do perceive, more impulsive, slower to react to risks, and less coordinated. Even consuming one drink—enough to raise the blood alcohol content to about 0.03%, depending on body weight—increases the risk of a fatal crash about threefold.[39] In the United States, 30% of deaths from automobile crashes involve a driver who is alcohol-impaired.[40] Other **psychoactive drugs** can also impair drivers' judgment and slow their reaction time. In a study from five cities, about 50% of people

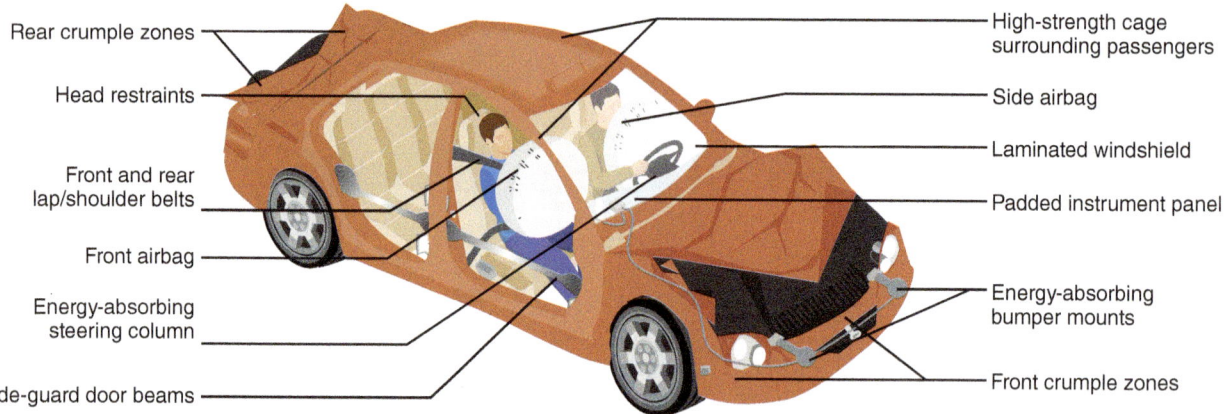

Figure 6.8 Safety Features in New Cars.

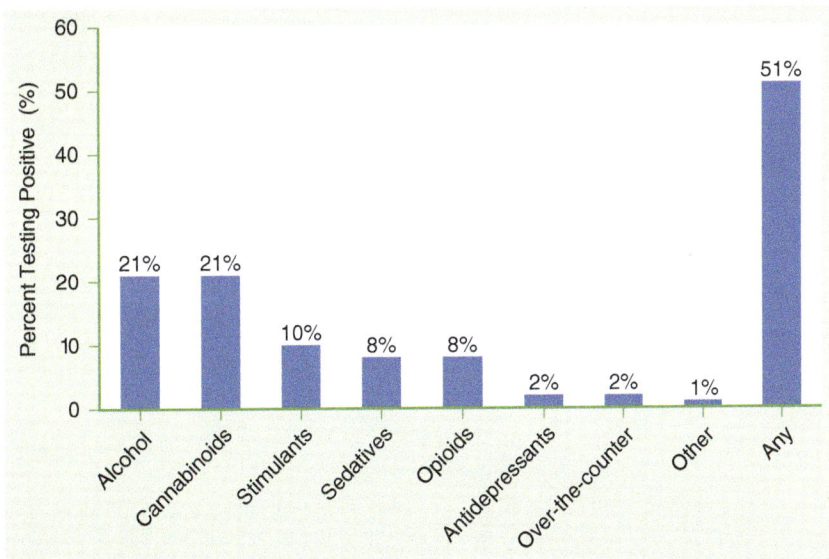

Figure 6.9 **Percent of Persons Killed and Seriously Injured in Motor Vehicle Crashes Found to Have Drugs in Body, United States, 2019.**

Data from Thomas F, Berning A, Darrah J, et al. Drug and Alcohol Prevalence in Seriously and Fatally Injured Road Users Before and During the COVID-19 Public Health Emergency. National Highway Traffic Safety Administration (Report No. DOT HS 813 018).

killed or seriously injured in a crash were found to have drugs in their systems.[41] The most common drugs were alcohol and marijuana, but the testing found many other street drugs and pharmaceutical drugs (**Figure 6.9**), and many people had been using more than one drug.[41]

- *Failure to follow traffic laws.* Traffic laws are meant to protect people, but many people ignore them. NHTSA estimates that **speeding**, that is, driving faster than the legal speed limit, contributes to nearly 30% of fatal crashes in the United States.[42] In addition, some driver and bicyclists run through red lights and stop signs, and some pedestrians jaywalk or cross intersections against the signals.
- *Behaviors of drivers, riders, and pedestrians that increase injuries from a crash.* Some people do not use equipment that can protect them:
  - *Failure to use seat belts.*[23] Of all the automobile safety features, the one that currently saves the most lives—by far—is the seat belt. Even with air bags, seatbelts are estimated to reduce deaths in a crash by about 50%–60%.[31] With mandatory seat belt laws, 92% of Americans now use them, but that leaves 8% who put themselves at risk by not wearing them. In 2021, 50% of U.S. vehicle occupants who were killed were not wearing seat belts.[43]
  - *Failure of motorcyclists and bicyclists to wear helmets.* Motorcycle helmets reduce head injuries by about 70% and reduce deaths by about 40%, but only about two-thirds of motorcyclists wear them.[44,45] Helmets are about equally protective of bicyclists, and bicyclists are even less likely to wear them.[46]

Preventive Interventions

The World Health Organization, the U.S. Department of Transportation, and many states and cities have similar strategies for reducing MVC injuries.[47,48] They consider even a single death or serious injury from a MVC unacceptable, so in many places MVC plans use the title **Vision Zero**. These plans are grounded in the **Safe System Approach**, which recognizes that people make mistakes and that the transportation system should protect them when they do.[47-49]

Interventions to address the risk factors for MVC injuries include:

- *Transportation and land-use systems that reduce dependence on private vehicles.* Injuries would be less frequent if people were to drive less, more often using other **modes of transportation**— walking, bicycling, and using buses, trains, and transit systems. People have the option to use these other modes with *higher-density, mixed land-use development* and *infrastructure for walking, bicycling, and public transit*, like sidewalks, bike lanes, and tram systems. The World Health Organization calls these changes **multi-modal transport and land use planning**.[47]

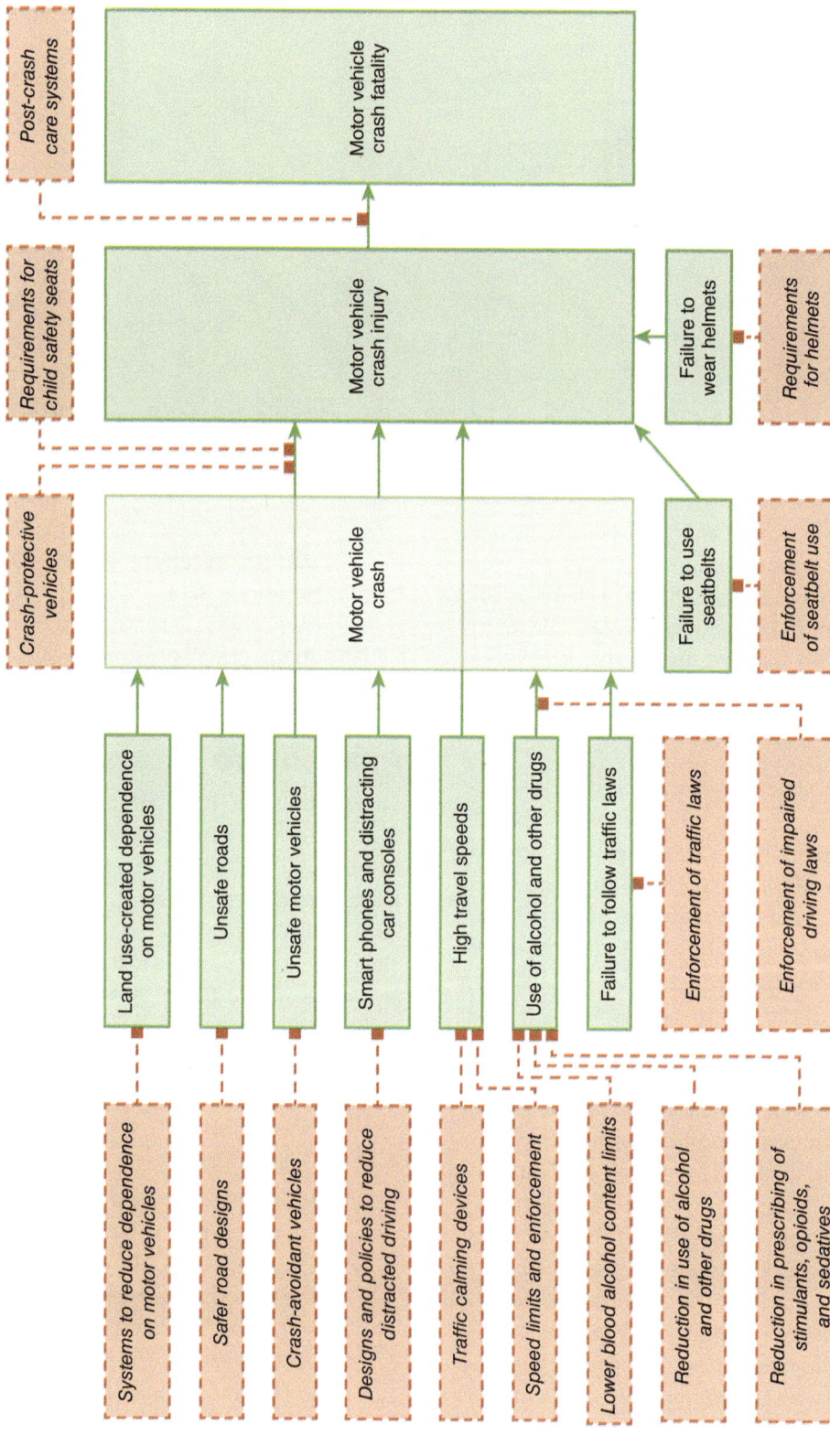

Figure 6.10 Cause-and-Effect Diagram for Motor Vehicle Crash Injuries, with Preventive Interventions.

- *Safer road designs.* Roads can incorporate safety features like median barriers to separate high-speed traffic, turn lanes, reduction of access driveways, conversion of intersections into circular **roundabouts**,[50] sidewalks, crosswalks, and protected bicycle lanes.[47] In countries with large numbers of motorcycle crashes, the World Health Organization recommends separate motorcycle lanes.[51]

- *Safer vehicles.* Vehicle safety standards must be continuously strengthened as technology advances. Most safety features today are what might be called *crash-protective*, that is, they are designed to protect vehicle occupants in a crash (event phase). Examples are collapsing steering columns and air bags. But increasingly, safety features are *crash-avoidant*, that is, they reduce the risk that a crash will occur (pre-event phase). Crash-avoidant technology that is already required on new vehicles is **electronic stability control**, which helps prevent cars at high speeds from steering too little or too much, reducing both single-vehicle and rollover crashes.[52] Technology that is appearing on new vehicles includes systems that sense an impending front crash and sound an alarm and (for some systems) automatically apply the brakes (**automatic emergency braking**).[53] Because most fatal crashes involve an impact from the front, these systems have great potential. Another crash-avoidant safety feature that could be required is **intelligent speed assistance**, which warns drivers or reduces power to the engine if drivers go faster than the speed limit.[54] Other safety features protect those hit by vehicles, such as "pop-up hoods" that help protect pedestrians from a head injury.[25] And future safety devices may include those that prevent people who are impaired from alcohol or drugs from driving.[55]

- *Designs and policies to reduce distracted driving.* Laws can prohibit people from holding electronic devices while driving. These laws are already in effect in some, but far from all, U.S. states.[35] Smart phones have a "do not disturb" feature that disables nonemergency calls and texting. Smartphone manufacturers can turn on this feature by default while the user is driving.[56] And car makers could be prohibited from building cars with consoles that are overly complex or that can show videos to drivers.[56]

- *Reduction of vehicle speeds with:*
  - *Traffic-calming devices.* Cars drive slower where there are **traffic-calming devices** built into roads. These include not just speed bumps

and speed humps but also roundabouts, road narrowing, **rumble strips** (a series of small road bumps that causes vibrations in a vehicle passing on top), and **chicanes** (curves deliberately added).[49]

- *Speed limits and their enforcement.* Lower speed limits let drivers know what speeds are considered safe. To reduce injuries, some cities in the United States are lowering default speed limits, for example, from 30 to 25 mph. The World Health Organization's plan encourages communities to consider limits of 50 km/h (16 mph) in urban areas and 30 km/h (10 mph) in areas with high numbers of pedestrians and cyclists.[49]

- *Safer traveler behavior:*
  - *Reduction in use of alcohol.* Any intervention that reduces alcohol consumption should reduce injuries from alcohol-related MVCs (see Chapter 12. Alcohol Use). For example, a modest increase in alcohol taxes in Illinois in 2009 was followed by a 26% reduction in alcohol-related crash deaths.[57]
  - *Lower blood alcohol content limits.* Nearly all high-income countries other than the United States prohibit driving with a blood alcohol level above 0.05%.[28] In the United States, 49 states and the District of Columbia have a higher limit of 0.08%, despite the higher risk of fatal crashes even at 0.05%.[28,39] After Utah lowered its limit to 0.05 percent, MVC fatalities fell by about 15%.[55]
  - *Enforcement of impaired driving laws.* **Sobriety checkpoints** involve the police stopping drivers at high-risk locations and times to identify drivers who are alcohol-and drug-impaired and take their keys away. When these checkpoints are visible and publicized, they reduce drunk driving.[55] Also, some people make a habit of drinking and driving. This repeated risky behavior can be reduced by fines, sentences for community service, and revocation of their driver's license. Most states also require offenders to use **ignition interlock devices**, which prevent vehicles from being started by people who have high breath alcohol levels.[55]
  - *Reduction in use of other psychoactive drugs.* It is clear from Figure 6.9 that alcohol is not the only drug involved in MVC deaths. Steps that reduce use of other recreational drugs (particularly marijuana, cocaine, and methamphetamine) and the prescribing of

psychoactive drugs (particularly stimulants, opioids, and sedatives) should reduce these injuries.

- *Enforcement of traffic laws.* To get the full protective benefit of traffic laws, they need to be enforced. In particular, although nearly all U.S. states require people in cars to wear seat belts, many still do not allow police to pull over drivers solely for not wearing them. Those states have lower seat belt use.[58] Crash fatalities can also be reduced by enforcement of laws prohibiting jaywalking and requiring drivers or bicyclists to stop at red lights. Automatic cameras at intersections can simplify this enforcement.[59]

- *Promotion of and requirements for child safety seats.* Child safety seats greatly reduce the risk of injury in a motor vehicle crash.[60] Use of these safety seats can be increased by distribution of safety seats and by laws requiring their use.[60]

- *Requirements for helmets.* Most U.S. states and many countries do not require motorcyclists to wear helmets,[61] even though these laws greatly increase helmet use.[24] Almost no jurisdictions require adult bicyclists to wear helmets. Requirements would substantially reduce serious head injuries and fatalities in both motorcyclists and bicyclists.[62]

Box 6.2 Summary—Prevention of MVC Injuries

- Transportation and land-use systems that reduce dependence on private vehicles
- Safer road designs
- Safer vehicles
  - Crash-avoidant
  - Crash-protective
- Designs and policies to reduce distracted driving
- Reduction of vehicle speeds
  - Traffic-calming devices
  - Speed limits and their enforcement
- Safer traveler behavior
  - Reduction in use of alcohol
  - Lower blood alcohol content limits
  - Enforcement of impaired driving laws
  - Reduction in use of other psychoactive drugs
  - Enforcement of traffic laws
  - Promotion of and requirements for child safety seats
  - Requirements for helmets
- Post-crash care systems

Box 6.3 Key Words—Motor Vehicle Crash Injuries

Arterial roads
Automatic emergency braking
Chicanes
Collector roads
Component cause
Driveway access points
Electronic stability control systems
Ignition interlock devices
Intelligent speed assistance
Median barriers
Mode(s) of transportation
Multi-modal transport and land use planning
Psychoactive drugs
Roundabouts
Rumble strips
Safe System Approach
Sobriety checkpoints
Speeding
Traffic-calming devices
Vision Zero

- *Post-crash care systems.* Of people who die from MVCs in the United States, an estimated 40% were alive when ambulances arrived. Better post-event systems of ambulances and qualified trauma centers to quickly transport victims for expert treatment may be able to save some of those who are injured.[48]

Resources—Motor Vehicle Crash Injuries

- The National Highway Traffic Safety Administration (NHTSA) maintains a website with extensive data on motor vehicle crashes, as well as analytic reports under the title *Traffic Safety Facts* at https://www.nhtsa.gov/data

- The Insurance Institute for Highway Safety and the Highway Loss Data Institute provide easy-to-understand, evidence-based reviews of the impact of motor vehicle technology and policies at https://www.iihs.org

- The Federal Highway Administration of the U.S. Department of Transportation supports the UNC Highway Safety Research Center to maintain a huge clearinghouse of studies on features of roadways that influence crash risks. The results of these studies are summarized as "crash mitigation factors" used by transportation departments in designing or redesigning roads. These summaries are available at www.cmfclearinghouse.org

- The World Health Organization's *Global Plan: Decade of Action for Road Safety 2021-2030* and *Save LIVES: A Road Safety Technical Package* are available at www.who.int/publications. Also available at this link from the WHO are a series of manuals for policymakers on specific topics, such as pedestrian safety and two-and three-wheeler safety.

Firearm Injuries

Introduction

As with injuries from motor vehicle crashes, injuries from firearms were long considered a problem caused by individual people. Suicides were viewed as caused by people with mental illnesses, homicides by criminals, and unintentional gun shots by careless gun owners. Since the late 1900s, though, public health experts have argued that firearm injuries are a social problem with many **component causes** that can be prevented with a public health approach.[63] Just as interventions to reduce injuries from motor vehicle crashes can be directed at people, motor vehicles, or roads, interventions to reduce injuries from firearms can be directed at the people, firearms themselves, or the environments in which guns are used. And many public health solutions apply regardless of the intent—for example, interventions to reduce firearm suicides will also prevent some homicides and unintentional injuries.

The United States has well-funded government and non-governmental organizations that analyze data on motor vehicle crashes and design safer roads and safer cars. If it had a similar effort on firearms, many firearm injuries might be prevented. As with motor vehicle crashes, each individual intervention may prevent only a small fraction of injuries, but the combined impact of many different interventions could be large.

Firearms

Firearms can be either **handguns** (most of which are either **semiautomatic pistols** or **revolvers**) or **long guns** (**rifles** or **shotguns**). Rifles fire individual bullets at high speeds of about 3,000 feet per second accurately over long distances. Shotguns fire packets of metal pellets (shot) at lower speeds of about 1,200 feet per second. Handguns fire individual bullets at lower speeds of about 1,000 feet per second and are less accurate. People shooting handguns often do not hit an intended target; the main advantages of these guns are that they can be easily carried and concealed.[64]

Nearly 90% of handguns sold in the United States are semiautomatic pistols.[65] These guns store ammunition **cartridges** (each composed of a bullet, a powdered **propellant**, and a **primer** in a metal **casing**) in a **magazine** within the pistol's grip (**Figure 6.11**). The user loads the first cartridge from the magazine into the **chamber** at the base of the gun's barrel by pulling back the **slide** on top of the gun. Then when the **trigger** is pulled, the hammer strikes the **firing**

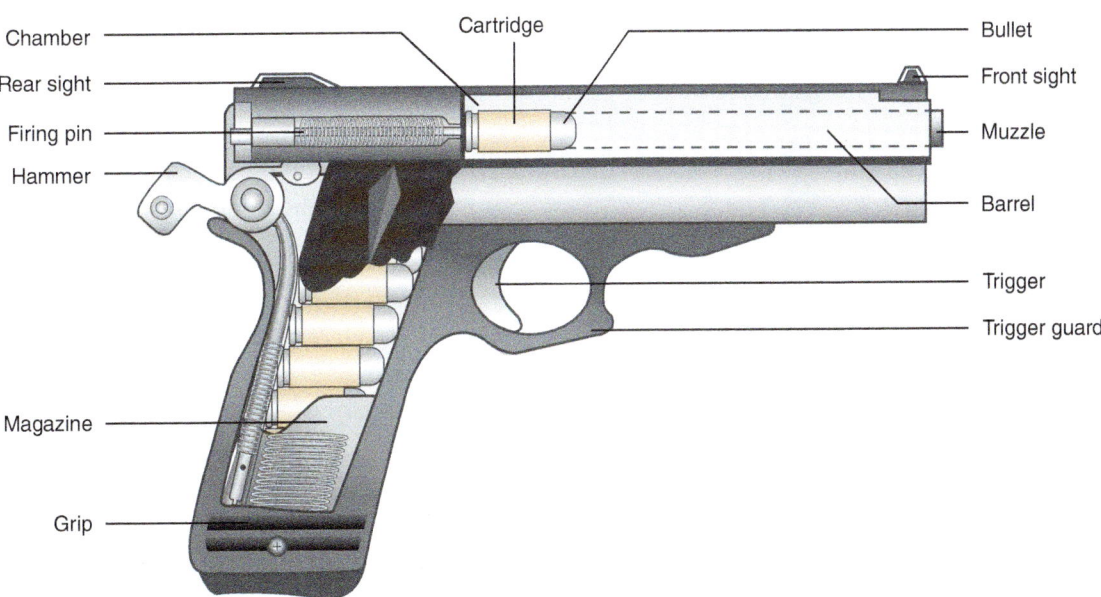

Figure 6.11 Anatomy of a Semiautomatic Pistol. Semiautomatic pistols store ammunition cartridges in a magazine within the pistol's grip. When the trigger is pulled, the hammer strikes the firing pin, which ignites the cartridge's propellant, sending the bullet down the barrel. The recoil pushes the slide backwards, which then loads another cartridge into the chamber.

pin, which ignites the cartridge's propellant, sending the bullet down the **barrel** and out of the gun's **muzzle**. The recoil from the firing of the bullet pushes the slide backwards, which then loads another cartridge into the chamber.

Firearm Injuries

In the 2020s, firearms kill about 43,000 Americans each year.[2] About twice that number are shot but survive. When combining fatal and nonfatal shootings, assaults and unintentional injuries are the most common intents (**Figure 6.12**). The outcomes differ greatly by intent though, with 89% of self-harm, 26% of assault, and 1% of unintentional shootings fatal.[66] Those shootings lead to about 25,000 firearm suicides, 17,000 firearm homicides, and 500 unintentional firearm deaths per year in the United States.[2]

Common Mechanisms of Gun Violence

There are many circumstances in which a gun can harm someone. But, as with injuries from motor vehicle crashes, a few circumstances are particularly common:

- *Self-harm.* Victims of self-harm shootings often are under psychological stress by conflicts with their intimate partners, physical health problems, or use of alcohol or drugs.[67] Their decisions are often impulsive. For example, in one study of people who survived suicide attempts, 70% said they had made the decision less than an hour before the attempt and 24% had made the decision less than 5 minutes before.[68] Those decisions are often heavily influenced by alcohol.[67] Most firearm suicides take place in the victims' homes,[67] using guns that are already owned by a household member (that is, not purchased just for the suicide), and most of them are handguns.

- *Neighborhood assaults.* Assaults with firearms often take place with teenage or young adult men as both perpetrators and victims, and disproportionately involve Black men in low-income neighborhoods.[69-71] Roughly half of both victims and perpetrators of violence have been violent perpetrators previously.[72] In most homicides, the shooter and the person shot know each other.[67] Some occur as part of another crime, such as a robbery or a burglary, and some are related to gang activity.[67] Often, the people involved are intoxicated with alcohol.[73] For men killed in homicides, shootings usually take place not at home, but outdoors or in a car, usually at night.[67,74] They almost all involve handguns, and usually the handguns were bought not directly from licensed gun retailers, but instead from other individuals, often illegally.[75-78]

- *Intimate partner violence.* Conflicts between intimate partners can lead to shootings. Women are far less likely to be victims of firearm homicides than men, but for those who are, about half the time the shooter is their intimate partner.[67] (Intimate partner violence is not just a problem for women, though. Eight percent of male homicide victims are killed by their intimate partners.)[67] The shooting usually happens in the home,[67] often with a gun owned by one of the partners or another household member.[79]

Less common, though still very disturbing, circumstances for shootings include:

- *Mass shootings.* Sometimes horrific events occur in which one person (sometimes with a semiautomatic rifle and a magazine holding many cartridges) shoots numerous others in a public place, like a workplace, store, place of worship, or even a school. These events can be psychologically traumatizing to the entire nation. In the United States, shootings involving four or more persons account for about 4% of firearm homicides and 2% of total firearm deaths.[80]

- *Unintentional shootings.* There are about 500 unintentional firearm deaths per year in the United States.

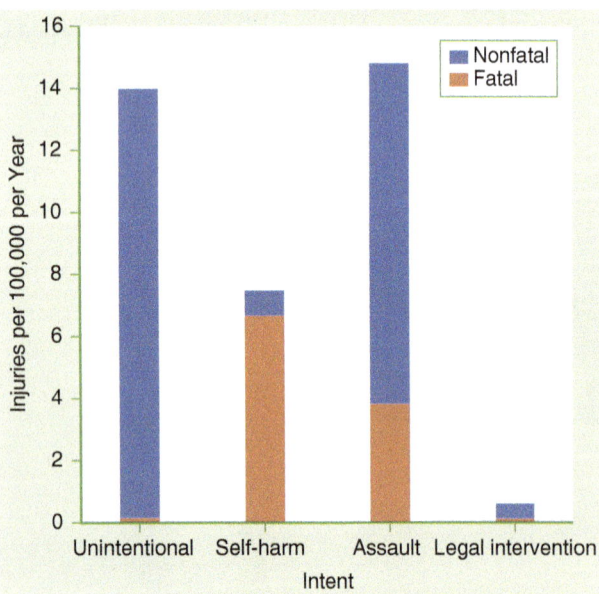

Figure 6.12 **Firearm injuries in the United States by Intent and Outcome, 2009–2017.** The most common intents are assaults and unintentional firearm injuries, but self-harm and assault injuries are much more likely to be fatal.

Data from Kaufman EJ, Wiebe DJ, Xiong RA, Morrison CN, Seamon MJ, Delgado MK. Epidemiologic Trends in Fatal and Nonfatal Firearm Injuries in the US, 2009-2017. JAMA Intern Med. 2021;181(2):237-244. doi:10.1001/jamainternmed.2020.6696

The most common explanations for the gun's firing are that a person pulled the trigger accidentally or believed that the gun was unloaded.[67] About one-fourth of victims are children.[2]

Common Mechanisms for Injury in a Shooting

The amount of damage to a body by a bullet depends on its speed, size, weight, and shape. When a bullet travels through tissue, it pushes the tissue aside, creating a temporary cavity much larger than the bullet itself. Higher-velocity bullets from rifles tear open larger cavities and cause more tissue damage. At any given speed, larger (that is, higher **caliber**) and heavier bullets cause more tissue damage. Some bullets, called **deforming rounds**, are designed to expand or break into fragments when they hit a target. These deforming rounds cause more tissue damage, but they are less likely to exit the body and hit another person.[81]

Epidemiology: Patterns and Trends

Firearm mortality rates vary by age, race, sex, and intent. Firearm suicides are about five times as frequent in men as in women, and rates are higher in White populations and older adults (**Figure 6.13**).[2]

Firearm homicides are also much more common in men, but rates are higher in Black populations and in younger adults (**Figure 6.14**).[2]

Rates of both firearm suicides and firearm homicides have fluctuated in recent decades, without obvious explanations (**Figure 6.15**). Firearm suicide rates have been rising since 2004 (see the suicide section later in this chapter).[2] Firearm homicide rates began to rise in 2014 but then spiked sharply with the social disruptions of the COVID-19 pandemic.[2]

Globally, mortality rates from firearms are much higher in some countries than others.[82] The United States has the highest firearm mortality rate of any high-income country,[63] but the countries with the

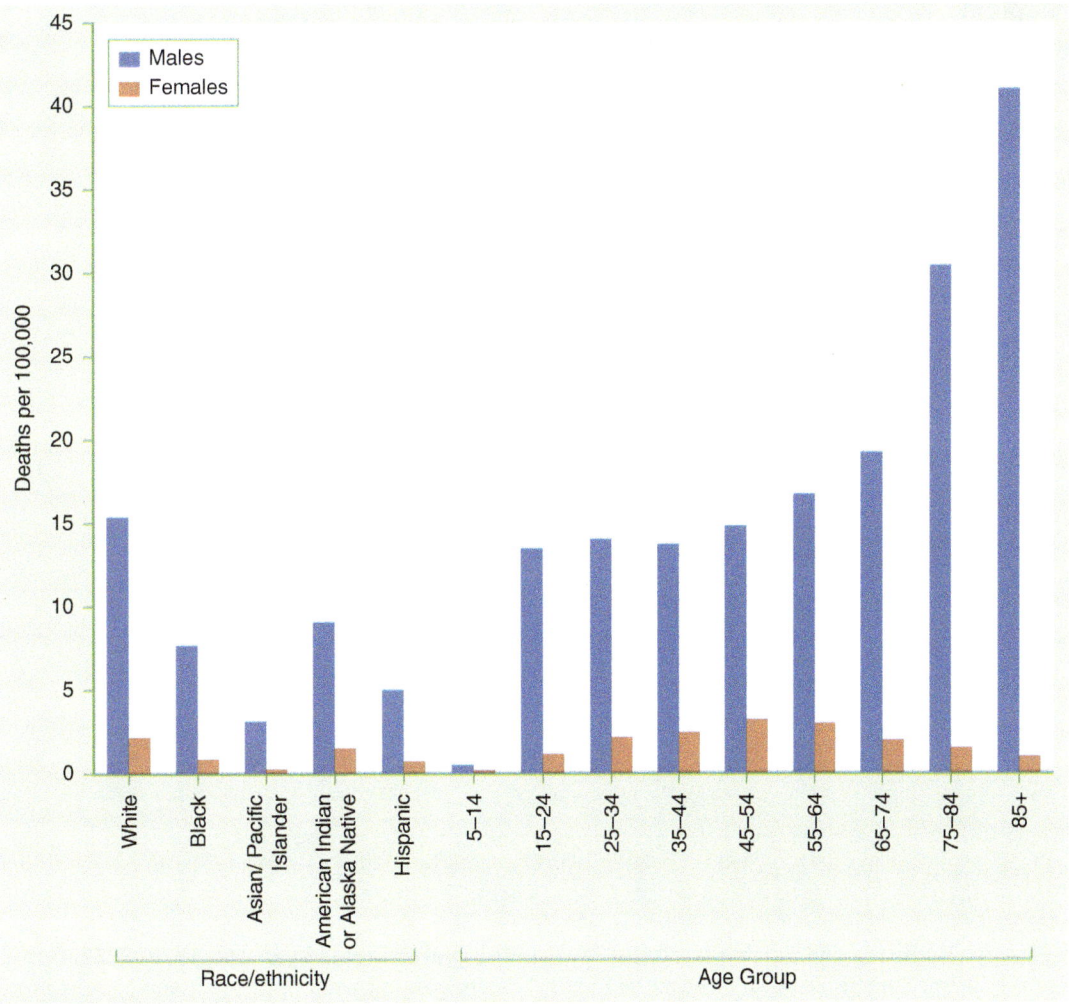

Figure 6.13 **Firearm Suicide Rates in the United States by Age, Race, and Sex, 2018–2021.**

Data from National Center for Health Statistics, Centers for Disease Control and Prevention. Underlying Cause of Death Data on CDC WONDER. Published 2023. Accessed June 12, 2024. https://wonder.cdc.gov/Deaths-by-Underlying-Cause.html

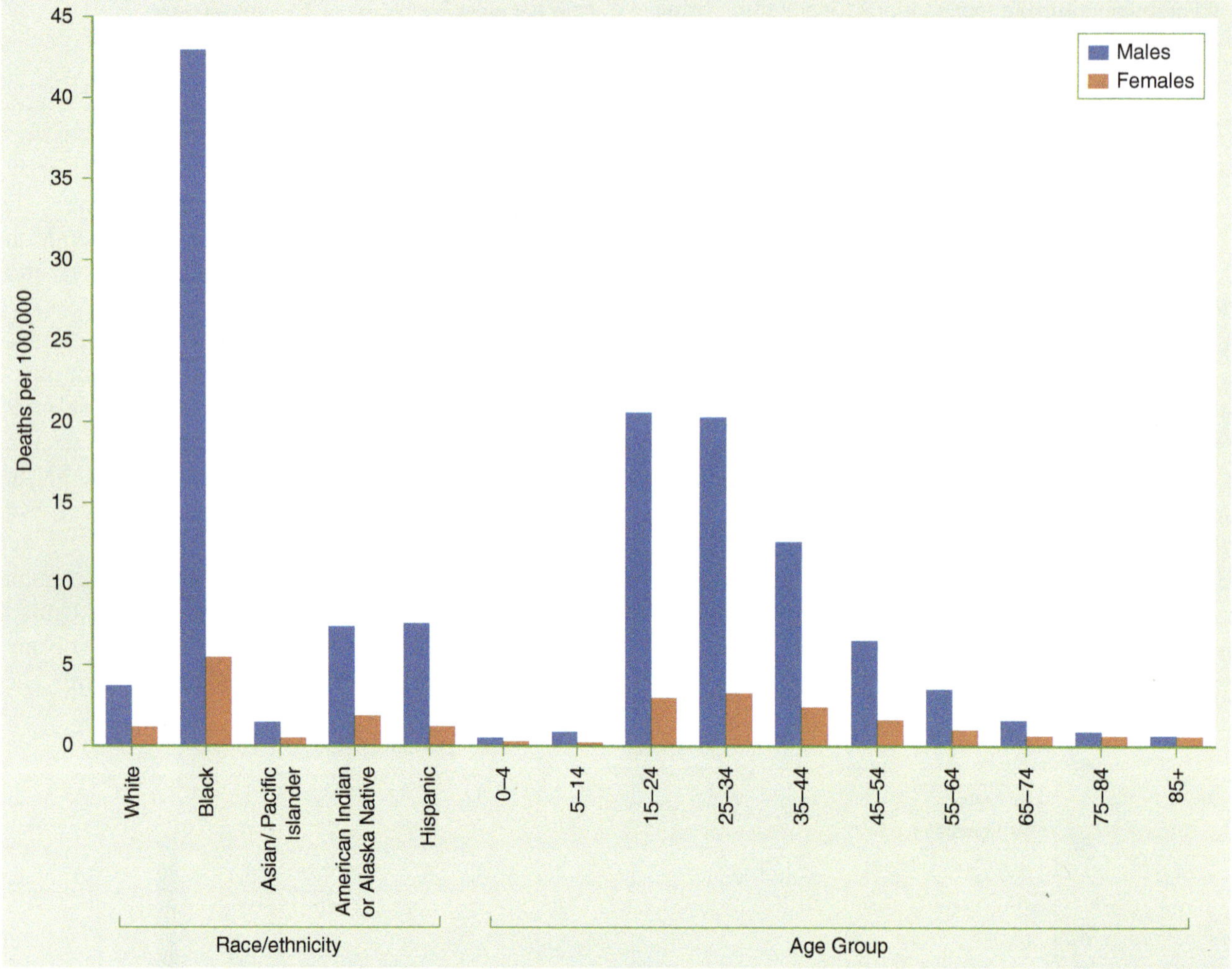

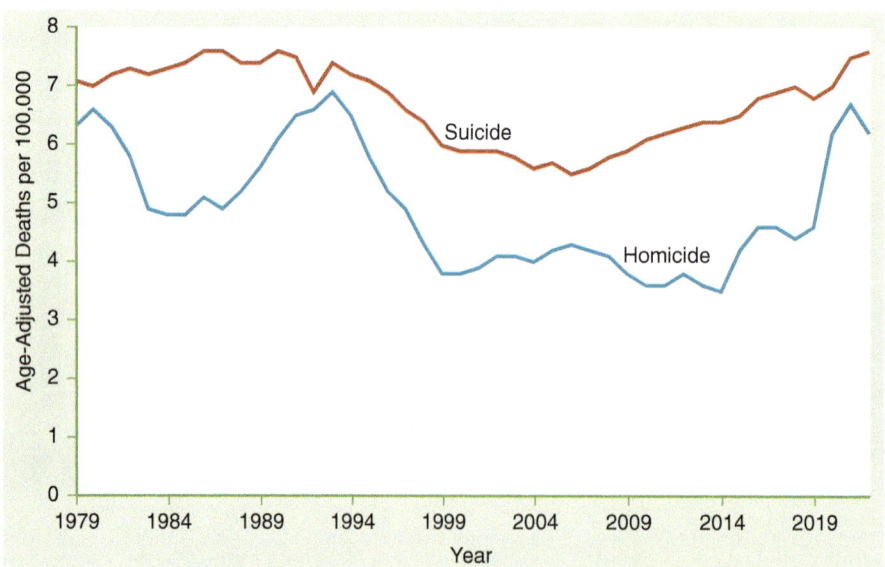

Figure 6.14 **Firearm Homicide Rates by Age, Race, and Sex, United States, 2018–2021.**

Data from National Center for Health Statistics, Centers for Disease Control and Prevention. Underlying Cause of Death Data on CDC WONDER. Published 2023. Accessed June 12, 2024. https://wonder.cdc.gov/Deaths-by-Underlying-Cause.html

Figure 6.15 **Firearm Homicide and Suicide Mortality Rates in the United States by Intent, 1979–2022.** Firearm suicide rates have been rising since 2004. Firearm homicide rates began to rise in 2014 but then spiked sharply with the social disruptions of the COVID-19 pandemic.

Data from National Center for Health Statistics, Centers for Disease Control and Prevention. Underlying Cause of Death Data on CDC WONDER. Published 2023. Accessed June 12, 2024. https://wonder.cdc.gov/Deaths-by-Underlying-Cause.html.; and from National Vital Statistics Reports for 1979-1998

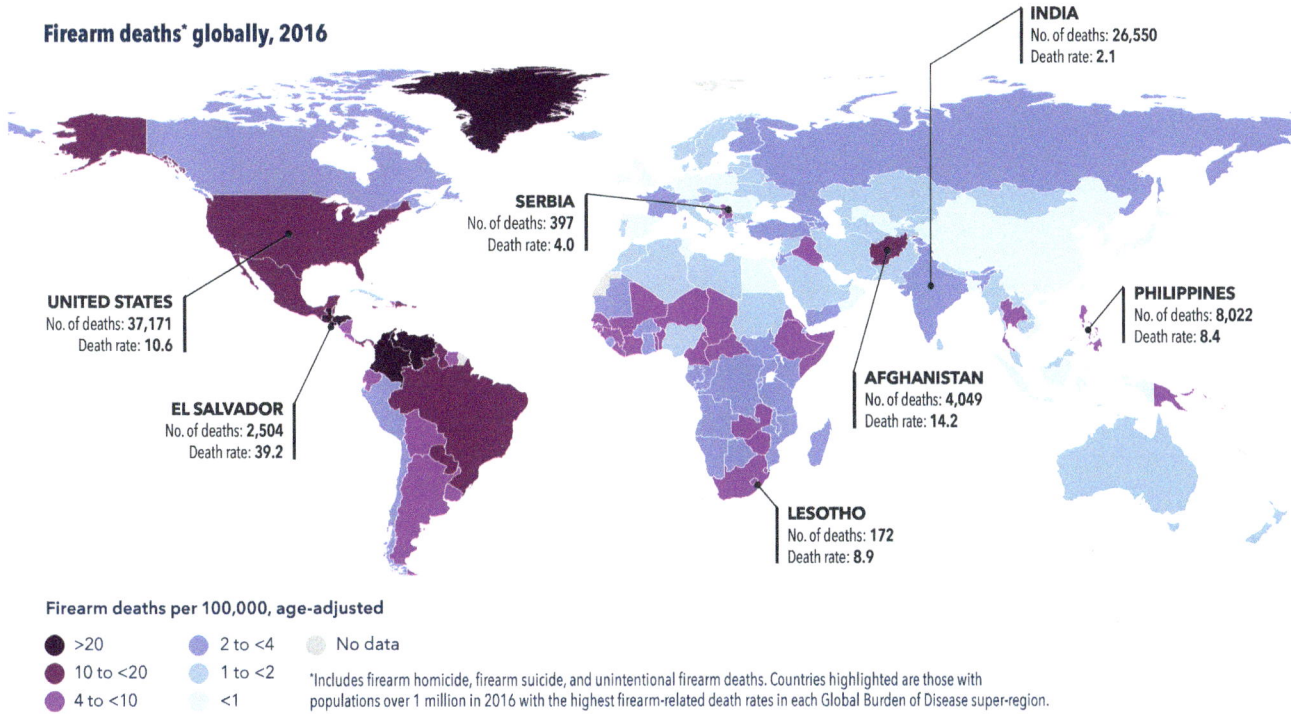

Firearm deaths* globally, 2016

INDIA
No. of deaths: 26,550
Death rate: 2.1

SERBIA
No. of deaths: 397
Death rate: 4.0

PHILIPPINES
No. of deaths: 8,022
Death rate: 8.4

UNITED STATES
No. of deaths: 37,171
Death rate: 10.6

EL SALVADOR
No. of deaths: 2,504
Death rate: 39.2

AFGHANISTAN
No. of deaths: 4,049
Death rate: 14.2

LESOTHO
No. of deaths: 172
Death rate: 8.9

Firearm deaths per 100,000, age-adjusted

- \>20
- 10 to <20
- 4 to <10
- 2 to <4
- 1 to <2
- <1
- No data

*Includes firearm homicide, firearm suicide, and unintentional firearm deaths. Countries highlighted are those with populations over 1 million in 2016 with the highest firearm-related death rates in each Global Burden of Disease super-region.

Figure 6.16 Firearm Deaths by Country, 2016.

Reproduced from Institute for Health Metrics and Evaluation. Firearm Deaths Around the World 2016. Accessed July 28, 2024. https://www.healthdata.org/sites/default/files/files/infographics/Infographic_Gun-Violence_2018.pdf

world's highest rates are in Latin America or the Caribbean (**Figure 6.16**).[82]

Risk Factors

There are modifiable risks of firearm injuries from the environments in which shootings take place, firearms themselves, and people (**Figure 6.17**).

Environment-related Risks

Firearm homicides tend to cluster in certain neighborhoods and locations within neighborhoods with these features:

- *Concentrated poverty.* Assault shootings are more common in neighborhoods in which a high percentage of residents live in poverty.[83-85]

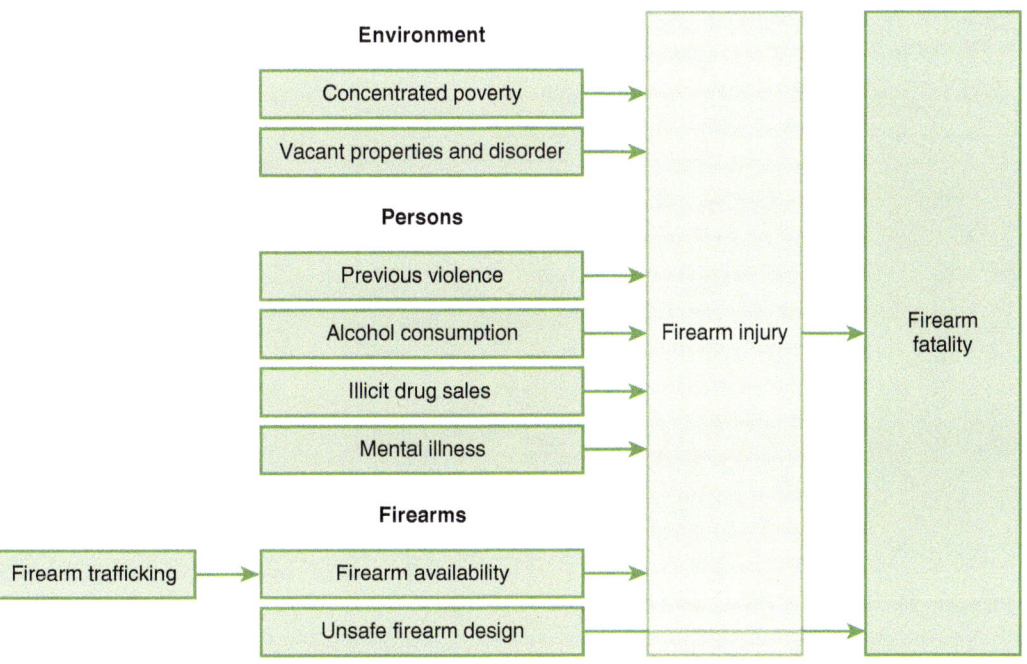

Environment
- Concentrated poverty
- Vacant properties and disorder

Persons
- Previous violence
- Alcohol consumption
- Illicit drug sales
- Mental illness

Firearms
- Firearm trafficking
- Firearm availability
- Unsafe firearm design

Firearm injury → Firearm fatality

Figure 6.17 Cause-and-Effect Diagram for Firearm Injuries.

- *Vacant properties and disorder.* Shootings are also more likely to happen near vacant properties and in areas where buildings and streets are in disrepair.[86] This has led to a theory that physical disorder conveys a message that the neighborhood is neglected, telling potential shooters that violence there is less likely to be caught or prosecuted.[85]

Firearm-related Risks

- *Firearm availability.* At the national, state, and city levels, where there are more guns, there are more firearm suicides and more firearm homicides.[63,82,87-89] One glaring example: Americans own about nine times as many guns per capita as people in western Europe, and the United States has a firearm mortality rate about eight times as high.[82,90] The gun-injury relationship is even true at the level of the home. That is, even though people usually buy guns to protect themselves, having a gun at home more than triples the risk of suicide and doubles the risk of being a victim of homicide.[91] This relationship does not just reflect people substituting guns for other weapons; the increase in risk is for total suicides and homicides, not just those by firearm.

- *Firearm trafficking.* The sources of nearly all firearms owned in the United States are American manufacturers, who sell their guns to federally-licensed distributors and retailers. Those retailers sell the guns to individual adults, but they are required to first conduct **background checks** to ensure that customers are not legally prohibited from purchasing guns.[75,92] There are many opportunities for these prohibited people to buy guns, though, through **firearm trafficking** (**Figure 6.18**). Some unscrupulous retailers do not conduct background checks. (A small percentage of dealers sell a large fraction of guns used in crimes.)[75] Some people called "traffickers" routinely buy guns from retailers just to resell them to others. Other individuals buy guns from retailers as **straw purchasers**—for example, one person purchasing a gun for another who has a criminal record.[75] Most guns used in crimes were bought on the secondary market rather than from federally-licensed retailers.[75,76,93]

- *Unsafe firearm design.* Guns are designed to harm people, but because they are not well designed, they often harm people in ways that are not intended. For example, semiautomatic pistols may have a cartridge loaded in the chamber when the magazine is removed, leading people to pull the trigger thinking that the gun was not loaded. Also, triggers can be pulled by children playing with guns. And most importantly, guns can be taken from their owners and then used against them or others.

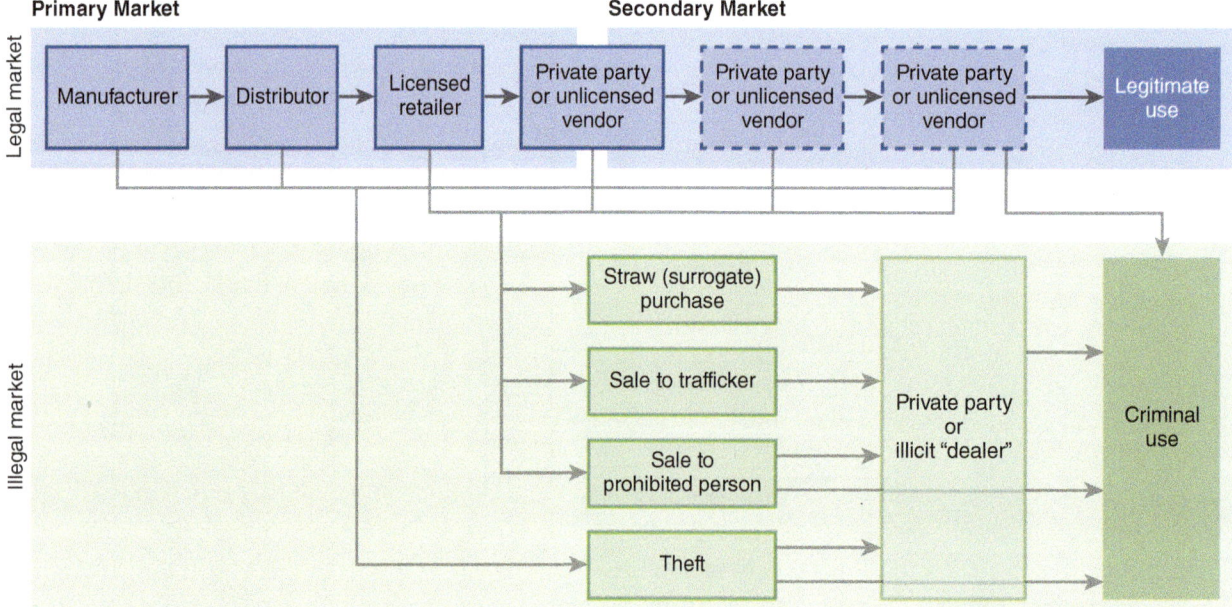

Figure 6.18 **Firearm Markets and How Legal Guns Enter the Illegal Market.** The sources of nearly all firearms owned in the United States are American manufacturers, who sell their guns to federally-licensed distributors and retailers. There are many opportunities for legally prohibited people to buy guns through firearm trafficking.

Person-related Risks

- *Alcohol consumption.* Drinking alcohol increases the risk of all types of gun injuries because it impairs people's judgment, makes them more aggressive, and reduces their physical coordination.[63] More than one-third of people who die by homicide, homicide perpetrators, and people who die by suicide drank alcohol before the shooting, as did nearly 50% of unintentional firearm injury victims.[73] In one pair of studies, heavy alcohol use increased the risk of firearm homicide sixfold and both firearm suicide and unintentional injury more than tenfold.[73]

- *Illicit drug sales.* The use of illicit drugs has not been consistently linked to firearm injuries, but the selling of illicit drugs has.[94]

- *Mental illnesses.* Not surprisingly, having a mental illness is a strong risk factor for firearm suicide.[95] People with mental illnesses are also at greater risk for being assaulted.[96] And while the overwhelming majority of people with mental illnesses are not violent toward others, mental illnesses (especially when combined with drug use) do increase the risk of being a perpetrator of violence.[96,97]

- *Previous violence.* People who have been involved in violence in the past (as either a victim or a perpetrator) are at greater risk of being involved in firearm violence in the future (as either a victim or a perpetrator). Likewise, people who have attempted suicide in the past are at greater risk for firearm suicide.[95]

Preventive Interventions

Interventions are available and already used in some states and localities to address most of these risk factors (**Figure 6.19**).

Environment-related Risks

- *Mixed-income development.* Chapter 16. Social Disadvantage discusses the reduction of poverty and income inequality, which may prevent disease and injuries. In addition, if the concentration of poverty within neighborhoods is a key factor increasing gun violence, then integrating neighborhoods by income should reduce gun violence. In the 1900s, governments built large public housing developments for low-income families, which led to concentrations of extreme poverty. In many cities, those housing developments experienced high levels of gun violence.

Since then, governments have shifted to smaller, "scattered-site" public housing and vouchers that subsidize rent in private housing. Some studies suggest that this mixed-income approach has reduced violence and crime, but more research is needed.[83]

- *Repair or demolition of vacant properties* and *cleaning/greening of vacant lots.* In some cities, in an attempt to reduce violence, city agencies and community groups repair or demolish blighted buildings and "clean and green" vacant lots so that the neighborhood looks cared-for. This work has been followed by reductions in gun violence in the immediate areas, without displacing it to nearby areas.[85,98]

- *Emergency medical services.* Maintaining emergency medical teams that respond extremely quickly to shootings is far from an ideal solution, but it may prevent some deaths. Researchers have estimated that about 15% of deaths from shootings may be prevented by emergency medical care.[99]

Firearm-related Risks

- *Limits on the availability of firearms and ammunition.* Firearm injuries can be prevented by reducing the number of guns that are purchased or owned—especially by people at high risk.
  - *Firearm sales reporting* and *universal background checks.* Currently, the federal government does not require background checks at gun shows and for sales between private individuals.[93] Some states require background checks for all sales, but without a national system, guns flow in illegally to those states from other states.[92,100] Trafficking can be reduced by requiring that all gun sales, including those between private individuals, be recorded and reported to a law enforcement agency,[92] tied to requirements for **universal background checks**, that is, background checks regardless of who sells the firearm.[63,75,92,93,100] Adding background checks for ammunition sales can help prevent prohibited persons from using illegal firearms that they already own.[92,101] One study suggested that universal firearm and ammunition background checks may be able to cut firearm mortality in the United States by more than half.[101]
  - *Firearm registration and owner licensure.* To legally drive a car in the United States, a person

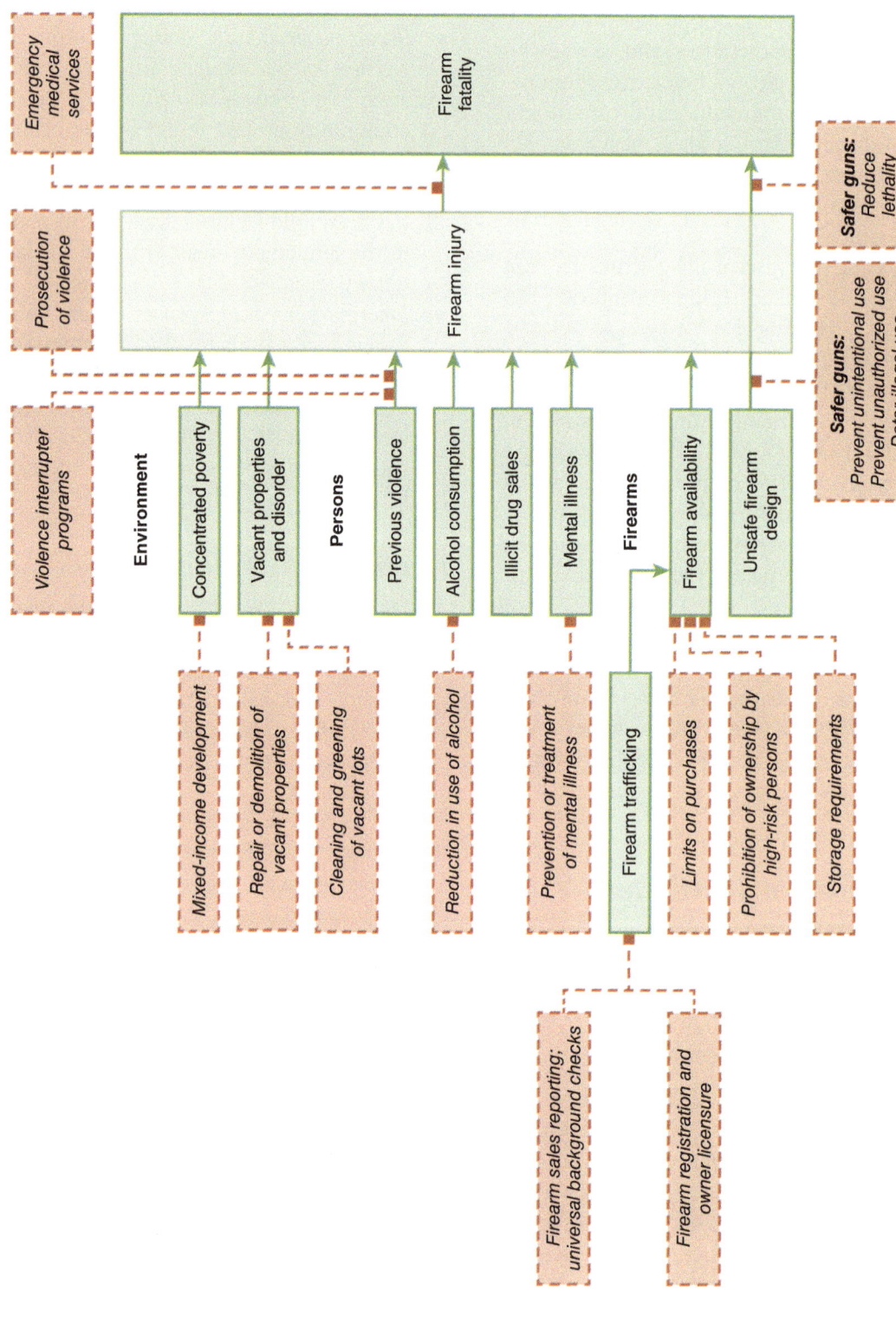

Figure 6.19 Cause-and-Effect Diagram for Firearm Injuries, with Preventive Interventions.

must have a valid driver's license, and the vehicle must be registered with the state. Governments can likewise require that all firearm owners be licensed and all firearms be registered.[75,100,102] Today, some states require people to have licenses or permits to purchase firearms. These **permit-to-purchase laws** work like universal background checks.[92] The preventive potential of laws requiring owner licensure and permit-to-purchase can be seen in New York City, which requires both. Legal gun ownership in New York City is very low—estimated at less than one percent of residents.[103] The firearm suicide rate in New York City is less than one-seventh that of other large U.S. cities (**Figure 6.20**), and the gun homicide rate is also much lower (**Figure 6.21**).

- *Limits on purchases.* Other limits on firearm purchases can reduce trafficking and injuries. For example, some states limit a person to buying no more than **one gun a month**, which makes gun trafficking less profitable.[75,93] And some states have a mandatory

waiting period between when a person requests a firearm and when they can receive it.[75,100] This gives enforcement agencies time to ensure that the purchaser is not prohibited, and the "cooling off" time may prevent some homicidal or suicidal shootings that are impulsive.[92]

- *Prohibition of ownership by persons at high risk.* Federal law already prohibits purchases or ownership of guns by those who have been committed to a mental institution, who are "addicted to any controlled substance," who are under a restraining order for threatening an intimate partner, and who have been convicted of a felony.[104] This list could be expanded, for example, to include people convicted of violent misdemeanors and people addicted to alcohol or with convictions related to alcohol use.[63,75,100]

- *Storage requirements.* Laws can require that guns be stored locked and unloaded to prevent children from accidentally shooting themselves and to reduce the number of guns

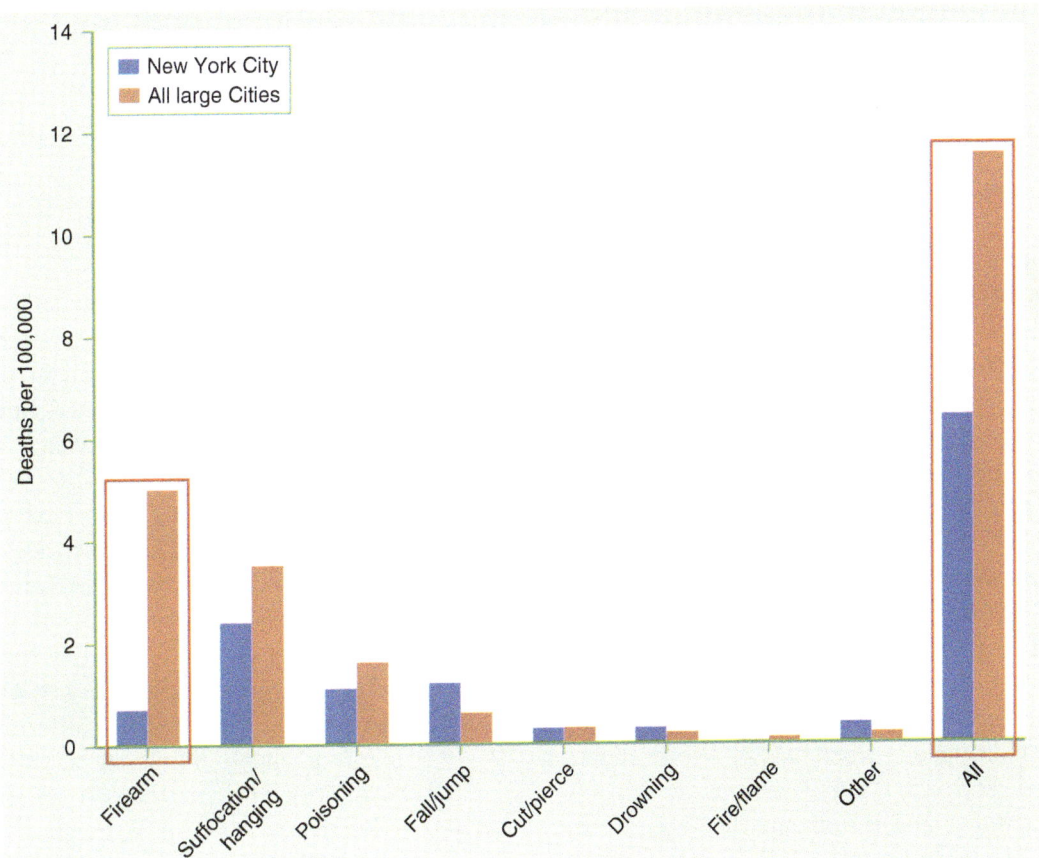

Figure 6.20 Rates of Suicide by Mechanism, New York City Versus Other Large U.S. Cities, 2018–2021. In New York City, the firearm suicide rate in is less than one-seventh and the overall suicide rate is about one-half that of other large U.S. cities. These differences may be caused by low rates of gun ownership in New York City.

Data from National Center for Health Statistics, Centers for Disease Control and Prevention. Underlying Cause of Death Data on CDC WONDER. Published 2023. Accessed June 12, 2024. https://wonder.cdc.gov/Deaths-by-Underlying-Cause.html

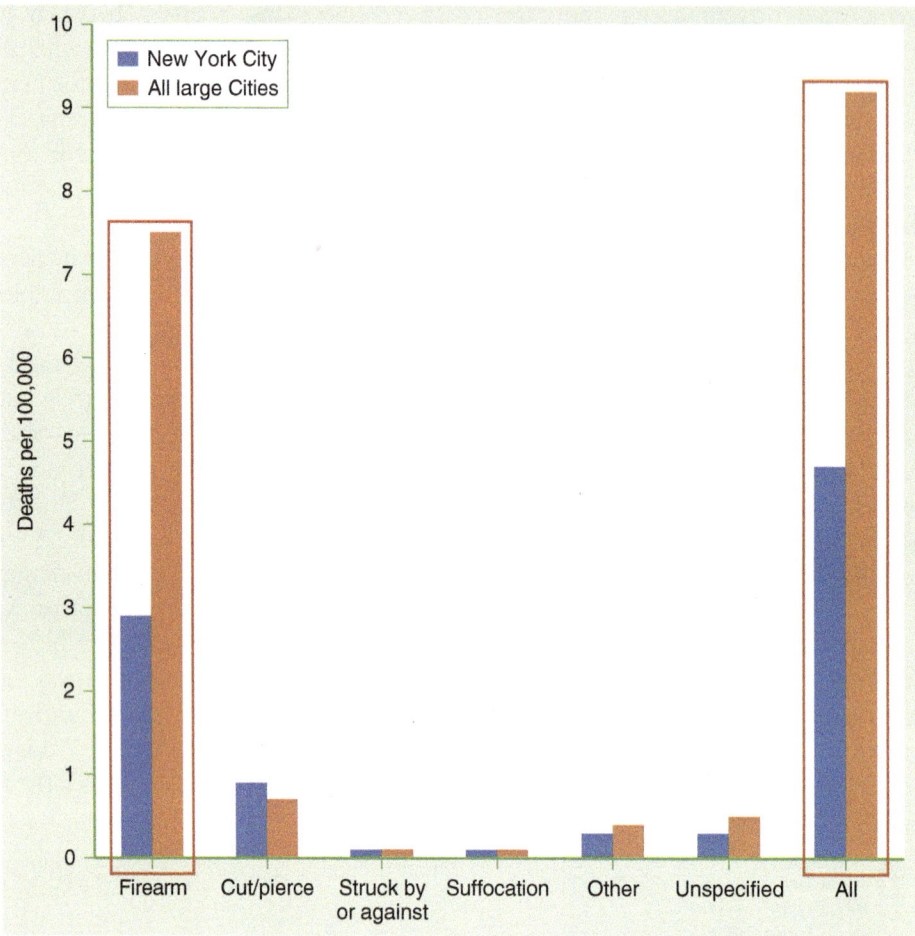

Figure 6.21 **Homicide Rates by Mechanism, New York City versus Other Large Cities, 2018–2021.** Firearm homicide rates and total homicide rates are also much lower in New York City than in other large cities.

Data from National Center for Health Statistics, Centers for Disease Control and Prevention. Underlying Cause of Death Data on CDC WONDER. Published 2023. Accessed June 12, 2024. https://wonder.cdc.gov/Deaths-by-Underlying-Cause.html

that are stolen.[102] These laws have been linked to fewer suicidal and unintentional firearm deaths in young people.[92,105]

- *Safer guns.* Just as cars are now required to have safer designs, guns can be required to have safer designs. Safety features could be designed:
  - *To prevent unintentional use.* For example, semiautomatic pistols can have a **magazine disconnect safety**, which blocks the gun from firing if the magazine has been removed.[102] A **grip safety**, which prevents the gun from firing if a lever on the grip is not squeezed, would prevent the gun from firing when dropped or when held by a young child. These and other safety features are already built into many pistols and are required by some states.[92]
  - *To prevent unauthorized use.* Shootings using guns that have been stolen could be prevented by features that prevent non-owners from firing a gun. Available today are **trigger locks** that require a key or combination to open. Manufacturers could make high-tech **personalized smart guns** that only fire if they recognize, for example, the owner's fingerprint or a microchip on the owner's wrist.[102]
  - *To track use and deter illegal use.* When police investigate a shooting, they have no reliable way to trace a bullet or a cartridge casing to a specific gun. **Firearm identification** technology exists that would put unique features into bullets or casings so that guns can be traced.[101] One example called **microstamping** is already required in California.[102]
  - *To reduce lethality.* While people shoot others to harm or deter them, they do not always want to kill them. Guns can be designed so that they are less likely to kill those who are shot. For example, one study found the fatality rate for people who were shot was 38% with small-caliber firearms, 47% with medium-caliber firearms, and 65% with large-caliber firearms.[106]

The researchers estimated that if all guns were small-caliber, the change would reduce gun deaths by 40%. Likewise, reducing the speed at which bullets travel or otherwise reducing the amount of tissue damage they cause could reduce gun deaths. Finally, regulations that limit the number of bullets that can be fired quickly (such as bans on high-capacity magazines) may reduce the number of mass shooting events or the number of people injured in these events.[107]

Person-related Risks

- *Reduction in alcohol consumption.* Alcohol is so strongly linked to firearm injuries that any intervention that reduces alcohol consumption should reduce firearm injuries. See Chapter 12. Alcohol Use.

- *Prevention or treatment of mental illnesses.* The treatment of mental illnesses can reduce the risk of suicide, but any impact of treatment on homicides is likely to be small. See Chapter 5. Mental Illnesses.

- *Intervention with people who use firearms.* Most efforts to reduce gun violence today focus on people who have already shot or been shot. Because gun violence is often a repeated behavior, in theory this could reduce future shootings. Specifically, steps today involve:
  - *Prosecution of people who commit firearm violence.* The potential value of prosecuting people who have shot others is to discourage violent behavior in everyone and to deter future violent behavior by the person charged or convicted. But that value is limited by two problems. First, prosecution is complicated, with many steps, and it often breaks down. Only an estimated 40%–75% of homicide perpetrators and 4%–8% of nonfatal assault perpetrators are identified, arrested, charged, and convicted.[108] Second, studies suggest that incarceration does not deter future criminal behavior.[109]
  - **Violence interrupter programs.** In many cities, organizations work with people who have been shot and those around them to prevent victims or others from retaliating. Some organizations more generally try to redirect young men involved in violence into school, jobs, or job training programs.[102] Evaluations of these programs have shown mixed results.[110]

Box 6.4 Summary–Prevention of Firearm Injuries

- Mixed-income development
- Repair or demolition of vacant properties and cleaning/greening of vacant lots
- Emergency medical services
- Limits on the availability of firearms and ammunition
  - Firearm sales reporting and universal background checks
  - Firearm registration and owner licensure
  - Limits on purchases
  - Prohibition of ownership by persons at high risk
  - Storage requirements
- Safer guns
  - To prevent unintentional use
  - To prevent unauthorized use
  - To track use and deter illegal use
  - To reduce lethality
- Reduction in alcohol consumption
- Prevention or treatment of mental illnesses
- Prosecution of people who commit firearm violence.
- Violence interrupter programs

Box 6.5 Key Words–Firearm Injuries

Background check
Barrel
Caliber
Cartridge
Casing
Chamber
Component cause
Deforming rounds
Firearm identification
Firearm trafficking
Firing pin
Grip safety
Handgun
Long gun
Magazine
Magazine disconnect safety
Microstamping
Muzzle
One gun a month laws
Permit-to-purchase laws
Personalized smart guns
Propellant
Primer
Revolver
Rifle
Semiautomatic pistol
Slide (on a pistol)

(continues)

Box 6.5 **Key Words–Firearm Injuries** *(continued)*

Shotgun
Straw purchase
Trigger
Trigger locks
Universal background check laws
Violence interrupter programs
Waiting period laws

Resources–Firearm Injuries

- Kaufman EJ, Wiebe DJ, Xiong RA, Morrison CN, Seamon MJ, Delgado MK. Epidemiologic trends in fatal and nonfatal firearm injuries in the US, 2009–2017. *JAMA Intern Med.* 2021;181(2): 237-244. doi:10.1001/jamainternmed.2020 .6696
- Nand D, Naghavi M, Marczak LB, et al. Global mortality from firearms, 1990–2016. *JAMA.* 2018; 320(8):792-814. doi:10.1001/jama.2018.10060
- Wilson RF, Liu G, Lyons BH, et al. Surveillance for Violent Deaths—National Violent Death Reporting System, 42 States, the District of Columbia, and Puerto Rico, 2019. *MMWR Surveillance Summaries.* 2022;71(6):1-40. doi:10.15585/mmwr .ss7106a1. This is a highly detailed analysis of extensive data collected on a large proportion of violent deaths in the United States.
- The Bureau of Alcohol, Tobacco, Firearms and Explosives (www.atf.gov) within the U.S. Department of Justice, conducts inspections of firearm retailers and traces firearms used in crimes to retailers. An extensive summary report on tracing of crime guns is available at https:// www.atf.gov/firearms/docs/report/nfcta-volume -ii-part-iii-crime-guns-recovered-and-traced-us /download
- Kondo MC, Andreyeva E, South EC, Macdonald JM, Branas CC. Neighborhood Interventions to Reduce Violence. *Annual Review of Public Health.* 2018;39:253-271. doi:10.1146/annurev -publhealth
- Smart R, Morral AR, Smucker S, et al. *The Science of Gun Policy: A Critical Synthesis of Research Evidence on the Effects of Gun Policies in the United States.* 2nd Edition. Santa Monica, CA: RAND Corporation; 2020. This book represents the most extensive review available on firearm-related policies and their effectiveness in reducing deaths.

Suicide

Introduction

This chapter is mainly organized around the mechanisms of injury rather than the intents, and firearm suicides are addressed in the firearm section. But just under half of suicides involve mechanisms other than firearms, so the topic of suicide itself deserves attention.

Suicide rates in the United States have been increasing since 1999.[111] It is not clear why. The rise may be related to use of the internet and social media, which appears to be causing a parallel increase in depression. Regardless, there are interventions available that can reduce suicide rates.

Common Mechanisms of Suicide

In the United States, the four most common mechanisms for suicide are firearms, suffocation (usually involving hanging), poisonings (usually involving drugs), and falls (usually jumps from a height).[67] The mechanisms used differ by gender (**Figure 6.22**). Men are more likely to die by firearm or suffocation, and women by poisoning.[67]

Epidemiology: Patterns and Trends

Rates of suicide vary by demographic group. They rise with age, with the highest rates in older adults.[2] Suicide rates are much higher in males, in White populations and American Indian/Alaska Native populations, and in rural areas.[2,112] And suicide rates are higher in people with less income or education and people who are unemployed.[113] These demographic differences are not well understood.

The increase in suicide rates that began in 1999 occurred in both men and women, and in all age groups except those over age 75.[2,111] And the rise has involved every common mechanism except poisoning (**Figure 6.23**)[2,111] Like the demographic differences, this increase in suicide is not well understood, but it may be tied to increases in depression during the same time period.

Risk Factors

Established risk factors for suicide include:

- *Mental illnesses.* Not surprisingly, people who are depressed are about 10 times as likely to die by suicide. People with schizophrenia have an equally high suicide risk. People with anxiety disorders are also at increased risk, though to a lesser

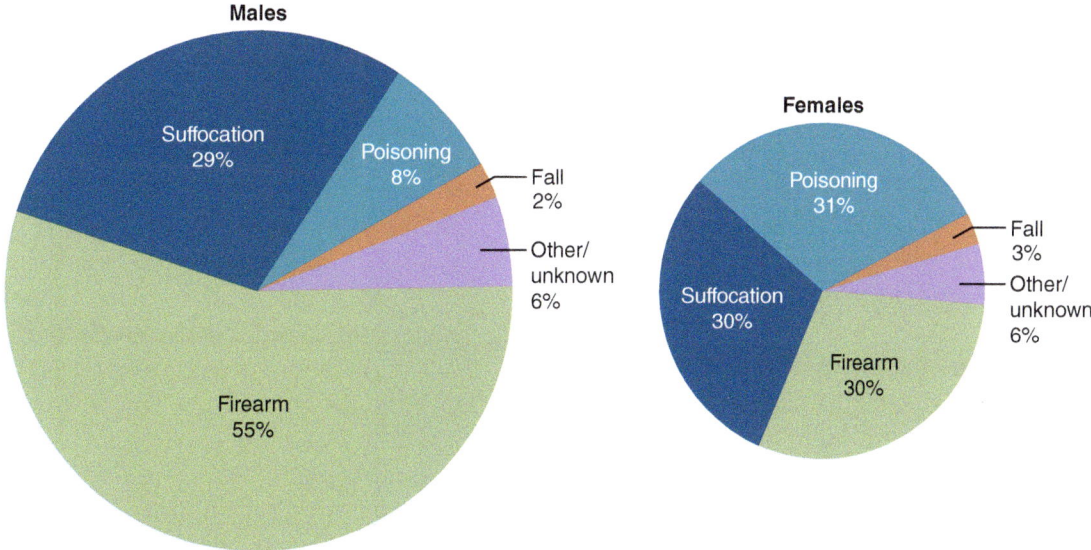

Figure 6.22 Mechanisms of Suicide in the United States by Gender, 2019.

Data from Wilson RF, Liu G. Lyons BH, et al. Surveillance for Violent Deaths — National Violent Death Reporting System, 42 States, the District of Columbia, and Puerto Rico, 2019. MMWR Surveillance Summaries. 2022;71(6):1-40. doi:10.15585/mmwr.ss7106a1

degree.[113] However, it is important to not equate suicide with mental illness. Most people with mental illness do not attempt suicide and about half of people who die by suicide do not have a diagnosed mental illness.[67]

- *Alcohol use.* People who have a diagnosed alcohol use disorder are about twice as likely to die by suicide.[114] But the more important risk is the immediate effect of alcohol. People who are intoxicated

from alcohol are, by different estimates, eight or more than 30 times as likely to die by suicide as people who have not been drinking.[115,116] Among those who die by suicide in the United States and are tested, about 40% have alcohol in their systems, usually at high levels.[67]

- *Drug use.* People who are diagnosed with drug use disorders are far more likely to die by suicide.[113,117] Heavy cannabis users, regardless of whether they

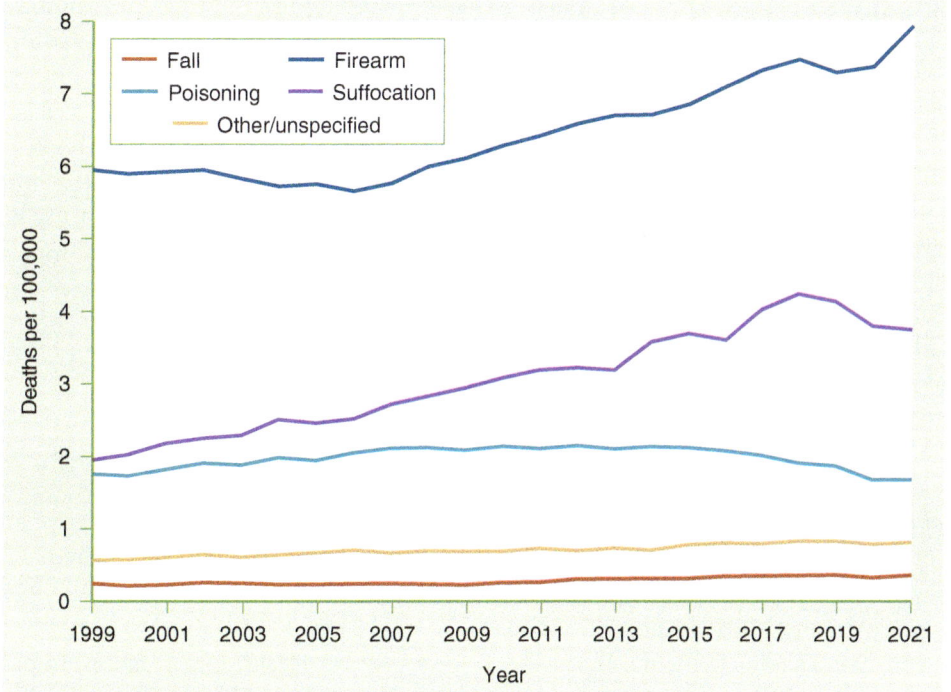

Figure 6.23 Suicide Rates by Mechanism in the United States, 1999–2021.

Data from National Center for Health Statistics, Centers for Disease Control and Prevention. Underlying Cause of Death Data on CDC WONDER. Published 2023. Accessed June 12, 2024. https://wonder.cdc.gov/Deaths-by-Underlying-Cause.html

are diagnosed with a disorder, are about three times more likely.[118]

- *Social isolation.* People who are socially isolated—having less contact with others to whom they can turn to for help—are more likely to die by suicide.[119] This may explain why the risk of suicide is about twice as high in adults who are unmarried as in those who are married.[120] And it may help explain why suicide rates are higher in rural areas.[112]

- *Access to lethal means.* Attempting suicide requires access to the means to kill oneself—like a gun, a bottle of pills, or a tall building from which to jump. People who have more access to these lethal means are more likely to die by suicide.[121]

- *Broadcast media reports of suicides.* Media reports about suicide, particularly suicides by celebrities, are sometimes followed for a few weeks by "copycat" suicides, often using the same method.[121,122]

- *Social media.* There appears to be a connection between use of social media and both suicide and nonfatal acts of self-harm, especially in adolescents.[123-125] This may be because using social media increases depression or anxiety or because it increases social isolation. Or it may simply be that people use social media to share information about how to die by suicide, which is similar to increasing access to lethal means.[126]

Preventive Interventions

Interventions to address these risk factors include:

- *Prevention and treatment of mental illnesses.* Medical treatment for depression or schizophrenia reduces the risk of suicide.[127] Treatment is particularly important for people who had survived an earlier suicide attempt.

- *School-based education programs.* Some school-based programs that teach children about mental health and how to manage stressful life events have been effective in reducing teen suicides.[127]

- *Reduction of alcohol use.* The extremely strong connection between alcohol use and suicide argues that any step to reduce alcohol consumption should reduce suicide rates. See Chapter 12. Alcohol Use.

- *Reduction of drug use.* See Chapter 13. Drug Use.

- *Promotion of social connections.* The U.S. Surgeon General's report on *Our Epidemic of Loneliness and Isolation* provides many ideas on how to reduce social isolation. See Chapter 5. Mental Illnesses.

- *Reduction in access to lethal means.* Reducing access to lethal means of suicide reduces suicide rates.[121] In the United States, the most important lethal means is firearms. Steps to reduce access to firearms can reduce suicides overall, as shown by the example of New York City earlier in this chapter (Figure 6.20). In addition, safer firearms that require the user to take specific actions before shooting (like unlock a lock) may deter some people in moments of crisis. At the same time, medicines with the potential for fatal overdose, such as opioids and tricyclic antidepressants, can be prescribed less frequently, or they can be sold in limited-size pill packs that require users to push out one pill at a time.[128] Barriers can be added to buildings and bridges to deter people from jumping.[121,129] And in developing, agricultural countries, substituting non-lethal pesticides for those that are lethal to humans can reduce suicidal poisonings.[121]

- *Helplines.* Many communities have suicide prevention helplines, in which trained staff give telephone support to persons in distress. However, at this point, there is not good evidence that these helplines reduce suicide rates.[127]

- *Promotion of responsible media reporting of suicides.* Broadcast media should be asked to cover suicides (if they cover them at all) responsibly. The World Health Organization has produced a media guide on this.[130] The organization recommends that outlets not "lead" with suicide stories, run them repeatedly, glamorize the suicide, or describe the suicide method used. Instead, media organizations should discuss ways for distressed people to cope with their problems and provide information on how people in distress can find help.

- *Promotion of responsible social media content.* Social media platforms like Facebook can be asked or required to block content that instructs people on how to attempt suicide. They can be also be required to attach advice about how to get support during stressful times to any suicide-related content.

Resources–Suicide

- Hedegaard H, Curtin SC, Warner M. Suicide Mortality in the United States, 1999–2019. *NCHS Data Brief.* 2021;(398):1-7.
- Zalsman G, Hawton K, Wasserman D, et al. Suicide prevention strategies revisited: 10-year systematic review. *Lancet Psychiatry.* 2016;3(7):646-659. doi:10.1016/S2215-0366(16)30030-X
- World Health Organization. Department of Mental Health and Substance Abuse. *Preventing Suicide: A Global Imperative.* World Health Organization; 2014. Available at https://www.who.int/publications

Falls in Older Adults

Introduction

When older adults fall to the ground, the impact can cause serious injury or death. In 2021, nearly 40,000 older adults in the United States died from falls.[2] According to estimates from the Global Burden of Disease group, falls are responsible for more disability-adjusted life-years (DALYs) lost than breast cancer, colorectal cancer, interpersonal violence, or self-harm.[131]

Mechanisms of Falls

A fall occurs when a person's center of gravity moves beyond the support provided by that person's feet. That can happen from a "slip"—in which a foot suddenly slides out of position—or a "trip"—in which a foot is caught or blocked from supporting an upper body that is moving. Falls from trips are far more common.[132,133] As people age, they are less able to sense a fall hazard or to limit the impact of a fall.[134]

Most falls take place at home, usually indoors, but sometimes on a porch or patio.[132,133,135] Within the home, the most common locations are living rooms and bedrooms, but those occurring in bathrooms are more likely to lead to injuries.[135,136] Most falls occur while a person is simply walking.[133] Objects that fallers commonly trip over are electrical cords, rugs, or carpets with upturned edges, clutter on the floor, and furniture that is out of the line of sight (**Figure 6.24**).

About one out of five falls causes a serious injury, such as a fracture or a concussion.[137] More than 95% of hip fractures are caused by falling, and falls are the most common cause of traumatic brain injuries.[138]

Epidemiology: Patterns and Trends

Falls in older adults are extremely common. In the United States, nearly 30% of adults above age 65 say they have fallen at least once in the previous 12 months, and 10% say they were injured from a fall.[139] The older the adult, the more often a fall leads to a serious injury.[139] Those aged 80-84 are more than 7 times as likely to have a fatal fall as those aged 65-69 (**Figure 6.25**).[140]

Rates of fatal falls differ markedly by race, with rates in White populations more than twice those in Black populations (**Figure 6.26**).[2] The reason for these racial differences is not clear, but it may have to do with differences in use of medicines that increase the risk of falls.

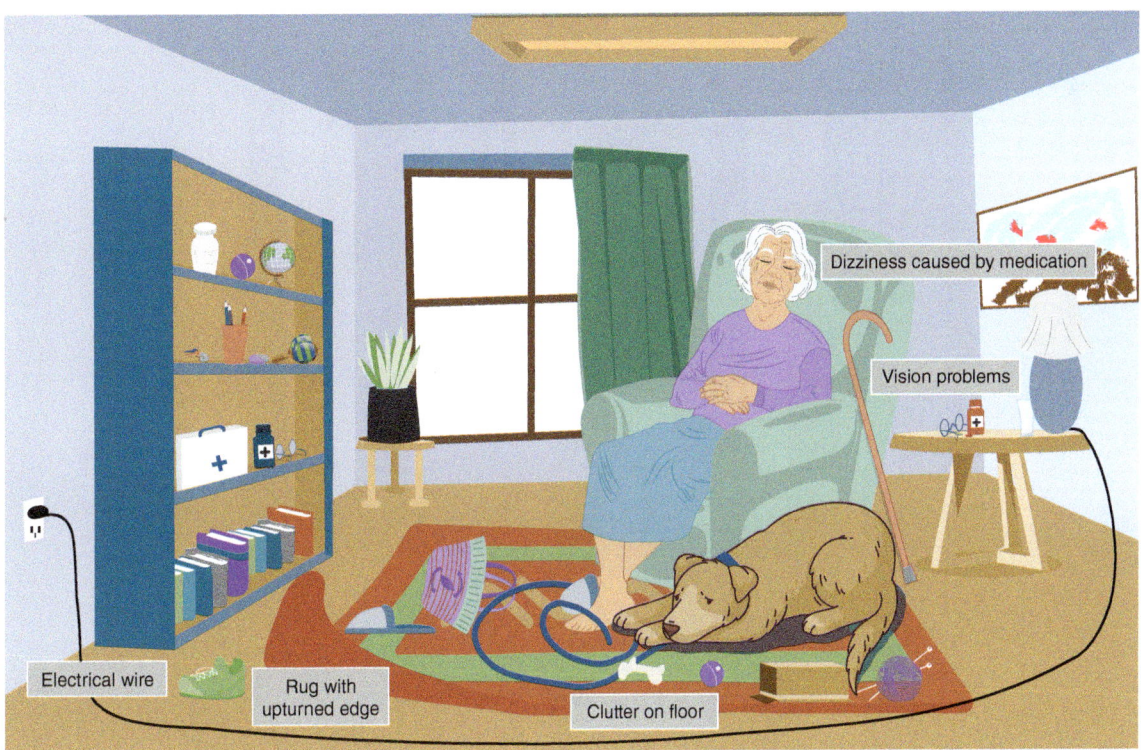

Figure 6.24 Common In-home Risks for Falls.

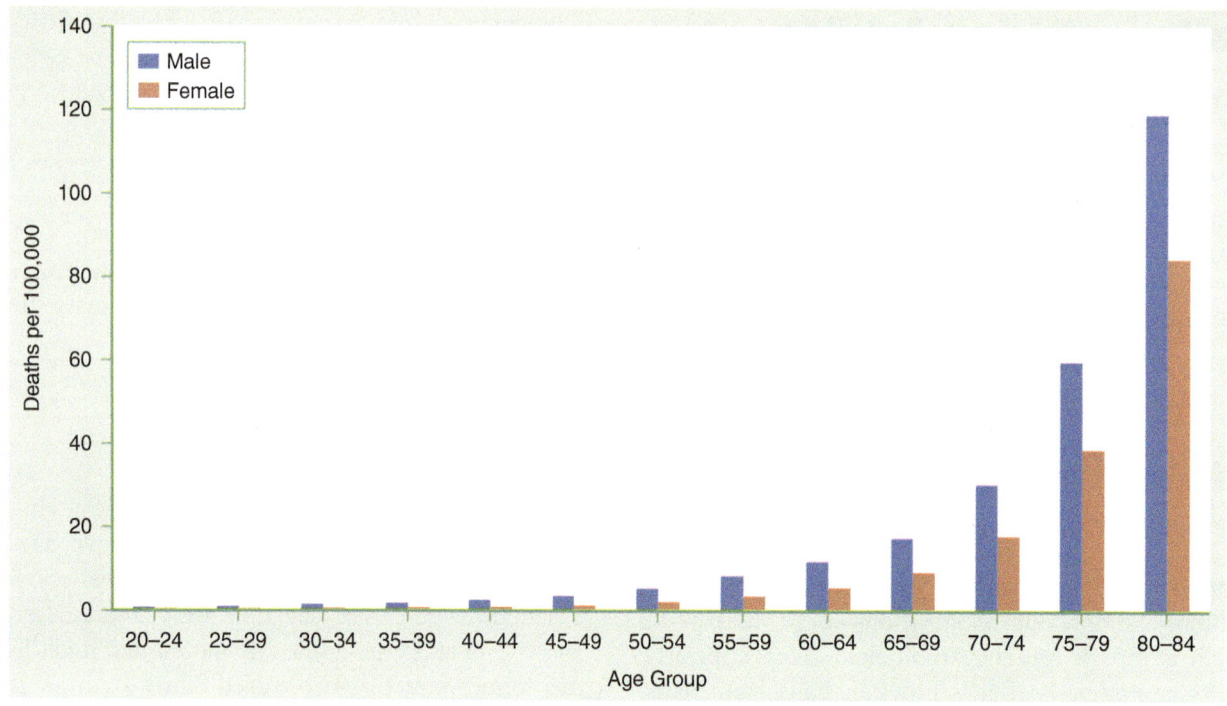

Figure 6.25 Mortality Rates from Unintentional Falls in United States by Age Group, 2018–2021.

Data from National Center for Health Statistics, Centers for Disease Control and Prevention. Underlying Cause of Death Data on CDC WONDER. Published 2023. Accessed June 12, 2024. https://wonder.cdc.gov/Deaths-by-Underlying-Cause.html

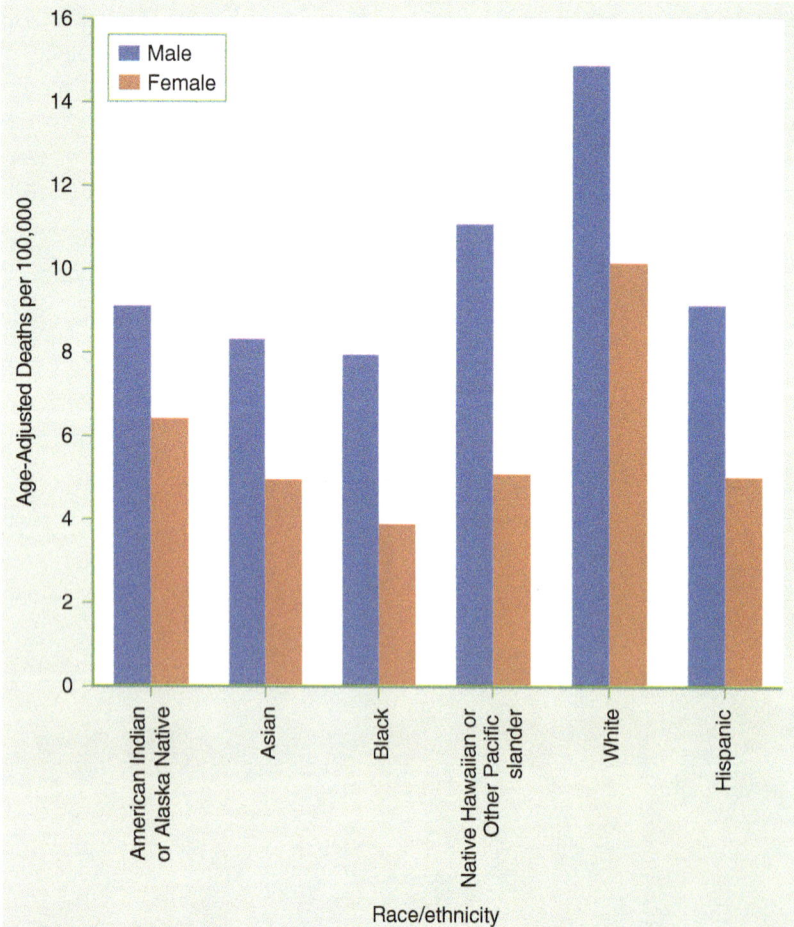

Figure 6.26 Mortality Rates from Falls By Race and Sex, 2022.

Data from National Center for Health Statistics, Centers for Disease Control and Prevention. Underlying Cause of Death Data on CDC WONDER. Published 2023. Accessed June 12, 2024. https://wonder.cdc.gov/Deaths-by-Underlying-Cause.html

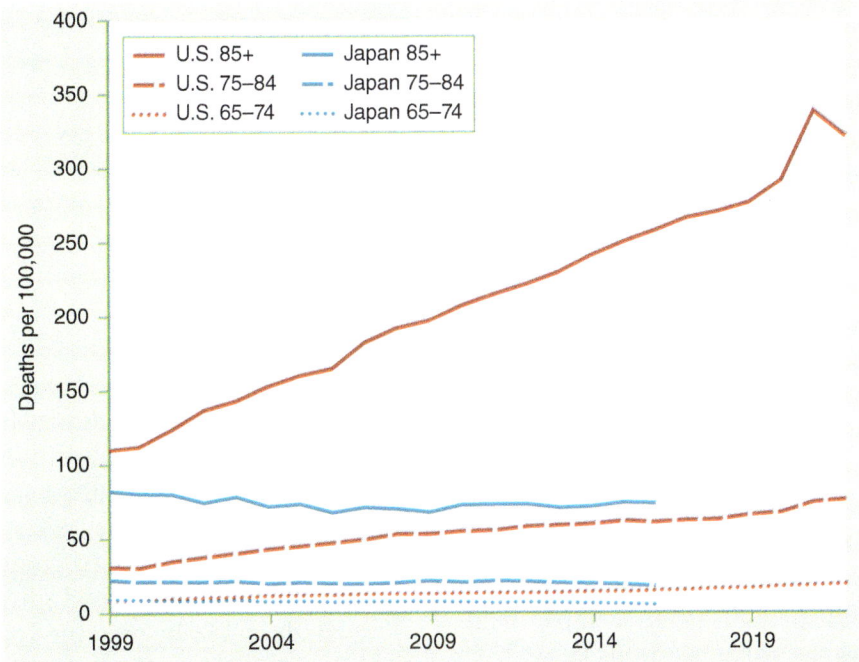

Figure 6.27 **Trends in Fall Mortality Rates, the United States and Japan, 1999–2022.** Mortality rates from falls in older adults tripled in the United States while they remained unchanged in Japan.

Data from National Center for Health Statistics, Centers for Disease Control and Prevention. Underlying Cause of Death Data on CDC WONDER. Published 2023. Accessed June 12, 2024. https://wonder.cdc.gov/Deaths-by-Underlying-Cause.html; and Hagiya H, Koyama T, Zamami Y, et al. Fall-related mortality trends in older Japanese adults aged ≥65 years: A nationwide observational study. BMJ Open. 2019;9(12). doi:10.1136/bmjopen-2019-033462

Disturbingly, death rates from falls in the United States nearly tripled between 1999 and 2022.[2] This surge in falls did not occur in other high-income countries.[141-145] For example, in 2016, fall death rates were more than three times as high in the United States as in Japan (**Figure 6.27**),[146] and roughly twice as high as in the United Kingdom and Australia.[141,147]

Risk Factors

Risk factors for fall injuries include those relating to a person and those relating to the environment (**Figure 6.28**):[148]

- *Muscle weakness in the lower body, balance problems, and difficulty walking. Everyone loses muscle*

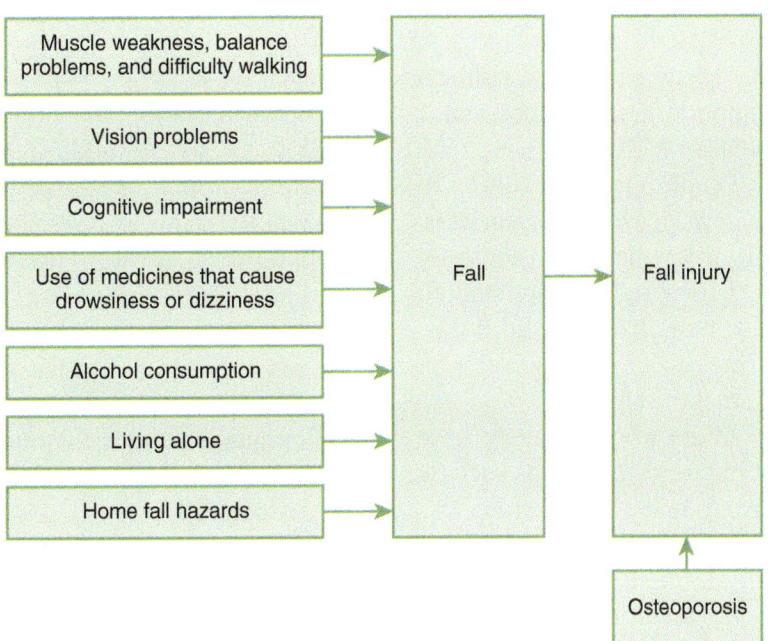

Figure 6.28 **Cause-and-Effect Diagram for Fall Injuries in Older Adults.**

strength as they age, and those with weaker muscles are less able to support themselves. By one estimate, older adults with muscle weakness were about five times as likely to have major falls.[148] Other limitations on walking, for example, caused by arthritis or problems with balance, may double or triple the risk of falls.[134,148]

- *Vision problems.* Vision problems, such as cataracts, are common in older adults may prevent them from seeing objects that they might trip over. Poor vision approximately doubles the risk of a serious fall.[134,148]

- *Cognitive impairment.* People with **dementia** have **cognitive impairment**, that is, they have difficulty learning and understanding their situations. They can become confused, increasing their risk of tripping. Cognitive impairment roughly doubles the risk of a serious fall.[134,148]

- *Use of medicines that cause drowsiness or dizziness.* People who are drowsy or dizzy are less likely to notice hazards and react more slowly if they trip over them. Drugs with this effect are called **fall risk-increasing drugs** or FRIDs. The drugs mostly strongly linked to serious falls are **opioids**, **benzodiazepines** (such as Xanax and Klonopin) and **antidepressants**.[149-152] A large majority of older Americans injured from falls had been taking at least one FRID, with many taking more than one.[153] The surge in fall-related deaths shown in Figure 6.27 occurred in parallel with a surge in the prescribing of opioids, benzodiazepines, and antidepressants to older adults.[154-157]

- *Alcohol consumption.* Several studies have shown that alcohol consumption among older adults increases the risk of falls.[158,159]

- *Home fall hazards.* People are more likely to trip if their homes have uneven floor surfaces, objects on the floor, or low lighting. People are more likely to slip if floor surfaces are smooth or wet. They are also more likely to slip if they are barefoot or wearing shoes that are loose, with high heels, or with smooth soles.[134,160]

- *Living alone.* Older adults who live alone have been found to be at higher risk, perhaps because they are less attentive to home fall hazards.[158]

- *Osteoporosis.* Not all falls result in serious injuries. But people who fall are more likely to fracture their bones if the bones are brittle from a condition called **osteoporosis**.

Preventive Interventions
Primary Prevention: Prevention of Falls

The difference in fall death rates between the United States and other countries, and the fact that fall rates were far lower 20 years ago, suggests that at least two-thirds of deaths due to falls can be prevented. Interventions to reduce falls include (**Figure 6.29**):[161-163]

- *Reductions in the prescribing of antidepressants, benzodiazepines, opioids, and other FRIDs to older adults.* Reducing medical providers' prescribing of FRIDs to older adults must be a central part of a prevention strategy. The American Geriatrics Society has detailed guidelines about which drugs to avoid.[164] Several studies have attempted to reduce falls by working with adults to reduce their FRID use. In general, these trials have not succeeded,[149,165] but that may be because most study participants did not actually reduce FRID use. However, two studies that successfully worked with primary care providers to "deprescribe" FRIDs in older adults were able to reduce falls.[162,166,167]

- *Reduction of alcohol consumption.* See Chapter 12. Alcohol Use.

- *Prevention of dementia.* The cognitive decline of dementia can be delayed. Interventions to delay dementia include those that reduce social isolation and those that reduce **atherosclerosis**, the condition of blood vessels that leads to heart disease and stroke. Dementia prevention is discussed in Chapter 5. Mental Illnesses.

- *Promotion of physical activity.* Physical activity helps maintain the lower-body muscle strength. See Chapter 15. Physical Activity.

- *Strength and balance exercise programs for older adults.* Many groups offer programs for older adults to improve lower-body strength and balance. These programs reduce fall rates by about 20%, with those lasting three or more hours per week the most effective, reducing falls by nearly 40%.[168,169] However, it is difficult to bring these programs to scale for entire populations.

- *Treatment of vision problems.* Cataract surgery reduces falls.[134]

- *Reduction in home fall hazards.* Programs to reduce home fall hazards reduce falls by about 25% overall, but by nearly 40% among those at greatest risk.[170] Some experts recommend

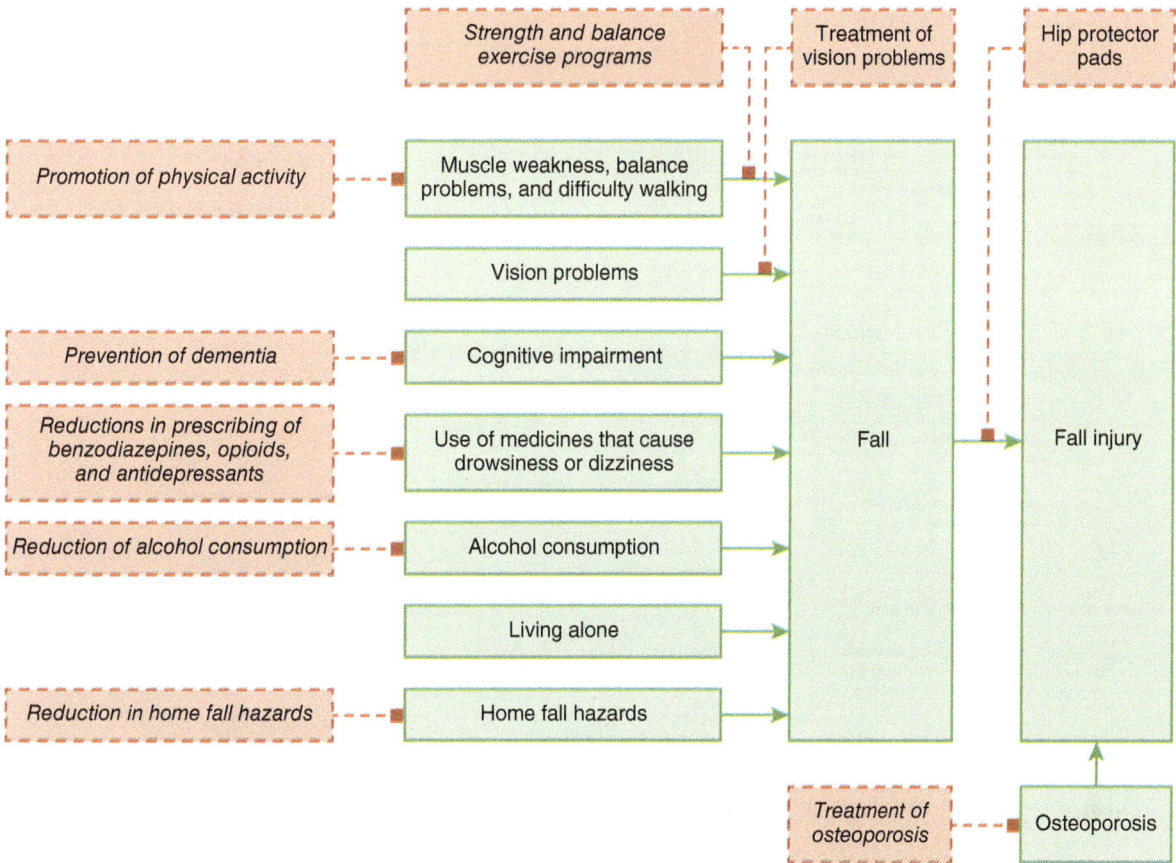

Figure 6.29 **Cause-and-Effect Diagram for Fall Injuries in Older Adults, with Preventive Interventions.**

that home hazards be assessed by an occupational therapist, but this may not be possible for entire populations. The CDC has created a checklist that enables people to assess their own home hazards and provides simple solutions (**Figure 6.30**).[171] Some of these solutions, such as grab bars in bathrooms, are required for people with disabilities under the Americans for Disability Act.

Expert groups have created guidelines for healthcare providers on how to assess risk of falls in older adults and how to help high-risk patients reduce that risk.[172,173] However, using these guidelines depends on people accessing primary care and their providers taking the time to go through the assessment, treatment plan, and referrals.

Secondary Prevention: Prevention of Injuries Among Persons Who Fall

In theory, injuries can be prevented by protecting or strengthening the body so that it can better withstand a fall, in the same way that seatbelts and airbags prevent injuries from car crashes. Exercise programs may reduce fall injuries in part by strengthening bones. In addition:

- *Hip protector pads* reduce fractures in people living in nursing homes. However, researchers have found it is difficult to get patients to wear them consistently.[174]
- *Treatment of osteoporosis* with calcium, vitamin D, and medications called **bisphosphonates** reduces hip fractures resulting from falls.[161]

Box 6.6 Summary–Prevention of Fall Injuries

- Reduction in the prescribing of benzodiazepines, opioids, and antidepressants for older adults
- Reduction of alcohol use
- Prevention of dementia
- Promotion of physical activity
- Strength and balance exercise programs for older adults
- Reduction in home fall hazards
- Treatment of vision problems
- Hip protector pads
- Treatment of osteoporosis

Use this checklist to find and fix hazards in your home.

STAIRS & STEPS (INDOORS & OUTDOORS)

Are there papers, shoes, books, or other objects on the stairs?

☐ Always keep objects off the stairs.

Are some steps broken or uneven?

☐ Fix loose or uneven steps.

Is there a light and light switch at the top and bottom of the stairs?

☐ Have an electrician put in an overhead light and light switch at the top and bottom of the stairs. You can get light switches that glow.

Has a stairway light bulb burned out?

☐ Have a friend or family member change the light bulb.

Is the carpet on the steps loose or torn?

☐ Make sure the carpet is firmly attached to every step, or remove the carpet and attach non-slip rubber treads to the stairs.

Are the handrails loose or broken? Is there a handrail on only one side of the stairs?

☐ Fix loose handrails, or put in new ones. Make sure handrails are on both sides of the stairs, and are as long as the stairs.

FLOORS

When you walk through a room, do you have to walk around furniture?

☐ Ask someone to move the furniture so your path is clear.

Do you have throw rugs on the floor?

☐ Remove the rugs, or use double-sided tape or a non-slip backing so the rugs won't slip.

Are there papers, shoes, books, or other objects on the floor?

☐ Pick up things that are on the floor. Always keep objects off the floor.

Do you have to walk over or around wires or cords (like lamp, telephone, or extension cords)?

☐ Coil or tape cords and wires next to the wall so you can't trip over them. If needed, have an electrician put in another outlet.

KITCHEN

Are the things you use often on high shelves?

☐ Keep things you use often on the lower shelves (about waist high).

Is your step stool sturdy?

☐ If you must use a step stool, get one with a bar to hold on to. Never use a chair as a step stool.

BEDROOMS

Is the light near the bed hard to reach?

☐ Place a lamp close to the bed where it's easy to reach.

Is the path from your bed to the bathroom dark?

☐ Put in a nightlight so you can see where you're walking. Some nightlights go on by themselves after dark.

BATHROOMS

Is the tub or shower floor slippery?

☐ Put a non-slip rubber mat or self-stick strips on the floor of the tub or shower.

Do you need some support when you get in and out of the tub, or up from the toilet?

☐ Have grab bars put in next to and inside the tub, and next to the toilet.

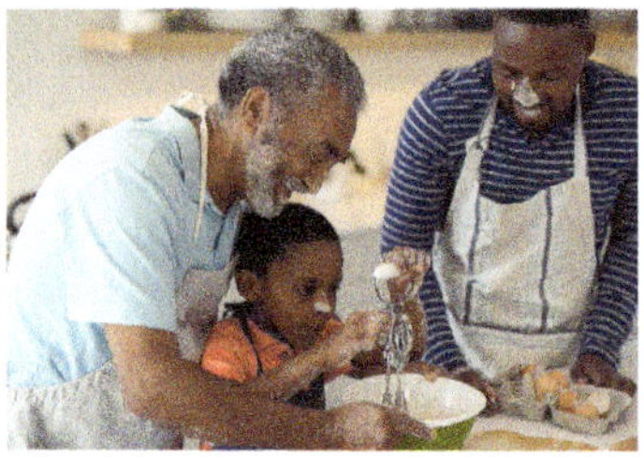

Figure 6.30 **CDC Fall Prevention Checklist.**

National Center for Injury Prevention, Centers for Disease Control and Prevention. Check for Safety: A Home Fall Prevention Checklist for Older Adults; 2017. www.cdc.gov/steadi

---

Box 6.7 **Key Words–Falls in Older Adults**

Antidepressants
Atherosclerosis
Benzodiazepines
Bisphosphonates
Cognitive impairment
Dementia
Fall risk-increasing drugs (FRIDs)
Opioids
Osteoporosis

- Centers for Disease Control and Prevention. Older adult fall prevention. Accessed March 17, 2025. Available at: www.cdc.gov/falls
- Centers for Disease Control and Prevention. *Check for Safety: A Home Fall Prevention Checklist for Older Adults*. Accessed March 17, 2025. Available at: www.cdc.gov/steadi
- Colón-Emeric CS, McDermott CL, Lee DS, Berry SD. Risk assessment and prevention of falls in older community-dwelling adults: A review. *JAMA*. 2024;331(16):1397-1406. doi:10.1001/jama.2024.1416

Resources–Falls in Older Adults

- American Geriatric Society. Beers Criteria for potentially inappropriate medication use in older adults. *J Am Geriatr Soc.* 2023;1-30 doi:10.1111/jgs.18372

References

1. Centers for Disease Control and Prevention. WISQARS: Web-based injury statistics query and reporting system. 2023. Accessed June 17, 2024. Available at: https://wisqars.cdc.gov/

2. National Center for Health Statistics, Centers for Disease Control and Prevention. Underlying cause of death data on CDC WONDER. CDC. 2023. Accessed June 12, 2024. Available at: https://wonder.cdc.gov/Deaths-by-Underlying-Cause.html

3. Haddon W. Advances in the epidemiology of injuries as a basis for public policy. *Public Health Rep.* 1980;95(5):411-421.

4. Centers for Disease Control and Prevention. Achievements in public health, 1900–1999 Motor-vehicle safety: A 20th century public health achievement. *MMWR.* 1999;48(18):369-379.

5. National Safety Council. Car crash deaths and rates. *NSC Injury Facts.* 2024. Accessed October 20, 2024. Available at: https://injuryfacts.nsc.org/motor-vehicle/historical-fatality-trends/deaths-and-rates/

6. Moynihan DP. Epidemic on the highways. *The Reporter.* Published online April 30, 1959:16-23.

7. Ker K, Roberts IG, Collier T, Beyer FR, Bunn F, Frost C. Post-license driver education for the prevention of road traffic crashes. *Cochrane Database Syst Rev.* Published online July 21, 2003. doi:10.1002/14651858.CD003734

8. Roberts IG, Kwan I. School-based driver education for the prevention of traffic crashes. *Cochrane Database Syst Rev.* Published online July 23, 2001. doi:10.1002/14651858.CD003201

9. Graham JD, Garber S. Evaluating the effects of automobile safety regulation. *J Policy Anal and Manage.* 1984;3(2):206-224. doi:10.1002/pam.4050030204

10. National Highway Traffic Safety Administration. *Traffic Safety Facts 2021: A Compilation of Motor Vehicle Traffic Crash Data.*; 2022. Accessed March 17, 2025. Available at: https://crashstats.nhtsa.dot.gov/

11. Williamson M, Zhou H, Fries RN. Safety effects of different driveway types defined in the *Highway Safety Manual.* 2018. Accessed June 19, 2024. Available at: https://trid.trb.org/View/1494787

12. Schultz GG, Braley KT, Boschert T. *Correlating Access Management to Crash Rate, Severity, and Collision Type.* 2008. Accessed June 19, 2024. https://trid.trb.org/View/847371

13. Khan SA, Afghari AP, Yasmin S, Haque MM. Effects of design consistency on run-off-road crashes: An application of a random parameters negative binomial Lindley model. *Accid Anal Prev.* 2023;186. doi:10.1016/j.aap.2023.107042

14. Liu C, Subramanian R, Chen CL, et al. Factors related to fatal single-vehicle run-off-road crashes. 2009. Accessed March 17, 2025. Available at: www.ntis.gov

15. National Highway Traffic Safety Administration, Department of Transportation. *Traffic Safety Facts-Pedestrians: 2021 Data DOT HS# 813458.* 2023. Accessed June 19, 2024. Available at: https://crashstats.nhtsa.dot.gov/

16. National Highway Traffic Safety Administration, Department of Transportation. *Traffic Safety Facts-Bicyclists and Other Cyclists: 2021 Data DOT HS# 813484.* 2023. Accessed June 19, 2024. Available at: https://crashstats.nhtsa.dot.gov/

17. Alrejjal A, Farid A, Ksaibati K. Investigating factors influencing rollover crash risk on mountainous interstates. *J Safety Res.* 2022;80:391-398. doi:10.1016/j.jsr.2021.12.020

18. Dischinger PC, Cushing BM, Kerns TJ. Injury patterns associated with direction of impact: Drivers admitted to trauma centers. *J Trauma Inj Infect Crit Care.* 1993;35(3). doi:10.1097/00005373-199309000-00020

19. Hazarika S, Willcox N, Porter K. Patterns of injury sustained by car occupants with relation to the direction of impact with motor vehicle trauma—evidence-based review. *Trauma.* 2007;9(3):145-150. doi:10.1177/1460408607084179

20. Fadl SA, Sandstrom CK. Pattern recognition: A mechanism-based approach to injury detection after motor vehicle collisions. *RadioGraphics.* 2019;39(3):857-876. doi:10.1148/rg.2019180063

21. Chen R, Gabler HC. Risk of thoracic injury from direct steering wheel impact in frontal crashes. *J Trauma Acute Care Surg.* 2014;76(6). doi:10.1097/TA.0000000000000222

22. O'Donovan S, van den Heuvel C, Baldock M, Byard RW. Causes of fatalities in motor vehicle occupants: an overview. *Forensic Sci Med Pathol.* 2022;18(4):511-515. doi:10.1007/s12024-022-00503-3

23. Bédard M, Guyatt GH, Stones MJ, Hirdes JP. The independent contribution of driver, crash, and vehicle characteristics to driver fatalities. *Accid Anal Prev.* 2002;34(6). doi:10.1016/S0001-4575(01)00072-0

24. Lepard JR, Spagiari R, Corley J, et al. Differences in outcomes of mandatory motorcycle helmet legislation by country income level: A systematic review and meta-analysis. *PLoS Med.* 2021;18(9). doi:10.1371/journal.pmed.1003795

25. Hu J, Lin YS, Boyle K, et al. Pedestrian safety: Assessment of crashworthiness test procedures. Accessed March 17, 2025. Available at: https://orcid.org/0000-0001-6477-0360

26. Kent T, Miller J, Shreve C, Allenback G, Wentz B. Comparison of injuries among motorcycle, moped and bicycle traffic accident victims. *Traffic Inj Prev.* 2022;23(1):34-39. doi:10.1080/15389588.2021.2004311

27. Global Burden of Disease Collaboration, Institute for Health Metrics and Evaluation. *GBD Results Tool.* July 12, 2023. Accessed July 11, 2023. Available at: https://vizhub.healthdata.org/gbd-results/

28. Yellman MA, Sauber-Schatz EK. Motor vehicle crash deaths—United States and 28 other high-income countries, 2015 and 2019. *MMWR Morb Mortal Wkly Rep.* 2022;71(26):837-843. doi:10.15585/mmwr.mm7126a1

29. World Health Organization. *Global Status Report on Road Safety 2023.* 2023. Accessed July 27, 2024. Available at: https://www.who.int/publications/i/item/9789240086517

30. UNC Highway Safety Research Center. *Crash Modification Factors Clearinghouse.* Federal Highway Administration, U.S. Department of Transportation. 2023. Accessed February 7, 2024. Available at: www.cmfclearinghouse.org

31. Kahane CJ. *Lives Saved by Vehicle Safety Technologies and Associated Federal Motor Vehicle Safety Standards, 1960 to 2012.* 2015. Accessed June 20, 2024. Available at: https://trid.trb.org/View/1341338

32. National Highway Traffic Safety Administration, Department of Transportation. *Traffic Safety Facts-Critical Reasons for Crashes Investigated in the National Motor Vehicle Crash Causation Survey DOT HS 812506.*; 2018. Accessed June 19, 2024. Available at: https://crashstats.nhtsa.dot.gov/

33. Voinea GD, Boboc RG, Buzdugan ID, Antonya C, Yannis G. Texting while driving: A literature review on driving simulator studies. *Int J Environ Res Public Health.* 2023;20(5). doi:10.3390/ijerph20054354

34. Choudhary P, Velaga NR. Mobile phone use during driving: Effects on speed and effectiveness of driver compensatory behaviour. *Accid Anal Prev.* 2017;106:370-378. doi:10.1016/j.aap.2017.06.021

35. Insurance Institute for Highway Safety, Highway Loss Data Institute. Distracted Driving. IIHS. December 2023. Accessed February 11, 2024. Available at: https://www.iihs.org/topics/distracted-driving

36. Boudette N. A new Tesla safety concern: drivers can play video games in moving cars. *The New York Times.* December 7, 2021. Accessed February 12, 2024. Available at: https://www.nytimes.com/2021/12/07/business/tesla-video-game-driving.html

37. Elvik R, Vadeby A, Hels T, van Schagen I. Updated estimates of the relationship between speed and road safety at the aggregate and individual levels. *Accid Anal Prev.* 2019;123:114-122. doi:10.1016/j.aap.2018.11.014

38. SWOV Institute for Road Safety. *The Relation Between Speed and Crashes.* 2012. Accessed June 20, 2024. Available at: https://safety.fhwa.dot.gov/speedmgt/ref_mats/fhwasa1304/Resources3/08%20-%20The%20Relation%20Between%20Speed%20and%20Crashes.pdf

39. Voas RB, Torres P, Romano E, Lacey JH. *Alcohol-Related Risk of Driver Fatalities: An Update Using 2007 Data.* Vol 73.; 2012.

40. National Highway Traffic Safety Administration. *Traffic Safety Facts: A Compilation of Motor Vehicle Crash Data (Table 13).* NHTSA. 2020. Accessed August 10, 2023. Available at: https://cdan.dot.gov/tsftables/tsfar.htm#

41. Thomas F, Berning A, Darrah J, et al. Drug and alcohol prevalence in seriously and fatally injured road users before and during the COVID-19 public health emergency. *National Highway Traffic Safety Administration* (Report No DOT HS 813 018). Published online October 2020. Accessed June 20, 2024. Available at: https://rosap.ntl.bts.gov/view/dot/50941

42. National Highway Traffic Safety Administration, Department of Transportation. *Traffic Safety Facts-Speeding: 2021 Data* (DOT HS 813473). 2023. Accessed June 19, 2024. Available at: https://crashstats.nhtsa.dot.gov/

43. National Highway Traffic Safety Administration, Department of Transportation. *Seat Belt Use in 2022-Use Rates in the States and Territories.* 2023. Accessed March 17, 2025. Available at: https://crashstats.nhtsa.dot.gov/

44. Liu BC, Ivers R, Norton R, Boufous S, Blows S, Lo SK. Helmets for preventing injury in motorcycle riders. *Cochrane Database of Syst Rev.* Published online January 23, 2008. doi:10.1002/14651858.CD004333.pub3

45. National Highway Traffic Safety Administration, Department of Transportation. *Traffic Safety Facts Research Note: Motorcycle Helmet Use in 2022* (DOT HS 813505). 2023. Accessed June 19, 2024. Available at: https://crashstats.nhtsa.dot.gov/

46. Olivier J, Creighton P. Bicycle injuries and helmet use: a systematic review and meta-analysis. *Int J Epidemiol.* Published online July 22, 2016:dyw153. doi:10.1093/ije/dyw153

47. World Health Organization. *Global Plan: Decade of Action for Road Safety 2021–2030.* 2020. Accessed June 20, 2024. Available at: https://www.who.int/publications/m/item/global-plan-for-the-decade-of-action-for-road-safety-2021-2030

48. United States Department of Transportation. *National Roadway Safety Strategy.* 2022. Accessed June 20, 2024. Available at: https://www.transportation.gov/NRSS

49. World Health Organization. *Save LIVES : A Road Safety Technical Package.* World Health Organization; 2017. Accessed June 20, 2024. Available at: https://www.who.int/publications/i/item/save-lives-a-road-safety-technical-package

50. Insurance Institute for Highway Safety, Highway Loss Data Institute. Roundabouts. IIHS. June 2023. Accessed February 12, 2024. Available at: https://www.iihs.org/topics/roundabouts

51. World Health Organization. *Powered Two-and Three-Wheeler Safety: A Road Safety Manual for Decision-Makers and Practitioners.* 2022. Accessed June 20, 2024. Available at: https://www.who.int/publications/i/item/9789240060562

52. National Highway Traffic Safety Administration, Department of Transportation. *Federal Motor Vehicle Safety Standards; Electronic Stability Control Systems.* NHTSA. 2023. Accessed February 14, 2024. Available at: https://www.nhtsa.gov/fmvss/federal-motor-vehicle-safety-standards-electronic-stability-control-systems-0

53. Insurance Institute for Highway Safety, Highway Loss Data Institute. *Advanced Driver Assistance.* IIHS. November 2023. Accessed February 12, 2024. https://www.iihs.org/topics/advanced-driver-assistance

54. Insurance Institute for Highway Safety, Highway Loss Data Institute. *In-Vehicle Alerts, Speed Limiters Needed to Curb Epidemic of Aggressive Driving.* IIHS. December 6, 2023. Accessed February 12, 2024. Available at: https://www.iihs.org/news/detail/in-vehicle-alerts-speed-limiters-needed-to-curb-epidemic-of-aggressive-driving

55. Insurance Institute for Highway Safety, Highway Loss Data Institute. *Alcohol and drugs.* IIHS. October 2023. Accessed February 12, 2024. Available at: https://www.iihs.org/topics/alcohol-and-drugs

56. Reagan I. *Smartphones lead to distraction. Could they also prevent it?* IIHS. July 25, 2023. Accessed February 12, 2024. Available at: https://www.iihs.org/news/detail/smartphones-lead-to-distraction-could-they-also-prevent-it

57. Wagenaar AC, Livingston MD, Staras SS. Effects of a 2009 Illinois alcohol tax increase on fatal motor vehicle crashes. *Am J Public Health.* 2015;105(9):1880-1885. doi:10.2105/AJPH.2014.302428

58. Insurance Institute for Highway Safety. *Seat Belts.* IIHS. July 2023. Accessed February 11, 2024. Available at: https://www.iihs.org/topics/seat-belts

59. Insurance Institute for Highway Safety, Highway Loss Data Institute. *Red Light Running.* IIHS. January 2024. Accessed February 12, 2024. Available at: https://www.iihs.org/topics/red-light-running

60. Zaza S, Sleet DA, Thompson RS, Sosin DM, Bolen JC. Reviews of evidence regarding interventions to increase use of child safety seats. *Am J Prev Med.* 2001;21(4):31-47. doi:10.1016/S0749-3797(01)00377-4

61. Insurance Institute for Highway Safety. *Motorcycle Helmet Use Laws.* IIHS. February 2024. Accessed February 11, 2024. Available at: https://www.iihs.org/topics/motorcycles/motorcycle-helmet-laws-table

62. Macpherson A, Spinks A. Bicycle helmet legislation for the uptake of helmet use and prevention of head injuries. *Cochrane Database of Syst Rev.* 2008;(3). doi:10.1002/14651858.CD005401.pub3

63. Wintemute GJ. The epidemiology of firearm violence in the twenty-first century United States. *Annu Rev Public Health.* 2015;36:5-19. doi:10.1146/annurev-publhealth-031914-122535

64. Utah Medicine. *Firearms Tutorial.* Utah Medical School Tutorial. Accessed February 20, 2024. Available at: https://webpath.med.utah.edu/TUTORIAL/GUNS/GUNINTRO.html

65. Bureau of Alcohol Tobacco and Firearms. *Annual Firearms Manufacturing and Export Report-Year 2022 Interim.* 2022. Accessed June 20, 2024. Available at: https://www.atf.gov/firearms/docs/report/2022-final-afmer/download

66. Kaufman EJ, Wiebe DJ, Xiong RA, Morrison CN, Seamon MJ, Delgado MK. Epidemiologic trends in fatal and nonfatal firearm injuries in the US, 2009–2017. *JAMA Intern Med.* 2021;181(2):237-244. doi:10.1001/jamainternmed.2020.6696

67. Wilson RF, Liu G, Lyons BH, et al. Surveillance for violent deaths—National Violent Death Reporting System, 42 states, the District of Columbia, and Puerto Rico, 2019. *MMWR Surveill Summ.* 2022;71(6):1-40. doi:10.15585/mmwr.ss7106a1

68. Pallin R, Barnhorst A. Clinical strategies for reducing firearm suicide. *Inj Epidemiol.* 2021;8(1). doi:10.1186/s40621-021-00352-8

69. Marineau LA, Uzzi M, Buggs SA, Ihenacho N, Campbell JC. Risk and protective factors for firearm assault injuries among Black men: A scoping review of research. *Trauma Violence Abuse.* 2024;25(3):2468-2488. doi:10.1177/15248380231217042

70. Dalve K, Gause E, Mills B, Floyd AS, Rivara FP, Rowhani-Rahbar A. Neighborhood disadvantage and firearm injury: Does shooting location matter? *Inj Epidemiol.* 2021;8(1). doi:10.1186/s40621-021-00304-2

71. Kegler SR, Dahlberg LL, Vivolo-Kantor AM. A descriptive exploration of the geographic and sociodemographic concentration of firearm homicide in the United States, 2004–2018. *Prev Med (Baltim).* 2021;153. doi:10.1016/j.ypmed.2021.106767

72. Reaves BA. *Felony Defendants in Large Urban Counties, 2009.* 2013. Accessed June 20, 2024. Available at: https://bjs.ojp.gov/library/publications/felony-defendants-large-urban-counties-2009-statistical-tables

73. Branas CC, Han S, Wiebe DJ. Alcohol use and firearm violence. *Epidemiol Rev.* 2016;38(1):32-45. doi:10.1093/epirev/mxv010

74. Klerman EB, Affouf M, Robbins R, et al. Characterizing gun violence by time, day of the week, holidays, and month in 6 US cities, 2015–2021. *J Biol Rhythms.* 2023;39(1):100-108. doi:10.1177/07487304231208469

75. Wintemute GJ. Where the guns come from: The gun industry and gun commerce. *Future of Children.* 2002;12(2):54-71.

76. Bureau of Alcohol Tobacco and Firearms, Department of Justics. *PART III: Crime Guns Recovered and Traced Within the United States and Its Territories.* 2023. Accessed June 20, 2024. Available at: https://www.atf.gov/firearms/docs/report/nfcta-volume-ii-part-iii-crime-guns-recovered-and-traced-us/download

77. Alper M, Glaze L. *Source and Use of Firearms Involved in Crimes: Survey of Prison Inmates, 2016.* 2019. Accessed June 20, 2024. Available at: https://bjs.ojp.gov/content/pub/pdf/suficspi16.pdf

78. Hargarten SW. Characteristics of firearms involved in fatalities. *JAMA.* 1996;275(1):42. doi:10.1001/jama.1996.03530250046025

79. Zeoli AM, Malinski R, Turchan B. Risks and targeted interventions: firearms in intimate partner violence. *Epidemiol Rev.* 2016;38(1):125-139. doi:10.1093/epirev/mxv007

80. Gun Violence Archive. 2024. Accessed October 17, 2024. Available at: https://www.gunviolencearchive.org/

81. Baum GR, Baum JT, Hayward D, Mackay BJ. Gunshot wounds: Ballistics, pathology, and treatment recommendations, with a focus on retained bullets. *Orthop Res Rev.* 2022;14:293-317. doi:10.2147/ORR.S378278

82. Nand D, Naghavi M, Marczak LB, et al. Global mortality from firearms, 1990–2016. *JAMA.* 2018;320(8):792-814. doi:10.1001/jama.2018.10060

83. Kondo MC, Andreyeva E, South EC, Macdonald JM, Branas CC. Neighborhood Interventions to Reduce Violence. *Annu Rev Public Health.* 2018;39:253-271. doi:10.1146/annurev-publhealth

84. Hohl BC, Wiley S, Wiebe DJ, Culyba AJ, Drake R, Branas CC. Association of drug and alcohol use with adolescent firearm homicide at individual, family, and neighborhood levels. *JAMA Intern Med.* 2017;177(3):317-324. doi:10.1001/jamainternmed.2016.8180

85. Gobaud AN, Jacobowitz AL, Mehranbod CA, Sprague NL, Branas CC, Morrison CN. Place-based Interventions and the epidemiology of violence prevention. *Curr Epidemiol Rep.* 2022;9(4):316-325. doi:10.1007/s40471-022-00301-z

86. Branas CC, Rubin D, Guo W. Vacant properties and violence in neighborhoods. *ISRN Public Health.* 2012;2012:1-9. doi:10.5402/2012/246142

87. Miller M, Warren M, Hemenway D, Azrael D. Firearms and suicide in US cities. *Inj Prev.* 2015;21(e1):e116-e119. doi:10.1136/injuryprev-2013-040969

88. Siegel M, Negussie Y, Vanture S, Pleskunas J, Ross CS, King C. The relationship between gun ownership and stranger and nonstranger firearm homicide rates in the United States, 1981–2010. *Am J Public Health.* 2014;104(10):1912-1919. doi:10.2105/AJPH.2014.302042

89. Miller M, Lippmann SJ, Azrael D, Hemenway D. Household firearm ownership and rates of suicide across the 50 United States. *J Trauma.* 2007;62(4):1029-1035. doi:10.1097/01.ta.0000198214.24056.40

90. Small Arms Survey. *Global Firearms Holdings.* Small Arms Survey. June 18, 2018. Accessed February 22, 2024. Available at: https://www.smallarmssurvey.org/database/global-firearms-holdings

91. Anglemyer A, Horvath T, Rutherford G. The accessibility of firearms and risk for suicide and homicide victimization among household members: A systematic review and meta-analysis. *Ann Intern Med.* 2014;160:101-110.

92. Smart R, Morral AR, Smucker S, et al. *The Science of Gun Policy: A Critical Synthesis of Research Evidence on the Effects of Gun Policies in the United States.* 2nd ed. RAND Corporation; 2020. Accessed June 20, 2024. Available at: https://www.rand.org/pubs/research_reports/RR2088.html

93. Vernick JS, Webster DW. Policies to prevent firearm trafficking. *Inj Prev.* 2007;13(2):78-79. doi:10.1136/ip.2007.015487

94. McGinty EE, Choksy S, Wintemute GJ. The relationship between controlled substances and violence. *Epidemiol Rev.* 2016;38(1):5-31. doi:10.1093/epirev/mxv008

95. Favril L, Yu R, Uyar A, Sharpe M, Fazel S. Risk factors for suicide in adults: systematic review and meta-analysis of psychological autopsy studies. *Evid Based Ment Health.* 2022;25(4):148-155. doi:10.1136/ebmental-2022-300549

96. Choe JY, Teplin LA, Abram KM. Perpetration of violence, violent victimization, and severe mental illness: Balancing public health concerns. *Psychiatr Serv.* 2008;59(2). doi:10.1176/ps.2008.59.2.153

97. Elbogen EB, Johnson SC. The intricate link between violence and mental disorder: Results from the National Epidemiologic Survey on Alcohol and Related Conditions. *Arch Gen Psychiatry.* 2009;66(2):152-161.

98. Branas CC, South E, Kondo MC, et al. Citywide cluster randomized trial to restore blighted vacant land and its effects on violence, crime, and fear. *Proc Natl Acad Sci U S A.* 2018;115(12):2946-2951. doi:10.1073/pnas.1718503115

99. Smith ER, Sarani B, Shapiro G, et al. Incidence and cause of potentially preventable death after civilian public mass

shooting in the US. *J Am Coll Surg*. 2019;229(3):244-251. doi:10.1016/j.jamcollsurg.2019.04.016

100. Collins T, Greenberg R, Siegel M, et al. State firearm laws and interstate transfer of guns in the USA, 2006–2016. *J Urban Health*. 2018;95(3):322-336. doi:10.1007/s11524 -018-0251-9

101. Kalesan B, Mobily ME, Keiser O, Fagan JA, Galea S. Firearm legislation and firearm mortality in the USA: A cross-sectional, state-level study. *Lancet*. 2016;387(10030): 1847-1855. doi:10.1016/S0140-6736(15)01026-0

102. Hemenway D, Miller M. Public health approach to the prevention of gun violence. *N Engl J Med*. 2013;368(21):2033-2035. doi:10.1056/nejmsb1302631

103. Gun ownership in New York City. NY Daily News. 2021. Accessed February 22, 2024. Available at: https://www .nydailynews.com/2021/05/16/staten-islanders-likeliest -in-nyc-to-own-legal-handguns-daily-news-analysis-of -nypd-data-shows/

104. Bureau of Alcohol Tobacco and Firearms, Department of Justice. *Identify Prohibited Persons*. ATF; 2020. Accessed February 21, 2024. Available at: https://www.atf.gov /firearms/identify-prohibited-persons

105. Santaella-Tenorio J, Cerdá M, Villaveces A, Galea S. What do we know about the association between firearm legislation and firearm-related injuries? *Epidemiol Rev*. 2016;38(1):140-157. doi:10.1093/epirev/mxv012

106. Braga AA, Cook PJ. The association of firearm caliber with likelihood of death from gunshot injury in criminal assaults. *JAMA Netw Open*. 2018;1(3):e180833. doi:10.1001/jamanetworkopen.2018.0833

107. The RAND Corporation. *The Effects of Bans on the Sale of Assault Weapons and High-Capacity Magazines*. RAND .org. March 2, 2018. Accessed October 20, 2024. Available at: https://www.rand.org/research/gun-policy/analysis/ban -assault-weapons.html

108. Baughman SB. How effective are the police: The problem of clearance rates and criminal accountability. *Ala Law Rev*. 2021;72(1). Accessed March 18, 2025. Available at: https://www.smithsonianmag.com/science-nature/myth -fingerprints-

109. Loeffler CE, Nagin DS. The impact of incarceration on recidivism. *Annu Rev Criminol*. 2022;5(1):133-152. doi:10 .1146/annurev-criminol-030920-112506

110. Buggs SA, Webster DW, Crifasi CK. Using synthetic control methodology to estimate effects of a Cure Violence intervention in Baltimore, Maryland. *Inj Prev*. 2022;28(1):61-67. doi:10.1136/injuryprev-2020-044056

111. Hedegaard H, Curtin SC, Warner M. Suicide mortality in the United States, 1999–2019. *NCHS Data Brief*. 2021;(398):1-7.

112. Fitzgerald B, Kenzie WR Mac, Rasmussen SA, et al. Suicide trends among and within urbanization levels by sex, race/ ethnicity, age group, and mechanism of death—United States, 2001–2015. *MMWR Surveill Summ*. 2018;66(18).

113. Li Z, Page A, Martin G, Taylor R. Attributable risk of psychiatric and socio-economic factors for suicide from individual-level, population-based studies: A systematic review. *Soc Sci Med*. 2011;72(4):608-616. doi:10.1016/j .socscimed.2010.11.008

114. Darvishi N, Farhadi M, Haghtalab T, Poorolajal J. Alcohol-related risk of suicidal ideation, suicide attempt, and completed suicide: A meta-analysis. *PLoS One*. 2015;10(5). doi:10.1371/journal.pone.0126870

115. Borges G, Bagge CL, Cherpitel CJ, Conner KR, Orozco R, Rossow I. A meta-analysis of acute use of alcohol and the risk of suicide attempt. *Psychol Med*. 2017;47(5):949-957. doi:10.1017/S0033291716002841

116. Kaplan MS, Huguet N, McFarland BH, et al. Use of alcohol before suicide in the United States. *Ann Epidemiol*. 2014;24(8). doi:10.1016/j.annepidem.2014.05.008

117. Richardson C, Robb KA, O'Connor RC. A systematic review of suicidal behaviour in men: A narrative synthesis of risk factors. *Soc Sci Med*. 2021;276:113831. doi:10.1016/j .socscimed.2021.113831

118. Borges G, Bagge CL, Orozco R. A literature review and meta-analyses of cannabis use and suicidality. *J Affect Disord*. 2016;195:63-74. doi:10.1016/j.jad.2016.02.007

119. Motillon-Toudic C, Walter M, Séguin M, Carrier JD, Berrouiguet S, Lemey C. Social isolation and suicide risk: Literature review and perspectives. *European Psychiatry*. 2022;65(1). doi:10.1192/j.eurpsy.2022.2320

120. Kyung-Sook W, SangSoo S, Sangjin S, Young-Jeon S. Marital status integration and suicide: A meta-analysis and meta-regression. *Soc Sci Med*. 2018;197:116-126. doi:10.1016/j .socscimed.2017.11.053

121. Sarchiapone M, Mandelli L, Iosue M, Andrisano C, Roy A. Controlling access to suicide means. *Int J Environ Res Public Health*. 2011;8(12):4550-4562. doi:10.3390/ijerph8 124550

122. Niederkrotenthaler T, Braun M, Pirkis J, et al. Association between suicide reporting in the media and suicide: Systematic review and meta-analysis. *BMJ*. 2020;368. doi:10 .1136/bmj.m575

123. Twenge JM. Why increases in adolescent depression may be linked to the technological environment. *Curr Opin Psychol*. 2020;32:89-94. doi:10.1016/j.copsyc.2019.06.036

124. Twenge JM, Martin GN, Campbell WK. Decreases in psychological well-being among American adolescents after 2012 and links to screen time during the rise of smartphone technology. *Emotion*. 2018;18(6):765-780. doi:10.1037/emo0000403

125. Twenge JM, Cooper AB, Joiner TE, Duffy ME, Binau SG. Age, period, and cohort trends in mood disorder indicators and suicide-related outcomes in a nationally representative dataset, 2005–2017. *J Abnorm Psychol*. 2019;128(3): 185-199. doi:10.1037/abn0000410

126. Nesi J, Burke TA, Bettis AH, et al. Social media use and self-injurious thoughts and behaviors: A systematic review and meta-analysis. *Clin Psychol Rev*. 2021;87. doi:10.1016/j .cpr.2021.102038

127. Zalsman G, Hawton K, Wasserman D, et al. Suicide prevention strategies revisited: 10-year systematic review. *Lancet Psychiatry*. 2016;3(7):646-659. doi:10.1016/S2215 -0366(16)30030-X

128. Emanuel EJ. A Simple Way to Reduce Suicides. *The New York Times*. June 2, 2013. Accessed February 27, 2024. Available at: https://archive.nytimes.com/opinionator .blogs.nytimes.com/2013/06/02/a-simple-way-to-reduce -suicides/

129. Pirkis J, Too LS, Spittal MJ, Krysinska K, Robinson J, Cheung YTD. Interventions to reduce suicides at suicide hotspots: a systematic review and meta-analysis. *Lancet Psychiatry*. 2015;2(11):994-1001. doi:10.1016/S2215-0366(15)00266-7

130. World Health Organization. Department of Mental Health and Substance Abuse. *Preventing Suicide : A Global Imperative*. WHO; 2014.

131. Global Burden of Disease Collaboration, Institute for Health Metrics and Evaluation. *GBD Results.* July 12, 2023. Accessed July 11, 2023. Available at: https://vizhub.healthdata.org/gbd-results/

132. Stevens JA, Mahoney JE, Ehrenreich H. Circumstances and outcomes of falls among high-risk community-dwelling older adults. *Inj Epidemiol.* 2014;1(1). doi:10.1186/2197-1714-1-5

133. Timsina LR, Willetts JL, Brennan MJ, et al. Circumstances of fall-related injuries by age and gender among community-dwelling adults in the United States. *PLoS One.* 2017;12(5). doi:10.1371/journal.pone.0176561

134. Colón-Emeric CS, McDermott CL, Lee DS, Berry SD. Risk assessment and prevention of falls in older community-dwelling adults: A review. *JAMA.* 2024;331(16):1397-1406. doi:10.1001/jama.2024.1416

135. Moreland BL, Kakara R, Haddad YK, Shakya I, Bergen G. A descriptive analysis of location of older adult falls that resulted in emergency department visits in the United States, 2015. *Am J Lifestyle Med.* 2021;15(6). doi:10.1177/1559827620942187

136. Stevens JA, Mahoney JE, Ehrenreich H. Circumstances and outcomes of falls among high-risk community-dwelling older adults. *Inj Epidemiol.* 2014;1(1). doi:10.1186/2197-1714-1-5

137. Centers for Disease Control and Prevention. *Facts about falls.* CDC; 2023. Accessed July 13, 2023. Available at: https://www.cdc.gov/falls/facts.html

138. Jager TE, Weiss HB, Coben JH, Pepe PE. Traumatic brain injuries evaluated in U.S. emergency departments, 1992–1994. *Acad Emerg Med.* 2000;7(2). doi:10.1111/j.1553-2712.2000.tb00515.x

139. Moreland B, Kakara R, Henry A. Trends in nonfatal falls and fall-related injuries among adults aged ≥65 years—United States, 2012–2018. *MMWR Morb Mortal Wkly Rep.* 2020;69(27). doi:10.15585/mmwr.mm6927a5

140. Garnett MF, Weeks JD, Spencer MR. Unintentional fall deaths among adults aged 65 and over: United States, 2020. *NCHS Data Brief.* 2022;(449):1-7.

141. Wu H, Mach J, Le Couteur DG, Hilmer SN. Fall-related mortality trends in Australia and the United Kingdom: Implications for research and practice. *Maturitas.* 2020;142. doi:10.1016/j.maturitas.2020.07.008

142. Hagiya H, Koyama T, Zamami Y, et al. Fall-related mortality trends in older Japanese adults aged ≥65 years: A nationwide observational study. *BMJ Open.* 2019;9(12). doi:10.1136/bmjopen-2019-033462

143. Kannus P, Niemi S, Sievänen H, Parkkari J. Declining incidence in fall-induced deaths of older adults: Finnish statistics during 1971–2015. *Aging Clin Exp Res.* 2018;30(9). doi:10.1007/s40520-018-0898-9

144. Majdan M, Mauritz W. Unintentional fall-related mortality in the elderly: Comparing patterns in two countries with different demographic structure. *BMJ Open.* 2015;5(8). doi:10.1136/bmjopen-2015-008672

145. Padrón-Monedero A, Damián J, Pilar Martin M, Fernández-Cuenca R. Mortality trends for accidental falls in older people in Spain, 2000–2015. *BMC Geriatr.* 2017;17(1). doi:10.1186/s12877-017-0670-6

146. Hagiya H, Koyama T, Zamami Y, et al. Fall-related mortality trends in older Japanese adults aged ≥65 years: A nationwide observational study. *BMJ Open.* 2019;9(12). doi:10.1136/bmjopen-2019-033462

147. Drew JAR, Xu D. Trends in fatal and nonfatal injuries among older Americans, 2004–2017. *Am J Prev Med.* 2020;59(1):3-11. doi:10.1016/j.amepre.2020.01.008

148. Rubenstein LZ. Falls in older people: epidemiology, risk factors and strategies for prevention. *Age Ageing.* 2006;35-S2: ii37-ii41.

149. Hart LA, Phelan EA, Yi JY, Marcum ZA, Gray SL. Use of fall risk—increasing drugs around a fall-related injury in older adults: A systematic review. *J Am Geriatr Soc.* 2020;68(6). doi:10.1111/jgs.16369

150. Seppala LJ, van de Glind EMM, Daams JG, et al. Fall-risk-increasing drugs: A systematic review and meta-analysis: III. Others. *J Am Med Dir Assoc.* 2018;19(4). doi:10.1016/j.jamda.2017.12.099

151. Seppala LJ, Wermelink AMAT, de Vries M, et al. Fall-risk-increasing drugs: A systematic review and meta-analysis: II. Psychotropics. *J Am Med Dir Assoc.* 2018;19(4). doi:10.1016/j.jamda.2017.12.098

152. Laberge S, Crizzle AM. A literature review of psychotropic medications and alcohol as risk factors for falls in community-dwelling older adults. *Clin Drug Investig.* 2019;39(2). doi:10.1007/s40261-018-0721-6

153. Hart LA, Walker R, Phelan EA, et al. Change in central nervous system-active medication use following fall-related injury in older adults. *J Am Geriatr Soc.* 2022;70(1): 168-177. doi:10.1111/jgs.17508

154. Hwang CS, Kang EM, Kornegay CJ, Staffa JA, Jones CM, McAninch JK. Trends in the concomitant prescribing of opioids and benzodiazepines, 2002–2014. *Am J Prev Med.* 2016;51(2). doi:10.1016/j.amepre.2016.02.014

155. Paulozzi LJ, Jones C, Mack K, Rudd R. Vital signs: overdoses of prescription opioid pain relievers. *MMWR Morb Mortal Wkly Rep.* 2011;60(43).

156. Shaver AL, Clark CM, Hejna M, Feuerstein S, Wahler RG, Jacobs DM. Trends in fall-related mortality and fall risk increasing drugs among older individuals in the United States, 1999–2017. *Pharmacoepidemiol Drug Saf.* 2021;30(8). doi:10.1002/pds.5201

157. Innes GK, Ogden CL, Crentsil V, Concato J, Fakhouri TH. Prescription medication use among older adults in the US. *JAMA Intern Med.* Published online 2024. doi:10.1001/jamainternmed.2024.2781

158. Xu Q, Ou X, Li J. The risk of falls among the aging population: A systematic review and meta-analysis. *Front Public Health.* 2022;10:902599. doi:10.3389/fpubh.2022.902599

159. Sun Y, Zhang B, Yao Q, et al. Association between usual alcohol consumption and risk of falls in middle-aged and older Chinese adults. *BMC Geriatr.* 2022;22(1). doi:10.1186/s12877-022-03429-1

160. Hatton AL, Rome K. Falls, footwear, and podiatric interventions in older adults. *Clin Geriatr Med.* 2019;35(2):161-171. doi:10.1016/j.cger.2018.12.001

161. Tricco AC, Thomas SM, Veroniki AA, et al. Comparisons of interventions for preventing falls in older adults: A systematic review and meta-analysis. *JAMA.* 2017;318(17):1687-1699. doi:10.1001/jama.2017.15006

162. Gillespie LD, Robertson MC, Gillespie WJ, et al. Interventions for preventing falls in older people living in the community. *Cochrane Database of Syst Rev.* 2012;(9):CD007146. doi:10.1002/14651858.CD007146.pub3

163. Clemson L, Stark S, Pighills AC, et al. Environmental interventions for preventing falls in older people living

in the community. *Cochrane Database of Syst Rev.* 2023;(3):CD013258. doi:10.1002/14651858.CD013258 .pub2

164. American Geriatrics Society 2023 updated AGS Beers Criteria® for potentially inappropriate medication use in older adults. *J Am Geriatr Soc.* Published online 2023. doi:10.1111/jgs.18372

165. Lee J, Negm A, Peters R, Wong EKC, Holbrook A. Deprescribing fall-risk increasing drugs (FRIDs) for the prevention of falls and fall-related complications: a systematic review and meta-analysis. *BMJ Open.* 2021;11(2):e035978. doi:10.1136/bmjopen-2019-035978

166. Pit SW, Byles JE, Henry DA, Holt L, Hansen V, Bowman DA. A quality use of medicines program for general practitioners and older people: A cluster randomised controlled trial. *Med J Aust.* 2007;187(1). doi:10.5694/j.1326-5377.2007 .tb01110.x

167. Campbell AJ, Robertson MC, Gardner MM, Norton RN, Buchner DM. Psychotropic medication withdrawal and a home-based exercise program to prevent falls: A randomized, controlled trial. *J Am Geriatr Soc.* 1999;47(7). doi:10.1111/j.1532-5415.1999.tb03843.x

168. Sherrington C, Michaleff ZA, Fairhall N, et al. Exercise to prevent falls in older adults: An updated systematic review and meta-analysis. *Br J Sports Med.* 2017;51(24):1749-1757. doi:10.1136/bjsports-2016-096547

169. Sherrington C, Michaleff ZA, Fairhall N, et al. Exercise to prevent falls in older adults: An updated systematic review and meta-analysis. *Br J Sports Med.* 2017;51(24):1749-1757. doi:10.1136/bjsports-2016-096547

170. Clemson L, Stark S, Pighills AC, et al. Environmental interventions for preventing falls in older people living in the community. *Cochrane Database of Syst Rev.* 2023;(3): CD013258. doi:10.1002/14651858.CD013258.pub2

171. National Center for Injury Prevention, Centers for Disease Control and Prevention. *Check for Safety: A Home Fall Prevention Checklist for Older Adults.* 2017. Accessed March 18. 2025. Available at: www.cdc.gov/steadi

172. Montero-Odasso M, Van Der Velde N, Martin FC, et al. World guidelines for falls prevention and management for older adults: a global initiative. *Age Ageing.* 2022;51(9). doi:10.1093/ageing/afac205

173. Centers for Disease Control and Prevention. *STEADI -Older Adult Fall Prevention.* Accessed July 13, 2023. Available at: www.cdc.gov/steadi/index.html

174. Santesso N, Carrasco-Labra A, Brignardello-Petersen R. Hip protectors for preventing hip fractures in older people. *Cochrane Database of Syst Rev.* 2014;(3):CD001255. doi:10.1002/14651858.CD001255.pub5

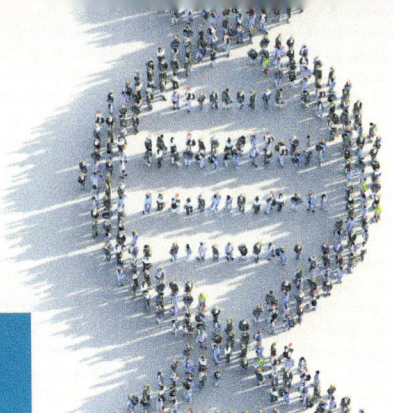

CHAPTER 7

Chronic Metabolic Diseases

The steady rise of obesity over the past few decades is driving increases in many other health problems worldwide. This chapter covers obesity and chronic metabolic diseases for which obesity is a key risk factor: type 2 diabetes, chronic kidney disease, and chronic liver disease.

Obesity and Diabetes

Introduction

Obesity is a metabolic condition in which the body stores too much fat. Type 2 diabetes is a closely-related chronic disease in which the body does not effectively use glucose, the main "sugar" in blood. This section covers both conditions, discussing our current understanding of excess fat storage, the regulation of glucose levels, the pathophysiology of obesity and diabetes, risk factors, and approaches to prevention.

Physiology: Fat, Carbohydrates, and Fat Regulation

Metabolic Fuels and Their Storage

Cells throughout the body need energy to do the work of metabolism. The storage forms of the two main fuels that the cells use are **fats** and **carbohydrates**.

- *Fats*, also known as **triglycerides**, are found in vegetable oils and the fatty parts of meat. Chemically, fats are large organic molecules in which three different **fatty acids** are linked to a backbone called **glycerol** (**Figure 7.1**). Cells in

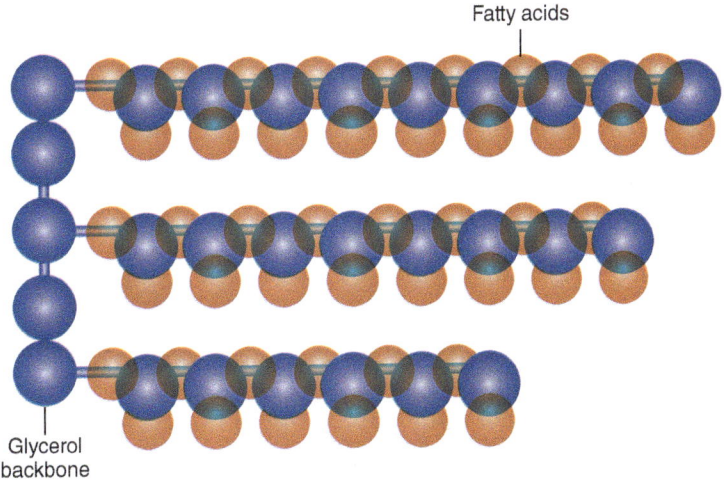

Figure 7.1 Triglycerides and Fatty Acids. Triglycerides, also known as fats, are molecules composed of three fatty acids connected to a molecule called glycerol.

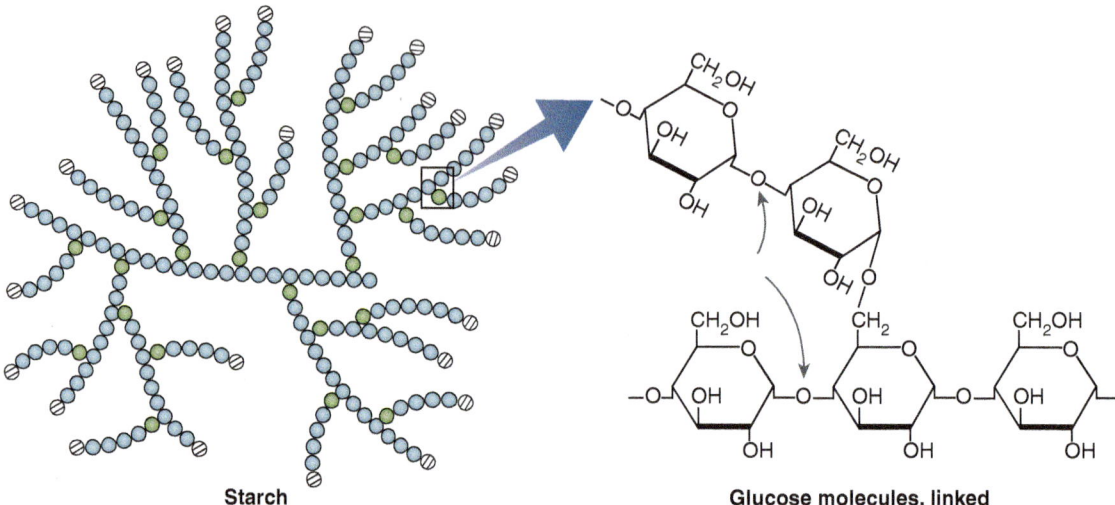

Starch

Glucose molecules, linked

Figure 7.2 Starch and Glucose. The main carbohydrate that humans eat is called starch. It is composed of extensive webs and chains of linked molecules of glucose.

the body separate fatty acids from this backbone and then metabolize the fatty acids, harvesting the energy in them. In particular, muscles use fatty acids for energy when they contract.

- *Carbohydrates* are found in grains; the main carbohydrate that humans eat is **starch**, which is in wheat, corn, rice and potatoes. Chemically, carbohydrates are organic compounds made up of carbon, hydrogen, and oxygen atoms in a ratio of 1:2:1. **Glucose** is a small hexagon-shaped molecule that is one of a group of carbohydrates called **monosaccharides**. Monosaccharides are informally known as "sugars" because most of them taste sweet. Starch and other "complex" carbohydrates that humans eat are long branching chains of glucose subunits (**Figure 7.2**). When

people consume starch and other complex carbohydrates, these carbohydrates are digested into glucose subunits. Glucose then circulates in the blood, supplying cells throughout the body. Cells in the brain require a constant supply of glucose for fuel, and muscle cells use glucose along with fatty acids for fuel during exercise.

The body adjusts the use and storage of these two fuels based on its needs and on their availability (**Figure 7.3**). Glucose levels in the blood fluctuate during the day. After a meal, when blood glucose levels are high, cells use glucose for energy, put some into excess storage in the form of a long-chain carbohydrate called **glycogen**, and convert the rest into fatty acids.[1] A few hours later, when blood glucose levels are low, the body burns mostly fatty acids for energy and breaks down the stored

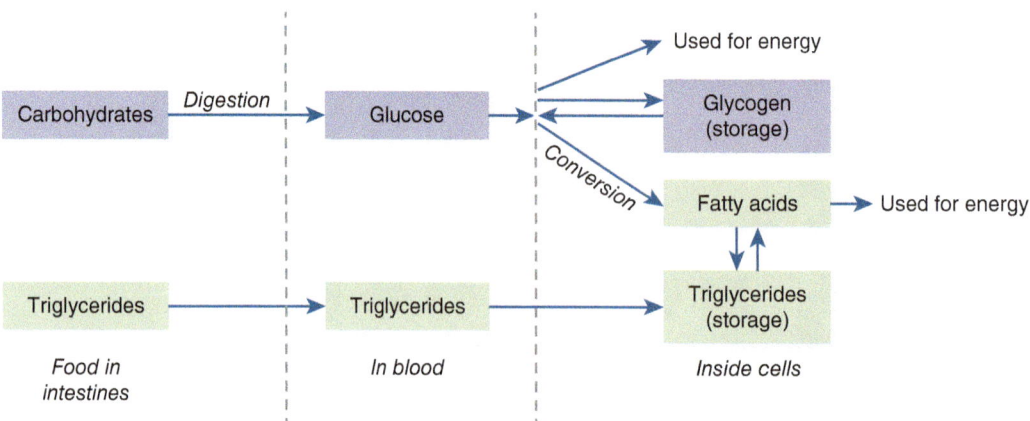

Figure 7.3 Use and Storage of Carbohydrates and Triglycerides (Fats). Both carbohydrates and triglycerides in foods can be either used by cells for energy or stored. First, carbohydrates are digested into glucose, and glucose and triglycerides are absorbed through the wall of the intestines into the blood. They then enter cells. Inside cells, glucose can be used for energy, stored as glycogen, or converted to fatty acids. Triglycerides can remain in storage or be broken down into fatty acids. Fatty acids can be used for energy or stored in the form of triglycerides. Thus, triglyceride storage can result from consumption of either triglycerides or carbohydrates.

glycogen into glucose. The glycogen that is stored is held mostly in the liver and muscles, but these organs can hold only about a 12- to 24-hour supply.[1]

The body has a much greater ability to store fats. Fatty acids can originate from either consuming fat-containing foods or the conversion of excess glucose (Figure 7.3). Those fatty acids can be either used for energy or stored as triglycerides in **adipocytes** (often called **fat cells**). When needed by muscles for energy, those triglycerides are broken down again into fatty acids.

Regulation of Fat Stores

All animals need stored fat to survive when food is not available, but having too much stored fat is harmful. Because of this, humans and other animals have many complex systems to keep body fat stores within a narrow range. These regulatory systems are coordinated by a part of the brain called the **hypothalamus**, and they constantly adjust both the appetite and how much energy the body expends.[2]

The systems involve signals from nerves in the stomach and the intestines, as well as several hormones released by the intestines and by adipocytes (**Figure 7.4**). For example, before a meal, the stomach

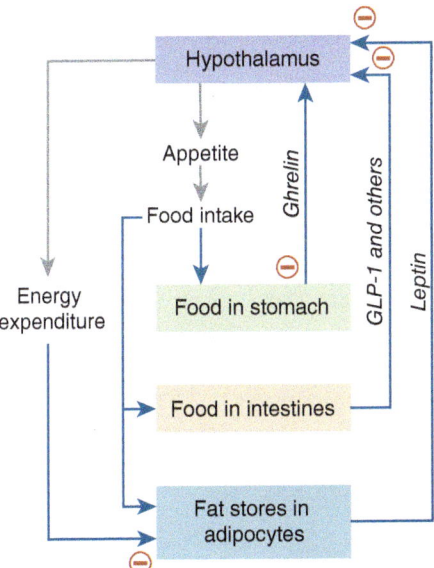

Figure 7.4 Regulation of Fat Storage. The body has complex systems to regulate the amount of fat stored in adipocytes, coordinated by the hypothalamus. Some of these systems are shown here. The hormone ghrelin is secreted by the stomach and stimulates appetite before a meal. After a meal, ghrelin levels drop and the intestines secrete several other hormones, including GLP-1, which suppress appetite. When body fat stores are high, the adipocytes secrete the hormone leptin, which suppresses appetite. The hypothalamus also adjusts the body's energy expenditure to maintain fat stores in the adipocytes.

secretes a hormone called **ghrelin**, which travels to the hypothalamus, where it stimulates appetite.[2] After a meal, the intestines secrete multiple hormones, including one called **glucacon-like peptide 1 (GLP-1)**, which suppress appetite. And when adipocytes are laden with fat, they secrete a hormone called **leptin**, which also suppresses appetite.[2] The actions of these hormones are the basis for drugs that treat obesity.

Insulin and Regulation of Blood Glucose Levels

If blood glucose levels fall below 70 mg per deciliter, the brain cells cannot function normally. If blood glucose levels rise above 140 mg per deciliter, the glucose can cause damage to organs. For these reasons, the body has even more carefully-calibrated systems to keep glucose levels in the blood in this narrow range.[3]

The hormone **insulin** is central to this regulation of blood glucose levels. Insulin is produced by the **beta cells** in the **pancreas**, which is an organ in the upper abdomen, behind the stomach. After a meal, carbohydrates in food are digested in the small intestine into glucose subunits. The glucose is then absorbed through the intestinal walls into the blood, causing glucose levels in the blood to rise.

When the beta cells of the pancreas sense higher glucose levels, they secrete insulin (**Figure 7.5**). Insulin then travels through the blood and fits into **insulin receptors** in the muscles and in the liver as a key would fit into a lock. When insulin fits into the receptors, it induces the muscles and liver to take up glucose from the blood and store it as glycogen. With glucose moving inside of cells, the amount of glucose left in the blood falls. This insulin response and the rise and fall in blood glucose levels happen within two hours after a meal.[3]

Insulin and Fat Storage

Although insulin's main role is regulation of blood glucose levels, the hormone also promotes the storage of fats. Insulin prompts liver cells to convert glucose into fatty acids and adipocytes to store fatty acids as triglycerides (**Figure 7.6**).[4,5]

Pathophysiology of Obesity and Diabetes

Obesity

In obesity, the adipocytes store more fat than is healthy.[2] The central question in the science of obesity is why the regulatory systems for fat storage fail.

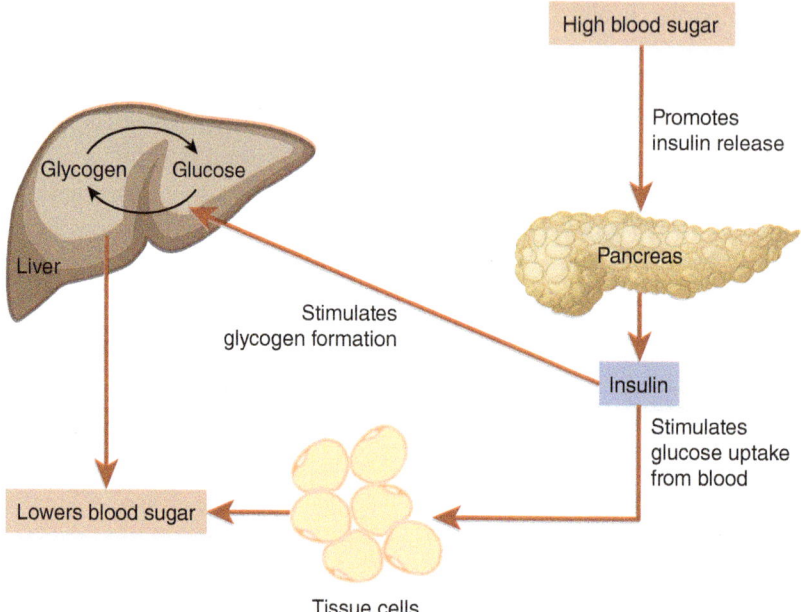

Figure 7.5 How Insulin Regulates Blood Glucose. The beta cells of the pancreas respond to high levels of glucose in the blood by secreting insulin. Insulin then induces the muscles and the liver to take up glucose from the blood and store it as glycogen. This lowers blood sugar back into a healthy range.

Despite decades of research on this question, not all experts agree on the answer.[2]

The most common view is that obesity is primarily a problem of energy balance, in which the body's regulatory systems, designed by evolution to survive famine more than excess, are simply overwhelmed by the amount of energy consumed.[6] In this view, an unhealthy "food environment" surrounds humans with foods that are tasty, in large portions. and **energy-dense**—that is, delivering a high number of calories per gram. It does not matter if the calories that are consumed are in the form of fats or carbohydrates because the body converts excess carbohydrates to fats. Fats chemically contain more energy than carbohydrates (9 versus 4 calories per gram), so high-fat foods are usually more energy-dense than low-fat foods. But refined carbohydrate foods (like white bread, crackers, and potato chips) are also energy-dense—in the range of 3–5 calories per gram.[7] On the other hand, fresh fruits and vegetables have a very low energy density of less than 0.6 calories per gram.

Some experts instead believe that obesity is primarily a problem of disordered metabolism, in which

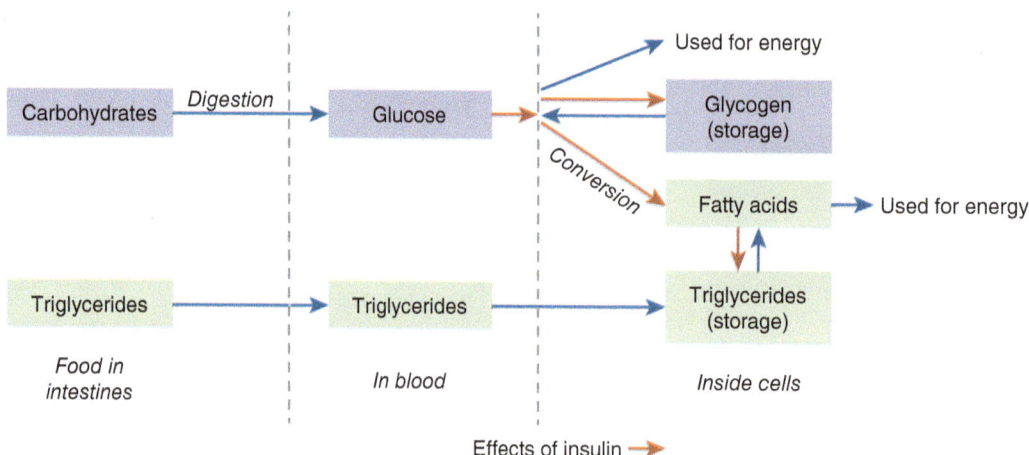

Figure 7.6 Effect of Insulin on the Use and Storage of Carbohydrates and Triglycerides (Fats). The hormone insulin: 1) enables glucose to enter cells from the blood, 2) promotes the storage of glucose as glycogen in muscle and liver cells, 3) promotes the conversion of glucose into fatty acids, and 4) promotes the storage of fatty acids as triglycerides in adipocytes. These effects are shown in red arrows.

certain foods cause the excess storage of fat in adipocytes.[8] This depletes the blood of fatty acids and glucose, and the hypothalamus responds with an increased appetite. In this model, overeating is a consequence of excess fat storage, not a cause of it. The main culprits in this theory are foods that cause a quick rise in blood glucose, which triggers a rapid spike in insulin levels (**Figure 7.7**), which in turn stores fat.[8,9] The insulin spike then rapidly lowers blood glucose levels, and the rapid fall in glucose levels leaves the person hungry.[9]

The **glycemic index** is a measure of how quickly blood glucose levels rise after eating different foods. Sugar-sweetened beverages like soft drinks cause a very rapid rise in glucose, so they have a very high glycemic index.[9] So do refined grains, like white bread.

It is possible that both theories are partly correct—humans overeat because tasty, energy-dense food is everywhere, *and* because some foods cause a rapid rise in blood sugar, which leads to excess fat storage. But neither theory explains all of the foods that have been linked to weight gain in epidemiologic studies.

And there are theories about additional factors contributing to excess fat storage. One theory is that exposure to **endocrine-disrupting chemicals** in food or the environment spurs excess growth of adipocytes in children.[10] Another theory is that the type of bacteria that live in the intestines, called the gut **microbiome** influences energy absorption, insulin levels, or appetite, and that persons who become obese have different microbiomes than those who do not.[11] More research is needed on these theories.

Experts do agree on a few key points, though.

First, humans' diet is central to the development of obesity—more so than physical activity. While physical activity can help limit weight gain, it is not a very effective way to do it.

Second, the obesity epidemic is not caused by individuals' lack of self-control. Some people tend to accumulate more excess fat than others, mainly because of the genes they inherited,[6] but the fact that entire populations are increasingly storing too much fat means that the epidemic cannot be explained by differences between individuals.

Third, certain foods are more likely to cause weight gain than others. In the past, experts argued about whether fats or carbohydrates were more responsible for weight gain. It is now clear that classifying foods or diets according to their fat or carbohydrate content is oversimplifying. The focus has now shifted to specific foods, how foods are processed, and people's complete dietary patterns.

Table 7.1 lists the foods and food components that studies have linked to obesity or to weight gain. The list of higher-risk foods includes those that are processed, energy-dense, and/or have a high sugar content, such as sugar-sweetened beverages, foods with added sugars (such as sweets and desserts), refined grains (such

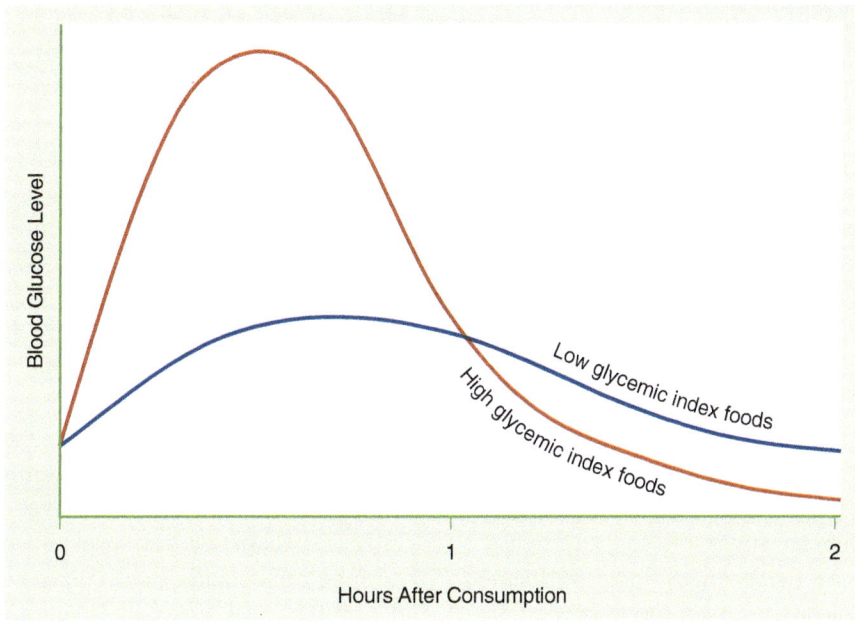

Figure 7.7 The Impact of Foods of Different Glycemic Index Levels on Blood Glucose Levels. Foods that cause a rapid rise in blood glucose after a meal are considered to have a high glycemic index. According to one theory of obesity, these foods trigger a rapid rise in insulin levels, which causes adipocytes to store too much fat, while also rapidly lowering blood glucose levels, leaving people both overweight and hungry.

Table 7.1 Foods and Food Components Associated with Higher or Lower Risk of Obesity or Weight Gain

Higher Risk	
	Sugar-sweetened beverages
	Foods with added sugars
	Refined grains
	Potatoes/fried potatoes
	Red meat
	Processed meat
	Saturated fats
	Sodium
Lower Risk	
	Vegetables
	Legumes
	Fruits
	Whole grains
	Seafood
	Low-fat dairy
	Unsaturated vegetable oils

Data From Dietary Guidelines Advisory Committee. Scientific Report of the 2020 Dietary Guidelines Advisory Committee Advisory Report to the Secretary of Agriculture and Secretary of Health and Human Services. Washington, DC; 2020. Accessed June 12, 2024. https://www.dietaryguidelines.gov/2020-advisory-committee-report

as crackers and white bread), and fried potatoes. Red meat, processed meat, saturated fats, and sodium have also been associated with weight gain, although the biologic reasons why are less clear.[12-14] The lower-risk foods that are not associated with weight gain are vegetables, fruits, legumes, whole grains, seafood, low-fat dairy products, and unsaturated fats and oils.[14,15]

In recent years, some experts have begun classifying foods according to the amount of processing involved to prepare them. **Ultra-processed foods** are those made industrially from wheat flour, corn syrup, vegetable oils and other food components, and that contain little or no whole foods.[16] Ultra-processed foods are usually full of fat, sugar, and sodium; are very energy-dense; and are designed by food companies to be tasty. Typical ultra-processed foods are cookies, pastries, breakfast cereals, sweet and savory packaged snacks, sugar-sweetened beverages, hamburgers, and sausages.[17] Ultra-processed foods make up most of the calories eaten by Americans and they are becoming increasingly popular in other countries.[17,18] Studies have shown that people who eat more ultra-processed foods over years gain more weight.[17] And one remarkable study conducted in a controlled environment found that when people were given ultra-processed foods, they consumed about 500 more calories per day than they did when given unprocessed foods.[19] Also, they gained about 2 pounds in just 2 weeks of the ultra-processed diet but lost about 2 pounds in 2 weeks of the unprocessed diet.

Diabetes

Diabetes mellitus is a pair of diseases involving high blood glucose and problems with insulin.[3]

In **type 1 diabetes** (formerly called juvenile-onset diabetes), the beta cells of the pancreas just stop producing insulin (**Figure 7.8**). With no insulin present, glucose cannot enter muscle or liver cells, so the glucose in the blood rises to extremely high levels.

In **type 2 diabetes**, the initial problem is not the production of insulin; it is the insulin receptors. At first, the insulin receptors become less "sensitive," so the insulin that is present is less effective. This condition is called reduced **insulin sensitivity** or **insulin resistance**. Like not having enough insulin, having faulty insulin receptors prevents glucose from entering cells, which causes blood glucose levels to rise, although to a lesser extent than in type 1 diabetes.

The Connection Between Obesity and Type 2 Diabetes

Obesity is the key risk factor for type 2 diabetes. The connection is this: excess triglyceride storage causes insulin resistance.[20] While the mechanisms are complex and not fully understood, it is known that the excess fat storage in obesity has a direct damaging effect on the insulin receptors on the muscle and liver cells.[20] The excess fat also harms adipocytes. The overloaded cells cannot store all of the triglycerides available; instead, triglycerides break down and spill fatty acids in blood.[20,21] These "free" fatty acids in the blood further promote insulin resistance (**Figure 7.9**).[3,22]

The body's initial response to insulin resistance in type 2 diabetes is just to secrete more insulin. For this reason, in the early stages of type 2 diabetes (unlike in type 1 diabetes), the levels of insulin in the blood may be abnormally high. Over years, the beta cells of the pancreas gradually cannot keep up with this abnormally high demand and "burn out."[3] As a result, people with longstanding type 2 diabetes have both insulin resistance and low levels of insulin in the blood. This further increases blood glucose levels.

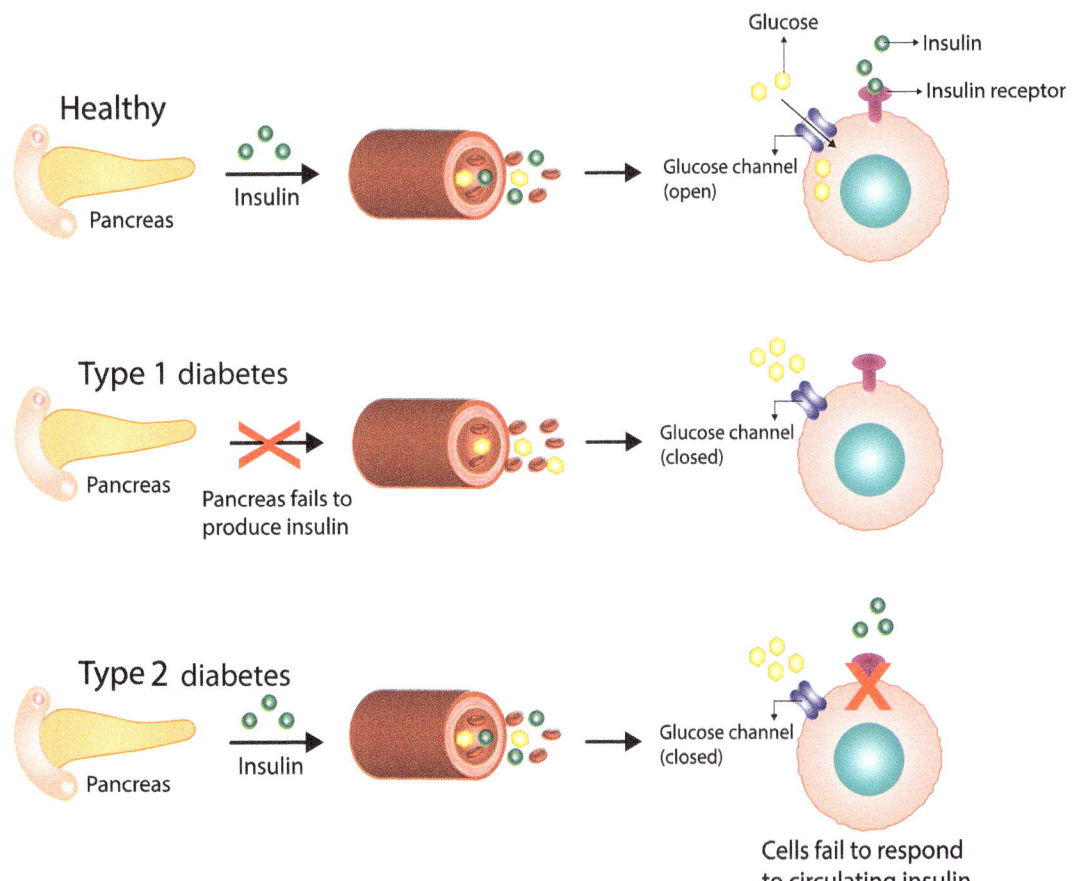

Figure 7.8 Functioning of Insulin and Insulin Receptors in Healthy Persons and Those with Diabetes. Insulin fits in an insulin receptor on cells, which opens a glucose channel, allowing glucose to enter cells. In Type 1 diabetes, the pancreas does not produce insulin, so the glucose channel remains closed and glucose cannot enter cells. In Type 2 diabetes, the initial problem is instead resistance to insulin that is present, which also causes the glucose channel to remain closed. Later, in Type 2 diabetes, the insulin-producing cells in the pancreas appear to "burn out" and produce less insulin.
© Ph-HY/Shutterstock

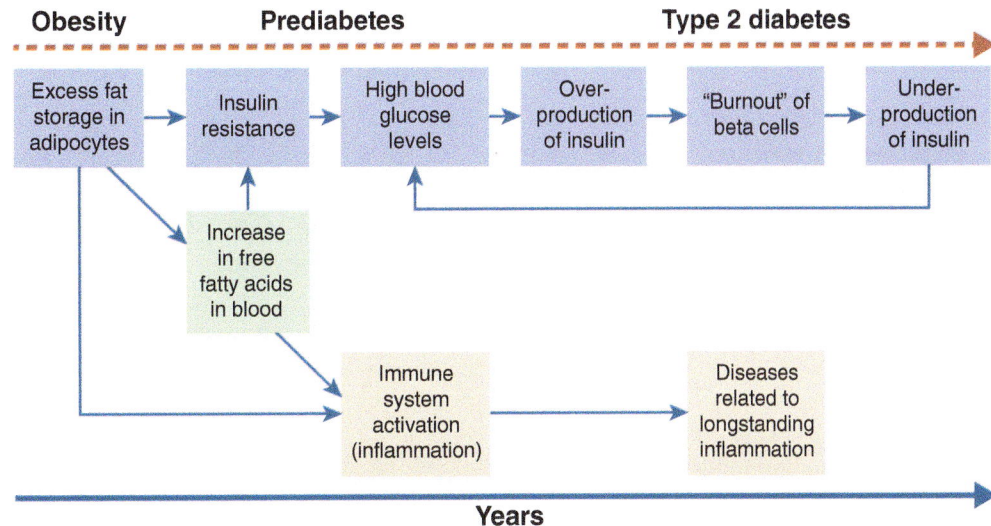

Figure 7.9 Links from Obesity to Type 2 Diabetes and to Other Long-term Health Effects. Obesity leads to diabetes by the excess fat storage causing insulin resistance. This causes high blood glucose levels, to which the beta cells respond by producing and secreting more insulin. Over time, the beta cells cannot keep up with this demand and "burn out." At the same time, the free fatty acids in the blood activate the immune system, causing inflammation that leads to many different diseases.

The overloaded adipocytes and free fatty acids in the blood in type 2 diabetes cause damage in another important way (Figure 7.9). They stimulate the body's immune system, causing **inflammation**.[3,22] Inflammation involves activation of immune cells, which try to defend the body against invading organisms. When there are no invading organisms, though, the inflammation harms the body's own tissues. In obesity and type 2 diabetes, a low-grade inflammation occurs throughout the body and continues for years, causing many other health problems, as discussed later in this chapter and in other chapters of this book.

Other exposures increase the risk of type 2 diabetes to a lesser degree than obesity does. Smoking and exposure to air pollution are two in particular. The connection is not entirely clear, but the lung damage from these also causes inflammation, and it may be that this inflammation increases insulin resistance.[23]

The Consequences of Type 2 Diabetes

Type 2 diabetes is a disease that people live with for decades. During that time, the disease gradually harms many organs throughout the body (**Table 7.2**). The damage is mainly due to its effects on large and small arteries, called the **macrovascular** and **microvascular complications of diabetes**.

Diabetes raises blood triglycerides and cholesterol, as well as damaging the cells lining the arteries, which leads to **atherosclerosis**—the narrowing of arteries by a buildup of cholesterol under the lining (see Chapter 2. Heart Disease and Stroke). When arteries are narrowed, not enough blood flows through them to supply tissues with oxygen and nutrients. Narrowed arteries supplying the heart can cause **ischemic heart disease** and narrowed arteries supplying the brain can cause an **ischemic stroke**.[3]

At the same time, the high levels of blood sugar damage the tiny arteries throughout the body. This microvascular damage harms a few organs in particular: (1) the kidneys, causing **chronic kidney disease**, (2) the retina (back of the eyes) and the lens (front of the eyes), causing cataracts and a gradual loss of vision, (3) many nerves, causing a partial loss of sensation, and 4) the brain, which is why people who have had diabetes for many years are more likely to develop **dementia** (see Chapter 5, Mental Illnesses).[24]

The macrovascular and microvascular complications combine to harm the feet of people with diabetes. People who have lost sensation in their feet because of nerve damage can get injured from shoes that do not fit or from stepping on sharp objects without noticing

---

Table 7.2 Consequences of Type 2 Diabetes

Atherosclerosis
Ischemic heart disease
Ischemic stroke
Peripheral artery disease
Dementia
Chronic kidney disease
Vision loss from damage to retina and/or lens
Nerve damage
Foot damage and infections

---

it. Because their feet do not get enough blood flow, people with diabetes can get foot infections after these minor injuries. If this happens, an amputation may be necessary to prevent the spread of the infection.[3]

Other Health Consequences of Obesity

Type 2 diabetes is the disease most closely linked to obesity. But people who are overweight or obese are also more likely to develop many other health problems, even if they do not develop diabetes.[25] The connection of obesity to many of these health problems is longstanding inflammation. The list of diseases and conditions for which obesity is a risk factor includes ischemic cardiovascular disease, chronic kidney disease, chronic liver disease, asthma, osteoarthritis, low back pain, many types of cancer, and depression.

Compared to people with a healthy weight, those who are overweight have only about a 10% increase in mortality, but those who are obese have a 40% increase and those who are severely obese about a doubling of their mortality rate.[26]

Measuring Obesity in Populations

Measuring obesity requires special equipment to accurately measure how much fat is in a person's body. But a simple way to estimate body fat is with the **body mass index (BMI)**, which is calculated as the weight in kilograms divided by the height in meters squared:

$$\text{Body Mass Index} = \frac{\text{Weight}}{\text{Height}^2}$$

For example, a person who is 5-feet 5-inches (1.65 meters) tall and weighs 150 pounds (68 kg) has a BMI of 24.96, which is at the top of the healthy range. For adults, CDC defines a healthy weight for height as a BMI between 18.5 and 24.9, **overweight**

Table 7.3 Definitions of Overweight and Obesity in Populations

Classification	BMI (Kg/m²)	Examples: Weight in Pounds	
		Height 5ft 2in	Height 5ft 10 in
Underweight	< 18.5	< 101	< 129
Healthy	18.5–< 25	101–< 136	129–< 174
Overweight	25–< 30	136–< 164	174–< 209
Obesity Class 1	30–< 35	164–< 191	209–< 244
Obesity Class 2	35–< 40	191–< 218	244–< 279
Obesity Class 3 or Severe Obesity	40+	218+	279+

Data from Expert Panel on the Identification Evaluation and Treatment of Overweight in Adults. Clinical Guidelines on the Identification, Evaluation, and Treatment of Overweight and Obesity in Adults: Executive Summary. Am J Clin Nutr. 1998;68(4):899-917. doi:10.1093/ajcn/68.4.899.

as a BMI between 25.0 and 29.9, and **obesity** as a BMI of 30.0 and above (**Table 7.3**).[27]

Body mass index is not a perfect measure for individuals. For example, football players who are very muscular may be inappropriately labeled by their BMI as overweight or obese. But BMI is the best available way to track patterns of obesity in populations and trends over time.

Children's BMIs change as they age. CDC has published growth charts showing healthy BMI ranges by age. A child is considered to have a healthy weight with a BMI between the 5th and 85th percentile for their age, overweight with a BMI between the 85th and 94th percentile, and obese with a BMI at the 95th percentile or above.

Measuring Diabetes in Populations

Tracking diabetes in populations is more complicated than tracking obesity because it requires measuring glucose levels in the blood. In the past, special laboratory equipment was needed for this, but now there are small devices that can do the testing.

Blood glucose is best measured when someone has not eaten any food in 12 or more hours (referred to as **fasting**) or two hours after someone drinks a standard amount of glucose dissolved in water (the **oral glucose tolerance test**, or **OGTT**). People are labelled as having diabetes if their fasting glucose is more than 126 mg/dl or their 2-hour oral glucose tolerance test is more than 200 mg/dL (**Table 7.4**).[28]

People who have fasting glucose just below this—100 to 125 mg/dL or 2-hr glucose 140-199 mg/dL on OGTT—are said to have **prediabetes**.[28] About one in three U.S. adults—or 96 million-has prediabetes.[29] Unless they reduce their risk in some way, about a third of these people will develop diabetes within 10 years.[30]

When blood glucose levels are high, glucose coats some of the hemoglobin carried by red blood cells. The percentage of hemoglobin that is coated

Table 7.4 Definitions of Diabetes and Prediabetes

Diagnosis	Hemoglobin A1C	Fasting Plasma Glucose	Oral Glucose Tolerance test	Random Plasma Glucose Test***
Normal	Below 5.7%	99 mg/dL or below	139 mg/dL or below	N/A
Prediabetes*	5.7% to 6.4%	100 to 125 mg/dL	140 to 199 mg/dL	N/A
Diabetes**	6.5% or above	126 mg/dL or above	200 mg/dL or above	200 mg/dL or above

* Prediabetes diagnosis = any one of these results and no result in the diabetes range
** Diabetes diagnosis = any one of these results
*** Combined with symptoms of diabetes

Data from American Diabetes Association. Diagnosis and classification of diabetes: Standards of care in diabetes. Diabetes Care. 2024;47:S20-S42. https://doi.org/10.2337/dc24-S002

by glucose is called the **Hemoglobin A1C** level (HbA1c), or just A1C or **glycosylated hemoglobin** level. This number is a convenient way to estimate a person's average blood glucose level over the previous 8–12 weeks. HbA1c is also used to classify people as having diabetes or prediabetes. A healthy person has HbA1c below 5.7%. A person with HbA1c above 6.5% has diabetes, and a person with HbA1c between 5.7% and 6.4% has prediabetes.[28] The higher HbA1c is, the more likely the person is to develop the severe health consequences of diabetes, so reducing HbA1c is a key goal of medical treatment of diabetes.[31]

Epidemiology: Patterns and Trends

Obesity

In the United States, obesity rates have been rising for decades (**Figure 7.10**). In 1960-62, 12% of American adults were obese. In 2017–2020, 42% were, and 74% of Americans were overweight.[32,33] In fact, the entire distribution of BMI is shifting upward—that is, everyone is gaining too much fat tissue (**Figure 7.11**).[34]

Figure 7.12 shows obesity rates by demographic group. While rates are lower in Asians and higher in Black women (patterns that are not understood), the most striking pattern is that obesity is very common in nearly every group.[33] Obesity begins early in childhood, with 14% of preschool children obese and 2% severely obese.[32]

Globally, about 40% of adults are overweight, including 13% who are obese.[35] Obesity rates are highest in the United States and high-income countries in Europe, the Americas, Oceania, and the Middle East, and lowest in the low-income countries of Southeast Asia and sub-Saharan Africa.[35] Many low-income countries now have a "double burden" of nutrition, with some of their population experiencing undernutrition and others obesity.

Diabetes

Fortunately, type 1 diabetes is relatively uncommon, affecting about 0.5% of people.[36] By contrast, there is the global epidemic of type 2 diabetes that is following in the footsteps of the global epidemic of obesity (**Figure 7.13**). As of 2017–2020, nearly 15% of adults in the United States had diabetes, nearly

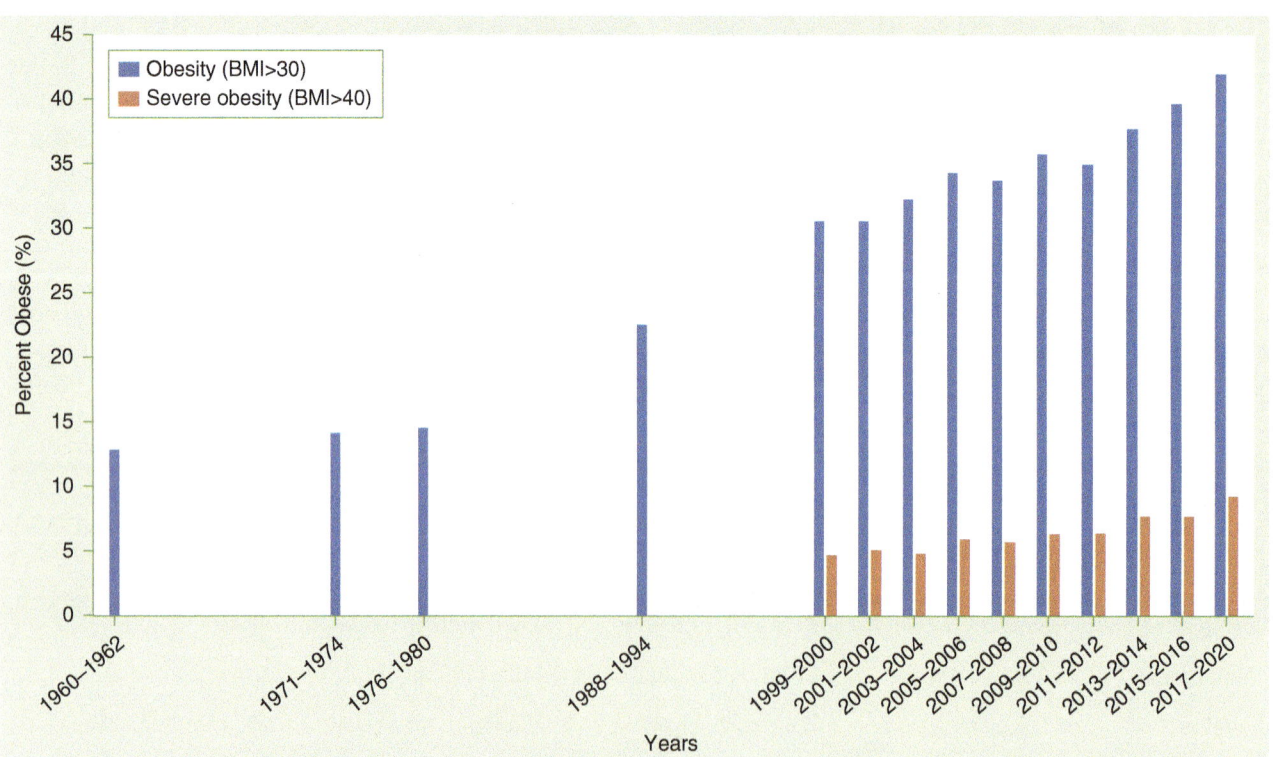

Figure 7.10 **Trends in the Prevalence of Obesity and Severe Obesity in U.S. Adults, 1960–2020.** The prevalence of obesity in the United States has been rising for at least the past 60 years.

Data from Flegal KM et al Overweight and obesity in the United States: Prevalence and Trends 1960-1994. Int J Obes Relat Metab Disord 1998;22:39-47 AND Hales DM. Prevalence of Obesity and Severe Obesity among Adults: United States, 2017-18, NCHS Data Brief 2020;360:1-8, and Stierman B, Afful J, Carroll MD, et al. National Health and Nutrition Examination Survey 2017-March 2020 Prepandemic Data Files-Development of Files and Prevalence Estimates for Selected Health Outcomes. Natl Health Stat Report. 2021;(158):1-21.

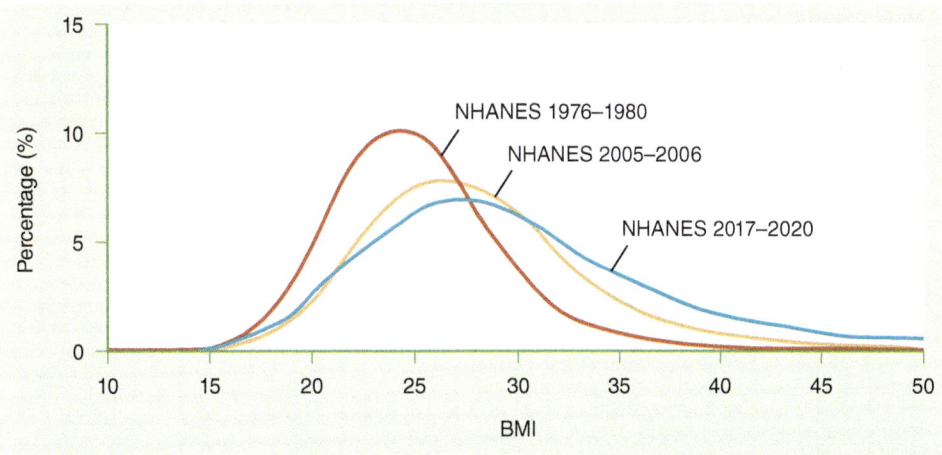

Figure 7.11 **Trends in the Distribution of Body Mass Index in U.S. Adults in the National Health and Nutrition Examination Survey (NHANES).** Underlying the increasing prevalence of obesity is a shift of the entire distribution curve of body mass index to higher values. That is, the obesity epidemic is having an impact on everyone.

Data from Ogden CL, Carroll MD, McDowell MA, Flegal KM. Obesity among adults in the United States--no statistically significant change since 2003-2004. NCHS Data Brief. 2007;(1):1-8, and author's analysis of data from National Center for Health Statistics, Centers for Disease Control and Prevention at https://wwwn.cdc.gov/nchs/nhanes/continuousnhanes/default.aspx?cycle=2017-2020

tripling from approximately 5% in 1976-80.[33,37,38] About one in four Americans with diabetes does not know that they have the disease—that is, they are "undiagnosed".

Diabetes is more common in Hispanic (21%), Black (19%) and Asian populations (18%) than in White populations (12%).[33] American Indians are at particularly high risk for type 2 diabetes, with rates of diagnosed diabetes higher than that for every other racial group in the United States.[39] Genetics underlies much of these racial differences. When people are compared to others with the same BMI, Blacks are about 30%, Hispanics about 90%, and Asians about 130% more likely than Whites to develop diabetes.[40]

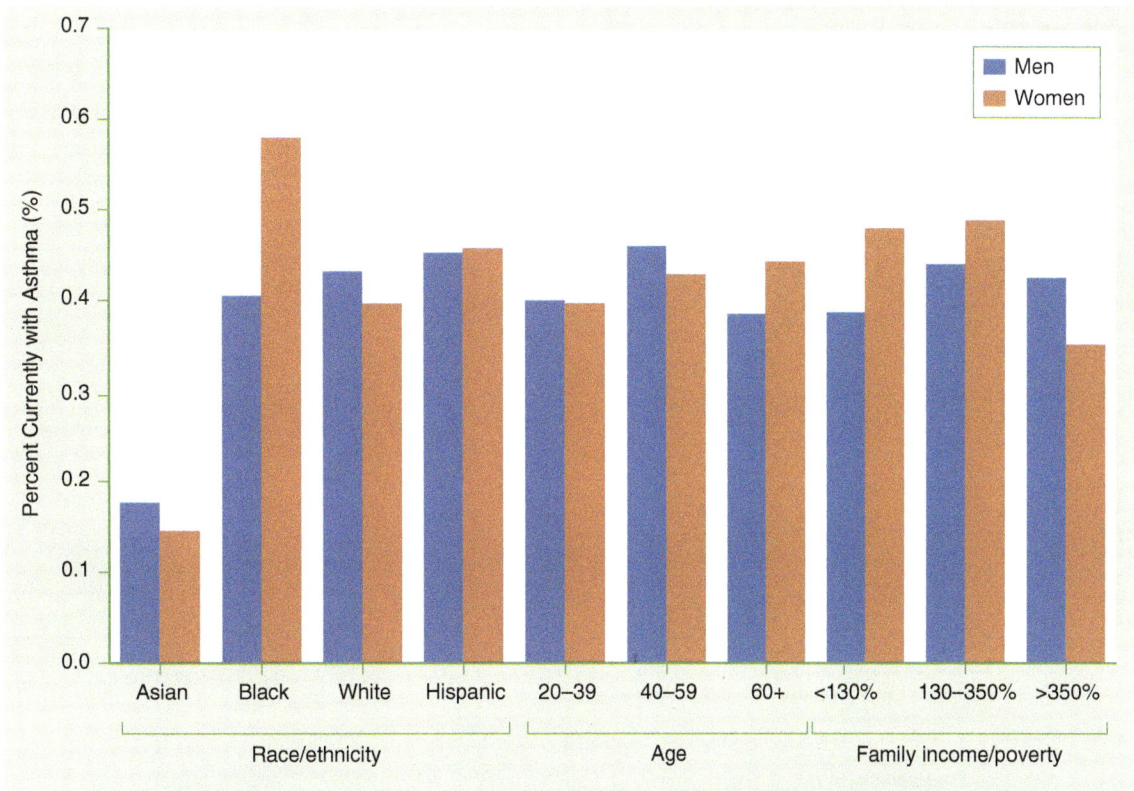

Figure 7.12 **Prevalence of Obesity in Adults in the United States by Demographic Group, 2017–2020.**

Data from Stierman B, Afful J, Carroll MD, et al. National Health and Nutrition Examination Survey 2017-March 2020 Prepandemic Data Files-Development of Files and Prevalence Estimates for Selected Health Outcomes. Natl Health Stat Report. 2021;(158):1-21.

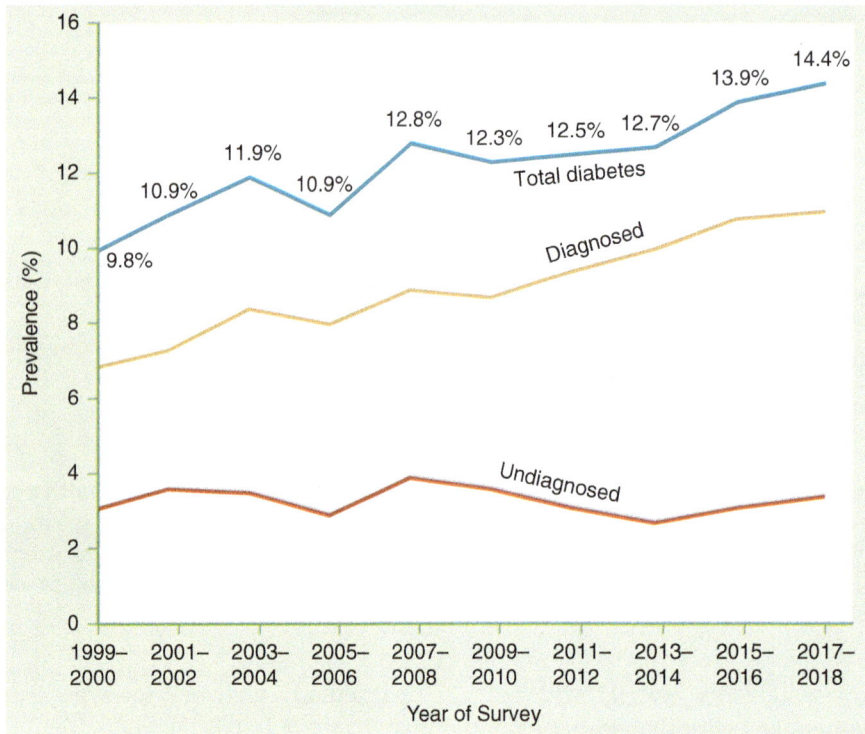

Figure 7.13 **Trends in the Prevalence of Diabetes in Adults in the United States, 1999–2018.** The obesity epidemic is causing a steady increase in the prevalence of diabetes.

Data from Wang L, Li X, Wang Z, et al. Trends in Prevalence of Diabetes and Control of Risk Factors in Diabetes among US Adults, 1999-2018. JAMA - Journal of the American Medical Association. 2021;326(8):704-716. doi:10.1001/jama.2021.9883.

Globally, about 5% of adults have type 2 diabetes, with rates rising rapidly in all regions of the world and the highest rates in the high-income countries of the Middle East.[41]

Risk Factors for Obesity

Modifiable risk factors for obesity are (**Figure 7.14**):

- *Lack of breastfeeding.* Children who are not breast fed in the first 6 months of life are more likely to develop obesity later.[14]

- *Unhealthy diet.* Consumption of high-risk foods and insufficient consumption of low-risk foods listed in Table 7.1 increase the risk of obesity.

- *Physical inactivity.* While exercising is not a very effective way to lose weight, people who get 150 minutes of moderate to vigorous activity per week are less likely to gain weight.[42,43] Also, sedentary behavior, such as time spent sitting or watching television, is associated with weight gain and obesity.

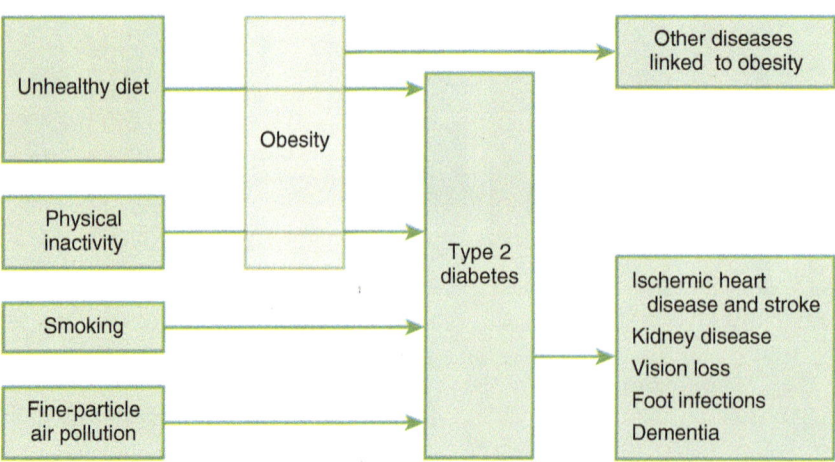

Figure 7.14 Cause-and-Effect Diagram for Obesity and Type 2 Diabetes.

Risk Factors for Type 2 Diabetes

Genetics strongly influences the risk of type 2 diabetes. People with close relatives who have type 2 diabetes are 5–10 times as likely to develop the disease themselves, even when compared to people with similar age and weight.[3]

Modifiable risk factors for type 2 diabetes are (Figure 7.14):

- *Obesity.* People who are overweight are about three times as likely and people who are obese about 7 to 10 times as likely as people with a healthy weight to develop diabetes.[44]
- *Unhealthy diet.* The dietary patterns linked to obesity listed above—including ultra-processed foods—are also associated with type 2 diabetes regardless of obesity.[45,46]
- *Physical inactivity* increases the risk of type 2 diabetes, independent of its effect on obesity, probably because physical activity increases insulin sensitivity.[47,48] In one study, people who did more than 150 minutes of aerobic activity per week had a nearly 50% lower risk of developing diabetes.[47]
- *Smoking* has been shown to increase insulin resistance and the risk of type 2 diabetes by about 40%.[45]
- *Fine-particle air pollution* increases the risk of diabetes, particularly in countries like India and China with high air pollution levels.[23] One study

estimated that 20% of the global burden of diabetes is attributable to air pollution.[23]

Preventive Interventions

Primary Prevention

Obesity and diabetes can be prevented by addressing these risk factors (**Figure 7.15**):

- *Promotion of breastfeeding.* Breastfeeding can be promoted by educating parents about its benefits, supporting mothers who breastfeed, and policies that restrict the marketing of infant formula.
- *Promotion of healthy diets.* Policies and programs can reduce the promotion of high-risk foods and increase the availability, accessibility, and promotion of lower-risk foods listed in Table 7.1. As one example, school policies to increase the availability of fruits, vegetables, and water and to restrict snack foods and sugary drinks have improved children's diets and reduced childhood obesity.[49] Promotion of healthy diets is discussed more in Chapter 14. Nutrition.
- *Promotion of physical activity.* See Chapter 15. Physical Inactivity.
- *Smoking prevention.* See Chapter 11. Tobacco Use.
- *Reduction in air pollution.* Air pollution and ways to reduce it are discussed in Chapter 8. Chronic Respiratory Diseases.

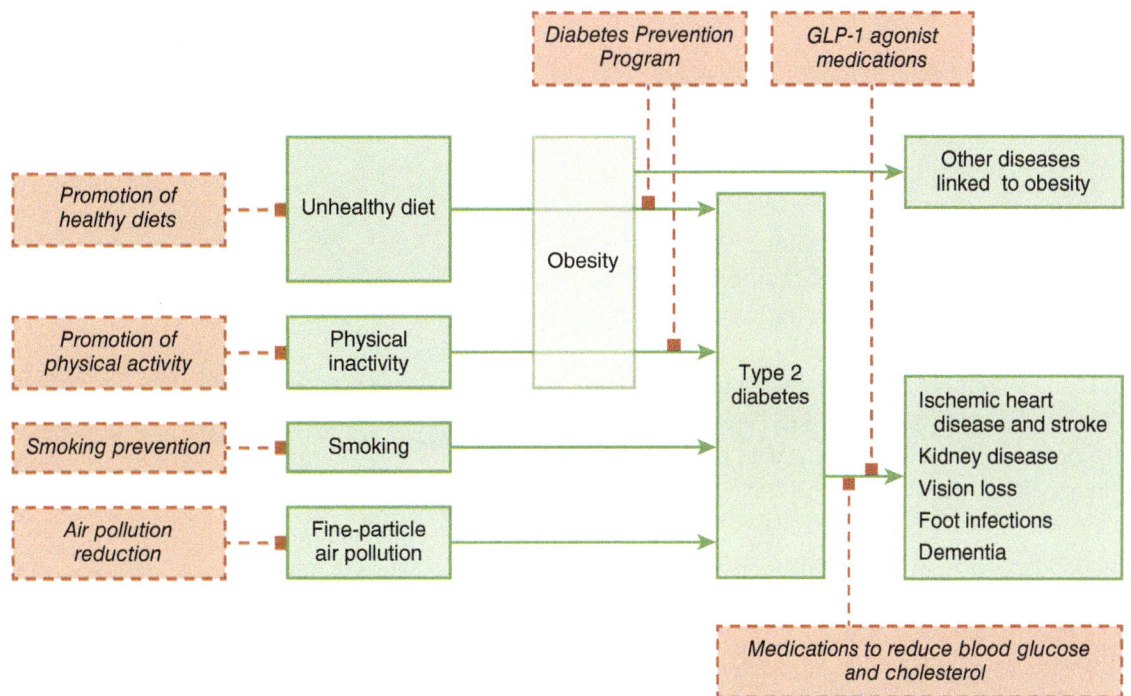

Figure 7.15 Cause-and-Effect Diagram for Obesity and Type 2 Diabetes, with Preventive Interventions.

Secondary Prevention

General diet and exercise programs for people who are overweight are not very effective. In most studies of weight loss programs, regardless of the diets people are given, participants lose a modest amount of weight in the first few months, but then regain most of that weight in the next year or two.[50,51] And these programs are even less successful outside of research studies.[52]

One exception is the Diabetes Prevention Program (DPP), an intensive year-long program for people with prediabetes, which involves 16 sessions of individual coaching and supervised physical activity sessions, as well as other help. In 2002, this program caused excitement when a study showed that it reduced the number of participants risk for developing diabetes over the next three years by nearly 60%.[53] But the program's intensity, which is probably central to its success, makes people reluctant to enroll or stay in it.[54]

Treatment of prediabetes with a drug called **metformin** that lowers blood glucose levels also reduces the incidence of diabetes—although less than DPP.[55] Metformin is very commonly used as treatment for people who already have diabetes. While the American Diabetes Association recommends that physician "consider" prescribing metformin for people with prediabetes,[56] the FDA has not approved the drug for this purpose, and physicians rarely prescribe it.[57]

There is much recent interest in **GLP-1 agonist** medications that mimic the effect of the hormone GLP-1 on the brain, reducing appetite. People taking weekly injections of the GLP-1 agonists semaglutide (sold under the brand names Ozempic and Wegovy), or tirzepatide (Mounjaro, Zepbound) eat less and lose 10%–20% of their weight over about 12 months.[58,59] In those with diabetes, HbA1c levels fall dramatically.[58-60] However, if they stop taking these drugs, most people quickly gain most of their weight back, so using GLP-1 agonists effectively requires a lifelong commitment.[59]

The U.S. Preventive Services Task Force recommends screening for prediabetes and type 2 diabetes in adults over age 35 who are overweight,[61] so that people with these conditions can take preventive actions.

Experts recommend that people with diabetes take glucose-lowering medications to reduce their HbA1c levels to below 7%; this lowers their risk of kidney disease or vision loss and may also lower their risk of heart disease and stroke.[31,62] The medications used include insulin, metformin, and group

of drugs called **SGLT-2 inhibitors**.[63] The SGLT-2 inhibitors work in the kidneys to excrete the excess glucose into the urine, leaving lower glucose levels in the blood. These drugs are discussed more in the next section of this chapter. The medications used to reduce blood cholesterol levels are called **statins**.

Box 7.1 Summary–Prevention of Obesity and Diabetes

- Primary prevention
  - Promotion of breastfeeding
  - Promotion of healthy diets
  - Promotion of physical activity
  - Smoking prevention
  - Reduction in air pollution
- Secondary prevention
  - Screening to identify persons with prediabetes and diabetes
  - Diet and exercise training (Diabetes Prevention Program)
  - GLP-1 agonist medications
  - Medications to reduce blood glucose and cholesterol

Box 7.2 Key Words–Obesity and Diabetes

Adipocyte
Atherosclerosis
Beta cells
Body mass index (BMI)
Carbohydrates
Chronic kidney disease
Dementia
Endocrine-disrupting chemicals
Energy density
Fasting
Fat cells
Fats
Fatty acids
Ghrelin
GLP-1 agonist
Glucagon-like peptide 1 (GLP-1)
Glucose
Glycemic index
Glycerol
Glycogen
Glycosylated hemoglobin
Hemoglobin A1C (HbA1c)
Hypothalamus
Inflammation
Insulin
Insulin receptors
Insulin resistance

Insulin sensitivity
Ischemic heart disease
Ischemic stroke
Leptin
Macrovascular complications of diabetes
Metformin
Microbiome
Microvascular complications of diabetes
Monosaccharide
Nerves
Obesity
Oral glucose tolerance test (OGTT)
Overweight
Pancreas
Prediabetes
SGLT-2 inhibitor
Starch
Statin
Triglycerides
Type 1 diabetes
Type 2 diabetes
Ultra-processed foods

Resources–Obesity and Diabetes

- *U.S. Department of Agriculture and U.S. Department of Health and Human Services Dietary Guidelines for Americans 2020–2025,* available at dietaryguidelines.gov. This provides detailed advice on diets to prevent weight gain at each stage of life.
- *Scientific Report of the 2020 Dietary Guidelines Advisory Committee: Advisory Report to the Secretary of Agriculture and Secretary of Health and Human Services.* This report is a detailed summary of the scientific research underpinning the Dietary Guidelines for Americans. Available at https://www.dietaryguidelines.gov/2020-advisory-committee-report
- Mozaffarian D. Dietary and Policy Priorities for Cardiovascular Disease, Diabetes, and Obesity. *Circulation.* 2016;133(2):187-225. doi:10.1161/circulationaha.115.018585. This reviews the research on the relationship each major food or nutrient has to weight gain, diabetes, and cardiovascular disease.
- Cowie CC, Casagrande SS, Menke A et al., editors. *Diabetes in America.* 3rd ed. National Institute of Diabetes and Digestive and Kidney Diseases, 2018. Available at https://pubmed.ncbi.nlm.nih.gov/33651524/. This is a 42-chapter compendium of information about diabetes. Chapter 13: Risk Factors for Type 2 Diabetes explains the risk factors for diabetes listed above in detail.

- ElSayed NA, Aleppo G, Bannuru RR, et al. Diagnosis and Classification of Diabetes: Standards of Care in Diabetes—2024. *Diabetes Care.* 2024;47(Suppl 1):S20–S42. doi:10.2337/dc24-S002. This provides very specific guidance from the American Diabetes Association on the medical management of prediabetes and diabetes.

Chronic Kidney Disease

Introduction

Chronic kidney disease (CKD) is a very common problem—far more common than most people realize because it causes no symptoms until the kidneys fail entirely. But people with CKD are more likely to have a heart attack or a stroke, and in some people, CKD will deteriorate further into **end-stage kidney disease**, also called **end-stage renal disease** (ESRD). End-stage renal disease is much less common than CKD, but more than 800,000 Americans now have it, most of whom must undergo regular **dialysis**.

CKD has many contributing causes, but the most important ones in the United States are high blood pressure, obesity, and diabetes. The best way to prevent CKD and ESRD is to reduce the prevalence of these three conditions, but consistent medical treatment of the conditions can slow the kidney's deterioration.

Physiology of the Kidney

The kidney carries out several functions, but the two most important are: (1) maintaining healthy levels of water and electrolytes in the body, and (2) excreting waste products of metabolism and other potentially harmful chemicals. The kidney does this by continuously filtering the blood. In addition, the kidney secretes several hormones, some of which help regulate blood pressure.[64]

The kidney's filtering of blood is carried out by hundreds of thousands of tiny units called **nephrons** (**Figure 7.16**). Each nephron is composed of: 1) a tuft of **capillaries** called a **glomerulus**, 2) a structure that wraps around the glomerulus called **Bowman's capsule**, and 3) a **renal tubule** connected to this capsule.[64]

The capillaries in the glomerulus carry blood, supplied to the kidney by the body's **arteries**. The arteries branch into smaller and smaller vessels as they become closer to the tissues that they supply, and the tiniest branches are called **arterioles**. The

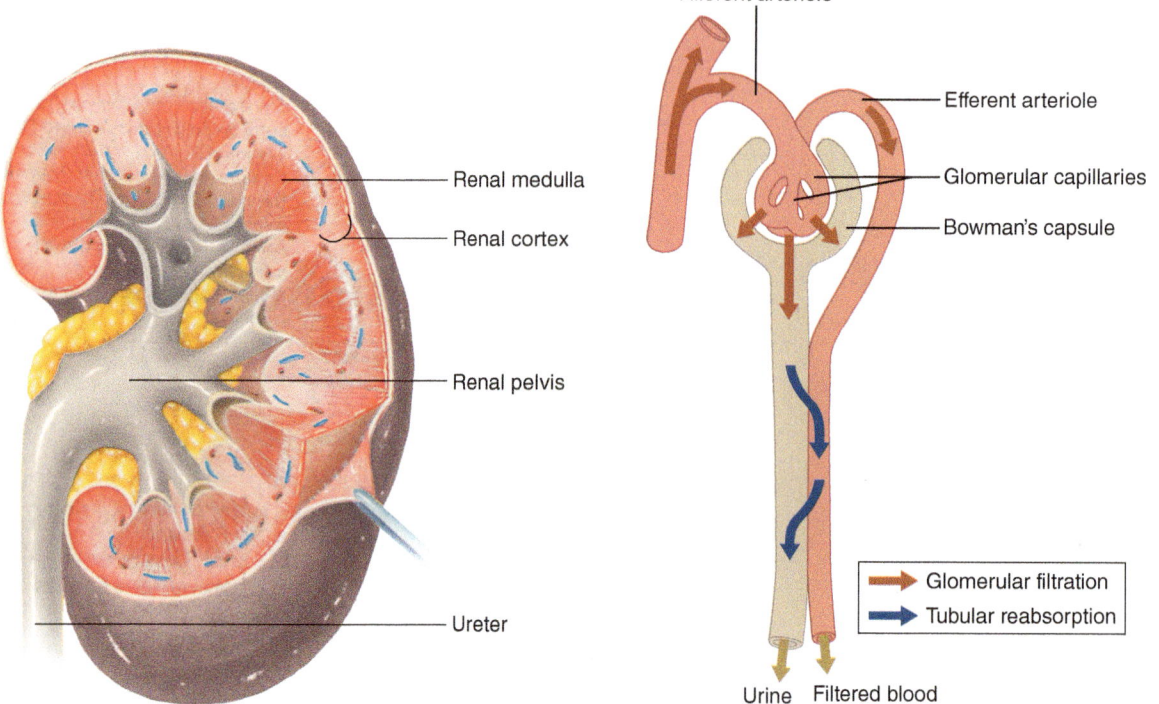

Figure 7.16 **The Kidney and the Nephron.** The nephron cleanses blood by filtering it through the glomerular capillaries into Bowman's capsule, and then reabsorbing the needed fluids and electrolytes from the renal tubule back into the blood. The remaining fluid and waste products of metabolism continue to flow down the renal tubule and are excreted as urine.

© Jones & Bartlett Learning

arterioles are connected to even smaller channels called capillaries.

The capillaries in the kidney's **glomeruli** are different from the capillaries elsewhere in the body. First, capillaries everywhere else connect arterioles to the tiniest veins, but capillaries in the glomerulus instead connect two different types of arterioles, the **afferent arterioles** and the **efferent arterioles** (Figure 7.16). The afferent arteriole directs blood *to* the nephron and the efferent arteriole directs blood *from* the nephron. Second, these glomerular capillaries have microscopic holes in their walls.

The nephron cleanses blood with two steps: **filtration** and **reabsorption**. In the filtration step, the components of blood that can fit through the holes in the capillaries flow into Bowman's capsule. The afferent arteriole and the efferent arteriole constantly adjust this flow by becoming narrower or wider, much like the valve on a faucet adjusts the flow of water into a sink.[65,66]

The fluid received by Bowman's capsule, called the **filtrate**, then flows into the renal tubule. The tubule runs alongside the efferent arteriole, which enables the second step of reabsorption. As the filtrate moves through the tubule, most of the fluid and

selected electrolytes and chemicals in the filtrate are reabsorbed—that is, they pass back into the blood. The filtrate that is not reabsorbed flows further down the tubule and leaves the body as urine.[64]

This two-step process is an ingenious mechanism, creating the default that any small compound that is unrecognized is flushed out of the body. This helps rid the body of a limitless number of potentially toxic chemicals, while allowing the body to selectively retain the compounds that it needs.

Table 7.5 summarizes how the filtration and reabsorption handle different components of blood. If the kidney is healthy, cells—particularly red blood cells—are not filtered, that is, they stay in the blood vessels. Nearly all proteins are likewise not filtered, and the smaller ones that fit through the holes are mostly reabsorbed back into the blood by the tubules.[65] Water and electrolytes, particularly sodium, potassium, chloride, and bicarbonate, are filtered, but the tubules reabsorb just the right amount of them to maintain healthy levels in the body.[67] Small chemical compounds are filtered and most are not reabsorbed. But a few crucial compounds needed for metabolism, particularly **glucose** and **amino acids**, are reabsorbed back into

Table 7.5 Summary of Filtration and Reabsorption of Blood Components by the Nephron

Blood Component	Filtered by Glomerulus?	Reabsorbed by Tubule?
Cells (mostly red blood cells)	No	–
Proteins	Mostly no	Yes
Small chemical compounds	Yes	Only selected ones
Electrolytes	Yes	Mostly, but regulated
Water	Yes	Mostly, but regulated

Data from Hall JE, Hall ME. Glomerular Filtration, Renal Blood Flow, and Their Control. In: Guyton and Hall Textbook of Medical Physiology. 14th ed. Philadelphia: Elsevier; 2021:331-342.

the blood. The reabsorption of glucose is handled by a very specialized protein embedded in the lining of the tubule called **sodium-glucose co-transporter-2 (SGLT-2)**. This protein is the target for some medications used to treat diabetes.

This work of the nephron is a continuous, high-volume process. About 1,700 liters (450 gallons) of blood flows through the kidneys each day.[65] The rate at which fluid from this blood is filtered is called the **glomerular filtration rate (GFR)**. For people who are young and healthy, the GFR is about 180 liters per day, or 125 ml per minute.[68] The GFR can be estimated in people by comparing levels in their blood and urine of a compound called **creatinine**, which is a normal waste product of muscle tissue, or with other blood tests.[67,69]

Pathophysiology: Biologic Mechanisms of Chronic Kidney Disease

Many different diseases, conditions, and exposures can damage the kidney's nephrons. And any damage is permanent; nephrons develop in a fetus in the third trimester of pregnancy, and after a child is born, the body cannot build new ones. Nephrons drop out naturally as people age.[64] Fortunately, the kidneys have much spare capacity. Each kidney contains between 800,000 and 1 million nephrons, which is more than twice what a human needs.[64] That is why a person can donate one kidney and live a healthy life with just the remaining one.[70] However, some conditions and exposures damage even more nephrons than people can spare.

Three common conditions are responsible for most of the damage to kidneys in the United States:

- *High blood pressure.* Normally, the afferent arterioles adjust to provide a consistent filtration through the glomerular capillaries.[66] But a blood pressure that is too high harms these afferent arterioles, reducing their ability to become narrower. This leads to the pressure becoming too high within the glomerulus, which damages it.[66] At the same time, chronic kidney disease tends to increase a person's blood pressure by releasing certain hormones. That sets up an unfortunate reinforcing feedback loop between high blood pressure and kidney damage.[66]

- *Diabetes.* Many features of diabetes can harm kidneys, but it appears that the most important is the high level of glucose in the blood.[71] When this happens, glucose molecules become attached to proteins or lipids, interfering with their normal function. These altered proteins and lipids damage the glomeruli, the tubules, and the tissues around them.[71]

- *Obesity.* Obesity causes both diabetes and high blood pressure, but it also damages the kidney directly. The biologic mechanism is not well understood, but it seems that the metabolic changes associated with obesity cause the afferent arterioles to open too widely.[72] At first, that wider "faucet" abnormally increases the blood flow through the glomerulus, causing an abnormally high GFR. But it also damages the glomerulus, damage that accumulates over years.[72]

After diabetes, high blood pressure, and obesity, the most common causes of kidney damage are infections or immune system diseases that cause **inflammation** in the glomeruli. This condition is called **glomerulonephritis**. It can happen suddenly, for example, after a "strep throat," when it is called **acute glomerulonephritis**. Or it can happen gradually, for example, in **autoimmune diseases** like **lupus**, in which the immune system mistakenly attacks the body's own cells.

Many different toxic chemicals and drugs can also damage the nephrons.

Damage to the nephrons from any cause appears as two problems that can be detected with medical tests.

First, the damaged glomeruli do not retain proteins well, so proteins "leak" into the urine. The protein that appears in the largest amounts in the urine is called **albumin**. The measurement of albumin in urine is usually expressed as the ratio of albumin to creatinine, which adjusts for how concentrated a person's urine is at the time of the test. The higher a person's urine **albumin-creatinine ratio (ACR)** is, the more kidney damage that person has. Healthy young adults usually have an ACR below 30 mg/g. An ACR above 30 mg/g is a sign of damaged glomeruli leaking protein, and an ACR above 300 mg/g reflects severe kidney damage.

Second, the damaged glomeruli filter less fluid, so the GFR is lower. Most healthy young adults have estimated GFRs above 90 ml/min (after adjustment for body size). Any number below 60 ml/min is considered chronic kidney disease, and a GFR below 15 m/min is considered kidney failure.

To assess the health of a person's kidneys, a healthcare provider will request both an ACR test and a GFR test. If either test result is abnormal, the person is labelled as having chronic kidney disease. The "stage" of the disease is labeled according to how abnormal these two tests are, as shown in **Table 7.6**.[73,74] In this table, all cells other than those that are colored green are considered to have chronic kidney disease. Persons in the yellow cells are considered to have low-risk disease, those in orange cells high-risk disease, and those in pink cells very high-risk disease.[73] These designations show how likely it is that a person will progress to complete kidney failure over time. For example, persons with low-risk disease are about four times as likely as healthy people to develop kidney failure, and those with high-risk disease are about 20–30 times as likely.[75]

Most people with chronic kidney disease have no symptoms, so they are not aware that they have the problem. But there are two severe consequences that may occur. First, having CKD roughly doubles the risk of having a heart attack, heart failure, or a stroke.[76] In fact, the main cause of death for people with CKD is not kidney disease itself but instead cardiovascular disease.[77] And second, over years, in some people CKD deteriorates into complete failure of the kidneys, called end-stage renal disease (ESRD).[73,78] Without kidneys to filter fluids, people with ESRD become overloaded with fluid, causing swelling in their legs. They also develop symptoms from a buildup of the waste products of metabolism, like constant itching, fatigue and weight loss. And they develop imbalances of electrolytes in their body fluids, which can cause abnormal heart rhythms. Unless their body fluids are restored to healthy levels and balances, they will die from the disease.[79]

Dialysis is a procedure in which the blood or body fluids are artificially filtered, doing the work of the kidneys. The most common form is **hemodialysis**,

Table 7.6 **Risk Criteria and Prevalence of Chronic Kidney Disease in U.S. Adults**

Chronic kidney disease (CKD) is defined as having either an estimated glomerular filtration rate (eGFR) below 60 or an albumin-creatinine ratio (ACR) above 30. All cells other than those that are colored green are considered to have CKD. Persons in the yellow cells are considered to have low risk disease, those in orange cells high risk disease, and those in pink cells very high-risk disease. The numbers in the cells show the percentage of American adults with test results in those ranges.

Estimated GFR (eGFR)	ACR < 30 (Normal)	ACR 30-299 (Moderately Increased)	ACR ≥ 300 (Severely increased)	Total
eGFR ≥90 (Normal)	59.8%	5.0%	0.7%	65.5%
eGFR 60–89	26.2%	2.4%	0.4%	28.9%
eGFR 45–59	3.1%	0.8%	0.1%	4.0%
eGFR 30–44	0.6%	0.3%	0.2%	1.1%
eGFR 15–29	0.1%	0.1%	0.2%	0.3%
eGFR <15 (Kidney failure)	0.0%	0.0%	0.1%	0.2%
Total	89.8%	8.6%	1.6%	100.0%

National Institute of Diabetes and Digestive and Kidney Diseases. United States Renal Data System 2023 Annual Data Report. National Institute of Diabetes and Digestive and Kidney Diseases, National Institutes of Health. Published 2023. Accessed February 29, 2024. https://usrds-adr.niddk.nih.gov/2023

in which blood flows out of a person's artery into a machine that exchanges the fluid in it, removing wastes and toxins. Hemodialysis is usually done over three to five hours, three times a week. Less common is **peritoneal dialysis**, in which fluid is inserted into a person's abdomen and withdrawn an hour or two later, removing the wastes and toxins. Peritoneal dialysis must be done several times a day. The better solution is a kidney transplant, but there are only enough donor kidneys to provide transplants to about a third of people with ESRD.

Epidemiology: Patterns and Trends

An estimated 14% of American adults have CKD, based on having either an abnormal GFR or an abnormal ACR test—that is, in the yellow, orange, or pink cells in Table 7.6. About 1% are considered at "very high risk"—that is, in the pink cells.[73]

Because damage to the kidneys accumulates over a lifetime, CKD becomes more common as people age (**Figure 7.17**). About one-third of people ages 65-79 and two-thirds of those over age 80 have CKD.[73] CKD is more common in Black people than White people,

perhaps in part because carrying the trait for sickle cell disease increases the risk of CKD.[73,79] CKD is slightly more common in people living in poverty.[73] Just over 20% of people with hypertension and nearly 40% of people with diabetes have CKD.[73]

Fortunately, most people with CKD do not go on to develop ESRD, but each year a small percentage do. In the United States, each year about 130,000 people are added to those who are already maintained on dialysis.[80] (Through a special program that is part of Medicare, the U.S. government covers the cost of providing dialysis for people with ESRD.) Today, more than 800,000 people in the United States—or about 2.4 per 1,000 persons—have ESRD.[73] The incidence rate of ESRD has been falling over the past 15 years, probably because of better treatment for people with earlier stages of CKD. However, the number of people living with ESRD continues to grow, both because the U.S. population is growing and because people with ESRD are living longer.[73]

The demographics of ESRD differ from those of CKD, perhaps reflecting varying quality of medical care received by people with CKD. The prevalence of ESRD is much higher in men than women, and about four times as high in Black people as in White people

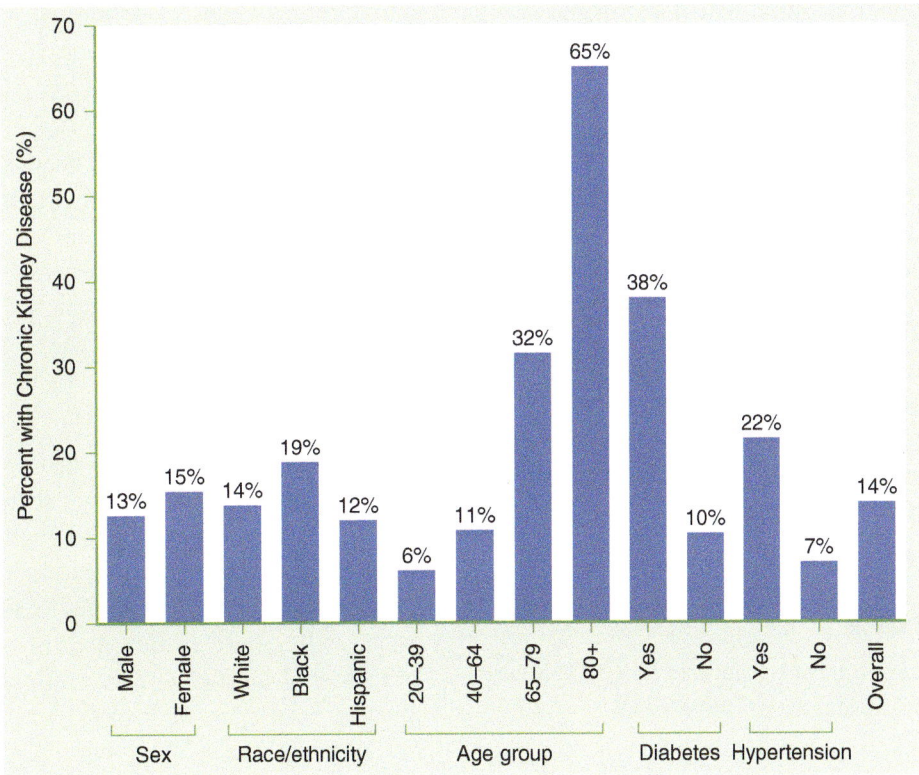

Figure 7.17 Prevalence of Chronic Kidney Disease in Adults in the United States by Demographics, Diabetes, and Hypertension. Chronic kidney disease is more common in people with diabetes or hypertension and rises sharply with age.

Data from National Institute of Diabetes and Digestive and Kidney Diseases. United States Renal Data System 2023 Annual Data Report. National Institute of Diabetes and Digestive and Kidney Diseases, National Institutes of Health. Published 2023. Accessed February 29, 2024. https://usrds-adr.niddk.nih.gov/2023. Age data are from 2011-12 and other data are from 2017-2020.

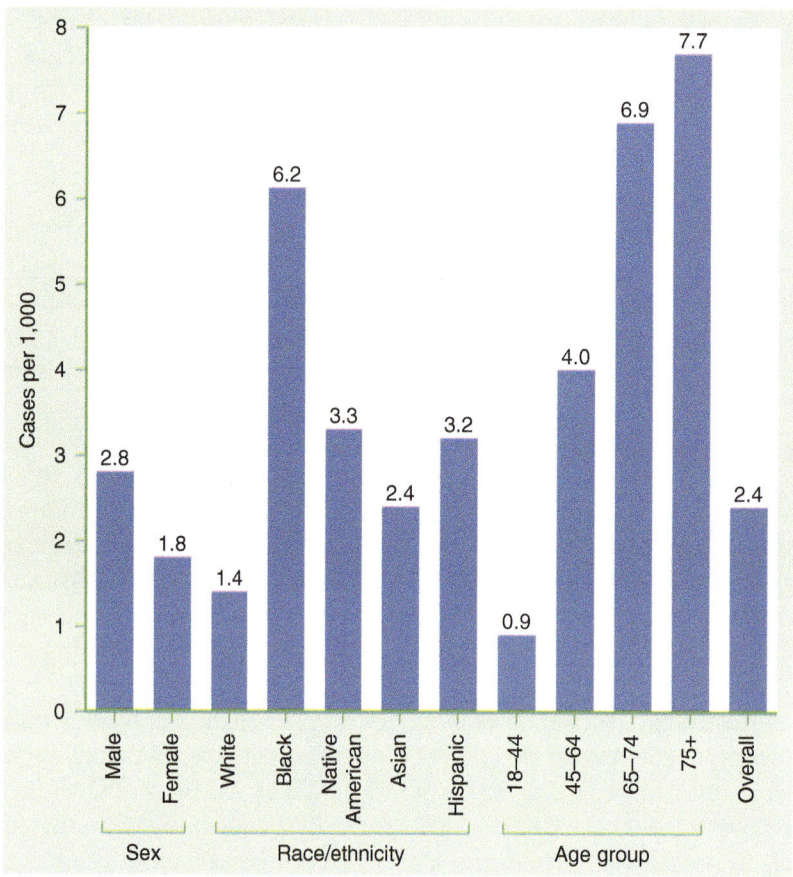

Figure 7.18 Prevalence of End-Stage Renal Disease in Adults in the United States by Demographic Group. End-stage kidney disease is more common in people who are Black than people in other racial or ethnic groups.

Data from National Institute of Diabetes and Digestive and Kidney Diseases. United States Renal Data System 2023 Annual Data Report. National Institute of Diabetes and Digestive and Kidney Diseases, National Institutes of Health. Published 2023. Accessed February 29, 2024. https://usrds-adr.niddk.nih.gov/2023

(**Figure 7.18**). Native Americans, Asians, and Hispanics also have a higher prevalence of the disease.[73]

Globally, CKD is generally less common in high-income countries and in Europe and more common in the lower-income countries of Africa, South Asia, and Southeast Asia.[76] Also, some individual countries like Mexico are hot spots for CKD, perhaps because they have very high rates of diabetes, high rates of infections causing glomerulonephritis, or high rates of exposure to toxic chemicals.[76] Globally, more people die from the consequences of CKD than from tuberculosis or HIV infection.[76]

Risk Factors

Three strong and common risk factors for CKD shown in epidemiologic studies are (**Figure 7.19**):

- *High blood pressure.* People with hypertension have more than twice the risk of CKD.[73]
- *Diabetes.* People with diabetes have nearly four times the risk of CKD.[73] Most of this risk at the population level comes from Type 2 diabetes, simply because it is so much more common than Type 1.

- *Overweight and obesity.* The risk of CKD related to body fat is not just in those who are obese, but also in those who are just overweight—that is, a large majority of Americans. Estimates are that those who are overweight (BMI between 25 and 30) have a 40% increase in risk of developing CKD and those who are obese (BMI above 30) have an 80% increase in risk.[72]

Of these three major risk factors, the Global Burden of Disease project estimates that the greatest fraction of CKD is attributable to high blood pressure, followed by diabetes and overweight/obesity.[81]

These three major risk factors very often overlap because they have common causes of *unhealthy diet* and *physical inactivity*. The relationship of diet and physical activity to high blood pressure is discussed in Chapter 2. Heart Disease and Stroke, and the relationship to overweight/obesity and to diabetes is discussed earlier in this chapter. Particularly important to blood pressure is the intake of sodium, and particularly important to obesity and diabetes is the intake of sugar and refined grains.

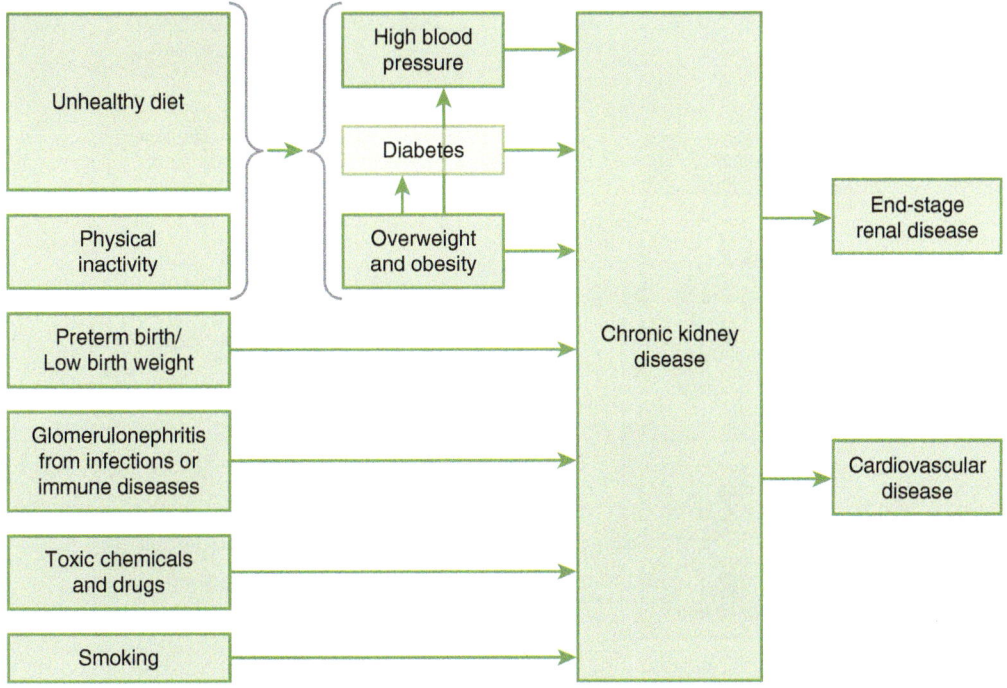

Figure 7.19 Cause-and-Effect Diagram for Chronic Kidney Disease.

Other risk factors include:

- *Preterm birth and low birth weight.* Several studies have now shown that children who were born prematurely or who had low birth weight are at substantially higher risk of developing CKD during childhood, and somewhat higher risk even in their adult years.[82,83] Experts speculate that this is because a baby who is born prematurely or who does not grow normally before birth does not build a normal number of nephrons, leaving the child vulnerable to any damage to the kidneys afterward.
- *Smoking.* Smoking is associated with a small increase in the risk of CKD, which is not surprising considering how many toxins circulate in the blood of people who smoke.[84]
- *Glomerulonephritis from infections or immune diseases.* Either acute or chronic glomerulonephritis can produce enough damage to cause CKD or ESRD.
- *Toxic chemicals and drugs.* A long list of chemicals and drugs have the potential to damage the kidneys. The list includes heavy metals like lead and arsenic, pesticides, air pollutants, some herbal medicines, certain antibiotics, and over-the-counter pain medicines.[85]

While glomerulonephritis and toxic chemicals and drugs are thought to be a relatively minor contributors to CKD in the United States, they may be more important contributors in lower-income countries, where the causes of CKD are less studied.[76]

Preventive Interventions
Primary Prevention

By the time that a person is recognized as having CKD, much permanent damage to the kidneys has already occurred. Primary prevention of that damage, whenever possible, is the best way to reduce CKD and ESRD. Primary prevention can be accomplished by reducing the prevalence of overweight/obesity, diabetes, and weight gain through (**Figure 7.20**):

- *Promotion of healthy diets,* with a particular focus on reducing intake of sodium, sugar, and refined grains. See Chapter 14. Dietary Risks.
- *Promotion of physical activity.* See Chapter 15. Physical Inactivity.

In addition, promoting healthy pregnancies to *prevent preterm birth and low birth weight* (as discussed in Chapter 10. Diseases of the Newborn) should reduce chronic kidney disease in children and perhaps in adults. Some additional reduction in CKD can occur from *reduction in smoking.* And in locations where it is clear that certain toxic chemicals or drugs are important causes, *reduction in exposure to toxic chemicals and drugs* should reduce population rates of CKD.

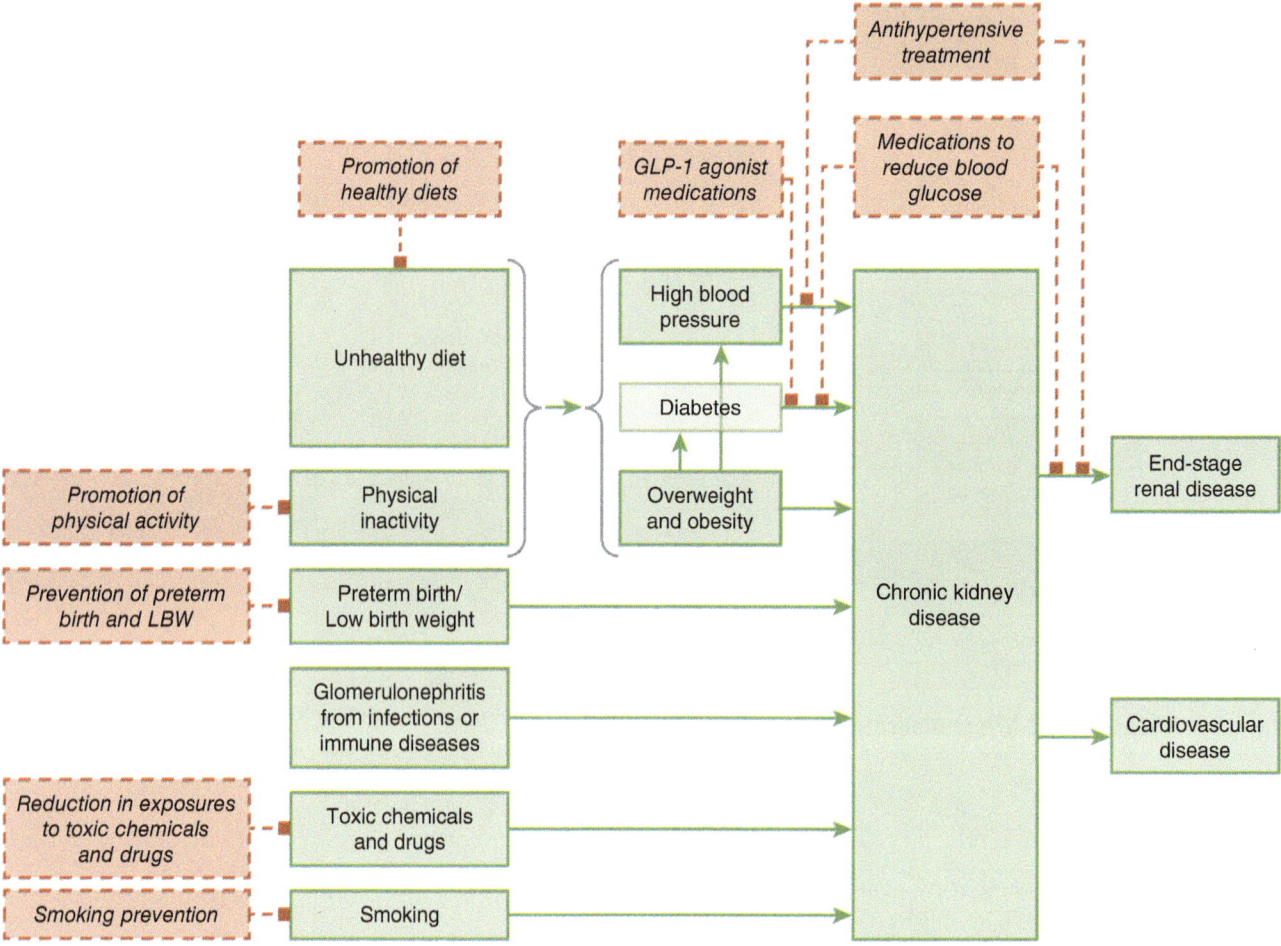

Figure 7.20 **Cause-and-Effect Diagram for Chronic Kidney Disease, with Preventive Interventions.**

Secondary Prevention

Medical treatment of the conditions that are known causes of CKD can reduce CKD or slow the deterioration of CKD to ESRD. The key treatments are:

- *Antihypertensive treatment* for people with high blood pressure. If medications lower blood pressure, they interrupt the feedback loop between high blood pressure and kidney damage.[74,86-88] Also, lowering of blood pressure reduces the consequences of cardiovascular disease, that is, heart attack, congestive heart failure, and stroke.[79] The antihypertensives most recommended are those that block the hormones secreted by the kidney to raise blood pressure.[66] These medications are usually referred to by their acronyms **ACE inhibitors** and **ARB antihypertensives**. Treatment of hypertension is discussed more in Chapter 2. Heart Disease and Stroke.
- *Medications to reduce blood glucose* for people with diabetes. Medications that reduce the abnormally high levels of glucose in the blood in diabetes can slow the damage to the kidneys caused by diabetes.[79]

One group of drugs blocks the specialized SGLT2 proteins that reabsorb glucose from the tubules into the blood. These drugs are called **SGLT-2 inhibitors**.[63] When these drugs are present, most of the glucose that has been filtered is not reabsorbed in the tubules, so it is flushed out in the urine. That leaves less glucose in the blood. In people with type 2 diabetes, these drugs reduce the deterioration of kidney disease from CKD to ESRD by 30%.[89-91]

- *GLP-1 agonist medications.* As discussed earlier in this chapter, GLP-1 agonist medications reduce appetite by mimicking the effect of the hormone **glucagon-like peptide 1 (GLP-1)** on the brain. In people with diabetes, these drugs reduce blood glucose levels and slow the progression of CKD.[92,93]

Resources–Chronic Kidney Disease

- National Institute of Diabetes and Digestive and Kidney Diseases, United States Renal Data System 2023 Annual Data Report. Available at: https://

- Primary prevention
  - Promotion of healthy diets
  - Promotion of physical activity
  - Prevention of preterm birth and low birth weight
  - Reduction in smoking
  - Reduction in exposure to toxic chemicals and drugs
- Secondary prevention
  - Antihypertensive treatment for people with high blood pressure
  - Medications to reduce blood glucose for people with diabetes
  - GLP-1 agonist medications for people with diabetes

Box 7.4 **Key Words–Chronic Kidney Disease**

ACE inhibitor
Acute glomerulonephritis
Afferent arterioles
Albumin
Albumin-creatinine ratio (ACR)
Amino acid
Antihypertensive
ARB antihypertensive
Arteries
Arterioles
Autoimmune diseases
Bowman's capsule
Capillaries
Chronic kidney disease
Creatinine
Dialysis
Efferent arterioles
End-stage kidney disease or end-stage renal disease (ESRD)
Filtrate
Filtration
Glomerular filtration rate (GFR)
Glomerulonephritis
Glomerulus (pl. glomeruli)
GLP-1 agonist
Glucagon-like peptide 1 (GLP-1)
Glucose
Hemodialysis
Inflammation
Lupus
Nephron
Peritoneal dialysis
Reabsorption
Renal tubule
SGLT-2 inhibitor
Sodium-glucose co-transporter-2 (SGLT-2)

usrds-adr.niddk.nih.gov/2023. This report, published annually, provides extensive data and facts about chronic kidney disease and end-stage kidney disease in the United States.

- Bikbov B, Purcell CA, Levey AS, et al. Global, regional, and national burden of chronic kidney disease, 1990–2017: A systematic analysis for the Global Burden of Disease Study 2017. *Lancet*. 2020;395(10225):709-733. doi:10.1016/S0140 -6736(20)30045-3
- Chen TK, Knicely DH, Grams ME. Chronic Kidney Disease Diagnosis and Management: A Review. *JAMA*. 2019;322(13):1294-1304. doi:10.1001/jama .2019.14745. This is an excellent guide for medical providers on how to treat people with CKD to slow its deterioration and prevent cardiovascular disease.

Chronic Liver Disease

Introduction

The liver serves as the body's first line of defense against many health threats, such as alcohol or toxic chemicals. That makes this organ vulnerable to damage from infections, toxins, and metabolic conditions like diabetes. Although the liver can repair itself, the repair mechanisms can become overwhelmed. The causes of **chronic liver disease** vary around the world, but in every region, chronic liver disease is both a major cause of early mortality and a cause of liver cancer. In the United States, while scientific breakthroughs have the potential to nearly eliminate **hepatitis viruses** as causes of liver failure, chronic liver disease continues to grow because of increases in alcohol use and obesity.

Physiology of the Liver

The liver is a large organ, tucked under the right ribcage in the upper abdomen, which works closely with the intestines. It has a unique blood supply, receiving blood through the **portal vein**, which runs from the intestines directly to the liver (**Figure 7.21**). The blood in the portal vein contains nutrients and other substances that have been eaten, digested, and absorbed through the intestinal walls. This design enables the liver to metabolize those nutrients and filter out toxins before they are distributed to the rest of the body.

The liver carries out many functions, most of which are related to handling the nutrients and other substances that people eat.[94] It metabolizes carbohydrates, fats, and proteins. For example, it stores excess **glucose** in the form of **glycogen**, and releases

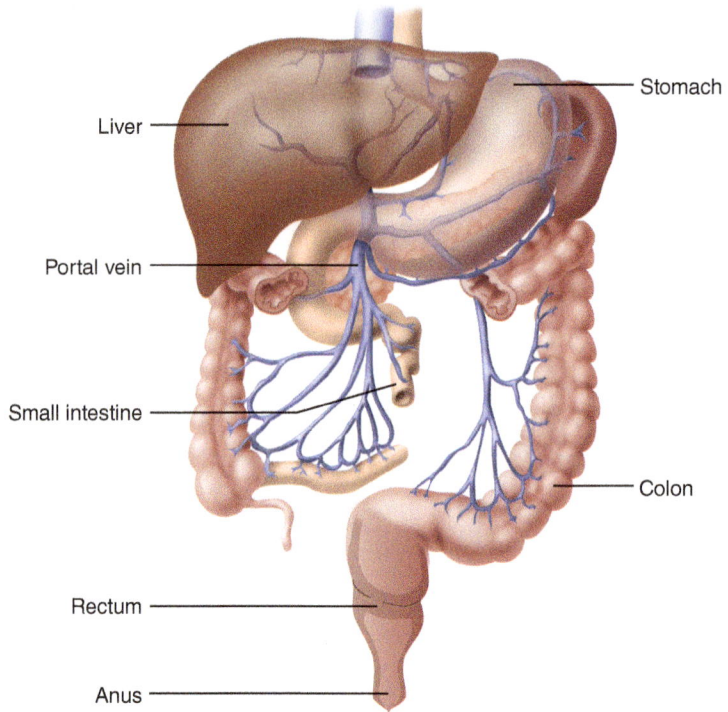

Figure 7.21 The Liver and the Portal Vein. The liver has a unique blood supply. It receives blood through the portal vein, which contains nutrients that have been digested by the intestines.

glucose into the blood when blood glucose levels become low. It converts glucose to fats and it metabolizes fatty acids to obtain energy. It stores vitamins and minerals—particularly vitamins A, D, and B12. And it redirects some metabolic waste products, such as ammonia, preventing them from damaging other organs. The liver also produces a liquid called **bile**, which is full of **bile acids**, and secretes it into the intestines to help absorb fats in foods.

A crucial function of the liver is to protect the rest of the body from toxic substances that are absorbed through the intestines. For example, some chemicals in food can be toxic to human cells; the liver metabolizes or disposes of them. Also, some bacteria and some toxic compounds inside of bacteria called **endotoxins** travel through the walls of the intestines and flow up the portal vein to the liver.[94] The liver can identify and remove these invading bacteria and endotoxins.

The functional unit of the liver is called the **liver lobule** (**Figure 7.22**). Each liver lobule is a hexagonal-shaped piece of tissue that surrounds a **central vein**. At each of the six points on the

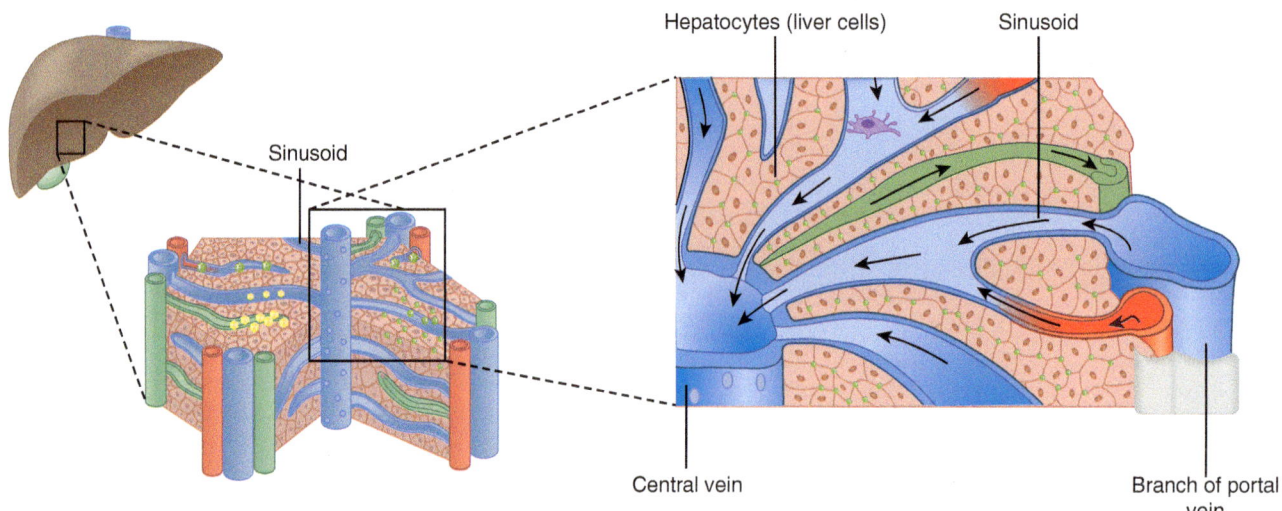

Figure 7.22 The Liver Lobule. In the liver lobule, blood from the portal vein flows through sinusoids alongside hepatocytes (liver cells). As the blood passes, the liver cells extract nutrients and toxins.

perimeter of the lobule is a small branch of the portal vein. Between the portal vein branch and the central vein are the cells called **hepatocytes**, arranged around the central vein like spokes in a wheel. Rows of hepatocytes are separated by open, specialized capillaries called **sinusoids**. Blood containing nutrients from the intestines flows from the portal vein branch through these sinusoids into the central vein.[94] Along the way, the hepatocytes extract nutrients and toxins from the blood and excrete the metabolized products into the blood.

Pathophysiology of Chronic Liver Disease

Chronic liver disease—a deterioration of liver function that lasts more than 6 months—is the result of long-term damage to the hepatocytes. Many different conditions and toxic exposures can inflict that damage, and for many people with chronic liver disease, more than one exposure is involved. Four conditions (alcohol, obesity, and two types of viral hepatitis) are responsible for about 85% of cases of chronic liver disease worldwide.[95] The remaining 15% are mostly caused by a wide variety of drugs and toxins.[96] Summarizing the main causes:

Alcohol Consumption

Despite how much people consume it, alcohol is not a compound that humans are biologically well-equipped to handle. When people drink, **ethanol** is rapidly absorbed through the walls of the intestines and flows up the portal vein to the liver. The hepatocytes quickly metabolize this ethanol to a chemical called **acetaldehyde**. Acetaldehyde changes how the hepatocytes metabolize **fatty acids** in ways that cause fatty acids and **triglycerides** to accumulate in the cells.[96] Also, acetaldehyde is toxic to hepatocytes and can kill the cells outright.[96,97] In addition, the presence of alcohol in the intestines allows more bacterial endotoxins to be absorbed and to reach the liver, which further damages the hepatocytes.[97] The hepatocytes killed by these combined effects are replaced with **scar tissue**—that is, non-liver cells connected by dense fibers.

After just a few days of heavy drinking, signs of significant damage to the liver can be seen under a microscope. The hepatocytes are filled with triglycerides, a condition called **hepatic steatosis** or **fatty liver** (**Figure 7.23**). Interspersed among them are immune cells, which is a sign that the immune system is responding to tissue damage; this condition is called **hepatitis**. The combination is called **steato-hepatitis**.[96] **Alcoholic liver disease** is the label used for either fatty liver or hepatitis occurring in a person who regularly drinks alcohol.

Unlike kidneys and most other organs, the liver has a remarkable ability to repair damage and rebuild itself. If surgeons remove 70% of a liver (for example, to treat cancer), the remaining 30% will regrow to restore the liver to its original size.[94] That self-repair ability helps the liver recover even after significant damage from alcohol. But with each bout of drinking, more hepatocytes are killed and replaced with scar tissue. This buildup of scar tissue is called **hepatic fibrosis** (Figure 7.23). And although

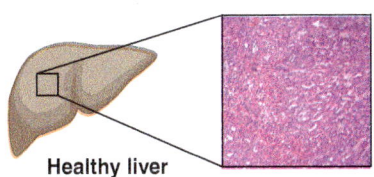

Healthy liver

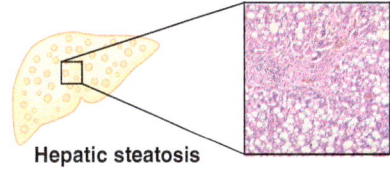

Hepatic steatosis

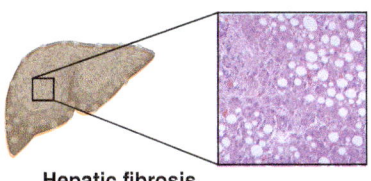

Hepatic fibrosis

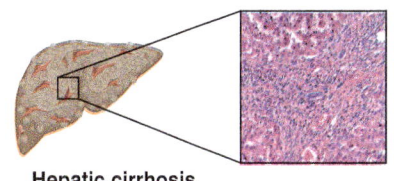

Hepatic cirrhosis

Figure 7.23 Types of Liver Disease. If the liver cells are filled with triglycerides, the condition is called hepatic steatosis or fatty liver. If the liver is damaged and accumulates scar tissue, the condition is called hepatic fibrosis. If this scar tissue replaces most of the liver, the condition is called cirrhosis.

new hepatocytes are constantly formed, when there is widespread damage, they are unable to re-create the normal hexagonal architecture of the liver lobule. Without the normal architecture, the liver cannot carry out its functions of cleansing the blood of toxins. When most of a liver has been replaced by scar tissue that separates small clusters of regrown hepatocytes, the condition is called **cirrhosis**.[94] Cirrhosis, unfortunately, is no longer reversible even if people stop drinking.[96]

The rapid growth of hepatocytes to restore the liver from the damage of alcohol has another unfortunate consequence. Any cell line in which the cells are dividing frequently can acquire mutations that leads to·cancer (see Chapter 3. Cancer). People with chronic liver disease from alcohol are more likely to develop cancer of the hepatocytes, called **hepatocellular cancer**.[96]

Obesity and Diabetes

Ordinarily, the liver is not a storage depot for fat. This is what **adipocytes** (fat cells) are for. But fatty acids and triglycerides do regularly flow in and out of hepatocytes.[98] That balance is disrupted in people who are overweight, who have excess triglycerides in their adipocytes, causing free fatty acids to "spill over" into the blood (see earlier section of this chapter on obesity and diabetes). Some of these fatty acids in the blood are taken up by the hepatocytes.[98] At the same time, people with type 2 diabetes have a combination of high levels in glucose and high levels of insulin in their blood; this combination stimulates the hepatocytes to convert glucose to additional fatty acids.[98] The joint result is an abnormal storage of triglycerides in the liver—again called **steatosis** or a fatty liver (Figure 7.23).[96,99] When people who do not drink alcohol have it, they are said to have **non-alcoholic fatty liver disease (NAFLD)**[96] NAFLD—like alcoholic liver disease—often causes the hepatocytes to die, triggering inflammation by the immune cells. When a person who does not drink alcohol has both excess fat and inflammation of the liver, that person is said to have **non-alcoholic steato-hepatitis (NASH)** .

With the epidemic of obesity, a shockingly high proportion of adults (nearly 40% and rising) have NAFLD, most of whom are not aware. Fortunately, the condition is reversible if people lose weight, and it does not cause major problems for most of those who do not lose weight.[96,99] However, in about 10%–20% of those affected, over 10–20 years NAFLD follows the course of alcoholic liver disease, ending in cirrhosis.[99] And like those who drink alcohol, people with NAFLD are more likely to develop hepatocellular cancer.[96]

Viral Hepatitis

Liver cells are vulnerable to many different **viruses**. When viruses infect the liver, the infection is called **viral hepatitis** or simply **hepatitis**. Researchers have assigned letters to hepatitis viruses according to the order in which they were discovered. The two viruses that are the greatest public health problems are type B and type C (generally just called hepatitis B and hepatitis C).

Viruses are small particles—much smaller than human cells—that contain only their genetic material (DNA or RNA) and a few proteins wrapped in an **envelope**. They cannot make copies of themselves, so they are not usually considered "alive." They thrive by hijacking the machinery of cells that they have infected to make copies of themselves. When they do, the immune system responds by attacking the viruses and the cells that are "hosting" them.

Most viruses cause a brief **acute infection**, after which they are killed by the immune system, never to return. The hepatitis B and hepatitis C viruses, in contrast, can cause **chronic infections**, persisting for years or even a lifetime, during which time they manage to evade the immune system.[96] People usually have no idea that they have a liver infection during this time. But over those years, these viruses and the immune response that they provoke gradually kill off a high proportion of hepatocytes. As with alcoholic liver disease or NAFLD, the killed hepatocytes are replaced with scar tissue. And as with those other conditions, this process can end in cirrhosis, and it increases the risk of hepatocellular cancer.[96]

The hepatitis B and C viruses are summarized in **Table 7.7**. In adults, hepatitis B usually causes only a temporary acute infection, but in children it usually causes a chronic infection and in infants it nearly always does.[100] Hepatitis C causes a chronic infection most of the time regardless of the age of the person infected. The viruses are spread from one person to another, through mechanisms covered in more detail in Table 7.7 and in the risk factor section below.

Epidemiology: Patterns and Trends

Figure 7.24 shows mortality rates of chronic liver disease by age, race, and sex in the United States. Rates rise with age, are higher in men than women, and are particularly high in American Indians/Alaska Natives, perhaps because they have higher rates of diabetes and heavy alcohol use.[39,101]

Mortality rates from chronic liver disease in the United States have risen by more than 60% since

Table 7.7 Characteristics of Two Major Causes of Viral Hepatitis

Characteristic		Hepatitis B	Hepatitis C
Genetic material		DNA	RNA
Fraction of infections that become chronic		Infants: 90%	>50%
		Children <5: 25–50%	
		Adults: 5%	
Fraction of chronic infections that lead to cirrhosis		15%–25%	5%–25%
Prevalence of infection in the United States		0.26%	0.7%
Prevalence of infection globally		4.1%	0.7%
High-prevalence areas		Western Pacific, Asia, Africa	Eastern Mediterranean, Eastern Europe
Transmission routes	Blood transfusion (if not tested)	++++	++++
	Needle reuse in medical care	+++	+++
	Needle sharing among drug users	+++	+++
	Sexual exposure	++	+
	Mother to infant during delivery	+++	+
	Mother to child and child to child	+	−
Prevention by vaccination		Yes	No
Curative treatment available		No	Yes

Plus and minus symbols indicate approximately how readily the viruses are transmitted by these routes.

Gill RM, Kakar S. The Liver and Bile Ducts. In: Kumar V, Abbas AK, Aster JC, Turner JR, eds. Robbins & Cotran Pathologic Basis of Disease. 10th ed. Philadelphia: Elsevier; 2021:823-846.

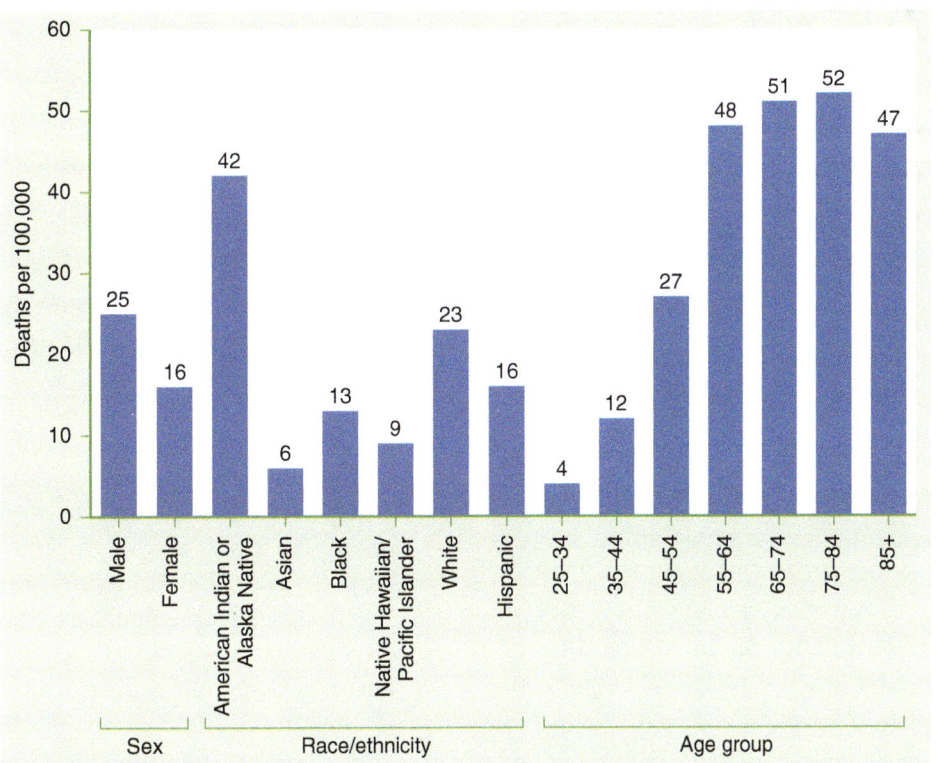

Figure 7.24 Mortality from Chronic Liver Disease in the United States by Demographic Group, 2018–2021.

Data from National Center for Health Statistics, Centers for Disease Control and Prevention. Underlying Cause of Death Data on CDC WONDER. Published 2023. Accessed June 12, 2024. https://wonder.cdc.gov/Deaths-by-Underlying-Cause.html

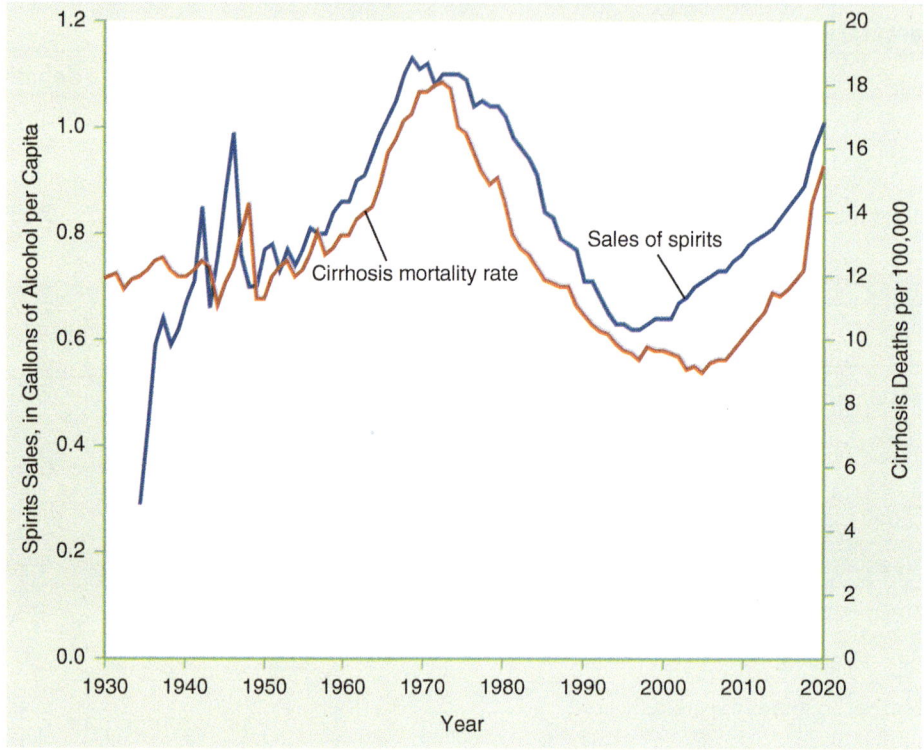

Figure 7.25 **Trends in Cirrhosis Mortality and Sales of Distilled Spirits, 1930–2021.** Mortality rates from cirrhosis of the liver closely parallel the sales of distilled spirits.

Data from Chen CM, Yoon YH. Surveillance Report #118. Liver Cirrhosis Mortality in the United States: National, State, and Regional Trends, 2000-2019. NIAAA Surveillance Reports. Published February 2022. Accessed March 8, 2024. https://www.niaaa.nih.gov/publications /surveillance-reports/surveillance118; and from Slater ME, Alpert HR. Surveillance Report #120 Apparent Per Capita Alcohol Consumption: National, State, and Regional Trends 1977-2021. NIAAA Research Surveillance Reports. Published April 2023. Accessed March 8, 2024. https://www.niaaa.nih.gov/publications/surveillance-reports/surveillance120

2000. This increase parallels increases in the prevalence of alcoholic liver disease and appears related to the increasing consumption of **distilled spirits**—that is, beverages like whiskey and vodka that have a very high alcohol content (**Figure 7.25**).[102-104]

The patterns of deaths from chronic liver disease reflect the combined patterns of the conditions that cause it:

- *Alcohol consumption* is discussed in more detail in Chapter 12. Alcohol Use. Heavy alcohol use peaks in the young adult years and falls with age after that, and men are more likely than women to drink heavily.[105]
- *NAFLD* is extremely and increasingly common, tracking rates of obesity and diabetes. The prevalence of the condition rose from 34% to 38% of U.S. adults just from 2011–2012 to 2017–2018.[106] The majority of American adults with obesity or diabetes have NAFLD, as do about one-third of American children who are obese.[99] The problem is not limited to the United States. An estimated 25% of people globally have this condition.[99,107]
- *Hepatitis B* rates vary markedly around the world and in racial groups in the United States

(Table 7.7). Globally, about 4% of people have chronic infection, which is more than 10 times the rate in the United States.[108] The hardest-hit areas are the Western Pacific and Africa, where 7% of people have chronic infection, and South-East Asia, where 3% of people do.[100] In these regions, the spread often occurs from mother-to-infant at the time of delivery or mother-to-child or child-to-child in early childhood.[108] In the United States, the prevalence of chronic hepatitis B infection is about 10 times as high in Asians (3%) and twice as high in Blacks (0.7%) as in Whites (0.3%).[108] These differences most likely reflect immigration from regions of the world with varying infection rates.

- *Hepatitis C* is estimated to chronically infect about 0.7% of people in the United States and globally.[109] Worldwide, rates are higher in areas where hospitals and clinics reuse (or have previously reused) hypodermic needles and where injection drug users share needles. In the United States, rates of chronic infection with hepatitis C among adults are estimated to be about twice as high in non-Hispanic Blacks as in people in other racial and ethnic groups

(1.8% vs. 0.8%). Also, rates are higher in "baby boomers" born between 1945 and 1969. Baby boomers are more likely to have received an HCV-infected blood transfusion before donated blood was tested for hepatitis C or to have shared needles to inject drugs when they were young adults.[110]

Risk Factors

The risk factors for chronic liver disease relate to the four major causes listed in the previous section (**Figure 7.26**):

- *Alcohol consumption.* The risk of developing cirrhosis is about twice as high among people who drink two drinks per day as nondrinkers. Heavier drinking sharply increases that risk: men who drink 5–6 drinks per day are nearly four times as likely to develop cirrhosis, and women about 12 times as likely.[111] As Figure 7.25 shows, the risk appears to be tied more strongly to consumption of distilled spirits than to consumption of beer or wine.[112,113]

- *Obesity or type 2 diabetes mellitus.* People who are overweight are about twice as likely to develop NAFLD, and those who are obese about four times as likely, even if they are considered metabolically healthy.[114] Even people in the higher end of the range of body mass index considered healthy (20-24.9 kg/m²) are at greater risk than those at the lower end.[115] For example, in one large study in China, 4% of those with a BMI below 23, 32% of those with a BMI between 23 and 25, and 32% of those with

a BMI above 25 had NAFLD.[115] Diabetes makes NAFLD worse.[116]

- *Viral hepatitis-related risk factors:* In people chronically infected with either hepatitis B or hepatitis C, active virus is present in blood and body fluids. These viruses can be transmitted if those body fluids enter the bloodstream of another person.[117] For hepatitis C, this spread mainly happens through sharing or reusing hypodermic needles, and for hepatitis B, this spread mainly happens from mother to child (Table 7.7). The risk factors for this transmission include:
  - *Medical care exposure.* Both hepatitis B and hepatitis C were once spread through transfusions, but testing of donated blood has now stopped this route of transmission.[96] But the viruses are still spread during medical care in some low- and middle-income countries where medical providers reuse hypodermic needles.[118]
  - *Injection drug use.* People who inject drugs often share hypodermic needles, syringes, or other injection equipment, spreading hepatitis viruses as they do. This appears to be the main route of the spread of hepatitis C today in the United States and perhaps globally.[96]
  - *High-risk sexual behavior.* Both hepatitis B and hepatitis C can be spread from a person with chronic infection to their sex partners. However, sexual transmission does not seem to happen very easily, especially for hepatitis C. Infection by this route is mainly in people with many sex partners or between men who

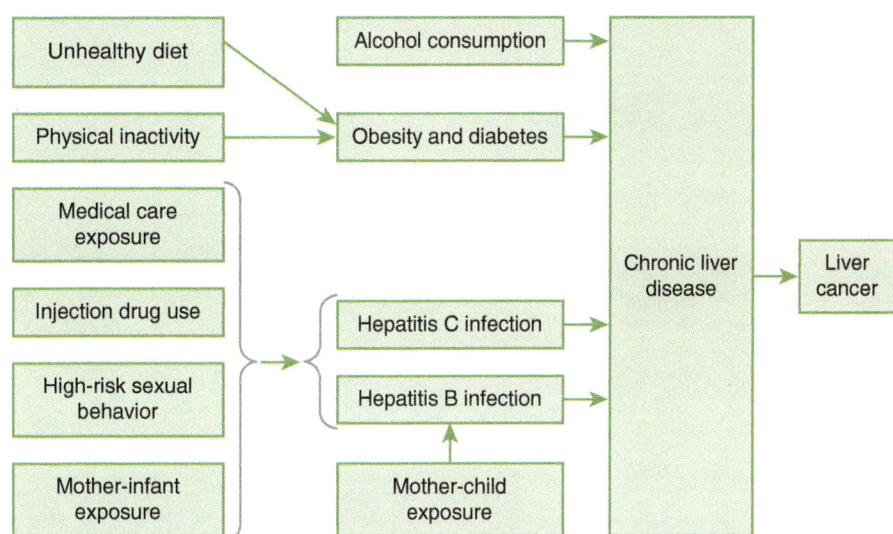

Figure 7.26 Cause-and-Effect Diagram for Chronic Liver Disease.

have sex with men (with anal sex perhaps increasing the risk).[119] Sexual spread of hepatitis C may be more common if one or the other partner is already infected with HIV. About 20%–30% of people with HIV infection worldwide also have chronic infection with hepatitis C.[117]

- *Mother-to-infant exposure.* During childbirth, the infant is covered with the mother's body fluids. This fluid contact enables hepatitis B to spread easily from mother to infant.[108,120] Hepatitis C can also be spread from mother to infant during delivery, but for unknown reasons it is much less likely to occur.[117]

- *Mother-to-child and child-to-child exposure.* Mothers usually have frequent skin-to-skin contact with their children. In areas of the world where the hepatitis B prevalence is high, such as some countries in the Western Pacific, this contact is an important route by which hepatitis B is spread—probably because of breaks in the skin or other exposure to body fluids.[96,120] It also appears that young children can spread hepatitis B to other children through skin-to-skin contact.[121] Hepatitis C is not believed to be spread this way.

Preventive Interventions

Rates of chronic liver disease and liver cancer can be reduced by addressing these risk factors (**Figure 7.27**):

- *Reduction of alcohol consumption*, especially distilled spirits. Figure 7.25 suggests that any action that reduces population-level consumption of spirits—such as tax increases—would reduce deaths from cirrhosis. Interventions to reduce alcohol consumption are discussed in Chapter 12. Alcohol Use.

- *Promotion of healthy diets* and *promotion of physical activity*. Any intervention that reduces people's fat stores or increases their insulin sensitivity should lead to a reduction in NAFLD and cirrhosis. The sort of dietary changes needed to reduce obesity is discussed earlier in this chapter, and interventions to promote these changes at a population level are discussed in Chapter 14. Dietary Risks. Physical activity is not a very effective way to reduce obesity, but it does increase insulin sensitivity, so it should help reduce NAFLD. The promotion of physical activity is discussed in Chapter 15. Physical Inactivity.

- *GLP-1 agonist treatment.* As of this writing, there is no scientific proof of this, but it is likely that NAFLD can be partially prevented if obese persons take the drugs that mimic the effect of the hormone **glucagon-like peptide-1 (GLP-1)** on

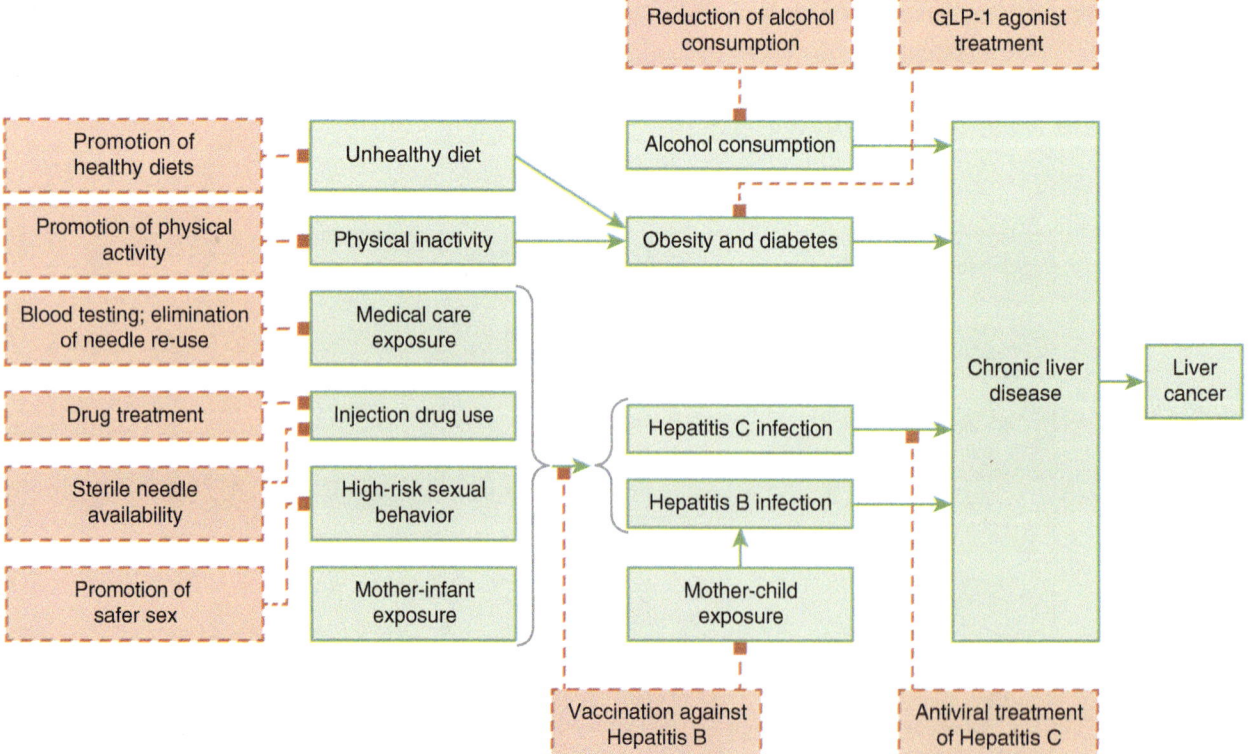

Figure 7.27 Cause-and-Effect Diagram for Chronic Liver Disease, with Preventive Interventions.

the brain. These medications reduce fat stores in adipocytes and blood glucose levels.

The World Health Organization has published a plan to eliminate viral hepatitis as a public health threat by 2030.[118] The plan emphasizes these interventions:

- *Blood testing before donation* and *elimination of the reuse of hypodermic needles*. The medical care system should no longer be a cause of a potentially fatal infection. The WHO estimates that 97% of samples of donated blood are tested for markers of hepatitis B and C before transfusion; that should occur 100% of the time. Likewise, the WHO estimates that 5% of injections given by medical providers use hypodermic needles that are not sterilized; that should never occur.
- *Sterile needle availability* and *drug treatment for drug users*. If drug users are given an adequate supply of sterile needles, for example, through needle exchange programs, they are much less likely to reuse needles and to spread hepatitis viruses. And drug users willing to undergo drug treatment are less likely to inject drugs at all. Primary *prevention of drug use* in theory can help, but this is not easy to achieve at a population level. Drug treatment and prevention of drug use are discussed in Chapter 13. Use of Addictive Drugs.
- *Vaccination against hepatitis B*. A highly effective vaccine against hepatitis B is widely available.[96] The vaccine is given in three doses over 6 months. In most but not all countries, this vaccine is recommended for all infants.[100] In the United States, about 80% of infants receive the first dose of hepatitis B vaccine within the first three days after birth. However, many other countries that routinely vaccinate infants against hepatitis B still do not administer the first dose at the time of birth. The WHO plan hopes to increase the proportion of babies who receive this birth dose from about 40% to 90% by 2030.[118] There is no vaccine currently available for hepatitis C.
- *Antiviral treatment of hepatitis C*. Medications can now cure chronic hepatitis C infection in just 8–12 weeks.[122] These medications represent an important breakthrough in the prevention of chronic liver disease. But the pharmaceutical companies have set very high prices for these medications, and those prices, combined with the need for testing to determine who should be treated, put treatment out of reach for some people in the United States and many around the world. Antiviral medications are also available to treat chronic hepatitis B infection, but unfortunately, these medications are much

less effective; they must be taken for 1–4 years and many people taking them relapse afterwards.[96,108]

In addition, the spread of hepatitis viruses can be reduced by:

- *Promotion of safer sex practices*. While it is difficult to achieve this, promotion of safer sex practices, particularly among men who have sex with men, should reduce spread of hepatitis B and C.[119]

Box 7.5 Summary–Prevention of Chronic Liver Disease

- Reduction in alcohol consumption
- Promotion of healthy diets
- Promotion of physical activity
- GLP-1 agonist treatment
- Blood testing before donation
- Elimination of reuse of hypodermic needles
- Sterile needle availability
- Drug treatment for drug users
- Vaccination against hepatitis B
- Antiviral treatment of hepatitis C
- Promotion of safer sex practices

Box 7.6 Key Words–Chronic Liver Disease

Acetaldehyde
Acute infection
Adipocyte
Alcoholic liver disease
Bile
Bile acids
Central vein (of the liver)
Chronic infection
Chronic liver disease
Cirrhosis
Distilled spirits
Endotoxins
Envelope (of a virus)
Ethanol or ethyl alcohol
Fatty acids
Fatty liver
Glucagon-like peptide 1 (GLP-1)
Glucose
Glycogen
Hepatic fibrosis
Hepatic steatosis
Hepatitis
Hepatitis viruses
Hepatocellular cancer
Hepatocyte
Liver lobule

(continues)

Box 7.6 Key Words–Chronic Liver Disease *(continued)*

Metabolic syndrome
Non-alcoholic fatty liver disease (NAFLD)
Non-alcoholic steato-hepatitis (NASH)
Portal vein
Scar tissue
Sinusoids
Steato-hepatitis
Steatosis
Triglycerides
Viral hepatitis
Virus

Resources–Chronic Liver Disease

- Powell EE, Wong VWS, Rinella M. Non-alcoholic fatty liver disease. *Lancet.* 2021;397(10290):2212-2224. doi:10.1016/S0140-6736(20)32511-3.

- Hosseini N, Shor J, Szabo G. Alcoholic Hepatitis: A Review. *Alcohol and Alcoholism.* 2019;54(4):408-416. doi:10.1093/alcalc/agz036.

- WHO. *Global Hepatitis Report 2017.* Geneva, 2017. Available at https://www.who.int/publications/i/item/9789241565455

- Chen CM, Yoon YH. Surveillance Report #118. Liver Cirrhosis Mortality in the United States: National, State, and Regional Trends, 2000–2019. *NIAAA Surveillance Reports.* Published February 2022. Accessed March 8, 2024. https://www.niaaa.nih.gov/publications/surveillance-reports/surveillance118

- Kim D, Alshuwaykh O, Dennis BB, Cholankeril G, Ahmed A. Trends in Etiology-based Mortality From Chronic Liver Disease Before and During COVID-19 Pandemic in the United States. *Clinical Gastroenterology and Hepatology.* 2022;22:2307-2316. doi:10.1016/j.cgh.2022.05.045.

- Sepanlou SG, Safiri S, Bisignano C, et al. The global, regional, and national burden of cirrhosis by cause in 195 countries and territories, 1990–2017: A systematic analysis for the Global Burden of Disease Study 2017. *Lancet Gastroenterol Hepatol.* 2020;5(3):245-266. doi:10.1016/S2468-1253(19)30349-8.

References

1. Hall JE, Hall MH. Metabolism and temperature regulation. In: *Guyton and Hall Textbook of Medical Physiology.* 14th ed. Elsevier; 2021:843-914.

2. Kumar V, Abbas AK, Aster JC, Turner JR. Obesity. In: Kumar V, Abbas AK, Aster JC, Turner JR, eds. *Robbins & Cotran Pathologic Basis of Disease.* 10th ed. Elsevier; 2021:444-449.

3. Maitra A. Diabetes mellitus. In: Kumar V, Abbas AK, Aster JC, Turner JR, eds. *Robbins & Cotran Pathologic Basis of Disease.* 10th ed. Elsevier; 2021:1099-1113.

4. Templeman NM, Skovsø S, Page MM, Lim GE, Johnson JD. A causal role for hyperinsulinemia in obesity. *J Endocrinol.* 2017;232(3):R173-R183. doi:10.1530/JOE-16-0449.

5. Hall JE, Hall ME. Insulin, glucagon, and diabetes mellitus. In: *Guyton and Hall Textbook of Medical Physiology.* 14th ed. Elsevier; 2021:973-989.

6. Hall KD, Farooqi IS, Friedman JM, et al. The energy balance model of obesity: beyond calories in, calories out. *Am J Clin Nutr.* 2022;115(5):1243-1254. doi:10.1093/ajcn/nqac031.

7. Vernarelli JA, Mitchell DC, Rolls BJ, Hartman TJ. Dietary energy density and obesity: how consumption patterns differ by body weight status. *Eur J Nutr.* 2018;57(1):351-361. doi:10.1007/s00394-016-1324-8.

8. Ludwig DS, Ebbeling CB. The carbohydrate-insulin model of obesity: Beyond "calories in, calories out." *JAMA Intern Med.* 2018;178(8):1098-1103. doi:10.1001/jamainternmed.2018.2933.

9. Mozaffarian D. Dietary and policy priorities for cardiovascular disease, diabetes, and obesity. *Circulation.* 2016;133(2):187-225. doi:10.1161/CIRCULATIONAHA.115.018585.

10. Darbre PD. Endocrine disruptors and obesity. *Curr Obes Rep.* 2017;6:18-27. doi:10.1007/s13679-017-0240-4.

11. Lee CJ, Sears CL, Maruthur N. Gut microbiome and its role in obesity and insulin resistance. *Ann N Y Acad Sci.* 2020;1461(1):37-52. doi:10.1111/nyas.14107.

12. Rohrmann S, Linseisen J. Processed meat: The real villain? *Proc Nutr Soc.* 2016;75(3):233-241. doi:10.1017/S0029665115004255.

13. Kim Y, Keogh J, Clifton P. A review of potential metabolic etiologies of the observed association between red meat consumption and development of type 2 diabetes mellitus. *Metabolism.* 2015;64(7):768-779. doi:10.1016/j.metabol.2015.03.008.

14. Dietary Guidelines Advisory Committee. *Scientific Report of the 2020 Dietary Guidelines Advisory Committee Advisory Report to the Secretary of Agriculture and Secretary of Health and Human Services.*; 2020. Accessed June 12, 2024. Available at: https://www.dietaryguidelines.gov/2020-advisory-committee-report

15. Liu X, Li Y, Tobias DK, et al. Changes in types of dietary fats influence long-term weight change in US women and men. *J Nutr.* 2018;148(11):1821-1829. doi:10.1093/jn/nxy183.

16. Monteiro CA, Cannon G, Levy RB, et al. Ultra-processed foods: What they are and how to identify them. *Public Health Nutr.* 2019;22(5):936-941. doi:10.1017/S1368980018003762.

17. de Deus Mendonça R, Pimenta AM, Gea A, et al. Ultra-processed food consumption and risk of overweight and obesity: The University of Navarra Follow-Up (SUN) cohort study. *Am J Clin Nutr.* 2016;104(5):1433-1440. doi:10.3945/ajcn.116.135004.

18. Poti JM, Mendez MA, Ng SW, Popkin BM. Is the degree of food processing and convenience linked with the nutritional quality of foods purchased by US households? *Am J Clin Nutr*. 2015;101(6):1251-1262. doi:10.3945/ajcn .114.100925.

19. Hall KD, Ayuketah A, Brychta R, et al. Ultra-processed diets cause excess calorie intake and weight gain: an inpatient randomized controlled trial of ad libitum food intake. *Cell Metab*. 2019;30(1):67-77.e3. doi:10.1016/j.cmet .2019.05.008.

20. Samuel VT, Shulman GI. The pathogenesis of insulin resistance: Integrating signaling pathways and substrate flux. *J Clin Invest*. 2016;126(1):12-22. doi:10.1172/JCI77812.

21. Yang A, Mottillo EP. Adipocyte lipolysis: From molecular mechanisms of regulation to disease and therapeutics. *Biochem J*. 2020;477(5):985-1008. doi:10.1042/BCJ20190468.

22. Boden G. Obesity and free fatty acids. *Endocrinol Metab Clin North Am*. 2008;37(3):635-646. doi:10.1016/j .ecl.2008.06.007.

23. Burkart K, Causey K, Cohen AJ, et al. Estimates, trends, and drivers of the global burden of type 2 diabetes attributable to PM2·5 air pollution, 1990–2019: An analysis of data from the Global Burden of Disease Study 2019. *Lancet Planet Health*. 2022;6(7):e586-e600. doi:10.1016/S2542-5196(22)0 0122-X.

24. Livingston G, Huntley J, Sommerlad A, et al. Dementia prevention, intervention, and care: 2020 report of the Lancet Commission. *Lancet*. 2020;396(10248):413-446. doi:10.1016/S0140-6736(20)30367-6.

25. Centers for Disease Control and Prevention. Health effects of obesity. CDC. Published September 24, 2022. Accessed September 18, 2023. Available at: https://www.cdc.gov /healthyweight/effects/index.html

26. Aune D, Sen A, Prasad M, et al. BMI and all cause mortality: Systematic review and non-linear dose-response meta-analysis of 230 cohort studies with 3.74 million deaths among 30.3 million participants. *BMJ*. 2016;353:i2156. doi:10.1136/bmj.i2156.

27. Expert Panel on the Identification Evaluation, and Treatment of Overweight in Adults. Clinical guidelines on the identification, evaluation, and treatment of overweight and obesity in adults: Executive summary. *Am J Clin Nutr*. 1998;68(4):899-917. doi:10.1093/ajcn/68.4.899.

28. ElSayed NA, Aleppo G, Bannuru RR, et al. Diagnosis and classification of diabetes: Standards of care in diabetes—2024. *Diabetes Care*. 2024;47(Suppl 1):S20-S42. doi:10.2337/dc24-S002.

29. National Institute of Diabetes and Digestive and Kidney Diseases. Insulin resistance and prediabetes. NIH.gov. Published May 2018. Accessed September 14, 2023. Available at: https://www.niddk.nih.gov/health-information/diabetes /overview/what-is-diabetes/prediabetes-insulin-resistance

30. Morris DH, Khunti K, Achana F, et al. Progression rates from HbA1c 6.0-6.4% and other prediabetes definitions to type 2 diabetes: A meta-analysis. *Diabetologia*. 2013;56(7):1489-1493. doi:10.1007/s00125-013-2902-4.

31. Gore MO, Mcguire DK. A Test in context: Hemoglobin A 1c and cardiovascular disease. *J Am Coll Cardiol*. 2016; 68(22):2479-2486.

32. Ogden CL, Fryar CD, Martin CB, et al. Trends in obesity prevalence by race and Hispanic origin—1999–2000 to 2017–2018. *JAMA*. 2020;324(12):1208-1210. doi:10.1001 /jama.2020.14590.

33. Stierman B, Afful J, Carroll MD, et al. National Health and Nutrition Examination Survey 2017-March 2020 prepandemic data files-Development of files and prevalence estimates for selected health outcomes. *Natl Health Stat Report*. 2021;(158):1-21.

34. Ogden CL, Carroll MD, McDowell MA, Flegal KM. Obesity among adults in the United States—no statistically significant change since 2003–2004. *NCHS Data Brief*. 2007;(1):1-8.

35. Chooi YC, Ding C, Magkos F. The epidemiology of obesity. *Metabolism*. 2019;92:6-10. doi:10.1016/j.metabol .2018.09.005.

36. Bullard KM, Cowie CC, Lessem SE, et al. Prevalence of diagnosed diabetes in adults by diabetes type—United States, 2016. *MMWR Morb Mortal Wkly Rep*. 2018;67(12):359-361. doi:10.15585/mmwr.mm6712a2.

37. Wang L, Li X, Wang Z, et al. Trends in prevalence of diabetes and control of risk factors in diabetes among US adults, 1999–2018. *JAMA*. 2021;326(8):704-716. doi:10.1001 /jama.2021.9883.

38. Gregg EW, Cadwell BL, Cheng YJ, et al. Trends in the prevalence and ratio of diagnosed to undiagnosed diabetes according to obesity levels in the U.S. *Diabetes Care*. 2004;27:2806-2812.

39. National Center for Health Statistics, Centers for Disease Control and Prevention. National Health Interview Survey: Summary health statistics. CDC.gov. Published September 21, 2023. Accessed June 25, 2024. Available at: https://www .cdc.gov/nchs/nhis/shs.htm

40. Shai I, Jiang R, Manson JE, et al. Ethnicity, obesity, and risk of type 2 diabetes in women. *Diabetes Care*. 2006;29(7):1585-1590. doi:10.2337/dc06-0057.

41. Tinajero MG, Malik VS. An update on the epidemiology of type 2 diabetes: A global perspective. *Endocrinol Metab Clin North Am*. 2021;50(3):337-355. doi:10.1016/j.ecl .2021.05.013.

42. Physical Activity Guidelines Advisory Committee. *2018 Physical Activity Guidelines Advisory Committee Scientific Report*. Accessed July 17, 2024. Available at: https://health .gov/healthypeople/tools-action/browse-evidence-based -resources/2018-physical-activity-guidelines-advisory -committee-scientific-report

43. Swift DL, Johannsen NM, Lavie CJ, Earnest CP, Church TS. The role of exercise and physical activity in weight loss and maintenance. *Prog Cardiovasc Dis*. 2014;56(4):441-447. doi:10.1016/j.pcad.2013.09.012.

44. Lee DH, Keum N, Hu FB, et al. Comparison of the association of predicted fat mass, body mass index, and other obesity indicators with type 2 diabetes risk: Two large prospective studies in US men and women. *Eur J Epidemiol*. 2018;33(11):1113-1123. doi:10.1007/sl0654-018-0433-5.

45. Ley SH, Schulze MB, Hivert MF, Meigs JB, Hu FB. Risk Factors for Type 2 Diabetes. In: Cowie CC, Casagrande SS, Menke A, Cissell MA, eds. *Diabetes in America*. 3rd ed. National Institute of Diabetes and Digestive and Kidney Diseases; 2018.

46. Srour B, Fezeu LK, Kesse-Guyot E, et al. Ultra-processed food consumption and risk of type 2 diabetes among participants of the NutriNet-Santé prospective cohort. *JAMA Intern Med*. 2020;180(2):283-291. doi:10.1001 /jamainternmed.2019.5942.

47. Grnøtved A, Rimm EB, Willett WC, Andersen LB, Hu FB. A prospective study of weight training and risk of type 2 diabetes

mellitus in men. *Arch Intern Med.* 2012;172(17):1306-1312. doi:10.1001/archinternmed.2012.3138.

48. Stocks B, Zierath JR. Post-translational modifications: The signals at the intersection of exercise, glucose uptake, and insulin sensitivity. *Endocr Rev.* 2022;43(4):654-677. doi:10.1210/endrev/bnab038.

49. Wethington HR, Finnie RKC, Buchanan LR, et al. Healthier food and beverage interventions in schools: four community guide systematic reviews. *Am J Prev Med.* 2020;59(1):e15-e26. doi:10.1016/j.amepre.2020.01.011.

50. Leblanc EL, Patnode CD, Webber EM, Redmond N, Rushkin M, O'connor EA. Evidence Synthesis Number 168: Behavioral and pharmacotherapy weight loss interventions to prevent obesity-related morbidity and mortality in adults: an updated systematic review for the U.S. Preventive Services Task Force Acknowledgments. Accessed March 18, 2025. Available at: https://www.ahrq.gov

51. Hall KD, Kahan S. Maintenance of lost weight and long-term management of obesity. *Med Clin North Am.* 2018;102(1):183-197. doi:10.1016/j.mcna.2017.08.012.

52. Kraschnewski JL, Kong L, Bryce CL, et al. Intensive behavioral therapy for weight loss in patients with, or at-risk of, type 2 diabetes: Results from the PaTH to health diabetes study. *Prev Med Rep.* 2023;31:102099. doi:10.1016/j.pmedr.2022.102099.

53. National Institute of Diabetes and Digestive and Kidney Diseases. Diabetes Prevention Program. Published May 2022. Accessed September 14, 2023. Available at: https://www.niddk.nih.gov/about-niddk/research-areas/diabetes/diabetes-prevention-program-dpp

54. Ackermann RT. From programs to policy and back again: The push and pull of realizing type 2 diabetes prevention on a national scale. *Diabetes Care.* 2017;40(10):1298-1301. doi:10.2337/dci17-0012.

55. Moin T, Schmittdiel JA, Flory JH, et al. Review of metformin use for type 2 diabetes prevention. *Am J Prev Med.* 2018;55(4):565-574. doi:10.1016/j.amepre.2018.04.038.

56. ElSayed NA, Aleppo G, Bannuru RR, et al. Prevention or delay of diabetes and associated comorbidities: Standards of care in diabetes—2024. *Diabetes Care.* 2024;47(Suppl 1):S43-S51. doi:10.2337/dc24-S003.

57. Shealy KM, Wu J, Waites J, Taylor NA, Blair Sarbacker G. Patterns of diabetes screening and prediabetes treatment during office visits in the US. *J Am Board Fam Med.* 2019;32(2):209-217. doi:10.3122/jabfm.2019.02.180259.

58. Wilding JPH, Batterham RL, Calanna S, et al. Once-weekly semaglutide in adults with overweight or obesity. *N Eng J Med.* 2021;384(11):989-1002. doi:10.1056/nejmoa2032183.

59. Aronne LJ, Sattar N, Horn DB, et al. Continued treatment with tirzepatide for maintenance of weight reduction in adults with obesity: The SURMOUNT-4 randomized clinical trial. *JAMA.* 2024;331(1):38-48. doi:10.1001/jama.2023.24945.

60. Frías JP, Davies MJ, Rosenstock J, et al. Tirzepatide versus semaglutide once weekly in patients with type 2 diabetes. *N Engl J Med.* 2021;385(6):503-515. doi:10.1056/nejmoa2107519.

61. U.S. Preventive Services Task Force. Prediabetes and type 2 diabetes: Screening. Published August 24, 2021. Accessed June 24, 2024. Available at: https://www.uspreventiveservicestaskforce.org/uspstf/recommendation/screening-for-prediabetes-and-type-2-diabetes

62. Davies MJ, Aroda VR, Collins BS, et al. Management of hyperglycemia in type 2 diabetes, 2022: A consensus report by the American Diabetes Association (ADA) and the European Association for the Study of Diabetes (EASD). *Diabetes Care.* 2022;45(11):2753-2786. doi:10.2337/dci22-0034.

63. de Boer IH, Khunti K, Sadusky T, et al. Diabetes management in chronic kidney disease: A consensus report by the American Diabetes Association (ADA) and Kidney Disease: Improving Global Outcomes (KDIGO). *Diabetes Care.* 2022;45(12):3075-3090. doi:10.2337/dci22-0027.

64. Hall JE, Hall ME. The urinary system: functional anatomy and urine formation by the kidney. In: *Guyton and Hall Textbook of Medical Physiology.* 14th ed. Elsevier; 2021:321-330.

65. Hall JE, Hall ME. Glomerular filtration, renal blood flow, and their control. In: *Guyton and Hall Textbook of Medical Physiology.* 14th ed. Elsevier; 2021:331-342.

66. Ku E, Lee BJ, Wei J, Weir MR. Hypertension in CKD: Core Curriculum 2019. *Am J Kidney Dis.* 2019;74(1):120-131. doi:10.1053/j.ajkd.2018.12.044.

67. Hall JE, Hall ME. Renal tubular reabsorption and secretion. In: *Guyton and Hall Textbook of Medical Physiology.* 14th ed. Elsevier; 2021:343-364.

68. Chang A, Laszik ZG. The kidney. In: Kumar V, Abbas AK, Aster JC, Turner JR, eds. *Robbins & Cotran Pathologic Basis of Disease.* 10th ed. Elsevier; 2021:896-952.

69. Inker LA, Eneanya ND, Coresh J, et al. New creatinine- and cystatin C–based equations to estimate GFR without race. *N Engl J Med.* 2021;385(19):1737-1749. doi:10.1056/nejmoa2102953.

70. Ibrahim HN, Foley R, Tan L, et al. Long-term consequences of kidney donation. *N Engl J Med.* 2009;360(5):459-469. doi:10.1056/NEJMoa0804883.

71. Agarwal R. Pathogenesis of diabetic nephropathy. *ADA Clin Compend.* 2021;2021(1):2-7. doi:10.2337/db20211-2.

72. Garland JS. Elevated body mass index as a risk factor for chronic kidney disease: Current perspectives. *Diabetes, Metab Syndr and Obes.* 2014;7:347-355. doi:10.2147/DMSO.S46674.

73. National Institute of Diabetes and Digestive and Kidney Diseases. United States Renal Data System 2023 Annual Data Report. National Institute of Diabetes and Digestive and Kidney Diseases, National Institutes of Health. Published 2023. Accessed February 29, 2024. Available at: https://usrds-adr.niddk.nih.gov/2023

74. Stevens PE. Evaluation and management of chronic kidney disease: synopsis of the Kidney Disease: Improving Global Outcomes 2012 clinical practice guideline. *Ann Intern Med.* 2013;158(11):825. doi:10.7326/0003-4819-158-11-201306040-00007.

75. Stevens PE, Ahmed SB, Carrero JJ, et al. KDIGO 2024 clinical practice guideline for the evaluation and management of chronic kidney disease. *Kidney Int.* 2024;105(4):S117-S314. doi:10.1016/j.kint.2023.10.018.

76. Bikbov B, Purcell CA, Levey AS, et al. Global, regional, and national burden of chronic kidney disease, 1990–2017: A systematic analysis for the Global Burden of Disease Study 2017. *Lancet.* 2020;395(10225):709-733. doi:10.1016/S0140-6736(20)30045-3.

77. Jankowski J, Floege J, Fliser D, Böhm M, Marx N. Cardiovascular disease in chronic kidney disease: pathophysiological insights and therapeutic options. *Circulation.* 2021;143(11):1157-1172. doi:10.1161/CIRCULATIONAHA.120.050686.

78. Centers for Disease Control and Prevention. CKD-related health problems. Centers for Disease Control and Prevention.

Published June 5, 2023. Accessed February 29, 2024. Available at: https://www.cdc.gov/kidneydisease/publications -resources/annual-report/ckd-related-health-problems .html

79. Chen TK, Knicely DH, Grams ME. Chronic kidney disease diagnosis and management: A review. *JAMA.* 2019;322(13):1294-1304. doi:10.1001/jama.2019.14745.

80. Centers for Disease Control and Prevention. Chronic kidney disease in the United States, 2023. Accessed March 18, 2025. Available at: https://www.cdc.gov/kidneydisease /publications-resources/CKD-national-facts.html

81. Global Burden of Disease Collaboration, Institute for Health Metrics and Evaluation. GBD Results Tool. Published July 12, 2023. Accessed July 11, 2023. Available at: https:// vizhub.healthdata.org/gbd-results/

82. Luyckx VA, Cherney DZI, Bello AK. Preventing CKD in developed countries. *Kidney Int Rep.* 2020;5(3):263-277. doi:10.1016/j.ekir.2019.12.003.

83. Crump C, Sundquist J, Winkleby MA, Sundquist K. Preterm birth and risk of chronic kidney disease from childhood into mid-adulthood: National cohort study. *BMJ.* 2019;365:l1346. doi:10.1136/bmj.l1346.

84. Xia J, Wang L, Ma Z, et al. Cigarette smoking and chronic kidney disease in the general population: A systematic review and meta-analysis of prospective cohort studies. *Nephrol Dial Transplant.* 2017;32(3):475-487. doi:10.1093 /ndt/gfw452.

85. Jayatilake N, Mendis S, Maheepala P, Mehta FR. Chronic kidney disease of uncertain aetiology: Prevalence and causative factors in a developing country. *BMC Nephrol.* 2013;14(1):180. doi:10.1186/1471-2369-14-180.

86. Emdin CA, Rahimi K, Neal B, Callender T, Perkovic V, Patel A. Blood pressure lowering in type 2 diabetes: A systematic review and meta-analysis. *JAMA.* 2015;313(6):603-615. doi:10.1001/jama.2014.18574.

87. Ettehad D, Emdin CA, Kiran A, et al. Blood pressure lowering for prevention of cardiovascular disease and death: A systematic review and meta-analysis. *Lancet.* 2016;387(10022):957-967. doi:10.1016/S0140-6736(15)01225-8.

88. Xie X, Atkins E, Lv J, et al. Effects of intensive blood pressure lowering on cardiovascular and renal outcomes: updated systematic review and meta-analysis. *Lancet.* 2016;387(10017): 435-443. doi:10.1016/S0140-6736(15)00805-3.

89. Aldafas R, Crabtree T, Vinogradova Y, Gordon JP, Idris I. Efficacy and safety of intensive versus conventional glucose targets in people with type 2 diabetes: a systematic review and meta-analysis. *Expert Rev Endocrinol Metab.* 2023;18(1): 95-110. doi:10.1080/17446651.2023.2166489.

90. ADVANCE group. Intensive blood glucose control and vascular outcomes in patients with type 2 diabetes. *N Engl J Med.* 2008;358(24):2560-2572. doi:10.1056 /nejmoa0802987.

91. Perkovic V, Jardine MJ, Neal B, et al. Canagliflozin and renal outcomes in type 2 diabetes and nephropathy. *N Engl J Med.* 2019;380(24):2295-2306. doi:10.1056/ nejmoa1811744.

92. Shaman AM, Bain SC, Bakris GL, et al. Effect of the glucagon-like peptide-1 receptor agonists semaglutide and liraglutide on kidney outcomes in patients with type 2 diabetes: Pooled analysis of SUSTAIN 6 and LEADER. *Circulation.* 2022;145(8):575-585. doi:10.1161/CIRCULATIONAHA.121.055459.

93. Marso SP, Bain SC, Consoli A, et al. Semaglutide and cardiovascular outcomes in patients with type 2 diabetes. *N Engl J Med.* 2016;375(19):1834-1844. doi:10.1056 /nejmoa1607141.

94. Hall JE, Hall ME. The Liver. In: *Guyton and Hall Textbook of Medical Physiology.* 14th ed. Elsevier; 2021:871-876.

95. Sepanlou SG, Safiri S, Bisignano C, et al. The global, regional, and national burden of cirrhosis by cause in 195 countries and territories, 1990–2017: A systematic analysis for the Global Burden of Disease Study 2017. *Lancet Gastroenterol Hepatol.* 2020;5(3):245-266. doi:10.1016 /S2468-1253(19)30349-8.

96. Gill RM, Kakar S. The liver and bile ducts. In: Kumar V, Abbas AK, Aster JC, Turner JR, eds. *Robbins & Cotran Pathologic Basis of Disease.* 10th ed. Elsevier; 2021:823-846.

97. Hosseini N, Shor J, Szabo G. Alcoholic hepatitis: A review. *Alcohol and Alcoholism.* 2019;54(4):408-416. doi:10.1093 /alcalc/agz036.

98. Kawano Y, Cohen DE. Mechanisms of hepatic triglyceride accumulation in non-alcoholic fatty liver disease. *J Gastroenterol.* 2013;48(4):434-441. doi:10.1007/s00535 -013-0758-5.

99. Powell EE, Wong VWS, Rinella M. Non-alcoholic fatty liver disease. *Lancet.* 2021;397(10290):2212-2224. doi:10 .1016/S0140-6736(20)32511-3.

100. Sheena BS, Hiebert L, Han H, et al. Global, regional, and national burden of hepatitis B, 1990–2019: A systematic analysis for the Global Burden of Disease Study 2019. *Lancet Gastroenterol Hepatol.* 2022;7(9):796-829. doi:10.1016 /S2468-1253(22)00124-8.

101. Substance Abuse and Mental Health Services Administration (SAMHSA). *National Survey on Drug Use and Health 2022—Detailed Tables.* Accessed March 31, 2025. Available at: https://www.samhsa.gov/data/data -we-collect/nsduh-national-survey-drug-use-and-health /national-releases/2022

102. Dang K, Hirode G, Singal AK, Sundaram V, Wong RJ. Alcoholic liver disease epidemiology in the United States: A retrospective analysis of 3 US databases. *Am J Gastroenterol.* 2020;115(1):96-104. doi:10.14309/ajg.0000000000000380.

103. Slater ME, Alpert HR. Surveillance Report #120 Apparent per capita alcohol consumption: National, state, and regional trends 1977–2021. *NIAAA Res Surveill Rep.* Published April 2023. Accessed March 8, 2024. Available at: https://www.niaaa.nih.gov/publications/surveillance -reports/surveillance120

104. Chen CM, Yoon YH. Surveillance Report #118. Liver cirrhosis mortality in the United States: National, state, and regional trendss, 2000–2019. *NIAAA Surveill Rep.* Published February 2022. Accessed March 8, 2024. Available at: https://www.niaaa.nih.gov/publications /surveillance-reports/surveillance118

105. Substance Use and Mental Health Services Administration. Key substance use and mental health indicators in the United States: Results from the 2020 National Survey on Drug Use and Health. Accessed June 17, 2024. Available at: https://www.samhsa.gov/data/sites/default/files/reports /rpt42731/2022-nsduh-nnr.pdf

106. Wong RJ, Cheung R. Trends in the prevalence of metabolic dysfunction-associated fatty liver disease in the United States, 2011–2018. *Clin Gastroenterol Hepatol.* 2022;20(3):e610-e613. doi:10.1016/j.cgh.2021.01.030.

107. Younossi ZM, Golabi P, de Avila L, et al. The global epidemiology of NAFLD and NASH in patients with type 2 diabetes: A systematic review and meta-analysis.

J Hepatol. 2019;71(4):793-801. doi:10.1016/j.jhep.2019.06.021.

108. Nguyen MH, Wong G, Gane E, Kao JH, Dusheiko G. Hepatitis B virus: Advances in prevention, diagnosis, and therapy. *Clin Microbiol Rev.* 2020;33(2):1-38.

109. Martinello M, Solomon SS, Terrault NA, Dore GJ. Hepatitis C. *Lancet.* 2023;402(10407):1085-1096. doi:10.1016/S0140-6736(23)01320-X.

110. Bradley H, Hall EW, Rosenthal EM, Sullivan PS, Ryerson AB, Rosenberg ES. Hepatitis C virus prevalence in 50 U.S. states and D.C. by sex, birth cohort, and race: 2013–2016. *Hepatol Commun.* 2020;4(3):355-370. doi:10.1002/hep4.1457/suppinfo.

111. Roerecke M, Vafaei A, Hasan OSM, et al. Alcohol consumption and risk of liver cirrhosis: A systematic review and meta-analysis. *Am J Gastroenterol.* 2019;114(10):1574-1586. doi:10.14309/ajg.0000000000000340.

112. Kerr WC, Fillmore KM, Marvy P. Beverage-specific alcohol consumption and cirrhosis mortality in a group of English-speaking beer-drinking countries. *Addiction.* 2000;95(3):339-346. doi:10.1046/j.1360-0443.2000.9533394.x.

113. Gruenewald PJ, Ponicki WR. The relationship of alcohol sales to cirrhosis mortality. *J Stud Alcohol.* 1995;56(6):635-641. doi:10.15288/jsa.1995.56.635.

114. Chang Y, Jung HS, Cho J, et al. Metabolically healthy obesity and the development of nonalcoholic fatty liver disease. *Am J Gastroenterol.* 2016;111(8):1133-1140. doi:10.1038/ajg.2016.178.

115. Chang M, Shao Z, Wei W, Shen P, Shen G. Sex-specific prevalence and risk factors of metabolic-associated fatty liver disease among 75,570 individuals in eastern China. *Front Endocrinol (Lausanne).* 2023;14:1241169. doi:10.3389/fendo.2023.1241169.

116. Jarvis H, Craig D, Barker R, et al. Metabolic risk factors and incident advanced liver disease in non-alcoholic fatty liver disease (NAFLD): A systematic review and meta-analysis of population-based observational studies. *PLoS Med.* 2020;17(4):1003100. doi:10.1371/JOURNAL.PMED.1003100.

117. Webster DP, Klenerman P, Dusheiko GM. Hepatitis C. *Lancet.* 2015;1124-1135. doi:10.1016/S0140-6736(14)62401-6.

118. World Health Organization. *Global Hepatitis Report 2017.* Accessed June 24, 2024. Available at: https://www.who.int/publications/i/item/9789241565455

119. Nijmeijer BM, Koopsen J, Schinkel J, Prins M, Bh Geijtenbeek T. Sexually transmitted hepatitis C virus infections: current trends, and recent advances in understanding the spread in men who have sex with men. *J Int AIDS Soc.* 2019;22(S6):e25348. doi:10.1002/jia2.25348/full.

120. World Health Organization. Hepatitis B vaccines: WHO position paper—July 2017. *WHO Wkly Epidemiol Rec.* 2017;92(27):369-392. Accessed March 19, 2025. Available at: http://www.who.int/wer

121. Franks AL, Berg CJ, Kane MA, et al. Hepatitis B virus infection among children born in the United States to Southeast Asian refugees. N Engl J Med. 1989;321(19):1301-1305. doi:10.1056/NEJM198911093211905.

122. Brunner N, Bruggmann P. Trends of the global hepatitis C disease burden: Strategies to achieve elimination. *J Prev Med Public Health.* 2021;54(4):251-258. doi:10.3961/JPMPH.21.151.

CHAPTER 8

Chronic Respiratory Diseases

This chapter discusses two chronic diseases of the lung: **asthma** and **chronic obstructive pulmonary disease (COPD)**. These diseases overlap, and at times they are indistinguishable. The main differences are that asthma affects children as well as adults, has temporary exacerbations called **asthma attacks**, and sometimes involves **allergy**. COPD is mostly a disease of adults and its symptoms do not fluctuate as much. Both diseases are caused by substances in the air that irritate the lung's airways.

The Lungs

The purpose of the lungs is to supply oxygen to the blood and remove carbon dioxide from it. The exchange of gases between the air and the blood occurs in hundreds of millions of tiny spherical sacs in the lungs called **alveoli** (**Figure 8.1**). These alveoli are connected to **bronchioles**, which are the smallest branches of the **bronchial tree**. The bronchial tree is a branching network of airways that starts with the **trachea** (windpipe) and that divides in each lung into ever-smaller branches of **bronchi** and bronchioles.

When a person inhales, the rib cage expands, which draws air in. This is called **inspiration**. When a person exhales, the rib cage contracts, which pushes air out. This is called **expiration**. The process of inspiration and expiration, repeated about 10–20 times per minute, replaces the gases inside the alveoli with outside air.

While this is happening, blood from the right side of the heart that is depleted of oxygen but full of carbon dioxide flows through capillaries that wrap around each alveolus. As the blood travels, carbon dioxide diffuses from the blood into the alveoli and oxygen diffuses from the alveoli into the blood (**Figure 8.2**). This exchanging of oxygen for carbon dioxide is called **gas exchange**.

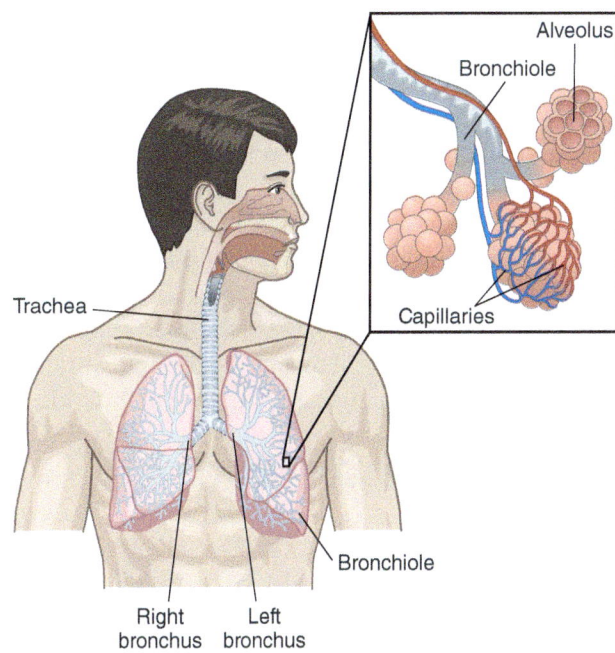

Figure 8.1 The Lung, Bronchioles, and Alveoli. The lung is composed of a branching network of large airways called bronchi and small airways called bronchioles, which end in tiny air sacs called alveoli.

197

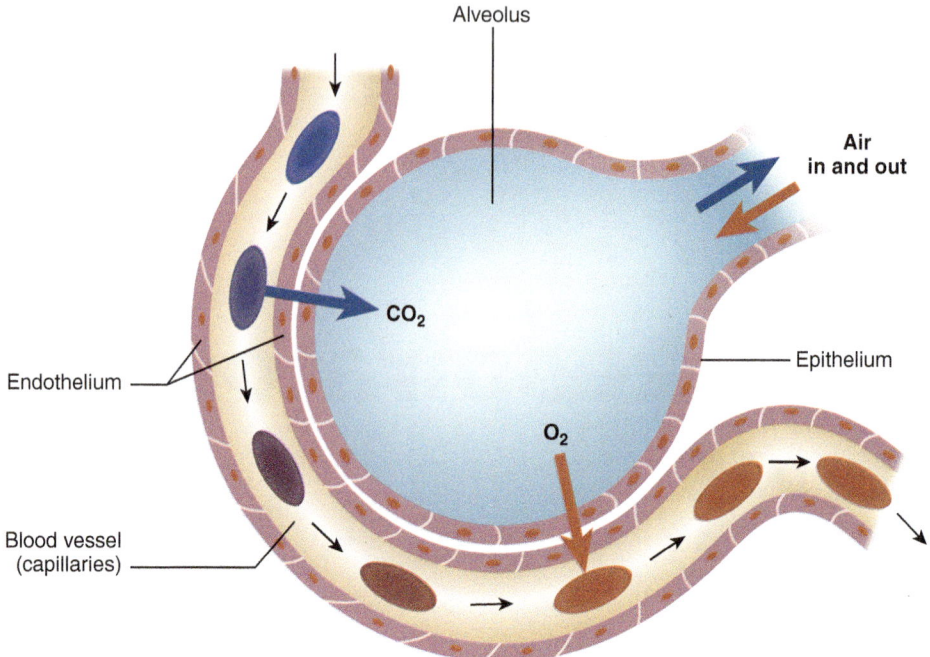

Figure 8.2 How Lung Alveoli Supply Oxygen to Blood and Remove Carbon Dioxide. The airways supply fresh air to the alveoli. Blood that is full of carbon dioxide and depleted of oxygen enters capillaries that wrap around the alveoli. As the blood passes the alveoli, carbon dioxide diffuses across the lining of the capillaries (endothelium) and the lining of the alveoli (epithelium) into the alveoli. Oxygen diffuses across the epithelium and endothelium in the opposite direction. This leaves the blood exiting the lungs full of oxygen and depleted of carbon dioxide.

The walls of the bronchioles contain specialized cells, called **smooth muscle cells** because they look smooth under a microscope. Like other muscles, these cells can contract (shorten) or relax (lengthen). When a person exercises and needs to obtain more oxygen and expel more carbon dioxide per minute, the smooth muscle cells in the walls relax. This increases the diameter of the bronchioles, like opening a spigot of a faucet, which allows more air to flow in and out. When a person breathes air containing irritating gases or particles, the smooth muscles contract. This shrinks the diameter of the bronchioles, like tightening the spigot of a faucet, which reduces air flow. This reduction of air flow can help protect alveoli from damaging gases and particles.

Pulmonary Function Tests

The health of the lungs can be measured with **spirometry** (**Figure 8.3**), which is a type of **pulmonary function test (PFT)**. Spirometry measures the maximum amount of air a person can breathe in or out, as well as how quickly the air moves. In spirometry, a person is asked to take in the deepest possible breath and then force the air out as quickly and completely as possible. The total volume of air that the person exhales is called the **forced vital capacity (FVC)**. The volume of air that is forced

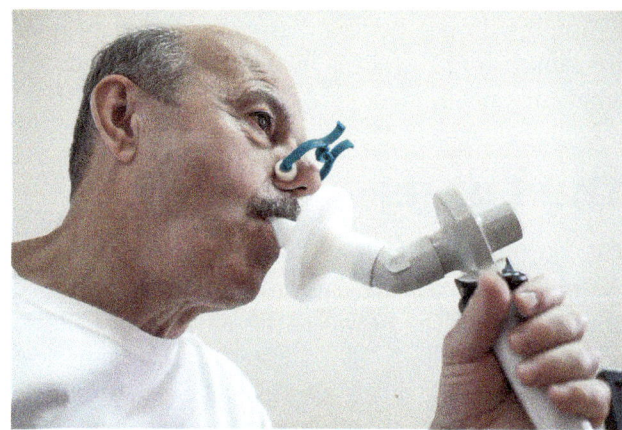

Figure 8.3 Spirometry. Spirometry measures the maximum amount of air a person can breathe in or out, as well as how quickly the air moves.
© Koldunov/Shutterstock

out in the first second is called the **forced expiratory volume 1** or FEV_1. The ratio FEV_1/FVC measures the fraction of that maximum breath that is expired in the first second. In a person with healthy lungs, the FEV_1/FVC ratio is above 0.70—that is, 70% of the air is exhaled in the first second. If a person's bronchioles are narrower than they should be, they slow the exhalation of air. With slower exhalation FEV_1 decreases and the ratio FEV_1/FVC drops below 0.70 (**Figure 8.4**).[1]

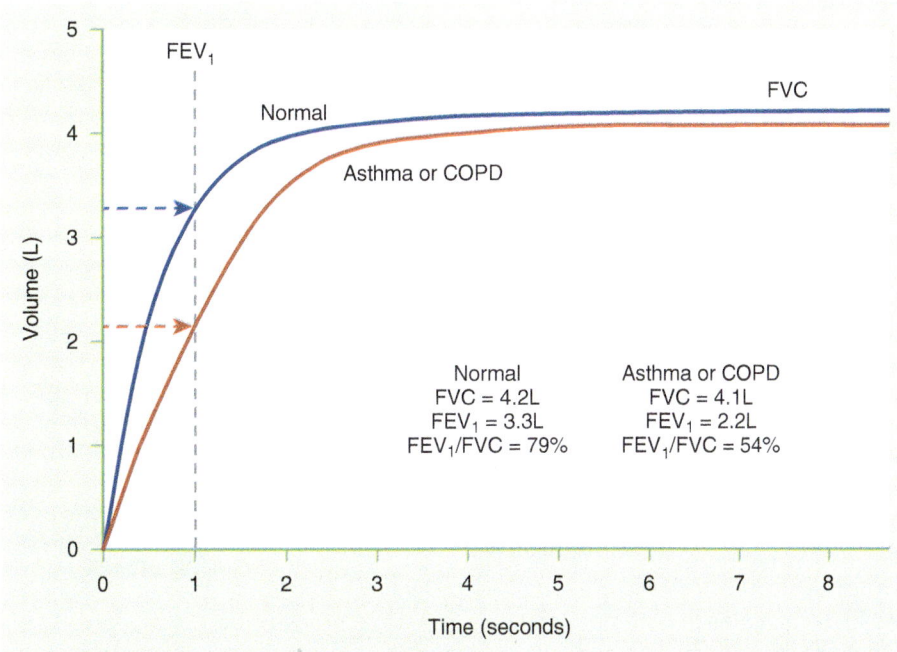

Figure 8.4 **Spirometry Results in Persons with Normal Lung versus Asthma or Chronic Obstructive Pulmonary Disease.** The graph shows the flow of air in a person with normal lungs and a person with asthma or chronic obstructive pulmonary disease (COPD). In a person with either of these diseases, the narrowed airways slow the flow of air (see red arrow), causing less air to be exhaled in the first second (FEV_1). That leads to an abnormally low FEV_1 and a low ratio of FEV_1 to the total air that is exhaled, called forced vital capacity (FEV_1/FVC).

Data from Louie, Samuel; Claudia M. Vukovich; Kivler, Celeste, 'Spirometry: Why, How, and When?', November 2015, Volume 55, Issue 11.

Asthma

Introduction

Asthma is an extremely common chronic disease of the lung in which the bronchi and bronchioles become inflamed and narrowed, causing those with the disease to cough and have difficulty breathing. It is characterized by periodic **asthma attacks**—episodes in which airways become narrower and symptoms worsen. Between asthma attacks, people with the disease may have only mild symptoms or no symptoms at all. Unlike most other chronic diseases, asthma often begins in early childhood, and it involves a distinct response of the immune system called **allergy**, which is discussed below. Many young children "outgrow" asthma—that is, the attacks disappear or become less common and less severe by the time the children start school.[2] On the other hand, some children develop asthma in their school-age years and some people develop the condition as adults.

Asthma rarely kills people, but it is a public health problem because so many people suffer from it. Despite extensive research, much about the causes of asthma is still not understood.

Pathophysiology of Asthma

Bronchioles in Asthma

The central problem with asthma is illustrated in **Figure 8.5**. Compared to normal bronchioles, the bronchioles of a person with asthma have thicker walls, and those walls contain immune cells, which is a sign of **inflammation**—that is, a response of the immune system to a perceived threat. The thicker walls make the internal channels of the bronchioles narrow. Then when a person has an asthma attack, the smooth muscles in the walls contract, making the bronchioles even narrower, and the cells lining the airways secrete mucus. With narrow bronchioles full of mucus, a person with asthma has difficulty inhaling air into the lungs, and even more difficulty exhaling air out. When air does move through the narrowed channels it makes a whistling sound called a **wheeze**.

If a person with an asthma attack is tested with spirometry, the difficulty in forcing air out of the lungs will cause both the FEV_1 and the ratio FEV_1/FVC to be abnormally low (Figure 8.4).[3,4]

A key characteristic of asthma is that the narrowed airways become wider again (the asthma attack is "reversed") if people are given medicines that cause the smooth muscles cells to relax. These medicines

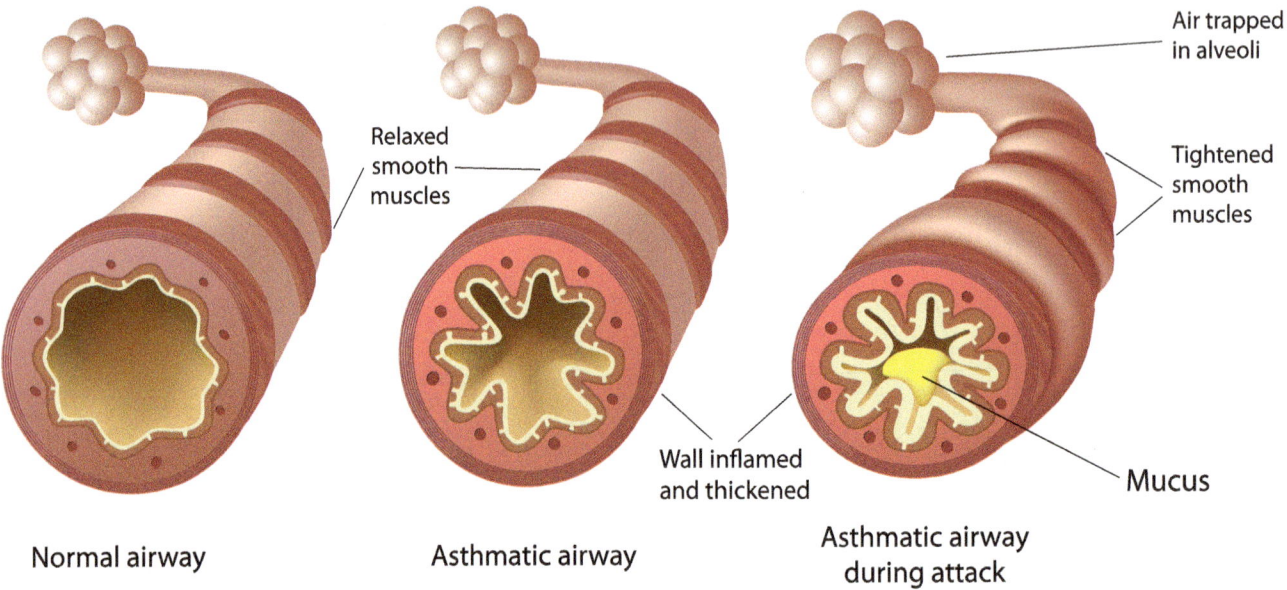

Figure 8.5 Changes in Bronchioles in Asthma. Compared to normal bronchioles, the bronchioles of a person with asthma have walls that are thicker and inflamed. The thicker walls make the internal channels of the bronchioles narrow. Then when a person has an asthma attack, the smooth muscles in the walls contract, making the bronchioles even narrower, and the cells lining the airways secrete mucus into the airways.

© Alila Medical Media/Shutterstock

are called **bronchodilators** because they **dilate** (expand the internal diameter of) the bronchioles. One way that doctors diagnose asthma, then, is to do a spirometry test before and after a patient is given bronchodilators to see if the results improve.[1]

Allergy and Asthma

The inflammation seen in asthma is often (but not always) caused by allergy.[3] Allergy is a condition in which cells in the immune system respond to even small amounts of biologic substances called **allergens**—such as tree pollen—with a disproportionate and unhealthy reaction. This **allergic** reaction typically involves symptoms such as itching, redness of the skin, a runny nose, sneezing, and coughing. People who have this reaction are said to be **sensitized** to the allergens that trigger them. In people with asthma, the allergic reaction causes the smooth muscles in the walls of bronchioles to contract and the lining of the bronchioles to secrete mucus.

The inflammation from allergy differs from the inflammation triggered by an infection. The immune system has many different branches and weapons. (The immune system is discussed in more detail in the section on HIV infection in Chapter 9. Infectious Diseases.) Among the immune system's weapons are **antibodies**, which are proteins shaped like the letter Y that can grab onto invading organisms to help kill them (**Figure 8.6**). There are several types

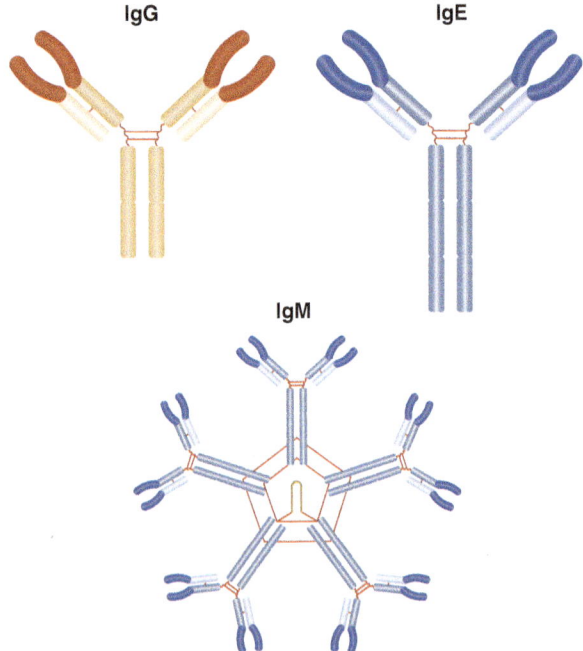

Figure 8.6 The Structure of Antibodies. Antibodies are specialized proteins shaped like the letter Y that grab onto foreign invading organisms. There are several types of antibodies, assigned different letters. People with allergies have an inappropriately strong response of IgE antibodies to allergens like pollen.

of antibodies, also called **immunoglobulins**, with names like IgE, IgG, and IgM as shorthand for immunoglobulin types E, G, and M. People with allergies have high levels of **IgE** antibodies. When these people are exposed to an allergen to which they are sensitized, IgE grabs onto the allergen and prompts certain immune cells to create the characteristic allergic inflammatory response.

Allergy and asthma are far more common today than they were 75 years ago. Many studies suggest a link between these conditions and being raised in a modern, non-agricultural environment. For example, children raised on farms have much lower rates of allergy and asthma than children raised in the suburbs or cities. A popular but still-unproven theory to explain this is called the **hygiene hypothesis**. According to this theory, children raised near animals are exposed early in life to many different bacteria and other microorganisms (**microbes**) that live with these animals; that exposure establishes a healthy, broad-based immune response to many biologic substances.[3-6] On the other hand, children raised in cleaner, non-agricultural environments do not develop this healthy immune response to microbes. When these children are later exposed to harmless substances like tree pollen, the IgE-using branch of their untrained immune systems overreacts in an unhealthy way.

The allergens most involved in asthma are commonly found inside homes. They include allergens shed by *house dust mites*, which are tiny insects (**Figure 8.7**) that live in house dust, bedding, upholstered furniture, and carpeting.[7] Pests like *cockroaches* and *mice* also leave allergens behind that many children with asthma are sensitized to. Other important allergens in asthma are *mold and other fungi*, which are present everywhere but are found in heavier concentration in homes with persistent *moisture*.[4]

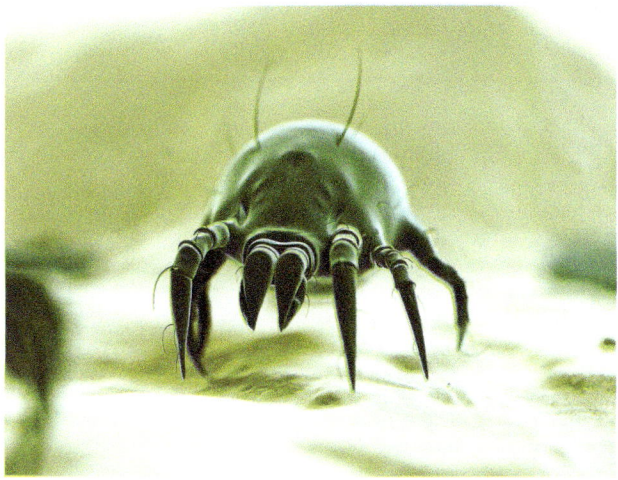

Figure 8.7 **House Dust Mite.** Many children with asthma are allergic to indoor insects like the tiny house dust mite.

© 3dMediSphere/Shutterstock

Causes Other Than Allergy

Allergy and the hygiene hypothesis may explain why asthma is much more common today than in the past, but they do not explain all cases of asthma. Many children with asthma are not particularly allergic and many substances other than allergens can increase the risk of asthma.

Other exposures that cause or exacerbate asthma include:

- *Respiratory viruses.* Some viruses tend to infect the cells lining the bronchial tree. Infection with these viruses increases airway inflammation. Viruses that have been linked to asthma include **respiratory syncytial Virus (RSV), rhinovirus**, and **influenza virus**.[4,5] It is too early to know if infection with SARS-CoV-2 (the virus that causes COVID-19) has a long-term effect on asthma.
- *Household or ambient air pollution.* Gases and particles in the air can irritate the airways, exacerbating asthma and perhaps initiating the disease. Substances that irritate the airways are called **irritants**. Particles in the air that are small enough to enter the lungs are irritants and trigger asthma attacks. Certain gases in the air, like ozone or NO_2, and chemicals can likewise irritate the airways. Air pollution involves combinations of irritating particles and gases. Particularly harmful forms of air pollution are environmental tobacco smoke, and smoke from burning marijuana, candles, and wood in stoves and fireplaces.[4,23] **Box 8.1** contains more details on air pollutants, the sources of air pollution, and the health effects of air pollution.

In most children with asthma, there are many triggers involved—some of which are allergens and some of which are irritants.[3]

The Importance of Household Air

While there is good reason to be concerned about ambient air pollution, household air is particularly important in asthma, especially in children. In part, that just reflects where people spend their time. A study from the 1990s found that people spent 87% of their time indoors, 6% of their time in vehicles, and only 7% outdoors. Children under age 12 spent even more of their time (89%) indoors.[24] With the internet having arrived since this study was done, it is likely that people spend even more of their time indoors today.

Household air is different from outdoor air. Air pollutants and allergens that are produced outdoors

Box 8.1 Air Pollution

Air pollution is a term used to describe gases, liquid aerosols, or particles that are not commonly present in air and that have adverse effects on humans or the natural environment. When most people hear that term, they think of black smoke flowing from factory chimneys, but air pollution comes from many different sources. It is usually separated into **household** (indoor) **air pollution** and **ambient** (outdoor) **air pollution.** These two types of air pollution have very different sources, pollutants, and concentrations of pollutants.

Household air pollution includes second-hand tobacco smoke, dust generated from sweeping and vacuuming, and smoke produced by fires used for cooking, heat, and light. In some low-income areas of the world, families burn wood, charcoal, dung, or the branches and leaves from their crops indoors for heat or cooking. These are called **biomass** fuels, and burning them generates very high levels of household air pollution. People who cook with biomass fuels and people who spend much time indoors where biomass fuels are used for heat can be heavily exposed. While household air pollution is much more of a problem in low-income countries, it can still be a problem in the United States, with exposure to second-hand tobacco smoke, dust, and pollutants emitted from gas stoves.[8]

The sources of ambient air pollution are summarized in **Table 8.1**. Some air pollution is produced by humans (**anthropogenic**) and some by the natural environment. Anthropogenic sources include those that are stationary and those that are mobile. Stationary sources include **point sources**, which are usually large industrial operations like power plants, and **non-point sources**, like homes, farm operations, and small commercial operations like dry cleaners. Mobile sources are categorized as on-road (or on-highway) vehicles, off-road (or off-highway) vehicles and non-road mobile sources like airplanes, ships, and trains.

Indoor or outdoor sources emit very many different gases, liquid aerosols, and particles. The Clean Air Act designated six important pollutants as **criteria air pollutants**. The Environmental Protection Agency (EPA) sets limits for these criteria air pollutants in outdoor air and regulates outdoor sources so that those limits are met.

The criteria air pollutants are summarized in **Table 8.2**. They include three gases (ozone, sulfur dioxide, and nitrogen oxides), one metal (lead), and **particulate matter**, which is a term for small particles in the air. Particulate matter differs from the other criteria pollutants in that it is defined not by its chemical composition but instead just by its size. Particulate matter refers to solid or liquid particles that are small enough to remain suspended in the air and be inhaled by humans. PM_{10} are particles that are less than 10 micrometers in diameter, and $PM_{2.5}$ are particles that are less than 2.5 micrometers in diameter. For comparison, a human hair is 50–70 micrometers in diameter (**Figure 8.8**). $PM_{2.5}$ particles can be inhaled deep into the lung and cause damage to the smallest airways.

Table 8.2 summarizes key adverse health effects of the criteria air pollutants. The criteria pollutant that is believed to be most harmful is $PM_{2.5}$. However, because these pollutants are often mixed, it can be difficult to distinguish the adverse health effects of any single pollutant. Five of the six criteria air pollutants are associated with exacerbation of asthma and chronic obstructive pulmonary disease. Exposure to particulate matter in either ambient or household air has been identified as a risk factor for a much longer list of health problems, including the ones below that are covered in this book:

Table 8.1 Sources of Ambient Pollution

Anthropogenic	Stationary	Point sources	Power plants, factories, petrochemical plants, incinerators
		Non-point sources	Single-family and multi-family residential buildings, farm operations, small commercial operations
	Mobile	On-road vehicles	Cars, trucks, and buses
		Off-road vehicles	Construction equipment, farm equipment
		Non-road mobile sources	Airplanes, ships, trains
Natural	Wildfires, dust, volcanic ash, pollen, sea spray, emissions from soil		

Data from Environmental Protection Agency. EPA.gov

Table 8.2 Criteria Air Pollutants, Their Key Sources, and Key Known Adverse Health Effects

Pollutant	Key Sources	Key Adverse Health Effects
Particulate matter ($PM_{2.5}$ and PM_{10})	Power plants,* industrial plants, vehicles, incinerators, wildfires, burning of crop wastes	Heart disease, stroke, chronic respiratory diseases, lung cancer, lower respiratory infections, premature mortality, adverse birth outcomes
Nitrogen oxides (NO_x)	Vehicles and off-road equipment,* power plants	Chronic respiratory diseases
Ozone (O_3)	Chemical reactions in atmosphere from other pollutants	Chronic respiratory diseases
Sulfur dioxide (SO_2)	Coal-burning power plants	Chronic respiratory diseases
Carbon monoxide (CO)	Vehicles and off-road equipment,* building furnaces*	Aggravation of chronic heart or lung diseases
Lead	Leaded gasoline, paint, batteries, waste incinerators	Brain and kidney toxicity

*Those that burn fossil fuels

Data from Environmental Protection Agency. Adverse health effects of particulate matter are discussed in other chapters

- Chronic respiratory disease (asthma and chronic obstructive lung disease)[5,6,9,10]
- Heart disease and stroke[11,12]
- Lung cancer[13]
- Dementia[14]
- Type 2 diabetes[15]
- Lower respiratory infections (LRI)[16]
- Tuberculosis[17]
- Preterm birth & low birth weight[18,19]

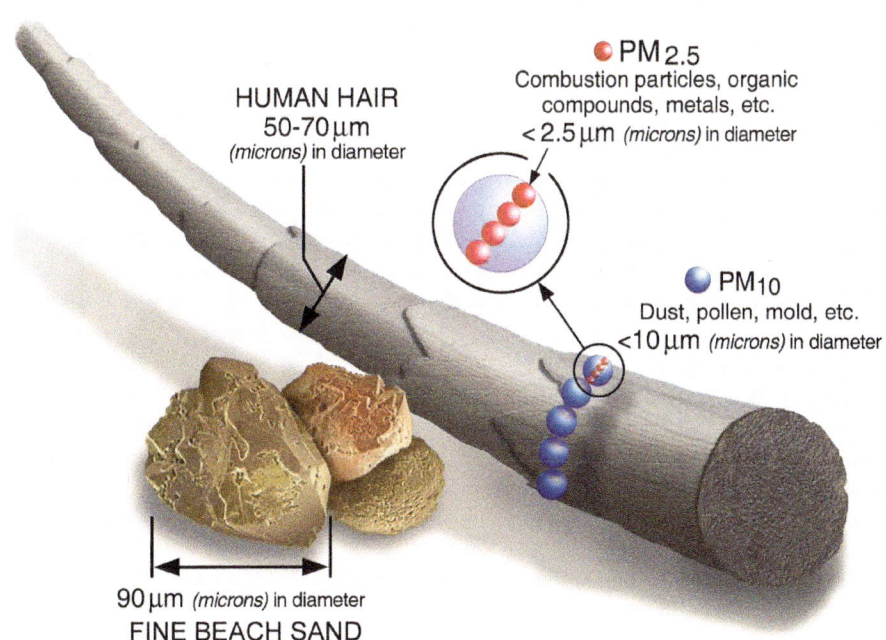

Figure 8.8 Size of Particulate Matter Compared to Human Hair and Grain of Sand.

Environmental Protection Agency. Particulate Matter (PM) Basics. Updated June 20, 2024. https://www.epa.gov/pm-pollution/particulate-matter-pm-basics

(continues)

Box 8.1 **Air Pollution** *(continued)*

Air pollution can be reduced by a combination of technological changes. Most air pollution is generated by burning some type of fuel. Switching to cleaner fuels can reduce the pollution that is emitted. For example, within households in low-income countries, substitution of biomass fuels with natural gas or liquefied petroleum gas (LPG) greatly reduces household $PM_{2.5}$ pollution.[20] Some countries have set up programs to substitute these cleaner fuels.[21]

Similarly, in buildings that burn oil for heat, switching from high-sulfur to low-sulfur fuel oils reduces sulfur dioxide emissions. Also, even if fuels are not changed, emissions of $PM_{2.5}$ from industrial plants can be reduced by various technologies, such as filters, scrubbers, and electrostatic precipitators.[22] Household air pollution can also be reduced by better-designed stoves and chimneys that direct smoke outdoors.[20] Finally, larger changes to how power is generated can virtually eliminate emissions. For example, using electricity for heating and cooking, and generating electricity by solar panels or wind turbines produces little air pollution. In any setting, then, there are steps that can be taken to reduce this health risk. These steps can be costly, though, so taking these steps often requires government programs, policies, and enforcement of these policies.

can certainly enter homes and contribute to asthma, but household sources contribute more. Levels of particulate matter ($PM_{2.5}$) are generally a little lower indoors than outdoors, but levels of these particles can be far higher indoors when people smoke, cook, or burn wood inside.[25] Also, levels of irritants can be higher indoors in housing that is crowded, deteriorated, or with malfunctioning appliances or systems for heating and ventilation.[26] And while levels of pollen are generally lower indoors than outdoors, levels of other asthma-triggering allergens, such as mold and those from house dust mites, cockroaches, and mice are likely to be much higher indoors.[27,28]

Epidemiology: Patterns and Trends

According to surveys of parents, about 6% of children in the United States have asthma.[29] The prevalence of asthma in children is shown in **Figure 8.9**. Rates are nearly twice as high in Black children as in White children. The reasons for this racial difference are not clear, but it may reflect a higher proportion living in deteriorated housing or exposure to environmental tobacco smoke.

About 9% of adults have asthma. Rates are higher in women than in men, and the condition is more strongly linked to poverty (**Figure 8.10**).[29]

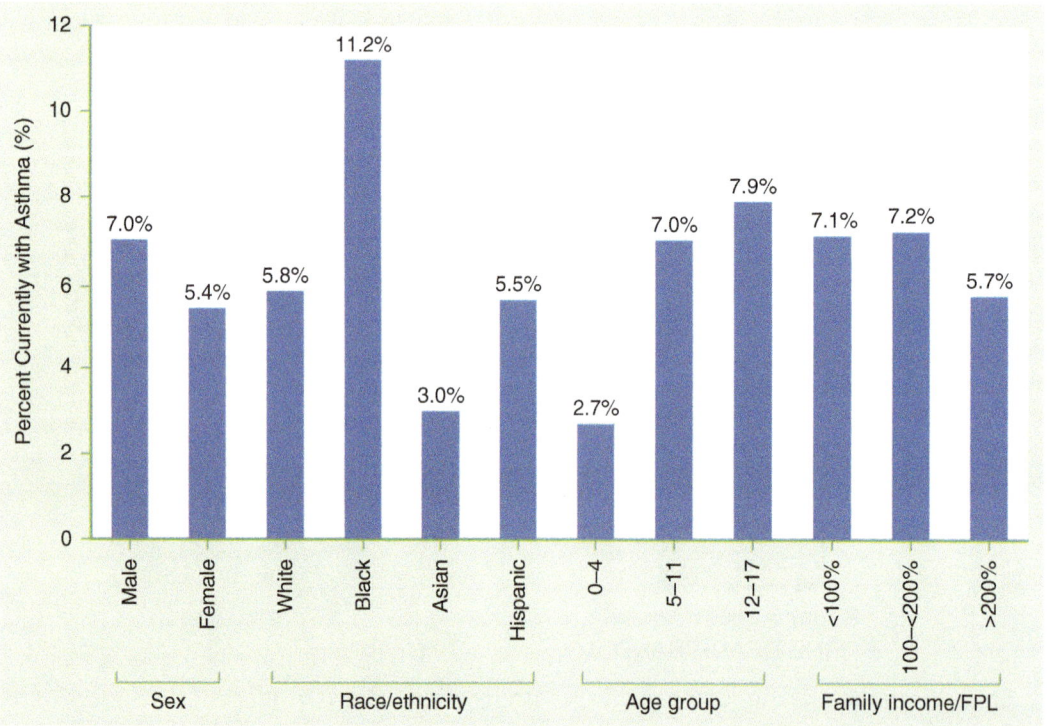

Figure 8.9 Prevalence of Asthma in Children in the United States, 2022.

Data from National Center for Health Statistics, Centers for Disease Control and Prevention. National Health Interview Survey: Summary Health Statistics. CDC.gov. Published September 21, 2023. Accessed June 25, 2024. https://www.cdc.gov/nchs/nhis/shs.htm

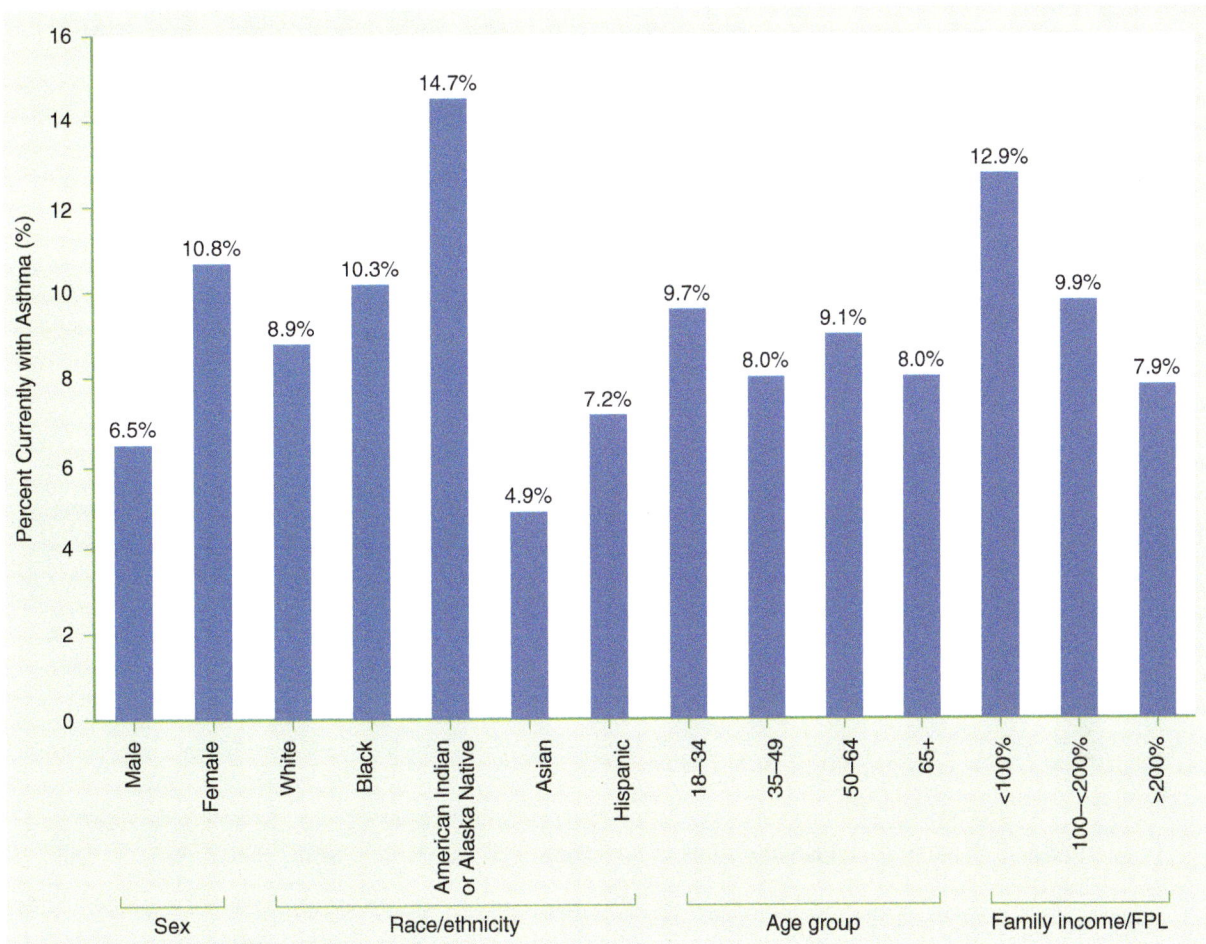

Figure 8.10 The Prevalence of Asthma in Adults in the United States, 2022.

Data from National Center for Health Statistics, Centers for Disease Control and Prevention. National Health Interview Survey: Summary Health Statistics. CDC.gov. Published September 21, 2023. Accessed June 25, 2024. https://www.cdc.gov/nchs/nhis/shs.htm

Asthma rates increased in the United States and Europe in the second half of the 20th century, and there have been increases in lower-income countries as they become more Westernized. This increase may be explained by the hygiene hypothesis as people in other countries move away from agriculture.[5]

In the United States, annual surveys by the National Center for Health Statistics—despite changes in how the questions were phrased—show big increases in asthma in children from the early 1980s until about 2010, followed by decreases into the 2020s (**Figure 8.11**). There is no proven explanation for either trend. We can only speculate that the increase in the late 20th century may relate to the hygiene hypothesis, and the decrease since 2010 might be caused by reductions in parents' smoking.[30,31]

Risk Factors

The key risk factors for asthma in children are (**Figure 8.12**):

- *Household allergens.* Children are much more likely to develop asthma if they are exposed during the first few years of life to house dust mites, cockroaches, mice, and mold/fungi.[5,6] The effect can last for many years. For example, children who are sensitized to dust mites at ages one and two are three to six times as likely to have asthma when they become teenagers.[5] Some, but not all, studies suggest that dog and cat dander also increase the risk of asthma.[5,6]

- *Environmental tobacco smoke.* In 1988-91, an astonishing 88% of nonsmokers in the United States were exposed to environmental tobacco smoke, also known as second-hand smoke.[31] That percentage has fallen dramatically since then. Still, in 2018, 25% of nonsmokers were exposed to second-hand smoke, making tobacco smoke a major source of asthma triggers today.[32] Environmental tobacco smoke also contributes to disparities in asthma, because children who are Black or from low-income families are 2–3 times

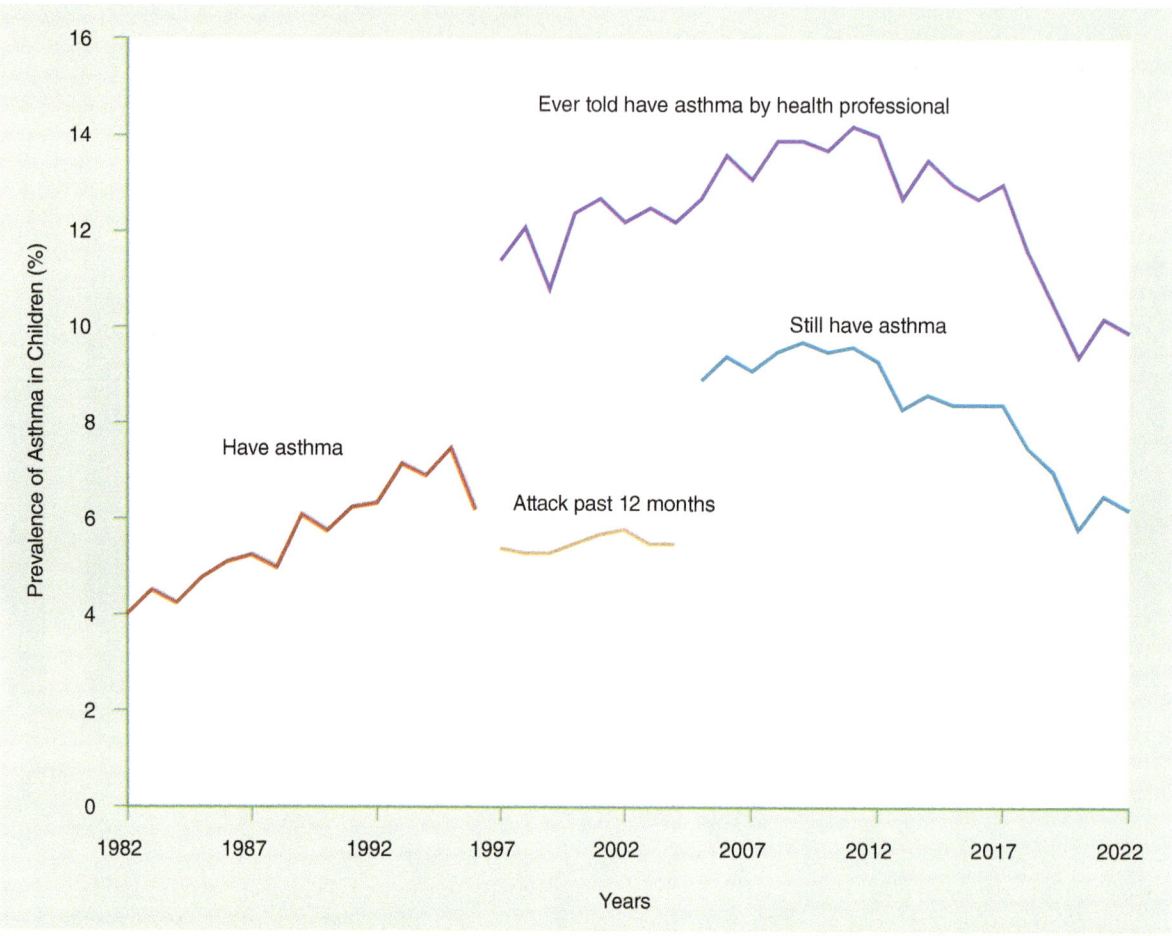

Figure 8.11 Trends in Asthma Among U.S. Children, 1982–2022.

Data from National Center for Health Statistics, Centers for Disease Control and Prevention. National Health Interview Survey: Summary Health Statistics. CDC.gov. Published September 21, 2023. Accessed June 25, 2024. https://www.cdc.gov/nchs/nhis/shs.htm

as likely to be exposed to second-hand smoke as other children.[33]

- *Other household air pollution.* Particles and gases that can trigger asthma can be produced by other household activities, including smoking other products like marijuana and burning candles and incense. Also, the use of biomass fuels in low-income countries creates very high levels of irritating particles and gases (Box 8.1).[9] Even in the United States, some people burn wood and coal for heat, and many use poorly functioning gas stoves and furnaces that emit air pollutants indoors.[9]

- *Deteriorated housing.* Housing that has deteriorated contributes to both household allergens and indoor air pollutants. In particular, leaky roofs or leaky plumbing can create high levels of moisture in homes; that moisture promotes the growth of mold/fungi, as well as pests. Moisture may by itself be a trigger for asthma.[6] Gaps in walls and floors allow pests to enter homes, and in multi-family buildings, they allow pests to move

between units. These gaps also allow pollutants to spread between units and allow outdoor pollutants to enter homes.

- *Ambient air pollution.* Some ambient (outdoor) air pollution enters homes even if the homes are modern and in good condition and can increase the risk of asthma.[5] A major source of these pollutants is exhaust from motor vehicles, and children living near major roadways are more likely to have asthma. By one estimate, 15% of asthma in European cities is attributable to traffic-related air pollution.[5,6]

- *Respiratory virus infections* increase the risk of asthma, particularly if children get the infections in their first year of life.[5,6]

- *Insufficient exposure to microbes in infancy.* If the hygiene hypothesis is correct, then infants raised in modern, "clean" environments face a greater risk of developing asthma. For example, in one study, children of the Hutterite religious group that live in modern, industrialized farms were about four times as likely to have asthma as

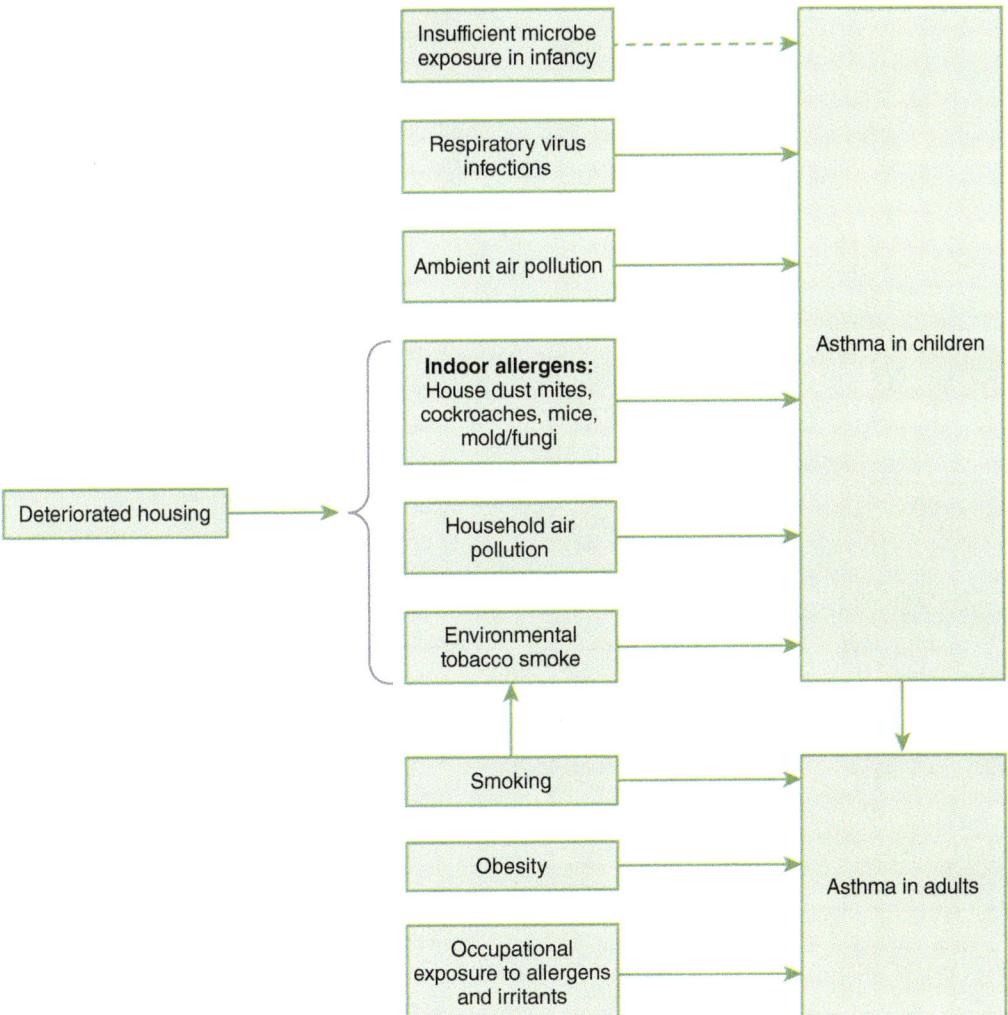

Figure 8.12 Cause-and-Effect Diagram for Asthma.

genetically-similar Amish children living on traditional, pre-industrial farms.[5,6] In theory, exposing infants to environments that contain microbes may prevent asthma. However, no one has turned that concept into a safe, proven, and practical preventive intervention.

Additional risk factors for asthma in adults are:

- *Smoking*, which gives a very heavy dose of irritants to the airways.
- *Obesity*. Adults are more than twice as likely to develop asthma if they are obese. The likely reason is that the body-wide inflammation seen in obesity also increases inflammation in the airways. This risk seems to affect women more than men.[5]
- *Occupational exposure*. Adults can be exposed to allergens or irritants as part of their jobs, and some of those who are exposed develop **occupational asthma**, also called **work-related asthma**. Hundreds of substances are known to cause

occupational asthma, including wheat flour, latex, wood dust, pesticides, solvents, and cleaning chemicals like bleach and ammonia.[5,34]

Preventive Interventions

Based on these risk factors, the prevalence of asthma or the frequency of asthma attacks can be reduced by (**Figure 8.13**):

- *Vaccination* against influenza and RSV.[4] Influenza vaccines do not eliminate the risk of influenza, but they do reduce it. Influenza vaccination must be repeated every year to keep up with the constantly-changing strains of the virus. While the influenza vaccine has been widely available for decades, it is under-used, especially in children. Vaccines against RSV are newly available. One vaccine, if given to women in the last few weeks of pregnancy, can prevent their infants from becoming infected. A different vaccine can

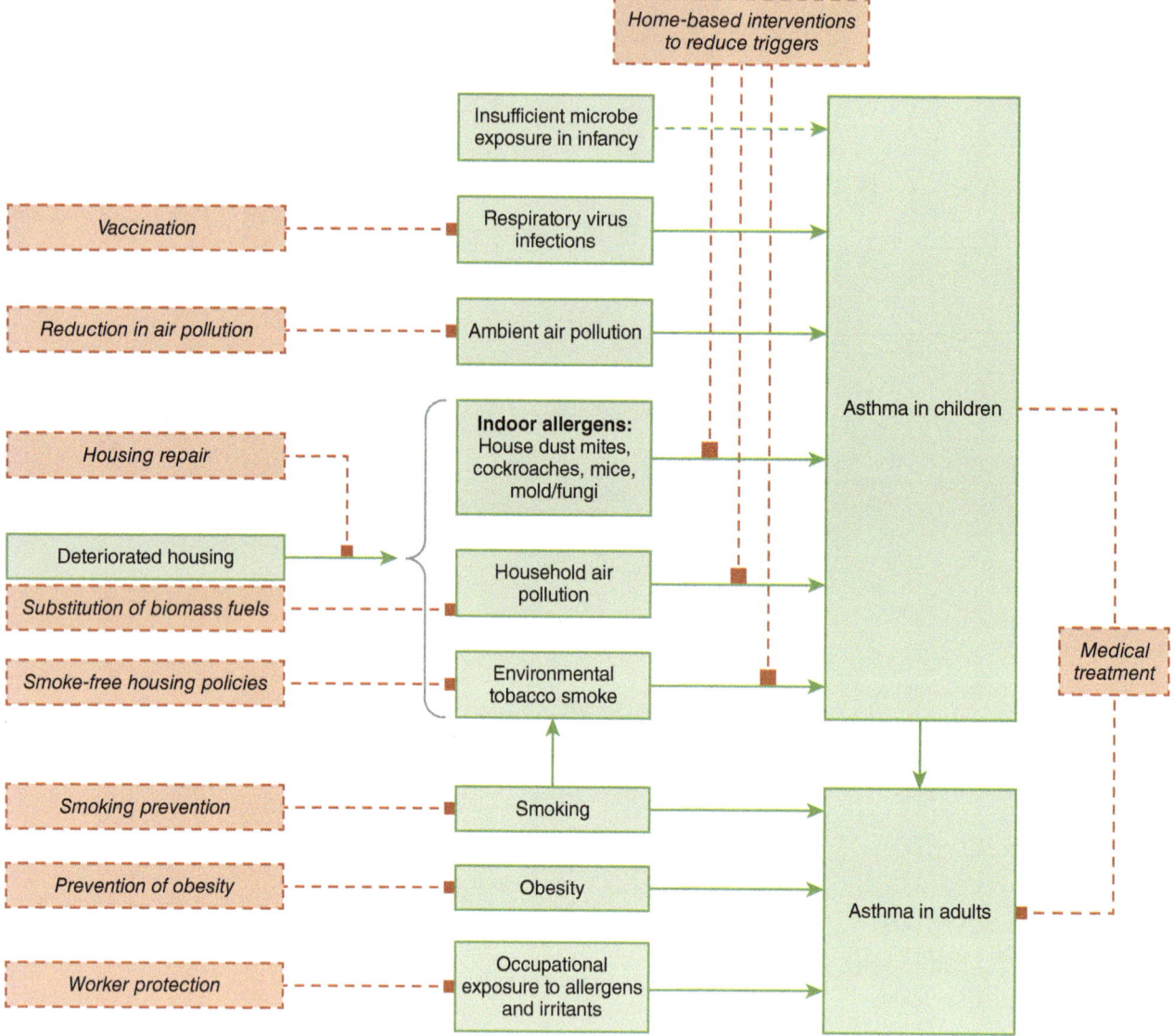

Figure 8.13 Cause-and-Effect Diagram for Asthma, with Preventive Interventions.

be given to very young infants to protect them for a single winter season. There are no available vaccines against rhinovirus.

- *Home-based interventions to reduce asthma triggers.* When families of children with asthma are educated about asthma risks and given help to reduce asthma triggers, the children have fewer and less severe asthma attacks.[35,36] These programs usually include:
  - Removing carpets and providing pillow and mattress covers to reduce exposure to house dust mites
  - Steps to reduce cockroaches and mice, such as providing sealed containers to store food and filling gaps in walls, which are often called **integrated pest management**
  - Fixing leaks to reduce moisture and mold/fungi
  - Education and help to quit smoking

  - Education to reduce other sources of household air pollution
  - Improvements in ventilation or filtration of indoor air[26,37]
- *Substitution of biomass fuels.* In low-income countries where biomass fuels are used, these fuels can be substituted with cleaner fuels like electricity, natural gas, and liquefied petroleum gas (LPG).[20]
- *Repair of deteriorated housing.*[38] Repairing housing conditions that contribute to asthma should reduce asthma exacerbations in children. Particularly important problems are roofs and plumbing that leak, gaps in walls and floors, and faulty heating, ventilation, and air conditioning systems. Families of children with asthma often cannot afford these repairs, so many communities have programs to help pay the cost. Also, when families rent their homes, it is landlords

who are in control of housing conditions, so public policies and programs for asthma-safe rental properties can help.

- *Smoking prevention.*[38] Preventing or reducing smoking has two benefits in reducing asthma—to people who smoke and to those around them. See Chapter 11 Tobacco Use.

- *Smoke-free housing policies.*[38] Policies that prohibit household smoking in multi-unit housing should reduce rates of asthma in residents.

- *Prevention of obesity.* See Chapter 7. Chronic Metabolic Diseases and Chapter 14. Dietary Risks.

- *Reduction of ambient air pollution.* Reductions in outdoor air pollution should reduce asthma exacerbations. Some (but not all) studies done where ambient air pollution has been reduced have found reductions in emergency department visits for asthma attacks.[39] Some public health officials in recent years have focused on replacing school buses that have highly-polluting diesel engines with those that emit less pollutants;[38] this is important because schoolchildren can be heavily exposed to emissions from these buses.

- *Worker protection.* Employers can prevent and reduce work-related asthma by reducing workers' exposure to allergens and irritants. The National Institute of Occupational Safety and Health has made recommendations on how to do this, and it emphasizes a "hierarchy of controls." In this hierarchy, the best action employers can take is to eliminate the hazardous substance, followed by engineering controls that prevent workers from breathing it in, followed by personal protective equipment such as masks.[40]

- *Medical treatment.* There is no cure for asthma, but medications can make asthma attacks less frequent and less severe. The medicine used the most are: 1) inhaled **corticosteroids**, which reduce inflammation in the airways and must be taken daily to prevent attacks, and 2) inhaled bronchodilators. The bronchodilators cause the smooth muscle cells in the bronchioles to relax, expanding the small airways. They should be taken only in response to asthma attacks. People with asthma tend to rely too much on bronchodilators, which can be dangerous. Overuse of these drugs has been linked to higher mortality rates from asthma. Much of the medical management of asthma involves helping people use the inhaled corticosteroids consistently so that they do not have asthma attacks.[41] To help children with asthma take these medicines, doctors and public health agencies use **Asthma Action Plans** that list which drugs are to be taken when and that authorize children to take their medications while at school.

Box 8.2 Summary–Prevention of Asthma

- Vaccination
- Home-based interventions to reduce asthma triggers
- Substitution of biomass fuels
- Repair of deteriorated housing
- Smoking prevention
- Smoke-free housing policies
- Prevention of obesity
- Reduction of outdoor air pollution
- Worker protection
- Medical treatment

Chronic Obstructive Pulmonary Disease

Introduction

Chronic obstructive pulmonary disease (COPD) is a leading killer and a major cause of disability in the United States and worldwide.[42] People with COPD have a persistent cough and difficulty breathing. Although COPD is related to asthma, it is almost exclusively a disease of adults and is far more deadly. Smoking is the dominant cause of COPD, but household and ambient (outdoor) air pollution also contribute, and exposures during early childhood can affect the development of COPD in the adult years.[3]

Pathophysiology of Chronic Obstructive Pulmonary Disease

COPD is mostly the result of damage to the lungs from years of inhaling fine particles (known as particulate matter—or $PM_{2.5}$ or PM_{10}, depending on their size) and irritating gases. These irritants flow into the bronchioles and alveoli and then damage the cells lining them. The lung responds to this damage with inflammation—that is, a migration of immune cells to the area, responding to what they perceive might be an infection. These immune cells are programmed to contain an infection by killing foreign cells and disposing of unrecognized substances. One unfortunate side effect of this response is that they produce additional damage to the lungs' own cells. The damage to lung tissues leads to two problems:

- *Narrowing of airways and secretion of extra mucus* (**Figure 8.14**). The inflammation causes the walls of the airways to swell and the smooth muscle cells wrapping around the airways to enlarge.[3] This swelling can only be accommodated by making

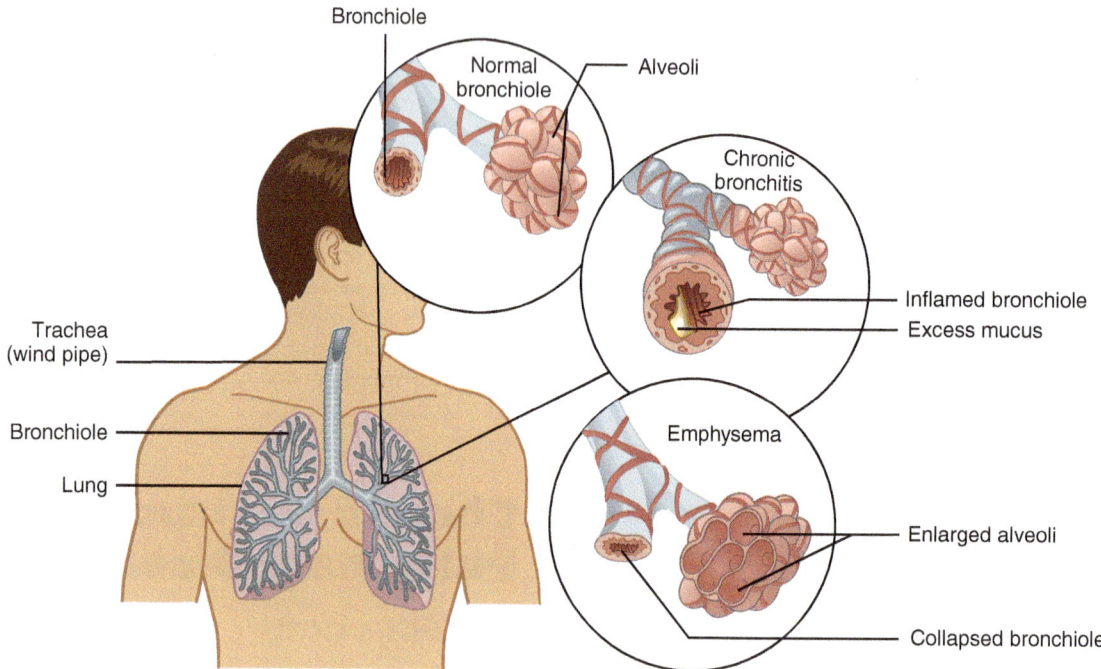

Figure 8.14 Damage to Lung in Chronic Obstructive Pulmonary Disease. Chronic obstructive pulmonary disease causes two types of damage to the lungs: 1) narrowing of airways and secretion of mucus, called chronic bronchitis, and 2) loss of tissue separating alveoli, called emphysema.

the internal channels of the airways narrower. At the same time, the inflamed airways secrete more mucus than normal. With narrower airways filled with mucus, it is difficult for the air to move through the airways, especially during expiration. When this condition is persistent, it is called **chronic bronchitis**.[3] This feature of COPD overlaps with the inflammation that occurs in asthma.

- *Loss of tissue separating the alveoli.* The tissue lining the alveoli is extremely thin and delicate—only about one cell thick—so it is easily destroyed. When a layer of tissue separating two alveoli is destroyed, the two coalesce into one larger alveolus, with less surface area than the two previously had. If this destructive process continues over years, the lungs have far fewer alveoli, each of which is much larger, like a sponge gradually transforming into a pack of balloons (**Figures 8.14–8.15**). With this change, the lungs have a much smaller total surface area for exchange of oxygen and carbon dioxide. This condition is called **emphysema**.[3]

COPD is usually a combination of chronic bronchitis and emphysema, although in some people one or the other problem predominates. With these two problems, people with COPD typically have a constant cough and feel short of breath, at first only when they exercise but later even at rest. The lungs cannot fully repair the damage from COPD, so after a certain point the symptoms become permanent.[43]

This damage also leaves the lungs less able to fight off infections. People with COPD occasionally have days or weeks when their symptoms get worse. Most of these exacerbations are thought to be caused by infections with bacteria or viruses.[43] The COVID-19 pandemic highlighted this problem: In the early waves, people with COPD were about twice as likely as people with healthy lungs to die from a COVID-19 infection.[44]

There is no cure for COPD, but medical treatment can help somewhat. Most important: if people with COPD quit smoking, the deterioration of their lung capacity slows markedly.[45] Antibiotics (bacteria-killing drugs) can help cure some infections. Bronchodilators can cause the smooth muscle cells in the walls of the bronchioles to relax somewhat, allowing for more air flow. Inhaled corticosteroids can reduce the inflammation. And breathing in extra oxygen can raise oxygen levels in blood.[3,43]

Pulmonary Function Tests in COPD

The spirometry tests in people with COPD, like those of people with asthma, show signs of narrowed airways, with a low FEV_1 and a low FEV_1/FVC ratio (see Figure 8.4 earlier in this chapter). However, unlike people with asthma, people with COPD do not show much improvement in their FEV_1/FVC ratio after taking bronchodilators. And if people with COPD have emphysema, their FVC may also be lower than normal.[3]

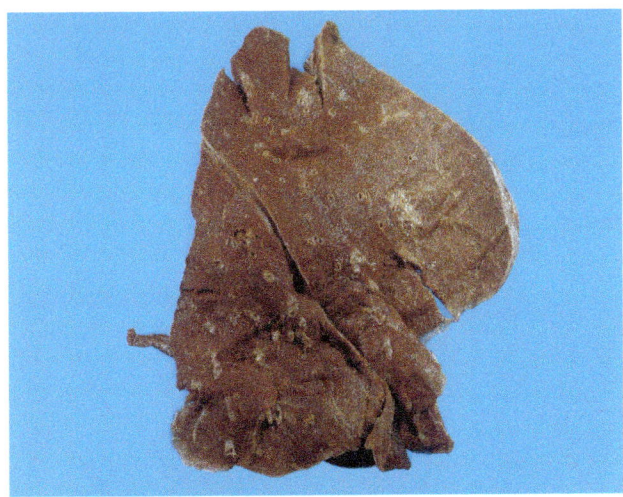

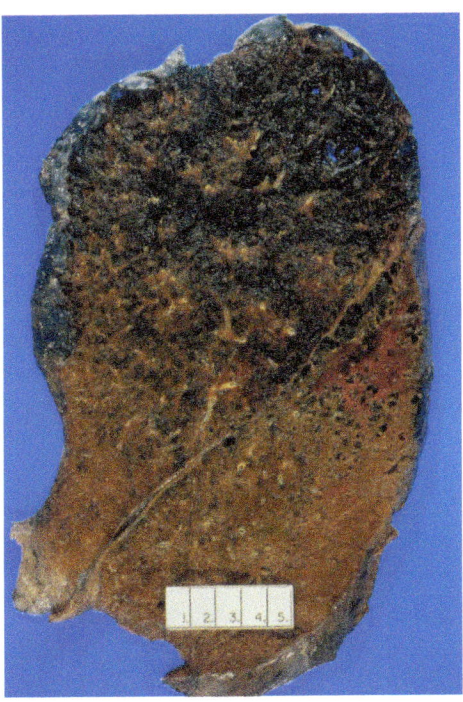

Figure 8.15 Normal Lung and Lung from a Smoker with Emphysema.
© Arthur Glauberman/Science Source; © Dr. E. Walker/Science Source

Experts use the FEV_1/FVC ratio to measure the prevalence of COPD in populations. To do that, some experts define COPD simply as an FEV_1/FVC ratio below 0.70, and others use a more tailored definition of FEV_1/FVC below the fifth percentile for healthy persons, adjusted for age, sex, and body size.[1,46]

Some people have much more severe COPD than others, with greater difficulty breathing after light physical activity or even at rest. The severity of COPD can be measured by how low the FEV_1 is. For example, one expert group labels COPD as "mild" if the FEV_1 is above 80% of average for a person's age, sex, and body size, "moderate" if the FEV_1 is between 50% and 80%, and "severe" if the FEV_1 is below 50%.[47]

Life Course of COPD

For many years, experts on COPD focused their attention almost solely on smoking and on adults. But in recent years they have begun to view COPD as a disease that begins in early childhood.

When a fetus is growing in the womb, the lungs are among the last organs to mature. At 36 weeks of gestation, the fetus is just developing alveoli, which is why the biggest problem of premature babies is low levels of oxygen in the blood.[48] After birth, the lungs continue to grow and develop new alveoli throughout childhood. The lungs' capabilities peak in people 20–25 years of age, after which the spirometry test results like FEV_1 gradually fall (**Figure 8.16**).[47,49-51] Smoking or other exposures in the adult years cause the lungs to deteriorate more quickly, leading to COPD.

But a second route to COPD, according to current thinking, is any exposure in childhood that interferes with the normal development of the lungs. This exposure reduces the lungs' peak capacity in the young adult years (shown in the red line in Figure 8.16), leaving them without enough reserve capacity later in life.[48] Or to put it another way, exposures that harm the lungs of infants and children have an outsized but delayed impact on their lifelong lung health. Those exposures could be environmental tobacco smoke or allergens in a child's home, outdoor air pollution, or viral infections of the lung.[10,43,47] They may even begin before a child is born, because several studies have found that adults who were born prematurely or with low birth weight are more likely to develop COPD.[52]

Epidemiology: Patterns and Trends

In the United States, about 6% of adults report on surveys that they have physician-diagnosed COPD. The prevalence rises sharply as people age, is higher in women than in men, and is especially high in American Indians/Alaska Natives (**Figure 8.17**).[53] COPD is also more common in people who have less income or education, probably tracking smoking rates.[53]

Most people with COPD do not die directly from the disease, but they have difficulty staying active, and they are more likely to get other health problems like infections. COPD itself kills about 150,000 Americans per year, a rate that surprisingly has not fallen in the past 20 years, even as smoking rates have dropped. Those who die from COPD are typically older adults; 85% of deaths occur in people over age 65.[54]

Globally, COPD is the third leading cause of death, after cardiovascular disease and cancer.[55] About

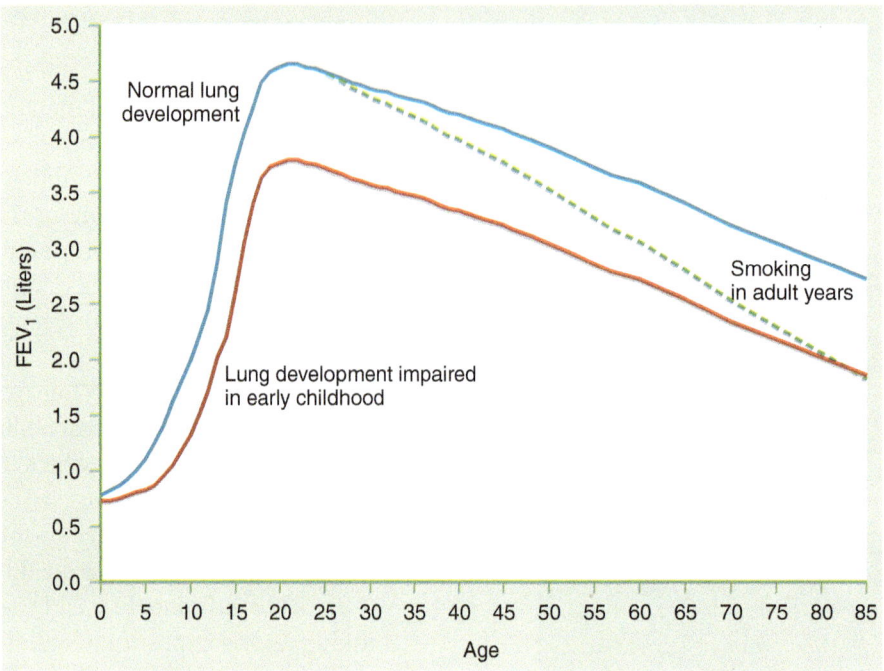

Figure 8.16 Theoretical Trajectories of Lung Function Across the Life Span. Lung capacity (measured by FEV, or FVC) increases throughout childhood, peaks in the young adult years, and then gradually falls in the adult years. Damaging exposures like smoking (dotted line) accelerate this fall in lung capacity. According to current thinking, any impairment of lung development prenatally or in childhood (shown in the red line) reduces the peak lung capacity, leaving less reserve capacity and causing chronic respiratory diseases in later adult years.

Data from Stanojevic S, Kaminsky DA, Miller MR, et al. ERS/ATS technical standard on interpretive strategies for routine lung function tests. Eur Respir J 2022; 60: 2101499. DOI: 10.1183/13993003.01499-2021

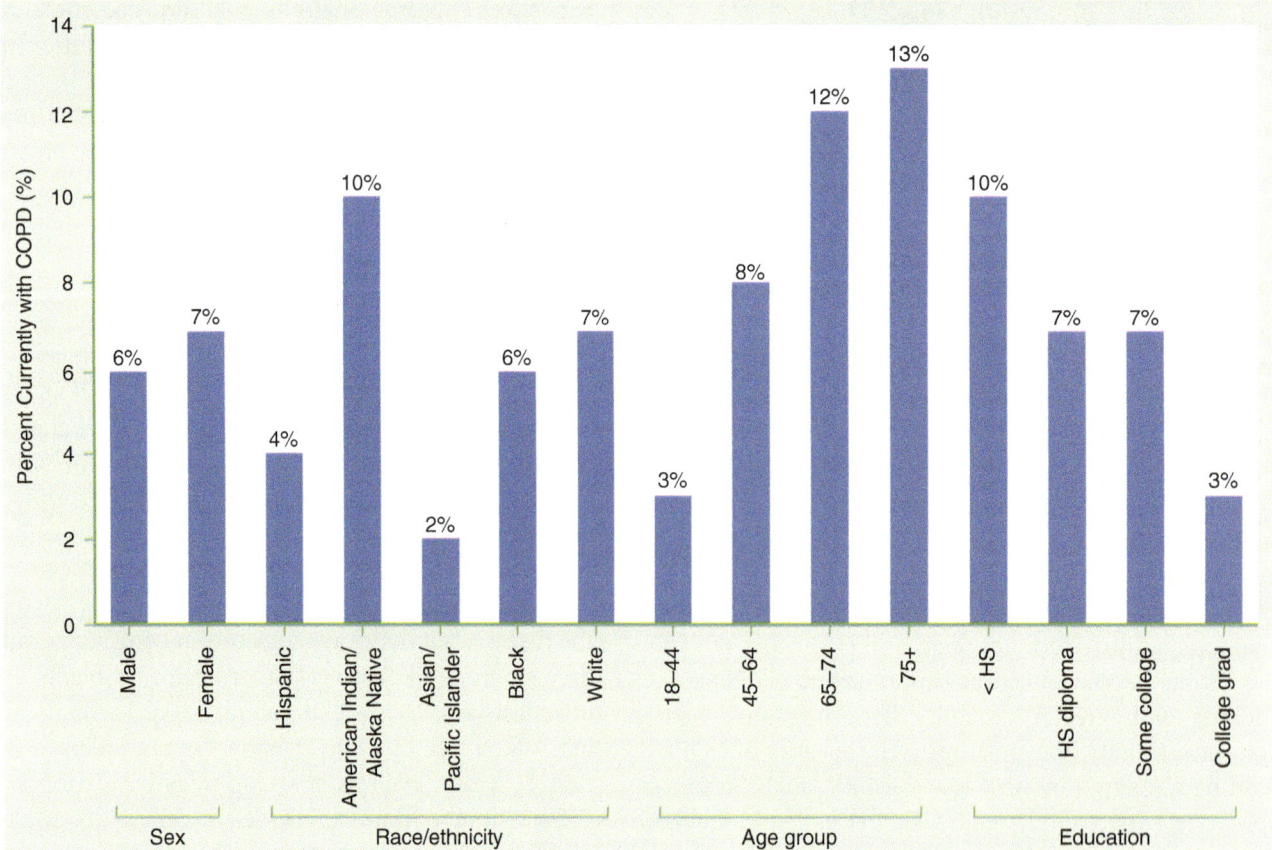

Figure 8.17 The Prevalence of Chronic Obstructive Pulmonary Disease (by Self-Report) in U.S. adults, 2021.

Data from Liu Y, Carlson SA, Watson KB, Xu F, Greenlund KJ. Trends in the Prevalence of Chronic Obstructive Pulmonary Disease Among Adults Aged ≥18 Years — United States, 2011–2021. MMWR Morb Mortal Wkly Rep. 2023;72(46):1250-1256. doi:10.15585/mmwr.mm7246a1

7%–10% of all adults have the disease (depending on the definition used), as do more than 25% of those older than 75 years. COPD is most common in areas of the world with high rates of both smoking and air pollution, including China and India.[46]

Risk Factors

Risk factors that are present before birth, during childhood, or in the adult years can lead to COPD (**Figure 8.18**).[55] All of these risk factors involve substances that are inhaled into the lungs:

- *Smoking.* The connection between smoking and COPD is extremely strong. For example, in surveys in the United States, 16.2% of people who smoke, 7.7% of people who formerly smoked, and 2.8% of adults who never smoked have physician-diagnosed COPD.[53] Only 25% of people with COPD in the United States do *not* smoke.[53] And people who smoke with COPD tend to have more severe symptoms than nonsmokers with COPD.[10] The relationship with smoking is less strong in other countries where people who do not smoke are exposed to more air pollution. Still, the Global Burden of Disease researchers estimate that about half of COPD globally is attributable to smoking (**Table 8.3**).[10,56]

- *Environmental tobacco smoke.* People who do not smoke but who regularly breathe in tobacco smoke in the environment are also at increased risk of COPD.[10,43] This risk is especially important in childhood, perhaps because it interferes with normal lung development.

- *Household air pollution.* Irritating particles and gases are produced not just by burning tobacco but also by burning biomass fuels (refer to Box 8.1 earlier in this chapter). This harms the lungs of both adults and young children,[9] and it is common. For example, in sub-Saharan Africa, more than 90% of rural households depend on biomass fuel for cooking.[46] That makes household air pollution a major risk factor for COPD in low-income countries and even on a global scale (Table 8.3).[10,20,43,46]

- *Ambient air pollution.* Outdoor (ambient) air pollution is thought to be the leading contributor to COPD after smoking, in the United States and globally (Table 8.3).[10,43,55,57] Most air pollution ultimately originates from burning something, like coal in a power plant or diesel fuel in a vehicle (refer to Box 8.1 earlier in this chapter for more on air pollution). The pollutants that irritate the lungs and increase the risk of COPD include particulate matter ($PM_{2.5}$ and PM_{10}), nitrogen dioxide,

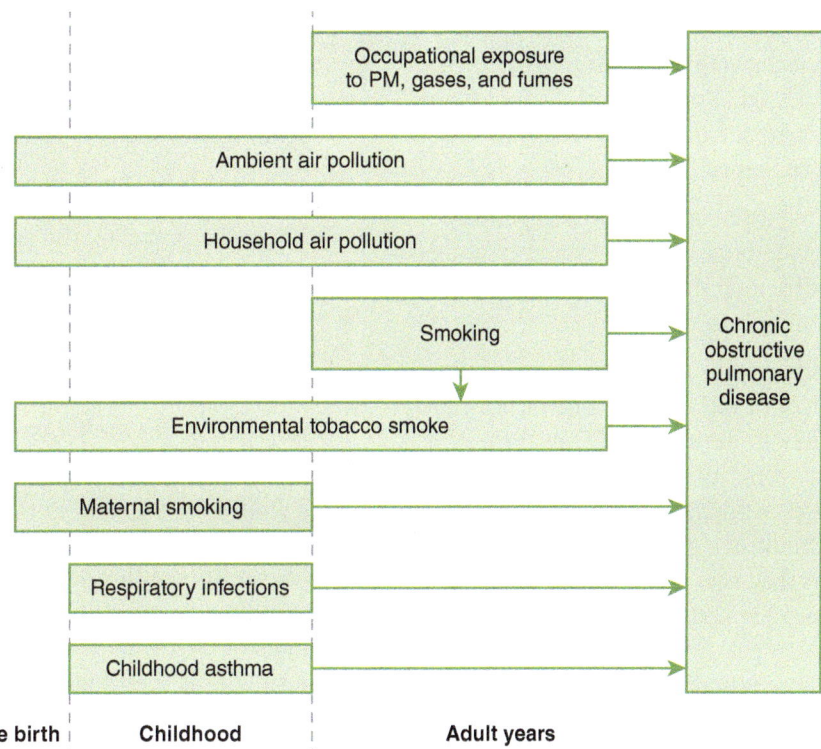

Figure 8.18 Cause-and-Effect Diagram for Chronic Obstructive Pulmonary Disease. Risk factors that are present before birth, during childhood, or in the adult years can ultimately lead to COPD.

Table 8.3 Attributable Risk for Chronic Obstructive Pulmonary Disease in the United States and Globally, 2019

Exposure	Attributable Risk	
	Global	US
Smoking	48%	56%
Air pollution (ambient and household)	40%	10%
Ambient particulate matter pollution	21%	4%
Ambient ozone pollution	11%	7%
Household air pollution from solid fuels	12%	0%
Occupational particulate matter, gases and fumes	16%	9%
Secondhand smoke	9%	4%

Data from Global Burden of Disease Collaboration, Institute for Health Metrics and Evaluation. GBD Results Tool. Published July 12, 2023. Accessed July 11, 2023. https://vizhub.healthdata.org/gbd-results/

sulfur dioxide, and ozone.[47] Levels of these pollutants are high enough in the United States to cause significant damage, but they are far higher and contribute far more to COPD in some other countries, particularly China, India, and countries in the Middle East and North Africa.[58]

- *Occupational exposure to particulate matter and gases.*[10,43,46] Machines and industrial processes produce particles and gases that can harm workers' lungs. For example, construction workers breathe in dust, transportation workers breathe in vehicle exhaust, and bartenders breathe in environmental tobacco smoke. One researcher estimated that 19% of cases of COPD overall and 31% of cases in non-smokers are attributable to these kinds of occupational exposures.[59]

The risk factors listed above impact people in their adult years or lifelong. But risk factors in childhood have also been linked to the development of COPD in adults many years later:

- *Maternal smoking.* People whose mothers smoked during pregnancy or around the time of birth are much more likely to develop COPD in their adult years.[50,51,60,61] It seems that having a mother who smokes interferes with the normal growth of the lungs during childhood, giving people less reserve capacity later as they age. It is not clear if the damage to their lungs happens during pregnancy, after birth, or both.
- *Severe childhood respiratory infections.* Adults who had severe infections in the lungs as children are more likely to develop COPD, probably because those infections interfere with the normal growth of the lungs.[10,46] Many severe infections can cause

this problem, but tuberculosis has been found in particular to predispose to COPD.[43,47] It is too early to know if children who had COVID-19 will be at risk for COPD when they become adults, but it is certainly possible.

- *Asthma in childhood.*[43,46] As the previous section pointed out, some children "grow out" of asthma. but others continue to have asthma in their adult years. And children who have asthma appear to be at greater risk of developing COPD as adults, either because the same exposures leading to asthma are causing COPD or because the inflammation present in asthma in children interferes with the lungs' growth.[46]

Preventive Interventions

COPD can be prevented by addressing these risk factors for adults (**Figure 8.19**):

- *Smoking prevention.* Preventing smoking or helping people quit smoking has the greatest potential to prevent COPD. It would address the risk factor responsible for most cases. Also, it would reduce the other risk factors of exposure to second-hand smoke and the effects of maternal smoking on their children's risk. See Chapter 11 Tobacco Use.
- *Smoke-free housing policies.*[38] Policies that prohibit smoking in multi-unit housing should reduce rates of COPD in adult residents, as well as child residents as they age.
- *Reduction in ambient air pollution.* Reducing ambient air pollution is particularly important because it affects everyone. See Box 8.1 for more on reduction of air pollution.

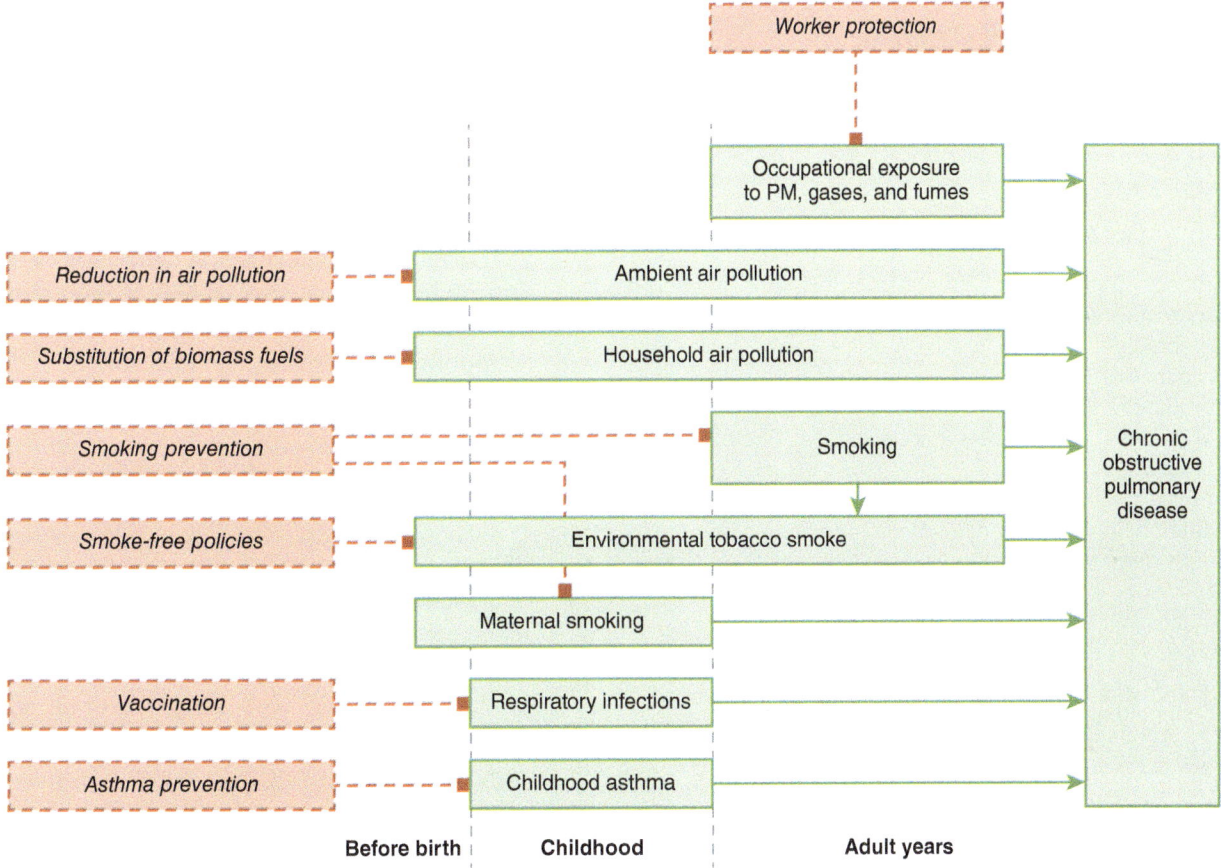

Figure 8.19 Cause-and-Effect Diagram for Chronic Obstructive Pulmonary Disease, with Preventive Interventions.

- *Substitution of biomass fuels.* The best way to reduce exposure to household air pollution from these fuels in low-income countries is to give people inexpensive access to cleaner fuels like electricity, natural gas, and liquefied petroleum gas (LPG).[20]
- *Worker protection.* Employers can take steps to protect workers from particulate matter and gases that can irritate the lungs, regardless of whether workers have symptoms. And, as with the prevention of occupational asthma, employers should follow the National Institute of Occupational Safety and Health "hierarchy of controls" recommendations, which set a priority on preventing workers from being exposed at all.[40]

Preventive interventions to protect children from damage that can interfere with lung development include:

- *Vaccination* against respiratory viruses, including influenza, RSV, and COVID-19.
- *Childhood asthma prevention.* The interventions listed in the previous section to reduce rates of childhood asthma should also reduce these children's risk of developing COPD as adults.

Box 8.3 Summary–Prevention of Chronic Obstructive Pulmonary Disease

- Smoking prevention
- Smoke-free housing policies
- Reduction in ambient air pollution
- Substitution of biomass fuels
- Worker protection
- Vaccination against respiratory viruses
- Childhood asthma prevention

Box 8.4 Key Words–Chronic Respiratory Diseases

Air pollution
Allergen
Allergic
Allergy
Alveoli (of the lung)
Ambient air pollution
Anthropogenic
Antibiotics

(continues)

Antibodies
Asthma
Asthma Action Plan
Asthma attack
Biomass
Bronchi
Bronchial tree
Bronchioles
Bronchodilators
Chronic bronchitis
Chronic obstructive pulmonary disease (COPD)
Corticosteroids
Criteria air pollutants
Dilate
Emphysema
Expiration
Forced expiratory volume 1 (FEV_1)
Forced vital capacity (FVC)
Gas exchange
Household air pollution
Hygiene hypothesis
IgE
Immunoglobulins
Inflammation
Influenza virus
Inspiration
Integrated pest management
Irritant
Microbes
Non-point sources (of air pollution)
Occupational asthma
Particulate matter
Point sources (of air pollution)
PM_{10}, $PM_{2.5}$
Pulmonary function test
Respiratory syncytial virus (RSV)
Rhinovirus
Sensitized
Smooth muscle cells
Spirometry
Trachea
Wheeze
Work-related asthma

Resources

Chronic Respiratory Diseases

- Soriano JB, Kendrick PJ, Paulson KR, et al. Prevalence and attributable health burden of chronic respiratory diseases, 1990–2017: A systematic analysis for the Global Burden of Disease Study 2017. *Lancet Respir Med.* 2020;8(6):585-596. doi:10.1016/S2213-2600(20)30105-3
- To address the problem of household air pollution in developing countries, the World Health Organization has developed science-based *Guidelines for household air quality: Household fuel combustion* (available at https://www.who.int/publications/i/item/9789241548885) and a *Clean Household Energy Solutions Toolkit (CHEST)* for public health planning (available at https://www.who.int/tools/clean-household-energy-solutions-toolkit).
- Resources for tobacco control are listed at the end of Chapter 11. Tobacco Use.

Asthma

- Hsu J, Sircar K, Herman E, Garbe P. EXHALE: A Technical Package to Control Asthma. Centers for Disease Control and Prevention. Atlanta; 2018. Available at: https://www.cdc.gov/asthma/exhale/index.htm. This is a guide from the CDC on a population-based strategy to prevent asthma and reduce asthma exacerbations.
- Kuruvilla ME, Vanijcharoenkarn K, Shih JA, Lee FEH. Epidemiology and risk factors for asthma. *Respir Med.* 2019;149:16-2. doi:10.1016/j.rmed.2019.01.014
- Murrison LB, Brandt EB, Myers JB, Khurana Hershey GK. Environmental exposures and mechanisms in allergy and asthma development. *J Clin Invest.* 2019;129(4):1504-1515. doi:10.1172/JCI124612

Chronic Obstructive Pulmonary Disease

- Christenson SA, Smith BM, Bafadhel M, Putcha N. Chronic obstructive pulmonary disease. *Lancet.* 2022;399(10342):2227-2242. doi:10.1016/S0140-6736(22)00470-6
- Liu Y, Carlson SA, Watson KB, Xu F, Greenlund KJ. Trends in the Prevalence of Chronic Obstructive Pulmonary Disease Among Adults Aged ≥18 Years—United States, 2011–2021. *MMWR Morb Mortal Wkly Rep.* 2023;72(46):1250-1256. doi:10.15585/mmwr.mm7246a1
- Yang IA, Jenkins CR, Salvi SS. Chronic obstructive pulmonary disease in never-smokers: risk factors, pathogenesis, and implications for prevention and treatment. *Lancet Respir Med.* 2022;10(5):497-511. doi:10.1016/S2213-2600(21)00506-3

References

1. Stanojevic S, Kaminsky DA, Miller MR, et al. ERS/ATS technical standard on interpretive strategies for routine lung function tests. *Eur Respir J*. 2022;60(1). doi:10.1183/13993003.01499-2021

2. Savenije OEM, Kerkhof M, Koppelman GH, Postma DS. Predicting who will have asthma at school age among preschool children. *J Allergy and Clin Immunol*. 2012;130(2):325-331. doi:10.1016/j.jaci.2012.05.007

3. Husain AN. Obstructive lung diseases. In: Kumar V, Abbas AK, Aster JC, Turner JR, eds. *Robbins & Cotran Pathologic Basis of Disease*. 10th ed. Elsevier ; 2021:678-687.

4. Patel SJ, Teach SJ. Asthma. *Pediatr Rev*. 2019;40(11):549-567.

5. Kuruvilla ME, Vanijcharoenkarn K, Shih JA, Lee FEH. Epidemiology and risk factors for asthma. *Respir Med*. 2019;149:16-22. doi:10.1016/j.rmed.2019.01.014

6. Murrison LB, Brandt EB, Myers JB, Khurana Hershey GK. Environmental exposures and mechanisms in allergy and asthma development. *J Clin Invest*. 2019;129(4):1504-1515. doi:10.1172/JCI124612

7. National Institute of Environmental Health Sciences. Dust mites and cockroaches. *National Institute of Environmental Health Sciences, NIH*. Published August 29, 2022. Accessed July 28, 2024. Available at: https://www.niehs.nih.gov/health/topics/agents/allergens/dustmites

8. Environmental Protection Agency. Indoor pollutants and sources. Published August 20, 2024. Accessed November 25, 2024. Available at: https://www.epa.gov/indoor-air-quality-iaq/indoor-pollutants-and-sources

9. Raju S, Siddharthan T, McCormack MC. Indoor air pollution and respiratory health. *Clin Chest Med*. 2020;41(4):825-843. doi:10.1016/j.ccm.2020.08.014

10. Yang IA, Jenkins CR, Salvi SS. Chronic obstructive pulmonary disease in never-smokers: Risk factors, pathogenesis, and implications for prevention and treatment. *Lancet Respir Med*. 2022;10(5):497-511. doi:10.1016/S2213-2600(21)00506-3

11. Lechner K, von Schacky C, McKenzie AL, et al. Lifestyle factors and high-risk atherosclerosis: Pathways and mechanisms beyond traditional risk factors. *Eur J Prev Cardiol*. 2020;27(4):394-406. doi:10.1177/2047487319869400

12. Münzel T, Miller MR, Sørensen M, Lelieveld J, Daiber A, Rajagopalan S. Reduction of environmental pollutants for prevention of cardiovascular disease: It's time to act. *Eur Heart J*. 2020;41(41). doi:10.1093/eurheartj/ehaa745

13. Bade BC, Dela Cruz CS. Lung Cancer 2020: Epidemiology, etiology, and prevention. *Clin Chest Med*. 2020;41(1):1-24. doi:10.1016/j.ccm.2019.10.001

14. Livingston G, Huntley J, Sommerlad A, et al. Dementia prevention, intervention, and care: 2020 report of the Lancet Commission. *Lancet*. 2020;396(10248):413-446. doi:10.1016/S0140-6736(20)30367-6

15. Burkart K, Causey K, Cohen AJ, et al. Estimates, trends, and drivers of the global burden of type 2 diabetes attributable to PM2.5 air pollution, 1990–2019: An analysis of data from the Global Burden of Disease Study 2019. *Lancet Planet Health*. 2022;6(7):e586-e600. doi:10.1016/S2542-5196(22)00122-X

16. Kyu HH, Vongpradith A, Sirota SB, et al. Age—sex differences in the global burden of lower respiratory infections and risk factors, 1990–2019: Results from the Global Burden of Disease Study 2019. *Lancet Infect Dis*. 2022;22(11):1626-1647. doi:10.1016/S1473-3099(22)00510-2

17. Kurmi OP, Sadhra CS, Ayres JG, Sadhra SS. Tuberculosis risk from exposure to solid fuel smoke: A systematic review and meta-analysis. *J Epidemiol Community Health (1978)*. 2014;68(12):1112-1118. doi:10.1136/jech-2014-204120

18. Younger A, Alkon A, Harknett K, Jean Louis R, Thompson LM. Adverse birth outcomes associated with household air pollution from unclean cooking fuels in low-and middle-income countries: A systematic review. *Environ Res*. 2022;204:112274. doi:10.1016/j.envres.2021.112274

19. Bekkar B, Pacheco S, Basu R, Basu R, Denicola N. Association of air pollution and heat exposure with preterm birth, low birth weight, and stillbirth in the US: A systematic review. *JAMA Netw Open*. 2020;3(6). doi:10.1001/jamanetworkopen.2020.8243

20. Gordon SB, Bruce NG, Grigg J, et al. Respiratory risks from household air pollution in low-and middle-income countries. *Lancet Respir Med*. 2014;2(10):823-860. doi:10.1016/S2213-2600(14)70168-7

21. United Nations. *Sustainable Development Goals*. UN.Org. Published 2024. Accessed March 27, 2024. Available at: https://sdgs.un.org/goals/goal7#targets_and_indicators

22. Friis RH. Air quality. In: *Essentials of Environmental Health*. 3rd ed. Burlington, MA: Jones & Bartlett Learning; 2019:241-271.

23. Akinbami LJ, Kit BK, Simon AE. Impact of environmental tobacco smoke on children with asthma. *Acad Pediatr*. 2013;13:508-516.

24. Klepeis NE, Nelson WC, Ott WR, et al. The National Human Activity Pattern Survey (NHAPS): A resource for assessing exposure to environmental pollutants. *J Exp Anal Env Epidemiol*. 2001;11:231-252. Accessed March 19, 2025. Available at: https://www.nature.com/jea

25. O'Dell K, Ford B, Burkhardt J, et al. Outside in: The relationship between indoor and outdoor particulate air quality during wildfire smoke events in western US cities. *Environ Res Health*. 2023;1(1):015003. doi:10.1088/2752-5309/ac7d69

26. Committee on Health Risks of Indoor Exposures to Fine Particulate Matter and Practical Mitigation Solutions. *Health Risks of Indoor Exposure to Fine Particulate Matter and Practical Mitigation Solutions*. National Academies Press; 2024. doi:10.17226/27341

27. Kanchongkittiphon W, Mendell MJ, Gaffin JM, Wang G, Phipatanakul W. Indoor environmental exposures and exacerbation of asthma: An update to the 2000 review by the Institute of Medicine. *Environ Health Perspect*. 2015;123(1):6-20. doi:10.1289/ehp.1307922

28. Burge HA, Rogers CA. Outdoor allergens. *Environ Health Perspect*. 2000;108(suppl 4):653-659. doi:10.1289/ehp.00108s4653

29. National Center for Health Statistics, Centers for Disease Control and Prevention. *National Health Interview Survey: Summary Health Statistics*. Published September 21, 2023. Accessed

June 25, 2024. Available at: https://www.cdc.gov/nchs/nhis/shs.htm

30. Caron KT, Zhu W, Bernert JT, et al. Geometric mean serum cotinine concentrations confirm a continued decline in secondhand smoke exposure among U.S. nonsmokers—NHANES 2003 to 2018. *Int J Environ Res Public Health.* 2022;19(10). doi:10.3390/ijerph19105862

31. Tsai J, Homa DM, Gentzke AS, et al. Exposure to secondhand smoke among nonsmokers—United States, 1988–2014. *MMWR Morb Mortal Wkly Rep.* 2018;67(48):1342-1346. doi:10.15585/mmwr.mm6748a3

32. Tsai J, Homa DM, Neff LJ, et al. Trends in secondhand smoke exposure, 2011–2018: Impact and implications of expanding serum cotinine range. *Am J Prev Med.* 2021;61(3):e109-e117. doi:10.1016/j.amepre.2021.04.004

33. Brody DJ, Lu Z, Tsai J. Secondhand smoke exposure among nonsmoking youth: United States, 2013–2016 Key findings Data from the National Health and Nutrition Examination Survey. *NCHS Data Brief.* 2019;(348):1-8.

34. Tiotiu AI, Novakova S, Labor M, et al. Progress in occupational asthma. *Int J Environ Res Public Health.* 2020;17(12):1-19. doi:10.3390/ijerph17124553

35. Crocker DD, Kinyota S, Dumitru GG, et al. Effectiveness of home-based, multi-trigger, multicomponent interventions with an environmental focus for reducing asthma morbidity: A community guide systematic review. *Am J Prev Med.* 2011;41(2 Suppl 1). doi:10.1016/j.amepre.2011.05.012

36. Morgan WJ, Crain EF, Gruchalla RS, et al. Results of a home-based environmental intervention among urban children with asthma. *N Engl J Med.* 2004;351(11):1068-1080. doi:10.1056/NEJMoa032097

37. Milligan KL, Matsui E, Sharma H. Asthma in urban children: Epidemiology, environmental risk factors, and the public health domain. *Curr Allergy Asthma Rep.* 2016;16(4). doi:10.1007/s11882-016-0609-6

38. Hsu J, Sircar K, Herman E, Garbe P. *EXHALE: A Technical Package to Control Asthma.* Atlanta; 2018. Accessed June 25, 2024. Available at: https://www.cdc.gov/national-asthma-control-program/media/pdfs/2024/06/EXHALE_technical_package-508.pdf

39. Gill I, Shah A, Lee EK, et al. Community interventions for childhood asthma ED visits and hospitalizations: A systematic review. *Pediatrics.* 2022;150(4). doi:10.1542/peds.2021-054825

40. National Institute for Occupational Safety and Health (NIOSH). *Preventing Work-Related Asthma.* Centers for Disease Control and Prevention. Published March 8, 2023. Accessed March 20, 2024. Available at: https://www.cdc.gov/niosh/topics/asthma/prevented.html

41. Naja AS, Permaul P, Phipatanakul W. Taming asthma in school-aged children: A comprehensive review. *J Allergy Clin Immunol Pract.* 2018;6(3):726-735. doi:10.1016/j.jaip.2018.01.023

42. Christenson SA, Smith BM, Bafadhel M, Putcha N. Chronic obstructive pulmonary disease. *Lancet.* 2022;399(10342):2227-2242. doi:10.1016/S0140-6736(22)00470-6

43. Decramer M, Janssens W, Miravitlles M. Chronic obstructive pulmonary disease. *Lancet.* 2012;379:1341-1351. doi:10.1016/S0140

44. Gerayeli F V., Milne S, Cheung C, et al. COPD and the risk of poor outcomes in COVID-19: A systematic review and meta-analysis. *EClinicalMedicine.* 2021;33:100789. doi:10.1016/j.eclinm.2021.100789

45. Willemse BWM, Postma DS, Timens W, ten Hacken NHT. The impact of smoking cessation on respiratory symptoms, lung function, airway hyperresponsiveness and inflammation. *Eur Respir J.* 2004;23(3):464-476. doi:10.1183/09031936.04.00012704

46. Adeloye D, Song P, Zhu Y, Campbell H, Sheikh A, Rudan I. Global, regional, and national prevalence of, and risk factors for, chronic obstructive pulmonary disease (COPD) in 2019: A systematic review and modelling analysis. *Lancet Respir Med.* 2022;10(5):447-458. doi:10.1016/S2213-2600(21)00511-7

47. Global Initiative for Chronic Obstructive Lung Disease. *Global Strategy for the Diagnosis, Management, and Prevention of Chronic Obstructive Pulmonary Disease.* 2024. Accessed June 25, 2024. Available at: https://goldcopd.org/2024-gold-report/

48. Deolmi M, Decarolis NM, Motta M, et al. Early origins of chronic obstructive pulmonary disease: Prenatal and early life risk factors. *Int J Environ Res Public Health.* 2023;20(3). doi:10.3390/ijerph20032294

49. Agustí A, Hogg JC. Update on the pathogenesis of chronic obstructive pulmonary disease. *N Engl J Med.* 2019;381(13):1248-1256. doi:10.1056/nejmra1900475

50. Bui DS, Lodge CJ, Burgess JA, et al. Childhood predictors of lung function trajectories and future COPD risk: A prospective cohort study from the first to the sixth decade of life. *Lancet Respir Med.* 2018;6(7):535-544. doi:10.1016/S2213-2600(18)30100-0

51. Dratva J, Zemp E, Dharmage SC, et al. Early life origins of lung ageing: Early life exposures and lung function decline in adulthood in two European cohorts aged 28-73 years. *PLoS One.* 2016;11(1). doi:10.1371/journal.pone.0145127

52. Lawlor DA, Ebrahim S, Smith GD. Association of birth weight with adult lung function: Findings from the British Women's Heart and Health Study and a meta-analysis. *Thorax.* 2005;60(10):851-858. doi:10.1136/thx.2005.042408

53. Liu Y, Carlson SA, Watson KB, Xu F, Greenlund KJ. Trends in the prevalence of Chronic obstructive pulmonary disease among adults aged ≥18 years—United States, 2011–2021. *MMWR Morb Mortal Wkly Rep.* 2023;72(46):1250-1256. doi:10.15585/mmwr.mm7246a1

54. National Center for Health Statistics, Centers for Disease Control and Prevention. *Underlying Cause of Death Data on CDC WONDER.* Published 2023. Accessed June 12, 2024. Available at: https://wonder.cdc.gov/Deaths-by-Underlying-Cause.html

55. Soriano JB, Kendrick PJ, Paulson KR, et al. Prevalence and attributable health burden of chronic respiratory diseases, 1990–2017: A systematic analysis for the Global Burden of Disease Study 2017. *Lancet Respir Med.* 2020;8(6):585-596. doi:10.1016/S2213-2600(20)30105-3

56. Global Burden of Disease Collaboration, Institute for Health Metrics and Evaluation. *GBD Results Tool.* Published July 12, 2023. Accessed July 11, 2023. Available at: https://vizhub.healthdata.org/gbd-results/

57. Guo C, Zhang Z, Yeoh MBBS E k, et al. Effect of long-term exposure to fine particulate matter on lung function decline and risk of chronic obstructive pulmonary disease in Taiwan: A longitudinal, cohort study. *Lancet Planet Health.* 2018;2:e114-25.

58. Cohen AJ, Brauer M, Burnett R, et al. Estimates and 25-year trends of the global burden of disease attributable to ambient

air pollution: An analysis of data from the Global Burden of Diseases Study 2015. *Lancet*. 2017;389(10082):1907-1918. doi:10.1016/S0140-6736(17)30505-6

59. Hnizdo E. Association between chronic obstructive pulmonary disease and employment by industry and occupation in the US population: A study of data from the Third National Health and Nutrition Examination Survey. *Am J Epidemiol*. 2002;156(8):738-746. doi:10.1093/aje/kwf105

60. Magnus MC, Henderson J, Tilling K, Howe LD, Fraser A. Independent and combined associations of maternal and own smoking with adult lung function and COPD. *Int J Epidemiol*. 2018;47(6):1855-1864. doi:10.1093/ije/dyy221

61. Perret JL, Walters H, Johns D, et al. Mother's smoking and complex lung function of offspring in middle age: A cohort study from childhood. *Respirology*. 2016;21(5):911-919. doi:10.1111/resp.12750

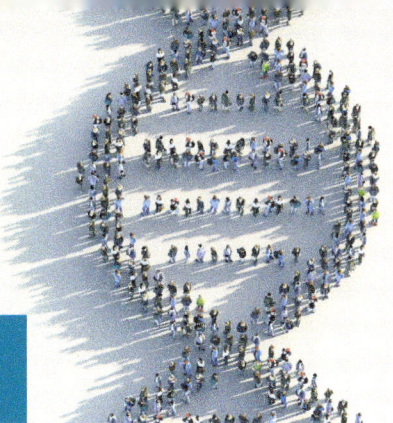

CHAPTER 9

Infectious Diseases

Humans live within an ecosystem of organisms. Some organisms are the plants and animals that we can easily see, but most are so small that they can only be seen with a microscope, so they are called **microorganisms** or **microbes**. For example, many bacteria live on or in humans' skin, lungs, and intestines. Together, the microorganisms that live in or on human tissues are called the human **microbiome**. Most of those microbes are harmless or even beneficial to humans. For example, bacteria in the intestines help extract nutrients from food. Most of the time, the humans' immune systems prevent these microbes from invading human tissues.

But, rarely, microbes invade, use the energy in human cells to make copies of themselves, and damage tissues. When microbes cause this damage, the condition is called an **infection** or an infectious disease. In 1850, the leading killers in the United States included many infectious diseases like cholera, dysentery, typhoid, pneumonia, and tuberculosis.[1] After the sanitary revolution and improvements in nutrition in the late 1800s, those diseases mostly dropped off the list of leading causes of death in the United States. But infectious diseases are still among the leading causes of death and disability globally. And as the COVID-19 pandemic showed, infectious diseases always have the potential to re-emerge as major public health threats everywhere.

This chapter discusses the infectious diseases responsible for the greatest public health burden worldwide. They are caused by several very different types of **infectious agents** or **pathogens**, including viruses, bacteria, fungi, and protozoa (**Table 9.1**).

Infectious Agents

Viruses

Viruses are extraordinarily simple packages of DNA or RNA that do not even qualify as independent life forms. They are very small—about 1/10 of a micron (a micron is 1/1,000 of a millimeter)—and can be seen only with an electron microscope. For most viruses, the DNA or RNA is contained within a coat of proteins called a **capsid**, and that capsid is itself wrapped in a membrane called an **envelope** that is studded with other proteins (**Figure 9.1**). The RNA or DNA in viruses codes for only a few to a few dozen different proteins. Viruses reproduce by inserting their DNA or RNA into host cells and hijacking the cells' machinery to make copies of themselves.

As simple as they are, viruses can cause extraordinary damage to humans. Viruses underlie several leading causes of death globally, including AIDS, lower respiratory infections, and diarrheal diseases. They can do this much damage in part because their simplicity allows viruses to mutate very quickly, enabling them to evade the defenses in humans' immune systems.

Bacteria

Bacteria are among the smallest independent life forms. They are about 1–2 microns in size, which is about 10–20 times as large as viruses and just large enough to be seen with a high-powered light microscope. Most are shaped either as tiny spheres called **cocci** or short rods called **bacilli** (**Figure 9.2**). Most

Table 9.1 Overview of Pathogens That Cause Human Diseases

Types		Examples		Related Diseases
Viruses	RNA Viruses	Orthomyxoviruses	Influenza virus	Influenza (LRI)
		Paramyxoviruses	Measles, Respiratory syncytial viruses	Measles, LRI
		Coronaviruses	"Cold" viruses, SARS-CoV-1, MERS-CoV, SARS-CoV-2	LRI
		Caliciviruses	Norovirus	Diarrheal diseases
		Reoviruses	Rotavirus	Diarrheal diseases
		Retroviruses	HIV	HIV/AIDS
	DNA Viruses	Adenoviruses	Human adenovirus type 40	Diarrheal diseases, LRI
		Herpes Viruses	Herpes simplex virus, Varicella zoster virus, Cytomegalovirus	Herpes, Varicella (Chicken pox)
		Papovaviruses	Human papillomavirus	Cervical cancer
Bacteria	Gram positive cocci		*Streptococcus pneumoniae, Staphylococcus aureus*	LRI
	Gram positive bacilli		*Listeria monocytogenes*	Listeria infection
	Gram negative cocci		*Neisseria gonorrheae*	Gonorrhea
	Gram negative bacilli		*Shigella sp., Escherichia coli, Haemophilus influenzae*	Diarrheal diseases, LRI
	Spirochetes		*Treponema pallidum*	Syphilis
	Mycobacteria		*Mycobacterium tuberculosis*	Tuberculosis
	Chlamydias		*Chlamydia pneumoniae*	LRI
	Mycoplasmas		*Mycoplasma pneumoniae*	LRI
Fungi		Candida	*Candida albicans*	Vaginal yeast infection
		Aspergillus	*Aspergillus flavus*	Infections in people with immune deficiency
		Pneumocystis	*Pneumocystis jirovecii*	PCP pneumonia
Protozoa		Plasmodium	*Plasmodium falciparum*	Malaria
		Cryptosporidium	*Cryptosporidium* sp.	Diarrheal diseases

are normal, healthful inhabitants of the human eco-system, but a few are pathogens that cause a wide range of diseases, including tuberculosis, gonorrhea, pneumonia, and dysentery. Bacteria can be killed by **antibiotics**, which are chemicals produced by other microorganisms to protect themselves.

ubiquitous, with mold spores normally in the air that we all breathe. It is rare for fungi to cause serious infections. However, vaginal yeast infections are common, and fungi can sometimes cause deadly infections in people with weakened immune systems, such as those with AIDS.

Fungi

Fungi can be single cells, clusters of cells, or multi-celled organisms.[2] The biologic kingdom of fungi includes yeast, mold, and mushrooms. Fungi are

Protozoa

Protozoa are the largest and most complex single-celled organisms. They are roughly 10–100 microns in size, or 10–50 times the size of bacteria. That makes

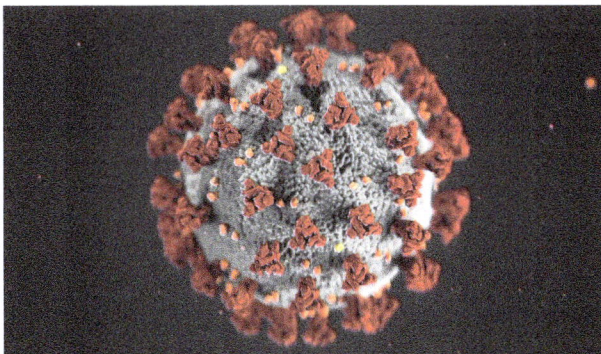

Figure 9.1 SARS-CoV-2, the Virus That Causes COVID-19 Illness. Viruses are simple packages of DNA or RNA wrapped in an envelope that is studded with proteins. The proteins on the surface of the SARS-CoV-2 virus are shown in red in this illustration.

Courtesy of Alissa Eckert, MSMI; Dan Higgins, MAMS/CDC.

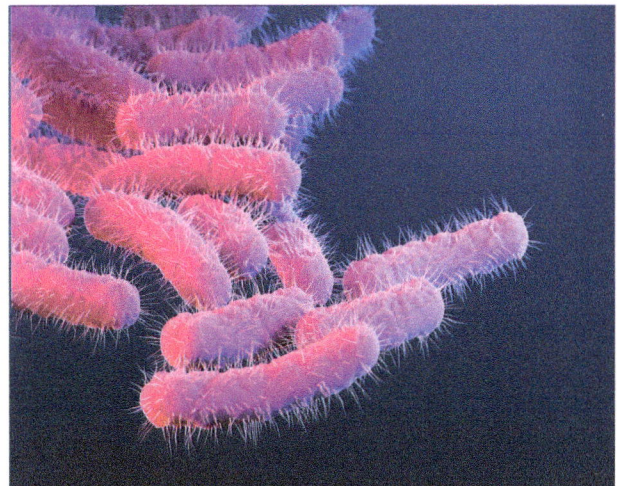

Figure 9.2 Shigella, the Bacteria That Causes Dysentery. Bacteria are about 10-20 times the size of viruses. They can be shaped like short rods (as in this photo) or spheres called cocci.

Courtesy of Stephanie Rossow/CDC.

them large enough to be seen under a low-powered light microscope.[3] Protozoa go through several stages in their life cycles, appearing in strikingly different forms in each stage. They can live within different "hosts" in different life stages. For example, *Plasmodium*, which causes malaria, lives within humans and within mosquitos at different stages of its complex life cycle. Protozoa can reproduce by simply dividing in two or sexually, with male and female forms joining their genes. While malaria is the protozoan disease with the greatest public health impact, diarrheal diseases are often caused by the protozoan *Cryptosporidium* (**Figure 9.3**).

HIV Infection

Introduction

In 1981, doctors in New York and Los Angeles raised alarms that they were seeing previously-healthy gay men with a rare form of cancer called **Kaposi**

Box 9.1 Key Words–Infectious Agents

Antibiotic
Bacillus, bacilli
Bacterium, bacteria
Capsid
Coccus, cocci
Envelope
Fungus, fungi
Infection
Infectious agents
Microbes
Microbiome
Microorganisms
Pathogen
Protozoan, protozoa
Virus

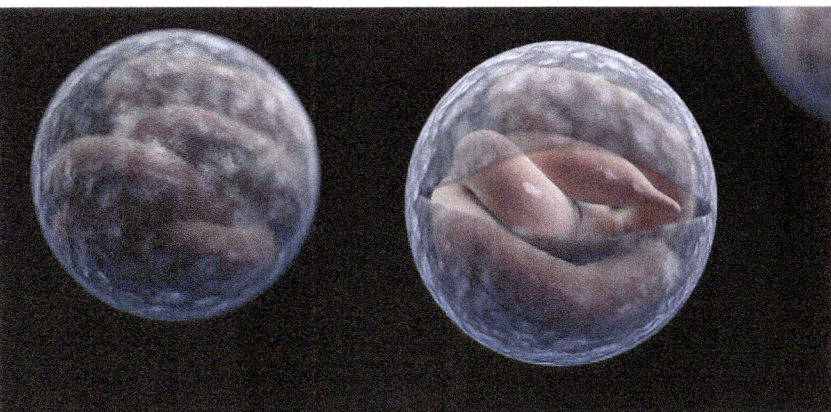

Figure 9.3 *Cryptosporidium*, **a Protozoan that Causes Diarrheal Disease**. Protozoa are 10-50 times the size of bacteria. They go through several stages in their life cycles and appear in strikingly different forms in each stage.

Centers for Disease Control and Prevention. About Cryptosporidiosis. https://www.cdc.gov/cryptosporidium/about/index.html

sarcoma and an even rarer type of pneumonia called **PCP**. These reports heralded the arrival of the pandemic of the acquired immunodeficiency syndrome (AIDS). At its peak, AIDS killed nearly 2 million people per year across the world. Since then, we have learned much about the **human immunodeficiency virus (HIV)**, the virus that causes AIDS, and antiviral drugs have put the pandemic into decline. But HIV still kills more than 600,000 people per year, mostly in low-income countries in sub-Saharan Africa.[4]

The body has an immune system that works to fight infections. Those battles take place mostly in the specific organ systems that the infectious agents are attacking. For example, SARS-CoV-2, the virus that causes COVID-19, attacks the lung, and the hepatitis B virus attacks the liver. HIV is unique in that it attacks the immune system itself. When it does, it weakens the immune system, leaving the person vulnerable to every other infectious agent. And that makes HIV infection particularly difficult to cure. This section will discuss the immune system, the effect of HIV on the immune system, the ways in which HIV is spread, and interventions to prevent HIV.

Physiology of the Immune System

The immune system is a network of different types of cells, scattered in tissues throughout the body, which work together to fight infections. Some cells have the job of recognizing an invading organism as "foreign," others have the job of killing organisms that are recognized as foreign, and others kill human cells that are infected.

The immune system has two main arms. The first arm, called **innate immunity**, recognizes invaders simply as unfamiliar, and responds quickly. The second arm, called **adaptive or acquired immunity**, recognizes specific foreign invaders and builds a stronger attack on them. This arm takes longer to respond.

Figure 9.4 summarizes how key cells work in these two arms.

Innate Immunity

Innate immunity is activated in minutes to hours after the arrival of a foreign invader. The responding immune cells attack any invader that, based on the proteins on its surface, does not look like the body's own cells. The two key immune cells involved are:

- **Macrophages,** which surround and then digest bacteria, viruses, other infectious agents, or foreign substances.[5] This process—essentially the macrophage "eating" invaders—is called **phagocytosis**.
- **Natural killer (or NK) lymphocytes,** which destroy damaged host (human) cells.[5] NK lymphocytes recognize and do not harm the body's own healthy cells, but they kill any host cell that appears stressed or abnormal, for example, one that is harboring a virus or that has been transformed into a cancer cell.

Adaptive Immunity

Adaptive immunity is tailored to specific invaders. It has a crucial feature of **memory**. It "remembers" an infection with a specific invader, which enables it to prevent a second infection with that same invader. This memory feature is why people do not get diseases like measles a second time. Adaptive immunity is the foundation for the biomedical tool that has saved more lives than any other: vaccination.

Adaptive immunity is a much more complex response than innate immunity, and it takes days to weeks to develop. Adaptive immunity recognizes a specific infectious agent and mounts a multi-celled attack on that agent. As it responds, it also produces specialized memory **lymphocytes** that remain on standby afterwards to kill that infectious agent if it reappears. Key cells involved in the adaptive immunity response include:

- **B lymphocytes.** These cells produce specialized proteins called **antibodies**. Antibodies are Y-shaped protein molecules (**Figure 9.5**) that attach to specific **antigens**—substances that elicit an immune response, such as proteins on the surface of invaders. The two arms of the Y grab onto the antigens; these antibodies and invaders then link up into one large clump that the body can dispose of. The production of antibodies is called **humoral immunity**. Also, the stem of the Y attaches to macrophages and prompts phagocytosis—that is, the antibody helps the macrophage "eat" the invader.
- **Cytotoxic T lymphocytes.** These cells recognize human cells that have been altered by specific foreign invaders and then kill them. This is called **cell-mediated immunity**.
- **Helper T lymphocytes.** These are the command-and-control cells of adaptive immunity. Helper T lymphocytes stimulate and assist other immune cells to attack invaders. Specifically, the helper T lymphocytes: 1) recruit more macrophages to the site of the infection and activate those macrophages to phagocytize the invaders,[5-7]

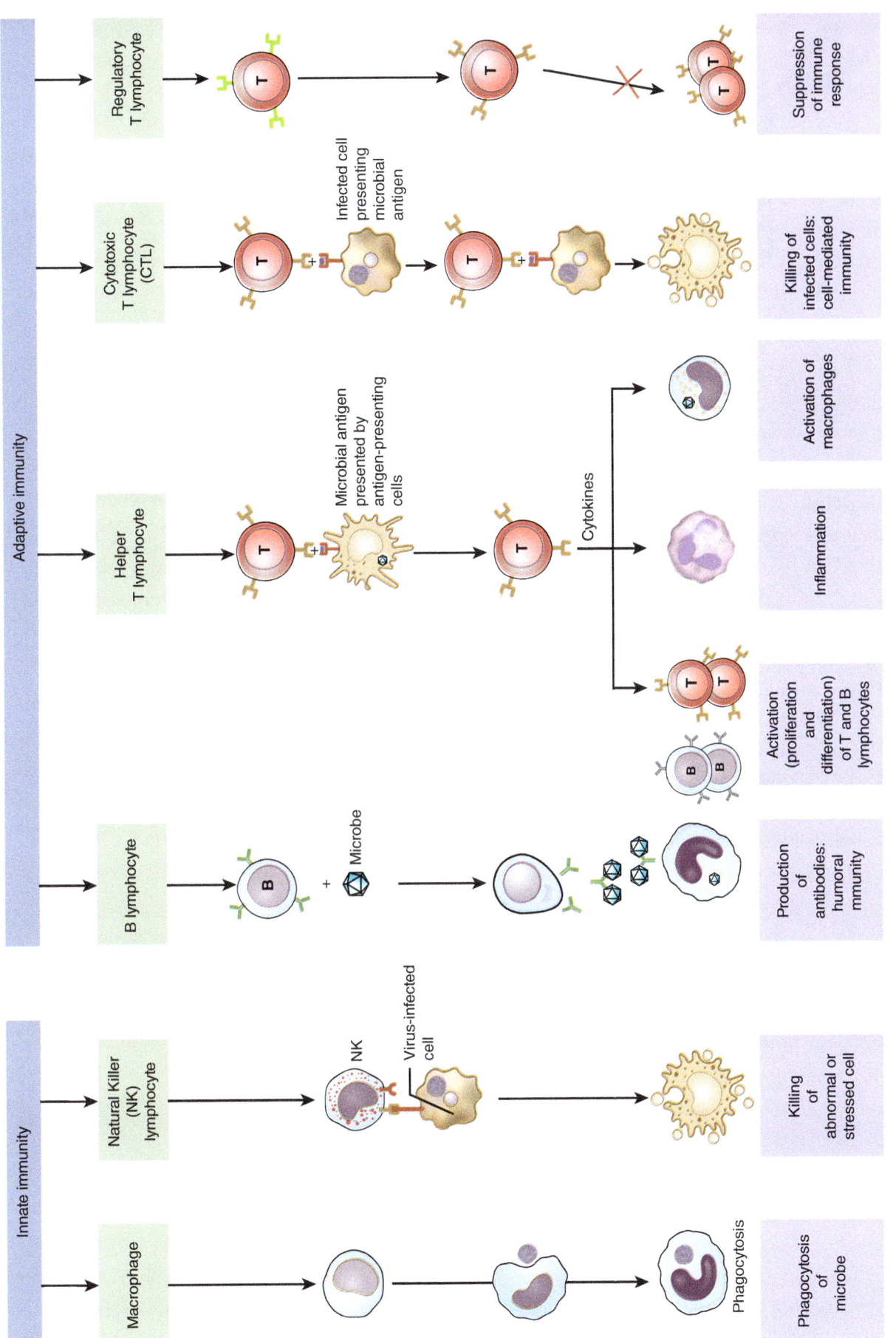

Figure 9.4 Function of Key Cells in Immune System. The immune system has two main arms: innate immunity and adaptive immunity. Innate immunity is a general, quick response, and adaptive immunity is a specific, slower response. In innate immunity, macrophages "eat" invading microbes and NK cells kill abnormal or stressed host cells. In adaptive immunity, B lymphocytes make antibodies, cytotoxic T lymphocytes kill invading organisms, helper T lymphocytes stimulate and assist other immune cells, and regulatory T lymphocytes suppress other immune cells.

Data from Kumar V, Abbas AK, Aster JC, Turner JR. The Normal Immune Response. In: Robbins & Cotran Pathologic Basis of Disease. 10th ed. Elsevier; 2021:190-203.

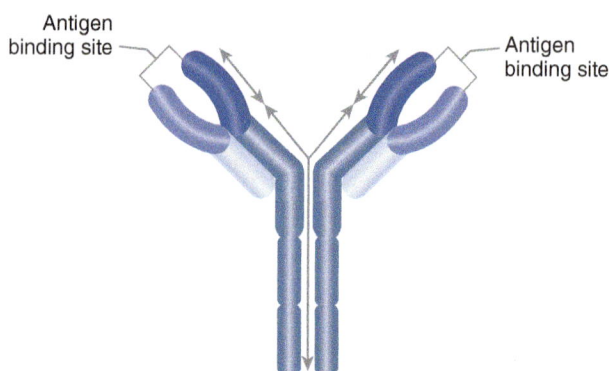

Figure 9.5 Structure of Antibodies. Antibodies are specialized Y-shaped proteins. The two arms of the Y grab onto antigens, and the stem of the Y attaches to macrophages and prompts phagocytosis.

2) stimulate B lymphocytes to make antibodies,[7,8] and 3) stimulate cytotoxic T lymphocytes to make copies of themselves.[7,8]

- *Regulatory T lymphocytes.* These cells *suppress* the activity of other immune cells. They are needed to keep the immune response from becoming overactive and harmful. Without regulatory T lymphocytes, the immune system could run amok, inappropriately attacking the body's own healthy cells. (When the immune system does attack the body's own cells, it produces **autoimmune diseases**, like rheumatoid arthritis and **lupus**.)

The helper T lymphocytes and regulatory T lymphocytes have a protein on their surface called CD4.[8] This **CD4 surface protein** is very important because it is the target of the HIV virus, as discussed below.

Pathophysiology of HIV/AIDS
The Human Immunodeficiency Virus

HIV is one of a group of viruses called **retroviruses.** For all the havoc that it causes, HIV is a remarkably simple virus, carrying just a few genes and producing just a few **enzymes** that it needs to make copies of itself.[5] (An enzyme is a specialized protein that acts to catalyze specific biochemical reactions.) The genes of HIV are surrounded by a **capsid** made of proteins, which is covered in the virus's **envelope** (**Figure 9.6**). The protein that makes up the capsid is called **p24.** This p24 protein can be found in the blood of people with HIV infection. The envelope of HIV is studded with **glycoproteins**, which are specialized proteins; these glycoproteins are what enable HIV to attach to and infect lymphocytes.[5]

HIV carries its genes as RNA. But when HIV gets inside human "host" cells, it copies ("reverse transcribes") that RNA into DNA and then integrates this DNA into the DNA of the human host cell (**Figure 9.7**).[5]

HIV uses three enzymes to do this work. **Reverse transcriptase** is the enzyme that copies the virus's RNA into DNA. **Integrase** is the enzyme that integrates that DNA from the virus into the DNA of the

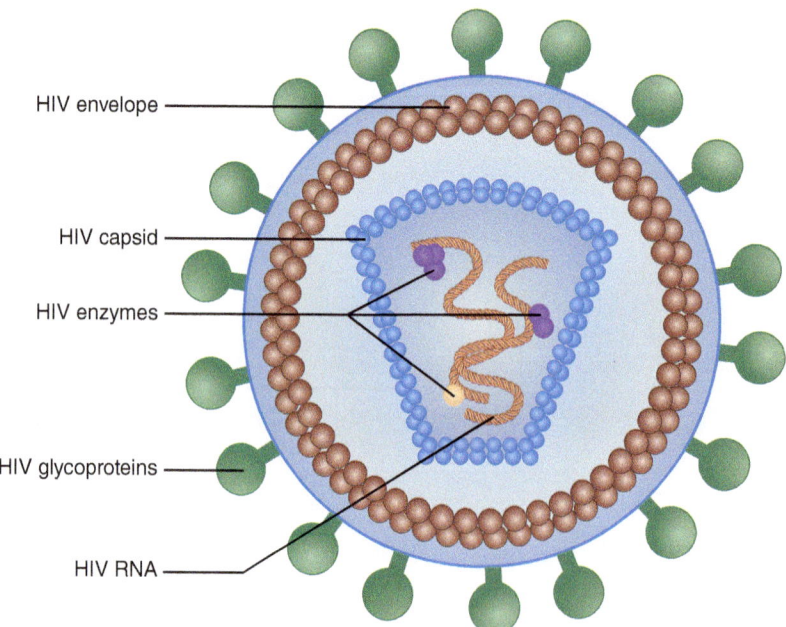

HIV envelope

HIV capsid

HIV enzymes

HIV glycoproteins

HIV RNA

Figure 9.6 The Structure of HIV. HIV is a virus that stores its genes as RNA. The RNA is surrounded by a capsid, which is itself covered by the virus's envelope. The envelope is studded with glycoproteins.

Office of AIDS Research, National Institutes of Health. Clinicalinfo. Accessed July 30, 2024. https://clinicalinfo.hiv.gov/en/glossary/human-immunodeficiency-virus-hiv

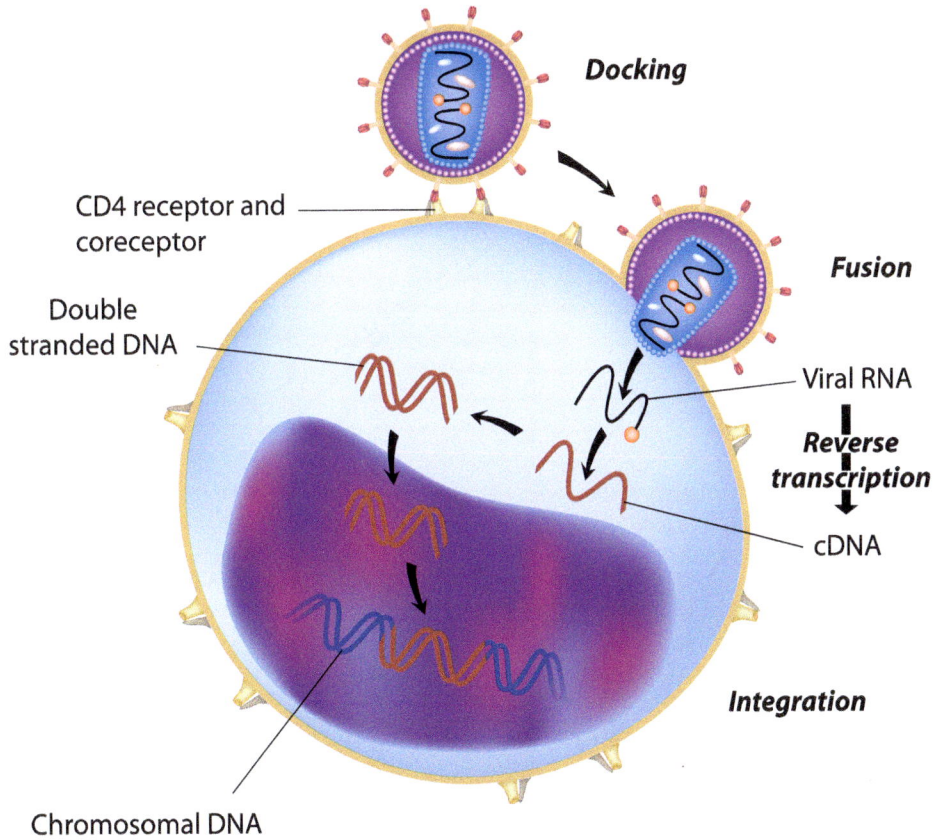

Figure 9.7 How HIV Infects a T Lymphocyte. HIV makes copies of itself by using the genetic machinery of a human T lymphocyte that has the CD4 protein on its surface. The virus uses CD4 to attach to the cell, inserts its RNA into the cell, "reverse transcribes" that RNA into DNA, and then integrates its DNA into the DNA of the host cell.
© Alila Medical Media/Shutterstock

human. And **protease** is an enzyme that helps produce the other two enzymes.[5] The antiviral drugs used to treat HIV infections work by interfering with these three enzymes.

How HIV Causes Disease

HIV does most of its damage by infecting lymphocytes that have the CD4 protein on their surface. Once it has entered a CD4 lymphocyte and integrated its genes, it uses the normal cellular machinery of the lymphocyte to make many copies of itself. This ultimately kills the lymphocyte and spills new copies of HIV into the surrounding fluid, where they infect more lymphocytes.[5]

Over many years, the body and HIV fight a battle over these CD4 lymphocytes (**Figure 9.8**). In the first few weeks of the infection, the number of copies of the virus in the blood (called the **viral load**) spikes to very high levels and the number of CD4 lymphocytes in the blood drops to low levels. During these early weeks, the person may have a fever or other symptoms, which is called **acute HIV infection**. Then the body rallies, greatly

increasing its production of CD4 lymphocytes and reducing the viral load to low levels. But over the next 2–10 years, the body gradually fails to produce enough new CD4 lymphocytes to replace those that are killed.[5] The CD4 count in the blood slowly falls and the viral load slowly rises.

Most CD4 lymphocytes are helper T lymphocytes— the leaders of the immune response.[5] When the body does not have enough of these helper T lymphocytes, other cells in the immune system fail. Macrophages are feeble at phagocytosis, B lymphocytes do not produce enough antibodies, and cytotoxic T cells do not kill enough infected cells.[5] That leaves a person with advanced HIV infection vulnerable to infections from nearly any organism, including those that normally cause humans no trouble.

The lower the CD4 count, the more vulnerable the person is to infections. A healthy person has about 1,000 CD4 lymphocytes per microliter of blood. An HIV-infected person with fewer than 500 CD4 lymphocytes has a weakened immune system and is susceptible to some infections. An HIV-infected person with fewer than 200 CD4 lymphocytes per microliter is highly

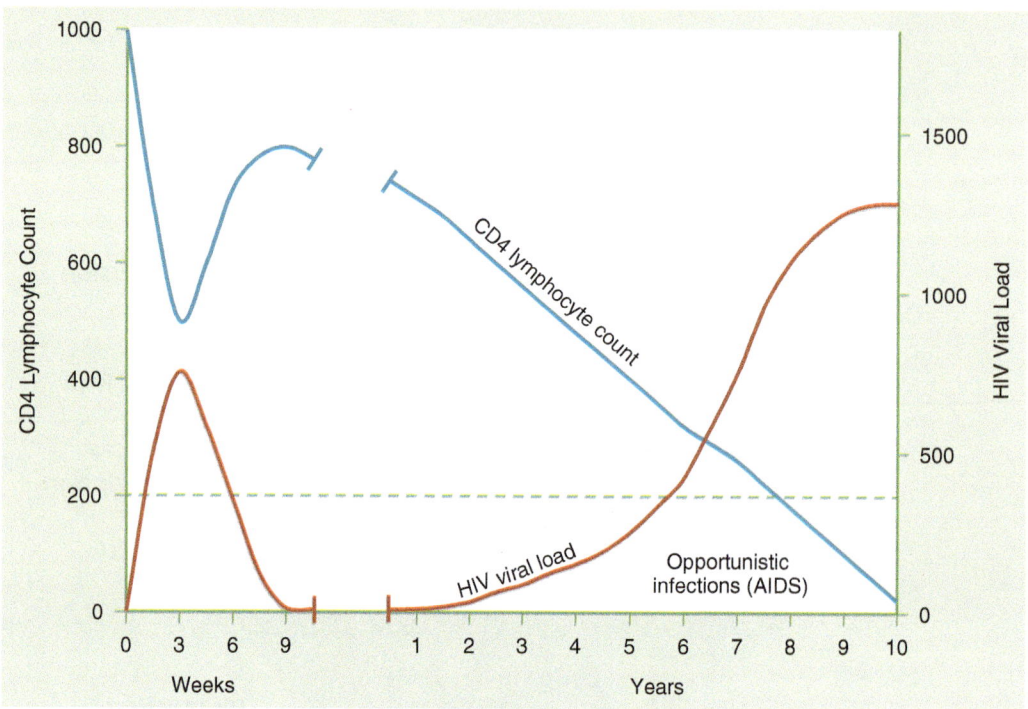

Figure 9.8 **Changes to CD4 Lymphocyte Count and Viral Load Over the Course of HIV illness.** The HIV illness unfolds over many years, during which there are changes in the number of CD4 lymphocytes and the number of virus particles (called the viral load) in the blood. In the first few weeks, the viral load (red line) spikes and CD4 lymphocytes (blue line) drops to low levels. Then the body rallies, greatly increasing its production of CD4 lymphocytes and reducing the viral load. But over the next 2–10 years, the CD4 lymphocytes fall and the viral load rises.

Data from Omari, M., & Ouifki, R. Oscillations in a Model for HIV Infection with Three Intracellular Delays and RTI: Delays Can Induce Viral Blips. 2010.

vulnerable to any infection and by definition has the **acquired immunodeficiency syndrome (AIDS)**.

People with AIDS get infections with organisms that ordinarily the immune system can contain. For example, the fungus *Pneumocystis jirovicii* often lives in the lungs of healthy people without causing problems, but in people with AIDS, it causes PCP pneumonia. The fungus *Candida* is everywhere in our environment, and it rarely causes anything more than a vaginal yeast infection, but in a person with AIDS, it can cause a severe infection of the esophagus. Infections caused by normally-harmless organisms are called **opportunistic infections**. When AIDS leads to death, it is generally opportunistic infections that are the final cause.

Tuberculosis is a particularly important infection in persons with HIV. Tuberculosis is an infection, usually involving the lungs, caused by a specific bacterium. While some people with healthy immune systems develop active tuberculosis, most can keep this bacterium under control. But people with immune systems weakened by HIV are much more likely to have a fast-moving, severe infection. Tuberculosis is discussed in depth later in this chapter.

A healthy immune system normally recognizes and kills cells that have been transformed into cancer cells, preventing them from growing into large, fatal cancers. Without a healthy immune system, people with HIV are more likely to develop many types of cancer, including **lymphoma** (cancer of the lymphocytes) and Kaposi sarcoma, the cancer that first signaled the arrival of AIDS.

Transmission of HIV

HIV is spread from one person to another when the viral particles from an infected person touch CD4 lymphocytes of another person (**Figure 9.9**). HIV viral particles are in many body fluids, including blood, semen, vaginal fluid, fluids in the rectum, and breast milk. CD4 lymphocytes live in tissues throughout the body. That means that whenever infected body fluids from one person enter the tissues of another person, HIV can be transmitted.[9,10] (HIV is not spread with sweat, tears, or saliva and does not penetrate intact skin. It is not spread by shaking hands, hugging, or kissing.) However, some types of contact are much more likely to transmit HIV than others. The important routes of spread of HIV are:

- *Sex.* HIV can be transmitted during sex when the viral particles in one partner's semen, vaginal fluid, or rectal fluid touch CD4 cells in the tissues of the

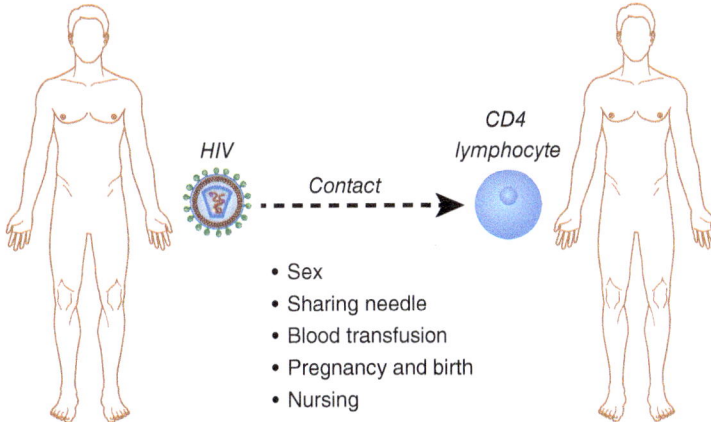

Figure 9.9 Transmission of HIV from One Person to Another. HIV is transmitted when the viral particles from an infected person touch the CD4 lymphocytes of another person.

other partner. Vaginal sex by itself is not a very efficient route of HIV transmission, with spread occurring only about once per 1,000 exposures.[11] But spread through vaginal sex happens much more often if the uninfected partner has an open sore in the genital area (called a **genital ulcer**) or a sexually transmitted disease like gonorrhea or herpes. These conditions open up much more contact with that partner's CD4 lymphocytes. Also, HIV is much more likely to spread to men who are uncircumcised, possibly because the lining of the foreskin contains many CD4 lymphocytes.[12] Finally HIV is much more likely to spread during anal sex (estimated at more than one per 100 exposures) because there are more CD4 lymphocyte targets in the rectum than the genitals.[11]

- *Needle sharing.* Blood is full of CD4 lymphocytes. Inserting hypodermic needles into blood vessels for an injection does not by itself pose a risk of transmitting HIV—it is routinely done safely in hospitals—but it does pose a risk if the needle or syringe contains even a microscopic amount of blood from an HIV-infected person. That happens when drug users share needles or syringes, or rarely in clinics or hospitals that reuse needles.
- *Transfusion.* If a pint of blood is transfused from a person who is infected with HIV to one who is not, the blood recipient almost always becomes infected.[11] Transfusion was a common route of spread of HIV in the very early days of the pandemic, but screening of blood donors has nearly eliminated this risk today.
- *Pregnancy and delivery.* Babies of mothers who are infected with HIV can themselves become infected when they are exposed to fluid from the mother's cervix or vagina. Most spread of HIV happens during delivery, when the baby is

heavily exposed to these fluids, but about a third of the time the transmission happens in the last 2 months of pregnancy.[13]
- *Breastfeeding.* HIV is present in breast milk and babies of HIV-infected mothers can become infected through breastfeeding.

Epidemiology: Patterns and Trends

In the United States, about 5,000 people per year die from HIV, which makes it a relatively uncommon cause of death today.[14] However, more than 1 million Americans are already infected with HIV and about 38,000 become infected each year.[15] The number of people newly infected each year in the United States has been falling slowly since about 2000.[15]

Of those newly infected, the CDC estimates that about two-thirds were infected through sexual contact between men, one-fourth were infected through heterosexual contact, and less than one in ten were infected through needle sharing during drug use.[15] The estimated rates of new HIV infections in different demographic groups are shown in **Figure 9.10**. New infections peak in young adult years, are four times more common in men than in women, and are more than seven times as high in Blacks/African-Americans as Whites or Asians.

Estimates of the global impact of HIV/AIDS are produced by the Joint United Nations Programme on HIV/AIDS (UNAIDS). UNAIDS estimates that in the early 2020s, 630,000 people died of AIDS and 1.3 million became infected with HIV every year worldwide.[4,16] HIV infections and HIV-related deaths are highest in sub-Saharan Africa, where most transmission is through heterosexual contact. A few other pockets around the world are also hit

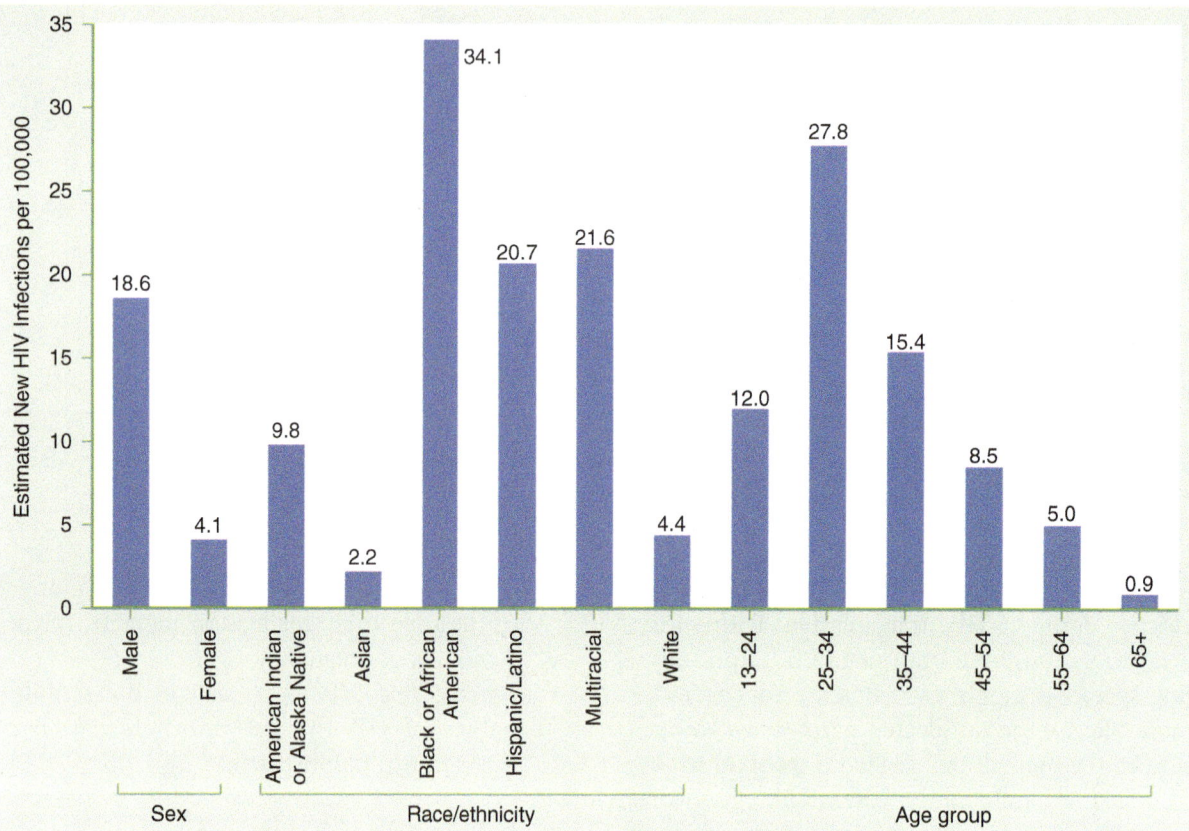

Figure 9.10 Estimated HIV Incidence in the United States by Demographic Group for 2022.

Data from National Center for HIV, Viral Hepatitis, STD, and Tuberculosis Prevention, Centers for Disease Control. AtlasPlus Accessed November 20, 2024. https://gis.cdc.gov/grasp/nchhstpatlas/charts.html

hard by AIDS. Those include Thailand and Russia, where the virus is mostly spread through injection drug use, and some countries in the Caribbean and South America, where transmission is through both sexual contact between men and heterosexual contact (**Figure 9.11**).

While the history of the AIDS epidemic is full of tragedy, the global AIDS response in recent decades has been a remarkable success story, with the number of annual AIDS deaths falling 48% and the number of people newly infected with HIV falling 38% from 2010 to 2022 (**Figure 9.12**).[16] The drop in new HIV infections in these years has been even more impressive—57%— in the hardest-hit areas of eastern and southern Africa.[16]

Risk Factors

Risk factors for HIV and AIDS are shown in **Figure 9.13**.

Sexual Transmission

Sexual exposure to HIV is more likely to occur where there are:

- *Connected sexual networks.* Individuals are more likely to be exposed to sexually transmitted diseases,

including HIV, if they have two or more sex partners. But their risk also depends on how many sex partners their partners have. At the population level, rates of STDs are higher where there are connected sexual networks, that is, when people have multiple sex partners, many of whom themselves have multiple other sex partners, as illustrated in **Figure 9.14**.[17,18]

- *Alcohol and drug use.* Alcohol use and use of drugs like cocaine (even if it is not injected) are associated with HIV/AIDS and other sexually transmitted diseases.[19-21] This is in part because people who drink alcohol and use drugs are more likely to take sexual risks.[22,23]

When a person is exposed to HIV during sex, the virus is more likely to be transmitted if any of these three **cofactors** are involved:

- *Anal sex.* When two partners regularly have anal sex, the risk of spread of HIV from an infected partner is very high—about 40%. The risk from anal sex is not just for gay men; about 5%–10% of adult women have anal sex at least once a year.[24]

- *Lack of circumcision.* Adult men who are uncircumcised are more than twice as likely to acquire

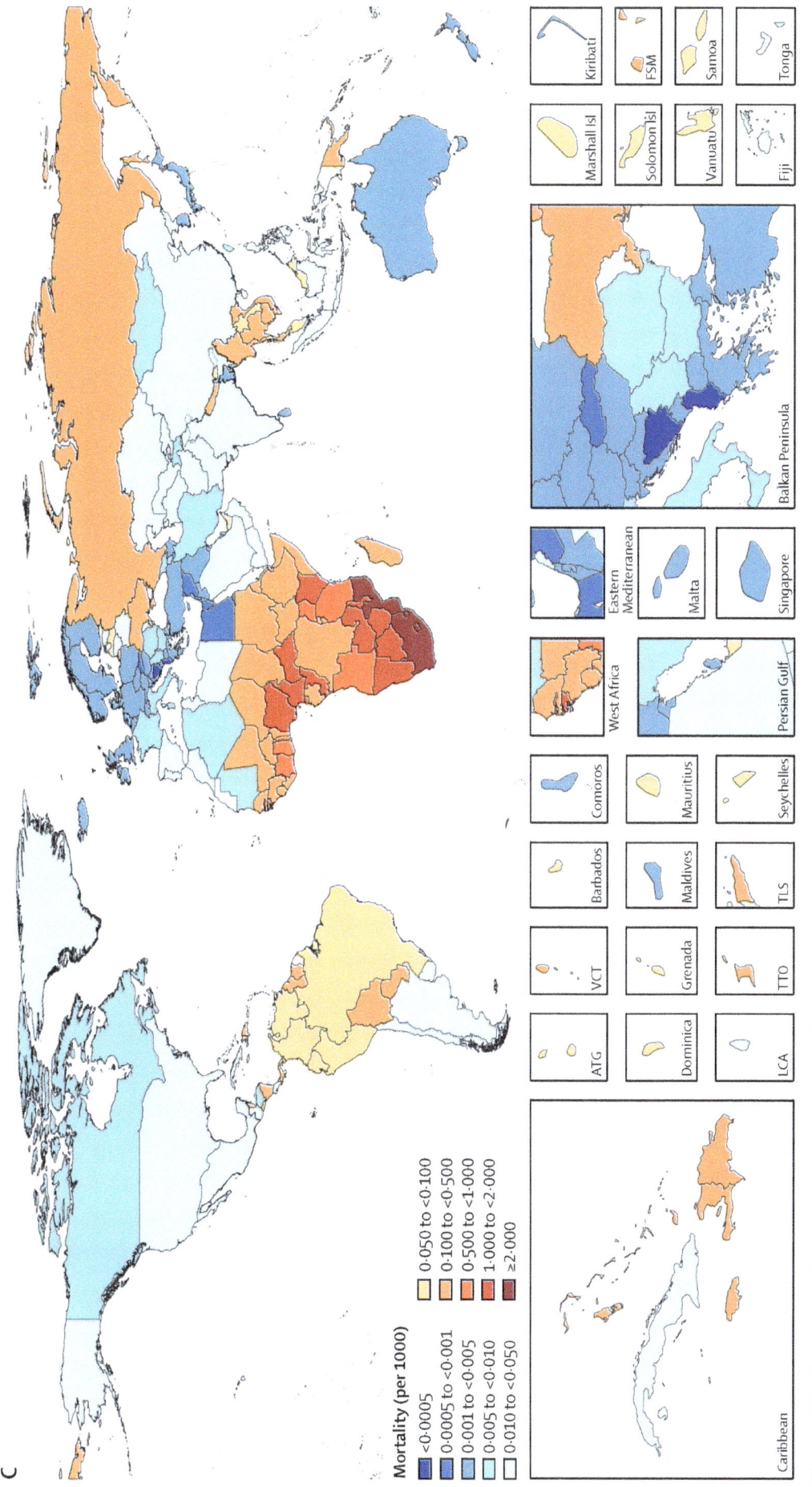

Mortality (per 1000)

- <0·0005
- 0·0005 to <0·001
- 0·001 to <0·005
- 0·005 to <0·010
- 0·010 to <0·050
- 0·050 to <0·100
- 0·100 to <0·500
- 0·500 to <1·000
- 1·000 to <2·000
- ≥2·000

Caribbean
ATG · Dominica · LCA
VCT · Grenada · TTO
Barbados · Maldives · TLS
Comoros · Mauritius · Seychelles
West Africa · Persian Gulf
Eastern Mediterranean · Malta · Singapore
Balkan Peninsula
Marshall Isl · Solomon Isl · Vanuatu · Fiji
Kiribati · FSM · Samoa · Tonga

Figure 9.11 Estimated HIV Mortality by Country, 2017.

Frank DT, Carter A, Jahagirdar D et al. Global, regional, and national incidence, prevalence, and mortality of HIV, 1980–2017, and forecasts to 2030, for 195 countries and territories: a systematic analysis for the Global Burden of Diseases, Injuries, and Risk Factors Study 2017. The Lancet HIV 2019;6,e831–59 https://doi.org/10.1016/S2352-3018(19)30196-1

C

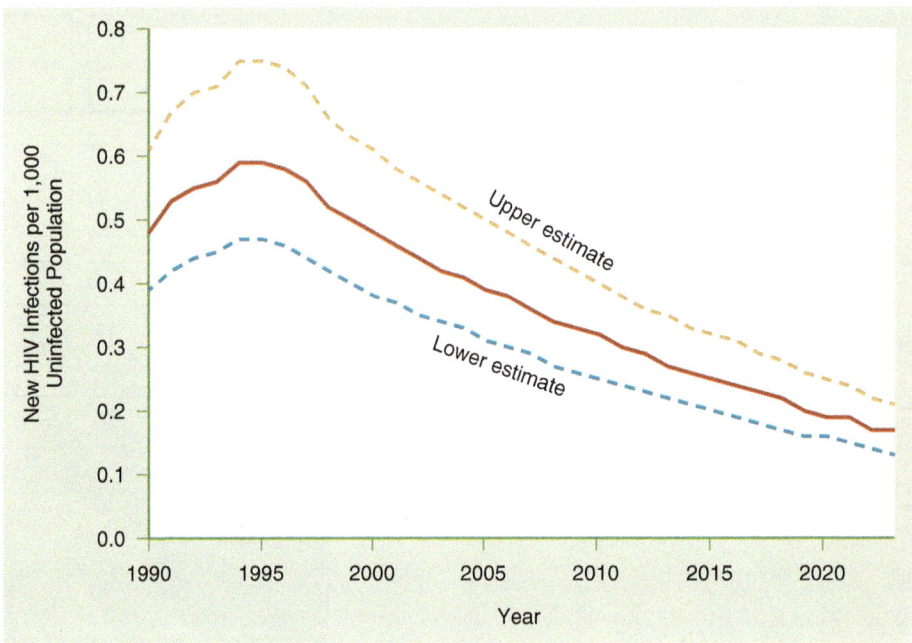

Figure 9.12 Trends in Estimated HIV Incidence Worldwide, 1990–2022.

Data from UNAIDS. AIDSinfo: Global data on HIV epidemiology and response. Accessed July 30, 2024. https://aidsinfo.unaids.org/

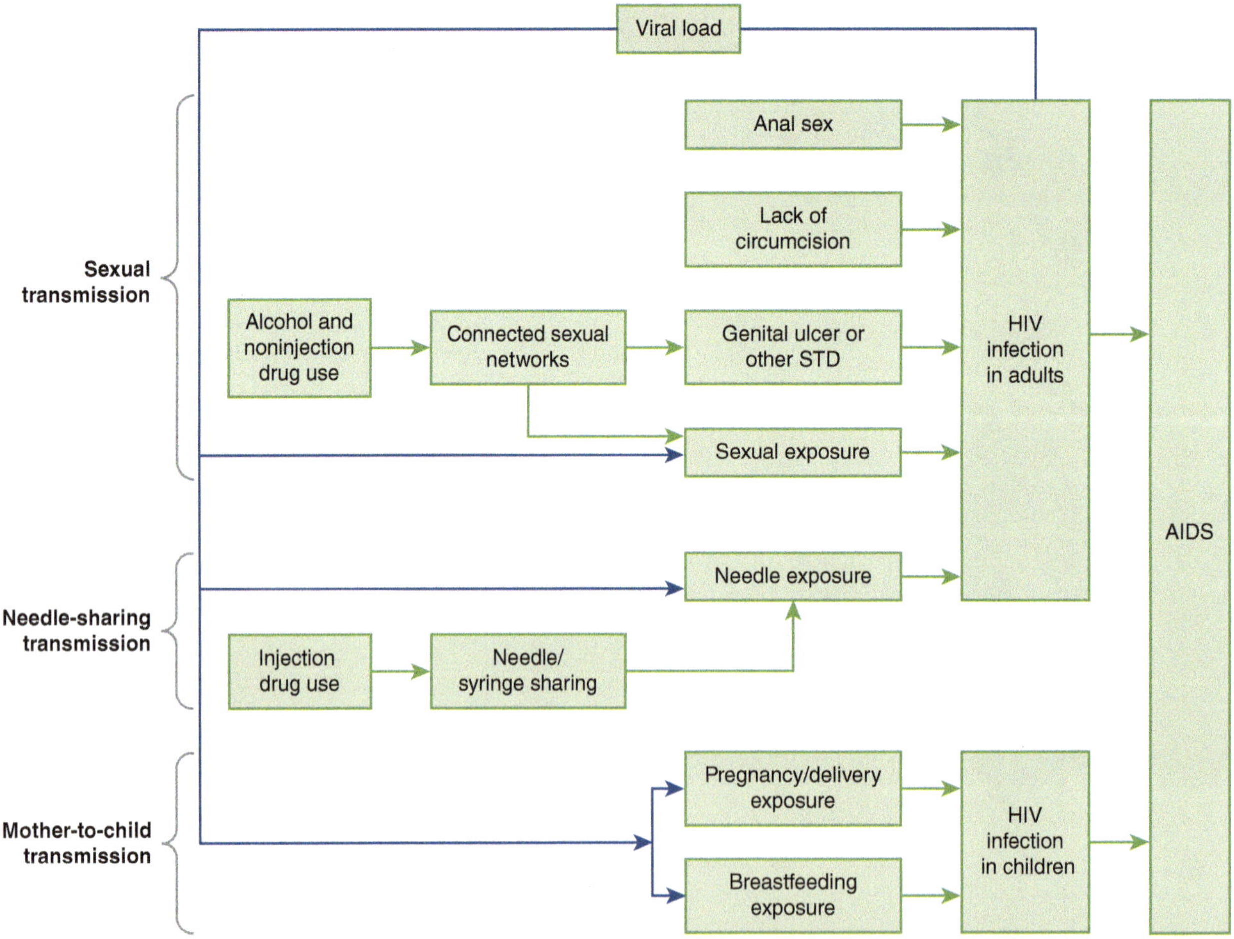

Figure 9.13 Cause-and-Effect Diagram for HIV/AIDS. The three main routes of transmission for HIV are sexual, needle-sharing, and mother-to-child. Each route has its own risk factors. However, for all of them, the viral load of the HIV-infected person involved is a key risk factor.

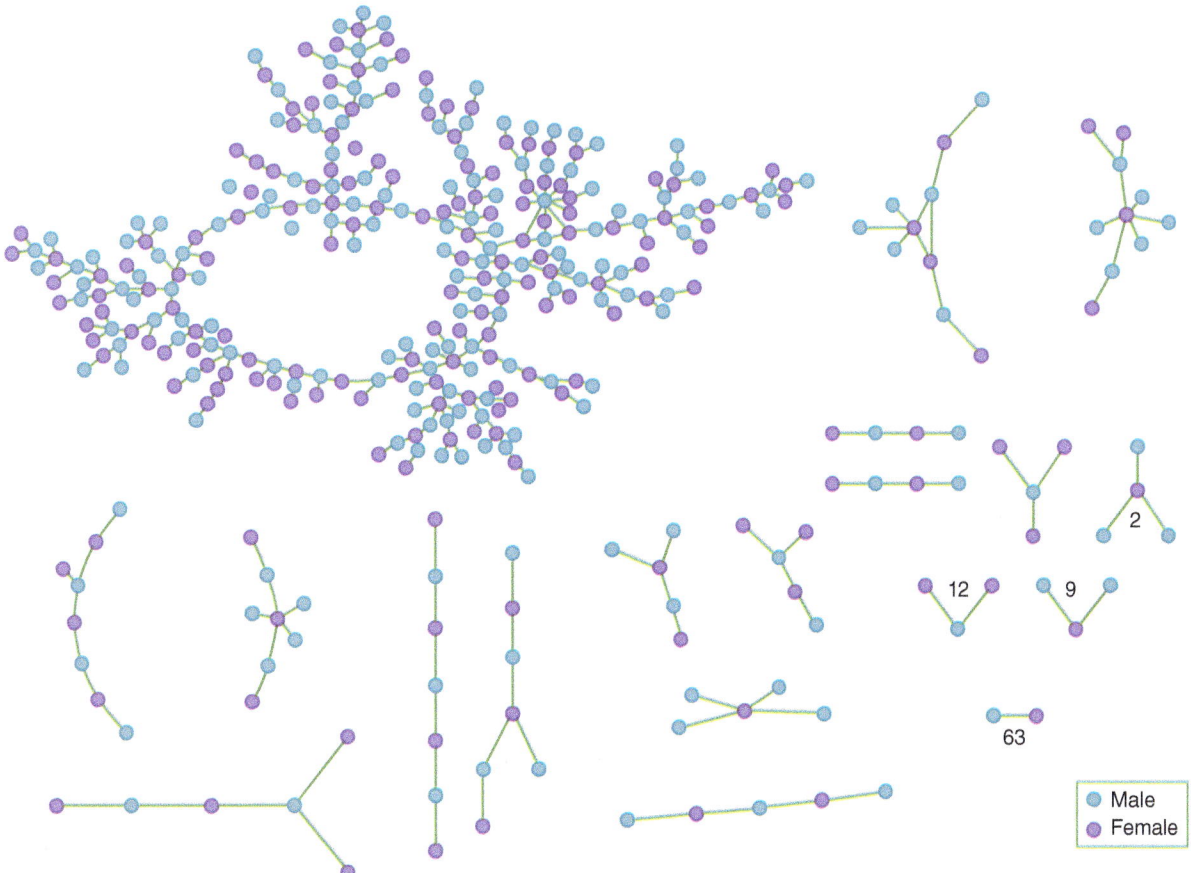

Figure 9.14 Romantic and Sexual Networks in a High School. Diagrams showing networks of romantic and sexual partnerships in a high school. Students in the unconnected networks (shown at the bottom and right) are less likely to acquire STDs than students with similar numbers of partners in the large connected network (shown at the top left).

Bearman PS, Moody J, Stovel K. Chains of Affection: The Structure of Adolescent Romantic and Sexual Networks. Am J Sociol 2004; 110:44-91 https://doi.org/10.1086/386272

HIV during sex as those who are circumcised. In Africa, studies show that areas with lower circumcision rates have higher HIV infection rates.[25] In some countries, because of religious traditions, nearly all men are circumcised, but in many countries in eastern and southern Africa, fewer than 20% are.[26]

- *Genital ulcer or other sexually transmitted diseases.* People who have genital ulcers (from syphilis, herpes, or other causes) or other sexually transmitted diseases like gonorrhea are nearly three times as likely acquire HIV during sex.[11,27]

Needle-Sharing Transmission

People can be exposed to HIV in hypodermic needles if they practice *needle or syringe sharing*. The CDC estimates that the risk of transmitting HIV from one injection drug user to another by needle sharing is about 6 per 1,000 exposures.[11] Because many drug users inject several times a day, though, people who share regularly are very likely to become infected eventually. And of course, people share needles because they are addicted to *injection drug use*.

Mother-to-Child Transmission

The main risk factor for HIV infection in children is *exposure to genital fluids during late pregnancy or delivery*. In a woman who is not receiving treatment for HIV infection, the risk of transmission during late pregnancy and delivery is quite high—about 23%.[11] The risk of transmission is higher if she has a genital ulcer or gonorrhea, which increase the number of viral particles in genital fluids.[28]

After birth, there is a risk of spread through *breastfeeding*. Current estimates are that, on average, just less than 1% of infants of HIV+ mothers who are not receiving antiviral treatment will become infected per month of breastfeeding (or about 9% over 12 months).[29]

For all routes of transmission, HIV is more likely to spread when persons with HIV have higher *viral loads*. In one study in Africa, every tenfold increase in viral load nearly tripled the risk of transmission of HIV.[27] Viral loads are high and people are more likely to transmit the infection in the first few weeks after HIV infection starts and again in the later years of HIV illness (Figure 9.8).[11] Today, the biggest influence on viral load is whether people are taking antiviral medications for their HIV infection.

Preventive Interventions

Primary Prevention of Risk Factors

The risk of HIV transmission through sex can be reduced by (**Figure 9.15**):

- *Reduction in the number of sex partners.* If people on average have fewer sex partners, sexual networks are less connected and everyone has a lower risk of sexually transmitted diseases, including HIV.[30]

- *Reduction of alcohol consumption.* Reducing population-level alcohol consumption should reduce the number of people having risky sexual encounters within connected sexual networks. See Chapter 12. Alcohol Use.

- *Promotion of condom use* among persons in connected sexual networks. If people use condoms consistently, they are much less likely to spread or catch HIV during sex.[11,27,31] Using condoms also greatly reduces the risks of catching other sexually transmitted diseases like herpes that are cofactors for HIV transmission. Unfortunately, according to estimates by UNAIDS, even when people have sex outside of steady partnerships, they use condoms only about 30% of the time.[4]

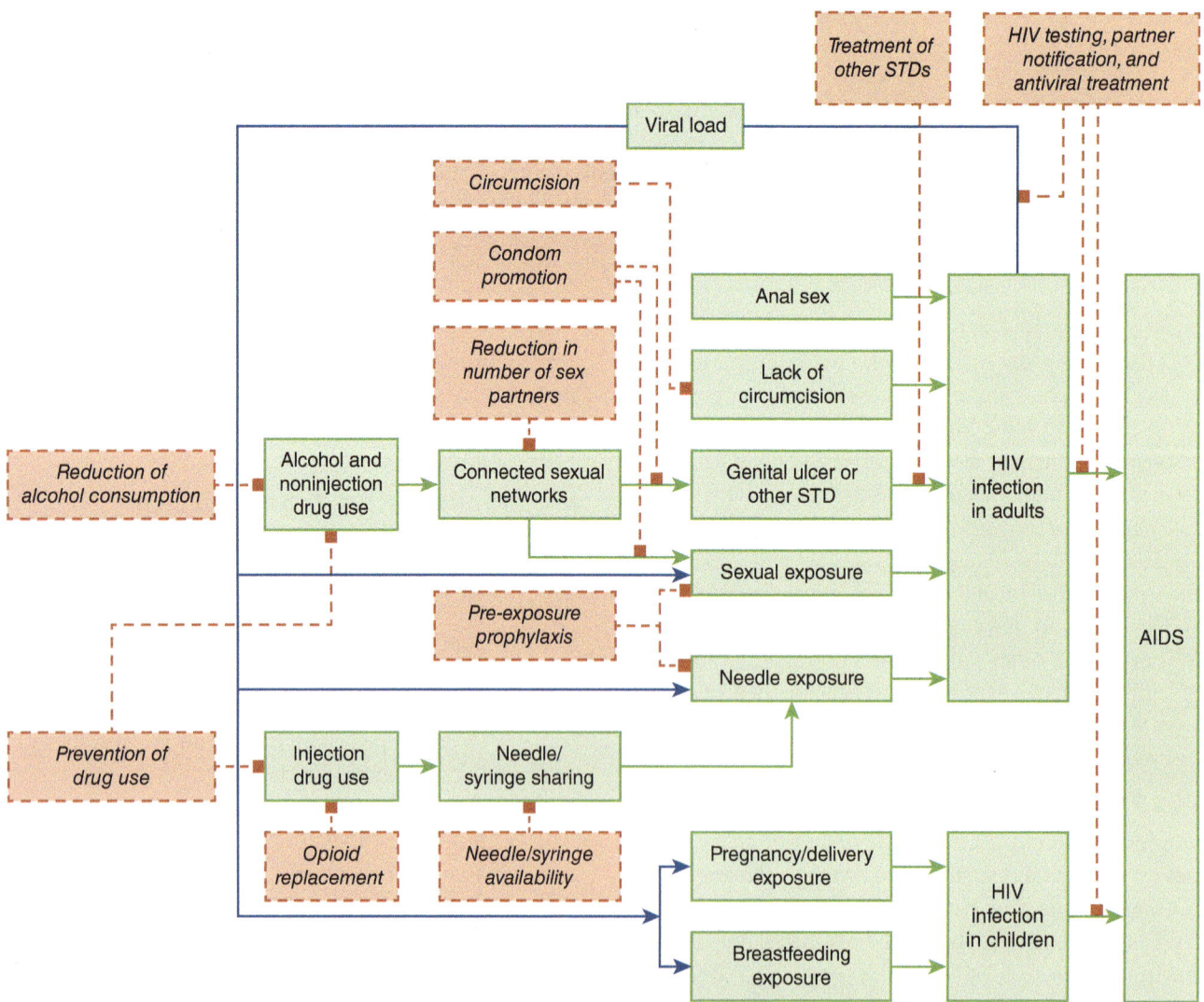

Figure 9.15 **Cause-and-Effect Diagram for HIV/AIDS, with Preventive Interventions.**

- *Male circumcision.* Research trials in Africa have shown that adult men who are circumcised reduce their risk of HIV infection by more than half.[32] To prevent HIV, 15 countries in eastern and southern Africa now offer voluntary circumcision to adult men and children. In these programs, almost 35 million males were circumcised between 2008 and 2022.[4]
- *Treatment of other sexually transmitted diseases.* Other sexually transmitted diseases like syphilis and gonorrhea that are cofactors for HIV spread can be cured by antibiotics, often with only a single dose.

The risk of HIV transmission through needle-sharing can be reduced by:

- *Prevention of drug use.* See Chapter 13. Use of Addictive Drugs.
- *Opioid replacement.* People who use heroin and other opioids sold on the street usually inject them. However, **methadone** and **buprenorphine** are opioids that prevent the symptoms of withdrawal and can be taken by mouth. If people who inject heroin or fentanyl switch entirely to these opioids, they will not spread HIV by needle sharing. This is called **opioid replacement**, and it is part of what is called **medication-assisted treatment** for drug addiction.
- *Availability of sterile needles and syringes.* Many drug users continue to inject drugs even when drug treatment programs are available to them. Providing sterile needles and syringes to these drug users reduces their need to reuse them, so they are less likely to spread HIV. Programs that give out needles and syringes (usually in exchange for returning used needles and syringes) reduce the risk of HIV by about half.[33]

Transmission of HIV by either sex or needle sharing can be greatly reduced by antiviral **pre-exposure prophylaxis (PrEP)**. This involves people who are uninfected but at high risk taking a daily pill that combines two antiviral drugs. Consistent use of PrEP reduces HIV transmission through sex by about 99% and through injection drug use by about 75%.[31,34] It is difficult to persuade people who are uninfected to take a daily pill for prevention for a long time.[34] Newer PrEP drugs that can be given by injection as infrequently as once every six months may get past this problem.[35]

For other viruses, the most successful intervention is vaccination. For decades, researchers have tried to develop a vaccine to prevent HIV infection.[36] So far, these vaccines have not succeeded, but research continues.

Antiviral Treatment

Antiviral treatment does not cure HIV, but it does stop the virus from damaging the immune system. That benefit in itself is awe-inspiring: UNAIDS estimates that just from 2001 to 2020, antiviral treatment prevented 16.5 million people from dying of AIDS. But at least as important, by reducing viral load, antiviral treatment has prevented millions of people from spreading HIV to others, and it has the potential to nearly eliminate HIV transmission.[34]

The antiviral drugs work by interfering with each of the three enzymes in HIV—reverse transcriptase, protease, and integrase. Typically, people with HIV are given a combination of two or three antiviral drugs, so the treatment is called **combination antiretroviral therapy or cART**.[34] When people take these drugs regularly, HIV slows or stops making copies of itself, and viral load levels drop so low that the virus cannot be detected by laboratory tests. Levels of CD4 lymphocytes rise back to normal, and people's immune systems are restored, so they can fight off infections again.

By reducing the viral load, the antiviral treatment reduces the risk of transmitting HIV by more than 90%.[11] In fact, studies have now confirmed that if the viral load is so low that it cannot be detected by laboratory tests, the risk of transmitting the virus through sex is zero.[37] That has led UNAIDS and the CDC to adopt the slogan "U=U" or "undetectable equals untransmittable."

Antiviral treatment also prevents pregnant women from spreading HIV to their babies during pregnancy, during delivery, or through breastfeeding. UNAIDS recommends that HIV-infected women take cART and continue to breastfeed. And antiviral treatment can help prevent transmission of HIV through needle sharing.

In theory, a particularly important time for people to take antiviral medications is in the first few weeks after they are infected, when they may have symptoms of acute HIV infection and they have very high viral loads (see Figure 9.8). In the future, more tools may be available to identify people with HIV in these early weeks so they can take antiviral treatment.

Antiviral treatment requires that people know that they are infected with HIV. That requires the ability to offer *HIV testing*. And the people who are most likely to be infected with HIV are those that are sexual partners or needle-sharing partners of people who themselves are infected. Finding those partners and offering HIV testing to them is called **partner notification** or just *partner services*.

The UNAIDS program has adopted a goal called 95/95/95, which is that 95% of people with HIV know that they are infected, 95% of those who know their status receive cART, and 95% of people receiving cART achieve **viral suppression**—that is, have an undetectable viral load.[4] If all three goals were met, at least 86% of all people with HIV infection would achieve viral suppression.

Antiviral treatment is a very complex intervention, involving widespread HIV testing, linkage of those who test positive to medical care, provision of medications, and repeated follow-up medical visits and laboratory tests.[34] Despite this complexity, this initiative has been a stunning success: as of 2022, 71% of people with HIV infection worldwide have achieved viral suppression. Perhaps even more surprising, the success has been even greater in the hardest-hit areas of southern Africa, where 77% achieved viral suppression.[4] And as of 2022, more than 80% of pregnant and breastfeeding women worldwide were receiving cART.

Still, antiviral treatment does not eradicate HIV from the body. Unless a radically new treatment is developed, the 39 million people with HIV infection around the world will have to take antiviral medications regularly for the rest of their lives. That points to the need to combine antiviral treatment with primary prevention.

Box 9.2 Summary–Prevention of HIV/AIDS

- Reduction in the number of sex partners
- Reduction of alcohol consumption
- Promotion of condom use among persons in connected sexual networks
- Male circumcision
- Treatment of other sexually transmitted diseases
- Prevention of drug use
- Opioid replacement
- Availability of sterile needles and syringes
- Pre-exposure prophylaxis (PrEP)
- HIV testing and partner notification
- Antiviral treatment

Box 9.3 Key Words–HIV/AIDS

Acquired immunity
Acquired immunodeficiency syndrome (AIDS)
Acute HIV infection
Adaptive immunity
Antibody, antibodies
Antigen
Autoimmune diseases
B lymphocytes
Buprenorphine
CD4 surface protein
Capsid
Cell-mediated immunity
Cofactor (for HIV transmission)
Combination antiretroviral therapy (cART)
Cytotoxic T lymphocytes
Envelope
Enzyme
Genital ulcer
Glycoproteins
Helper T lymphocytes
Human immunodeficiency virus (HIV)
Humoral immunity
Innate immunity
Integrase
Kaposi sarcoma
Lupus
Lymphocyte
Lymphoma
Macrophage
Medication-assisted treatment
Memory (in the immune system)
Methadone
Natural killer (NK) lymphocyte
Opioid replacement
Opportunistic infections
p24
Partner notification (for HIV)
PCP
Phagocytosis
Pre-exposure prophylaxis (PrEP)
Protease
Regulatory T lymphocytes
Retrovirus
Reverse transcriptase
Viral load
Viral suppression

Resources–HIV/AIDS

- Ghosn J, Taiwo B, Seedat S, Autran B, Katlama C. HIV. *Lancet*. 2018;392(10148):685-697. doi:10.1016/S0140-6736(18)31311-4. This is an excellent review of the biology, epidemiology, and treatment of HIV.

- The Joint United Nations Programme on HIV/AIDS (UNAIDS) maintains a portal of statistics on global HIV/AIDS at https://aidsinfo.unaids.org and publishes annual reports on its progress, such as *The Path that Ends AIDS: 2023 UNAIDS Global AIDS Update*. Geneva: Joint United Nations Programme on HIV/AIDS; 2023. Available at https://www.unaids.org/en/resources/documents/2023/global-aids-update-2023

- The CDC maintains a portal of statistics on HIV/AIDS in the United States called AtlasPlus at https://www.cdc.gov/nchhstp/atlas/index.htm. It also provides detailed scientific background on the effectiveness of strategies for preventing transmission of HIV at https://www.cdc.gov/hiv/risk/estimates/preventionstrategies.html

Diarrheal Diseases

Introduction

Diarrheal diseases (or diarrhoeal diseases, if you are British) are diseases characterized by frequent, liquid **stools** (feces). Although diarrhea can be a symptom of many different diseases, the term diarrheal diseases is usually used for infections of lining of the intestines, so a more accurate term might be intestinal infections. (A term that is often used is **gastroenteritis**, which means infection of the **gastrointestinal tract**, that is, the stomach or intestines.)

In high-income countries, diarrheal diseases are usually little more than a nuisance, but in low-income countries they are major killers of young children. Diarrheal diseases are closely linked to under nutrition. Many types of infectious agents cause diarrheal diseases, all of which are spread by the **fecal-oral route**—that is, by one person ingesting particles that are in the feces of another. The main environmental causes of diarrheal diseases are inadequate **sanitation** and unsafe sources of water.

Physiology of the Gastrointestinal Tract

The gastrointestinal tract (**Figure 9.16**) includes the mouth, esophagus, stomach, **small intestine**, and **large intestine** (including the **colon** and the **rectum**). The interior channel of this tract is called the **lumen**.

This organ system digests foods and absorbs nutrients. Solid food and liquids that are swallowed pass through the esophagus to the stomach, where they are partially broken down with acid, and then into the small intestine. The small intestine has three sections, the **duodenum**, the **jejunum**, and the **ileum**. In the lumen, food is broken down into digestible nutrients by enzymes produced by the pancreas and by **bile acids** produced by the liver. The nutrients are then absorbed through the small intestine's lining.[38]

The gastrointestinal tract also helps maintain healthy levels of water and electrolytes in the body. For solid food to be digested and absorbed, it must first

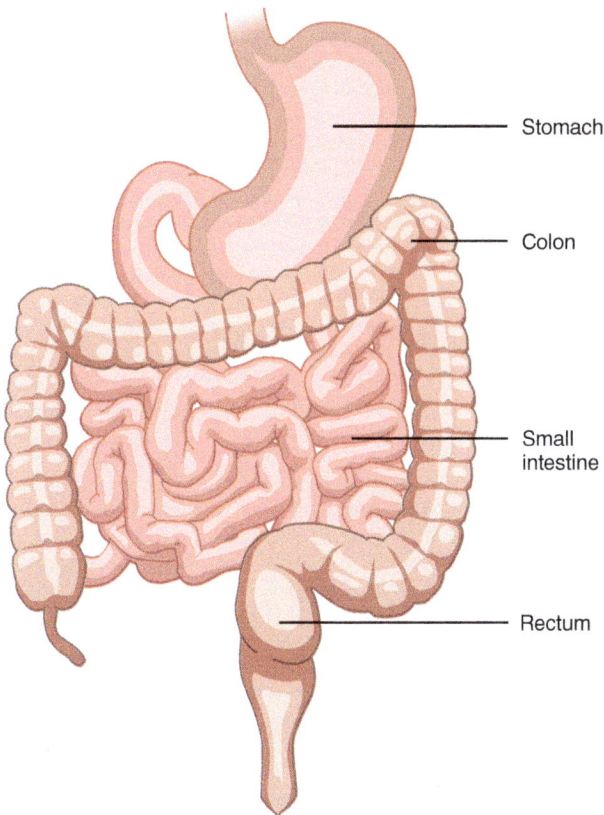

Figure 9.16 The Gastrointestinal Tract. The gastrointestinal tract includes the mouth, esophagus, stomach, small intestine (duodenum, jejunum, and ileum), and large intestine (including the colon and the rectum).

Alqahtani, M. S., Kazi, M., Alsenaidy, M. A., & Ahmad, M. Z. Advances in oral drug delivery. Frontiers in pharmacology, 2021; 12, 618411.

be liquified. To make that happen, the liver and the lining of the stomach and small intestine secrete some three to four liters of fluid per day into the lumen. If that fluid were lost to the body, a person would become dangerously dehydrated within a day. To prevent that, the small intestine reabsorbs large amounts of this fluid through its lining into the blood.[38]

The lining of the small intestine is dense with tiny finger-like peaks (called **villi**) and valleys (called **crypts**; **Figure 9.17**) that increase the surface area for absorption of nutrients and fluids. The tissue in the lining is called **epithelium** and its cells are called **epithelial** cells. The epithelial cells further increase the surface for absorption with microscopic hair-like **microvilli** that stick out from their membranes into the lumen.

The small intestine has several mechanisms to reabsorb water and electrolytes, but one is particularly important. The positive ion **sodium** (abbreviated Na+) is the main electrolyte in body fluids outside of cells; **glucose** is the main sugar that circulates in the blood. A protein embedded in the lumen side of the

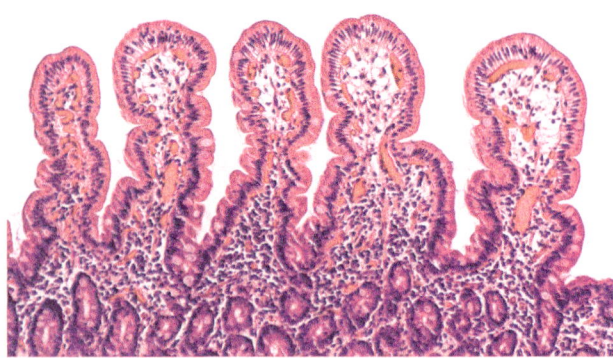

Figure 9.17 Normal Epithelium of Small Intestine. The lining of the small intestine is dense with finger-like peaks called villi and valleys called crypts that increase the surface area for absorption of nutrients and fluids.

© David A Litman/Shutterstock

epithelial cell membrane called **sodium-glucose co-transporter 1** (abbreviated **SGLT1**) actively finds both sodium and glucose in the intestinal fluid and pumps them into the cell (**Figure 9.18**). At the same time, another protein embedded in the other side of the epithelial cell pumps sodium from inside the cell to the blood, exchanging it for **potassium**. These two pumps tend to create a higher concentration of sodium in the blood than in the intestinal lumen. **Osmosis** is a word for the tendency for water to

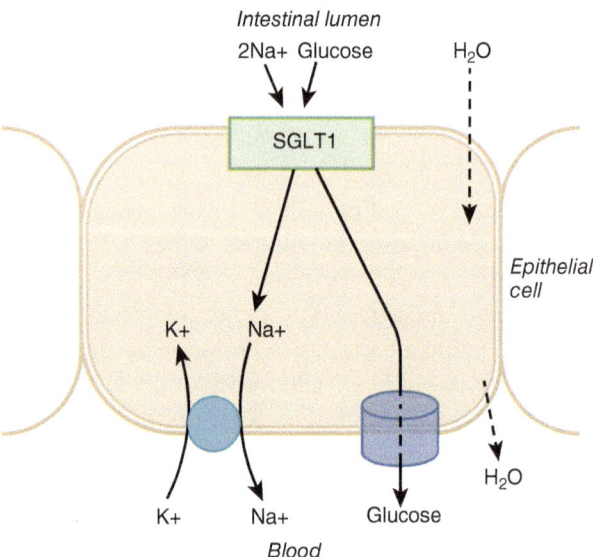

Figure 9.18 How the Sodium-Glucose Co-Transporter Causes Fluid to Be Reabsorbed Though Epithelial Cells. The sodium-glucose co-transporter 1 (SGLT1) transports sodium and glucose from the intestinal lumen into the cell. At the same time, another protein pumps sodium from the cell into the blood, exchanging it for potassium. Through osmosis, water follows sodium from the intestinal lumen into the cell and then into the blood.

equalize the concentration of solutions on either side of a membrane. Because of osmosis, water inside the intestines follows sodium across the cell membranes and into the blood.[38] This SGLT1 fluid absorption mechanism is used by oral rehydration solutions, discussed below.

At the end of the small intestine, about 1.5 liters of fluid remains in the lumen. This fluid then passes into the colon (the large intestine). If it is healthy, the colon does not secrete fluid into the lumen. Instead, it just reabsorbs most of the remaining fluid.[38]

Pathophysiology of Diarrheal Diseases

During an infection of the intestines, this system to maintain healthy fluid levels breaks down. Most infecting viruses, bacteria, or other organisms enter the epithelial cells of the small intestine and colon and multiply inside them.[38] This damages the epithelium and provokes **inflammation**, recruiting immune cells that try to kill the infecting agent. The damage from the infection and the immune response can flatten the villi and destroy the cells' microvilli.[39] This damage causes a loss of sodium and water into the intestinal lumen and reduces the ability of the epithelium to reabsorb fluid. The result is diarrhea—liquid feces and the loss to the body of water and electrolytes.[38]

In part, diarrhea can be helpful because it helps the body rid itself of the infecting organism. But that benefit carries with it two big risks. First, the loss of fluid can be large enough to cause dangerous **dehydration**—a condition in which the body does not have enough fluids to maintain healthy organ systems. Small children, whose bodies contain little fluid, are particularly vulnerable to dehydration. Second, the feces of persons with gastroenteritis contain very many infectious organisms, so the infection is easily spread to others.

Diarrheal diseases vary in how severe they are and how long they last. For collecting data in populations:

- **Diarrhea** is defined as the passage of three or more loose or liquid stools per day;
- **Acute watery diarrhea** is an episode of diarrhea that lasts several hours or days in which blood is not found in feces;
- **Acute bloody diarrhea**, also called **dysentery**, is an episode of diarrhea in which blood is present in feces; and
- **Persistent diarrhea** is an episode of diarrhea that lasts 14 days or longer.[40]

Pathogens That Cause Diarrheal Diseases

Many different **pathogens** can cause diarrheal diseases. **Table 9.2** lists the pathogens found most often in children with diarrhea in areas of the world with unsafe water and sanitation.[41-43] The connection between pathogens and symptoms is a little complicated: children with diarrhea in these areas often carry more than one pathogen, and many children without symptoms of diarrhea, if tested, are found to also carry these pathogens.[41,44] But the pathogens do follow some patterns:

- *Viruses* tend to cause acute watery diarrhea that lasts only a few days, and to cause less long-lasting damage than other types of pathogens.[45-47] Viruses are extremely easily spread from one person to another, so outbreaks occur even among groups

---

Table 9.2 Pathogens Causing Diarrhea in Low- and Middle-Income Countries

Most Common	
Viruses	Rotavirus
	Adenovirus 40/41
	Sapovirus
	Norovirus
	Astrovirus
Bacteria	Shigella
	Camplyobacter
	Escherichia coli (enteroinvasive)
	Escherichia coli (entertoxigenic)
	Escherichia coli (enterpathogenic)
Others	Cryptosporidium

Less Common	
Bacteria	Salmonella
	Aeromonas
	Helicobacter pylori
	Escherichia coli (enteraggregative)
Others	Giardia
	Cystoisospora
	Cyclospora
	Entamoeba

---

with excellent sanitation, water, and hygiene. Viruses can usually be eliminated from water with **hypochlorite**, the active ingredient in bleach. **Rotavirus** was an extremely common cause of winter or spring outbreaks of acute watery diarrhea in infants until the development of a rotavirus vaccine.[48] Other viruses, such as **norovirus** and **adenovirus types 40/41**, continue as common causes of diarrhea.

- *Shigella* is a bacterium that invades the epithelium and does more damage than viruses. Infection with shigella often causes bloody diarrhea.[47] While not as easily spread as viruses, *Shigella* is more readily transmitted than other bacteria, so it is the most frequent bacterial cause of childhood diarrhea in low-income countries. Outbreaks occur even in high-income countries in childcare centers.

- *Campylobacter* is a bacterium that can cause either watery diarrhea or bloody diarrhea. It is sometimes found in poultry or raw milk and occasionally causes outbreaks in high-income countries, but it is far more common as a cause of diarrhea in countries with inadequate sanitation.[43,47]

- *Escherichia coli* (commonly called *E. coli*) is an abundant species of bacteria that lives in everyone's gastrointestinal tract as part of the normal, healthy **gut microbiome**. However, rare strains of *Escherichia coli* produce toxins or damage the intestinal epithelium in other ways. These pathogenic strains are labeled by the damage they cause. **Enteroinvasive E. coli** invades the epithelium as *Shigella* does and is similar to *Shigella* in other ways. **Enterotoxigenic E. coli** does not invade the epithelium, but instead produces a toxin that stimulates secretion of fluid, causing a severe diarrhea; this is a common cause of "traveler's diarrhea." **Enteropathogenic E. coli** and **Enteroaggregative E. coli** each have other, unique ways of damaging the epithelial cells.[47]

- *Vibrio cholera* causes the disease called cholera.[47] In most times it is an uncommon cause of diarrheal diseases, but in areas with little sanitation it can periodically cause huge, deadly outbreaks. For example, the cholera outbreak that took place in Haiti after the earthquake of 2010 sickened 600,000 and killed at least 7,400 people.[49] *Vibrio cholera* does not invade the epithelial cells. Instead, it produces a toxin that causes the epithelial cells in the ileum and colon to secrete sodium and chloride into the lumen, leading to very watery diarrhea. People with cholera can lose 5-10 liters of fluid per day. Cholera is a rare diarrheal disease that can kill otherwise healthy adults through dehydration.[38]

- *Cryptosporidium* is a very common cause of diarrheal disease in low-income countries. The organism is a protozoan that has many stages in its life cycle. It survives well in water and is resistant to bleach, but it can be removed by filtering water. In high-income countries, outbreaks have been traced to contaminated swimming pools and public water systems.[50] Cryptosporidium invades the epithelial cells and interferes with sodium absorption, causing watery diarrhea that can last two weeks or more.[45-47,50,51]

Health Consequences of Diarrhea: Dehydration and Undernutrition

The two major consequences of diarrheal diseases are dehydration and undernutrition.

Dehydration occurs if so much fluid is lost that the blood volume is too low to supply fluid and nutrients to vital organs. Dehydration once was a common killer of young children in areas without good sanitation. Now, with the use of oral rehydration solution and other treatments, death from dehydration is much less common.[40]

The connection between diarrheal diseases and undernutrition remains strong, though, especially in children. The relationship goes in both directions (**Figure 9.19**). Children with undernutrition are more vulnerable to developing diarrhea because the weakened epithelial tissues and immune system are less able to fight off an infection. At the same time, diarrheal diseases cause undernutrition,[52] for three reasons. First, children feeling sick with diarrheal diseases often do not eat as much food. Second, the disease causes a breakdown of tissues throughout the body, which increases the need for nutrients. And third, the damage to the intestinal epithelium caused by infections— such as flattened villi and loss of microvilli—leaves the epithelium less capable of absorbing nutrients.[40,53] The undernutrition caused by intestinal infections involves both **macronutrients** (carbohydrates, fats, and proteins) and **micronutrients** like **vitamins** and essential **minerals**. (Vitamins are small organic compounds needed by human cells that must be obtained from food.)

Undernutrition from diarrhea can harm children permanently. Young children in low-income settings with diarrhea are more likely to become **stunted**, that is, short for their age.[54] Even children who do not have overt diarrhea but are found to carry the bacteria listed in Table 9.2 grow more slowly afterward.[55] For *Shigella*, antibiotic treatment has been shown to limit this damaging effect on growth.[56]

More important, children with diarrhea are much more likely to die afterward. In one study, children with even a single episode of diarrhea had a mortality rate about eight times that of children without diarrhea in the following three months.[44,56] In part, this is because diarrhea can cause or exacerbate a deficiency in Vitamin A, which is deadly (**Box 9.4**), but probably many other nutritional deficiencies contribute.[57]

Transmission of Diarrheal Pathogens

The pathogens listed in Table 9.2 are present in the feces of persons who have infections. They can be spread to other persons through several routes, as shown in **Figure 9.20**. Many of these routes involve words that start with the letter F, so this has been called the "F Diagram."

Spread of enteric pathogens can happen through:

- Fields that have been contaminated with feces when persons defecate on the ground;

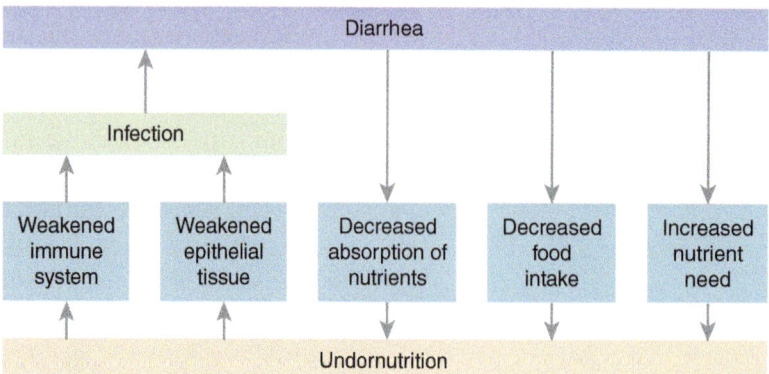

Figure 9.19 **Relationship Between Diarrheal Diseases and Undernutrition.** Diarrheal diseases can cause undernutrition and undernutrition increases the risk of diarrheal diseases.

Box 9.4 Diarrhea and Vitamin A deficiency

In the 1980s, researchers in Indonesia trying to prevent blindness made an astonishing discovery: children given large doses of Vitamin A were one-third less likely to die afterward.[58] Later, studies from other low-income countries confirmed this powerful benefit of Vitamin A supplements. Giving children Vitamin A is now estimated to reduce child mortality by 23%.[59]

Vitamin A is needed for chemical processes involved in growth, the immune system, vision, and maintaining a healthy epithelium. People who do not take in enough Vitamin A have weakened immune systems, **night blindness** (difficulty seeing in dim light), dry eyes, and damage to the membranes lining the respiratory tract and gastrointestinal tract. Children who do not consume enough Vitamin A grow slowly, have difficulty fighting off infections, and are more likely to die from many illnesses—especially from measles.[60,61] They are also more likely to have a serious bout of diarrheal disease.[53,62-64] And children with diarrhea are more likely to become deficient in Vitamin A.

Vitamin A is not a single chemical, but instead a group of compounds found in orange colored-vegetables (like carrots, sweet potatoes, and pumpkins), dark leafy greens (like kale and spinach), dairy products, liver, and fish. Breast milk contains just enough Vitamin A for babies' daily needs, but not enough for them to build up stores. Children in low- and middle-income countries with narrow diets often do not get enough of any Vitamin A-containing foods, so they become deficient in Vitamin A, especially in the months after they stop breastfeeding.

The percentage of children who are deficient in Vitamin A has been falling since 1990, but it is still a very common problem.[65] By current estimates, 20% of children aged 0-5 years in low- and middle-income countries are deficient in Vitamin A; in Africa, more than 30% are.[66]

If people take in large amounts of Vitamin A, the excess is stored in the liver, to be mobilized later when the body needs it. That is why Vitamin A deficiency can be treated by giving children infrequent, large doses of Vitamin A. Since the 1990s, many countries around the world have been giving Vitamin A supplements to all children twice a year.[61] UNICEF estimates that in 2022, 59% of children in low-and middle-income countries received two supplements.[67] Some countries also "fortify" commonly eaten foods like cooking oils, wheat flour, or refined sugar with Vitamin A.[61]

- Fluids (that is, water) that have been contaminated with feces;
- Flies that get pathogens on their legs when they rest on feces and then transport those pathogens to food, persons, or the objects that persons touch;
- **Fomites**, which are objects that people touch, like countertops, utensils, toys, or towels.
- Fingers (that is, direct contact); or
- Food that has been contaminated by contact with the previous Fs.[68]

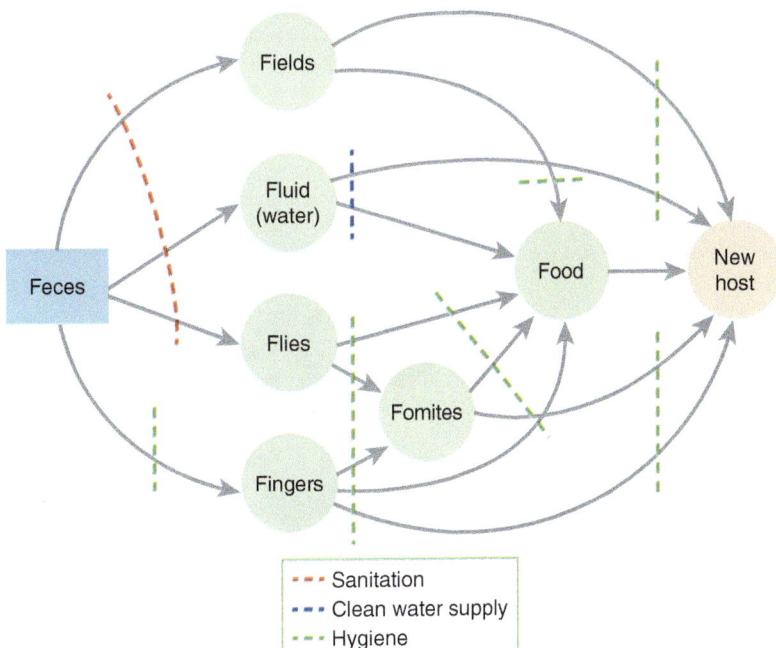

Figure 9.20 **"F-Diagram" Showing Possible Routes of Spread of Enteric Pathogens from One Person to Another.**
Enteric pathogens can be spread from an infected person to others through several routes, all of which involve words that start with the letter F. Sanitation, clean water, and hygiene (particularly handwashing) can each interrupt some of these routes, and the combination is most effective.

The importance of each route depends on which pathogens is involved and the circumstances in which people live.

Infection can be spread by extraordinarily small amounts of feces. For example, a person with diarrhea from *Shigella* infection may produce as many as 10^9 organism per gram in stool, and an infection can be caused by just a few hundred organisms.[47] That means that one *ten-millionth of a gram* of feces is enough to cause an infection. Even people who wash their hands thoroughly after defecating can leave this much behind.

Viruses are spread even more easily. For example, people with rotavirus infection may produce 10^{11} viral particles per gram of feces, and ingesting only 10 of these particles may be enough to cause an infection.[47] That means that, if one gram of stool is diluted with an Olympic-sized swimming pool's worth of (unchlorinated) water, the water is contaminated enough that a few drops can cause an infection.

With infection spread this easily, it is virtually impossible to prevent all diarrheal diseases. For example, there will always be some spread in high-risk situations, like villages without running water or toilets, or childcare centers among children who are not toilet trained. However, transmission can be greatly reduced by water, sanitation, and hygiene (**WASH**)—that is, providing safe water and sanitation and promoting hand washing with soap (Figure 9.20).

Epidemiology: Patterns and Trends

Diarrheal diseases kill about 400,000 children under age 5 each year around the world, ranking these diseases just below malaria and lower respiratory infections among the top three killers of young children in low-income countries.[69,70] Mortality rates are highest in sub-Saharan Africa and South Asia, but high rates persist in a few other areas (**Figure 9.21**). With economic development leading to improved water, sanitation, and hygiene, diarrhea-caused deaths are falling (**Figure 9.22**).

Risk Factors

Risk factors for diarrheal diseases in children in low-income areas are (**Figure 9.23**):

- *Unsafe disposal of feces.* Any situation in which even small amounts of human or animal feces can get on humans' hands is one in which diarrhea-causing pathogens can spread. The most unsafe practice is open defecation. **Pit latrines**, which are holes in the ground for deposition of human waste, are somewhat safer, but their safety depends on how well they are designed to protect users from exposure to feces.[71-75]

- *Unsafe water.* Water can easily become contaminated with pathogens from human feces at its source, during distribution, or during storage in the home.

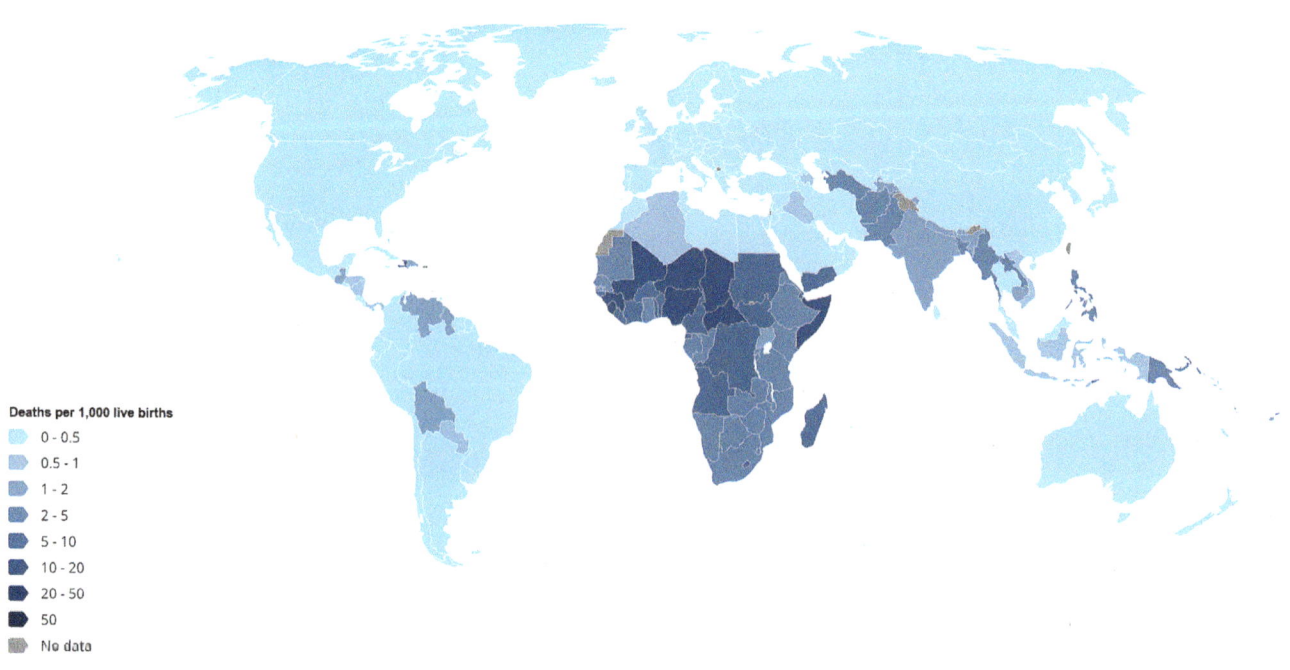

Deaths per 1,000 live births
- 0 - 0.5
- 0.5 - 1
- 1 - 2
- 2 - 5
- 5 - 10
- 10 - 20
- 20 - 50
- 50
- No data

Figure 9.21 **Mortality Rate for Children Under Age 5 from Diarrheal Diseases by Country, 2021.**

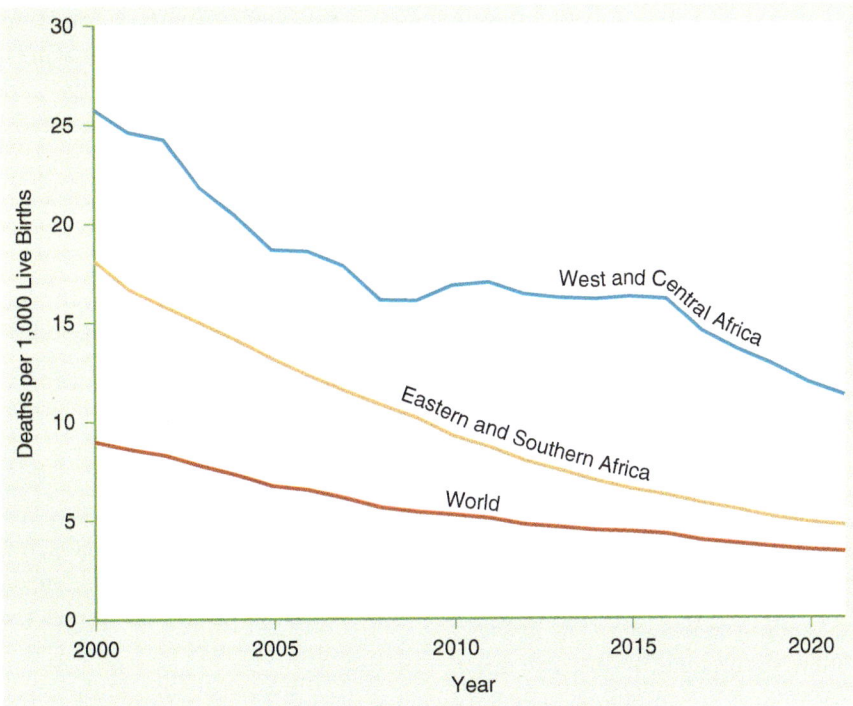

Figure 9.22 **Trends in Mortality from Diarrheal Diseases in Children Under Age 5.**

Data from United Nations Inter-Agency Group for Child Mortality Estimation. Accessed July 30, 2024. https://childmortality.org

In low-income communities, water is unsafe if is not treated to remove pathogens, not distributed to homes (for example, available only at a community tap or well), available only intermittently, or stored in open containers in the home.[71-77]

- *Insufficient handwashing.* When family members do not wash their hands with water and soap regularly (especially after defecation and before handling food), the risk of diarrheal diseases is higher.[71-73,78,79]
- *Undernutrition.* As described above, children who are malnourished are more likely to develop diarrheal diseases and to die from them.[71,80,81]

- *Suboptimal breastfeeding.*[71,73,74] Breastfeeding protects infants from diarrheal diseases in three ways. First, infants who feed only on breast milk are far less likely to ingest pathogens in water or food. Second, breast milk contains **antibodies** and other infection-preventing characteristics, so those who are exposed to pathogens are less likely to become infected.[82] And third, infants who breastfeed are less likely to become malnourished, so their immune systems are better able to combat an infection that does occur.[83] The risk from stopping breastfeeding early is very high. The World Health Organization (WHO)

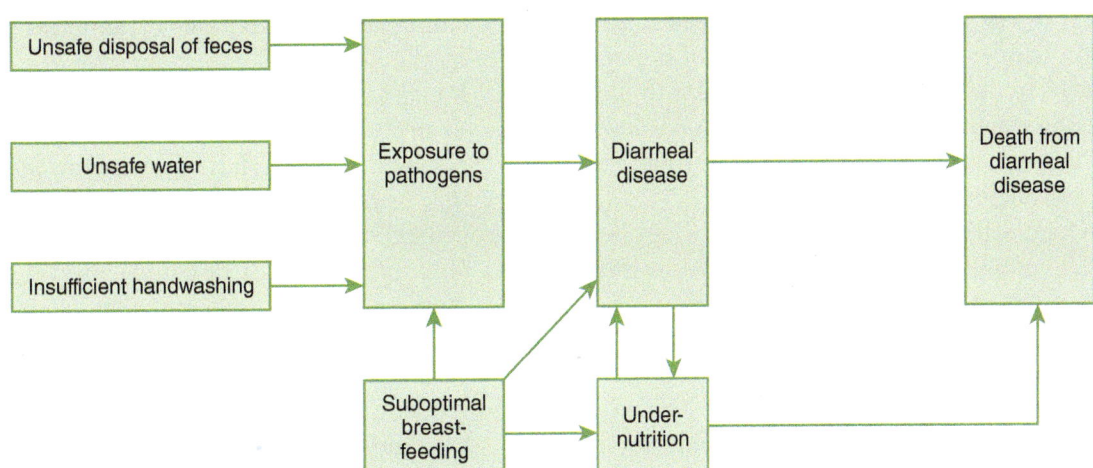

Figure 9.23 **Cause-and-Effect Diagram for Diarrheal Diseases.**

estimates that babies who are not exclusively breastfed for six months are about 10 times as likely to die from diarrheal diseases, and babies who do not continue breastfeeding from 6 to 24 months of age are about three times as likely to die from them.[84]

In addition, some studies have found that living with domestic animals increases the risk of diarrhea, probably because some human pathogens (for example, cryptosporidium and *Camplyobacter*) can be carried by those animals. And some studies have found that household crowding increases the risk.[72,73,77]

Finally, even in countries where nearly everyone has a low income by the U.S. standards, diarrhea is more common in families with lower socioeconomic status—for example, those with less income, mothers with less education, or fewer assets.[71-73,76,78,80] In these studies, socioeconomic status may be just a marker for especially unsafe water and sanitation, or it may reflect the "piling on" of the multiple risks of poverty. Socioeconomic risks to health are discussed in Chapter 16. Social Disadvantage.

Preventive Interventions

The WHO has adopted an integrated plan for diarrhea and pneumonia because these problems overlap so much.[84] For diarrheal diseases, the plan includes both primary prevention and secondary prevention.

Primary Prevention

Diarrheal diseases can be prevented by (**Figure 9.24**):

- *Safely-managed sanitation.*[84] Systems for safer disposal of human wastes are typically referred to as sanitation although the word "sanitation," is also used to describe cleanliness more broadly. The WHO and UNICEF have developed a "Sanitation Ladder" that ranks the safety of different types of facilities; the agencies use these to measure the quality of sanitation at national levels and to track progress.[85] The ranking, from least to most safe, is:
  - Open defecation
  - Unimproved pit latrines—that is, without barriers to human contact with feces
  - Limited improved latrines—that is, with barriers to human contact with feces, but facilities shared between households
  - Basic improved latrines—that is, with barriers to human contact with feces, and not shared between households

- Safely-managed sanitation. Safely-managed facilities are those that are improved, not shared between households, and in which feces are safely stored, transported, and treated.

  Building latrines reduces the rate of diarrheal diseases by about 20%, and installing toilets connected to sewers reduces the rate by about one-half.[75]

- *Provision of safe water.*[84] There are many ways water can be made safer, limited mainly by cost. The *quality* of the water can be improved by treating it chemically to kill pathogens, filtering it, and treating it with ultraviolet light.[86] Water *quantity* and the consistency of delivery can be increased because when more water is available, people use more for cleaning themselves and their households.[86] Water *distribution* can be improved by building pipes into homes instead of community taps. The ultimate goal should always be a continuous, cost-free, pathogen-free supply of water provided directly to each home. Interventions in which families have been given treated water piped directly into their homes have cut rates of diarrheal diseases in half.[75]

- *Promotion of handwashing with soap.* Promoting handwashing with soap reduces the incidence of diarrheal diseases by about 30%.[79,84] The best way to promote this is to provide a continuous supply of water to homes so that handwashing is easy to do.

- *Breastfeeding promotion.* The WHO recommends that all babies breastfeed exclusively for the first six months and continue to breastfeed until their second birthday.

- *Prevention or treatment of undernutrition.* Any actions that reduce undernutrition should also reduce the incidence and mortality from diarrheal diseases.[87] Chapter 14. Nutrition discusses causes and prevention of undernutrition in mothers and children.

- *Vitamin A supplementation.* Giving supplements to all children in countries where Vitamin A deficiency is a public health problem reduces their risk of dying from diarrheal diseases and other causes.[84]

- *Vaccination.* The list of pathogens that can cause diarrheal diseases is so long that vaccination will never be able to protect children entirely. However, vaccination against the most common causes can reduce rates of some diarrheal diseases. Vaccines are currently available and widely used to prevent rotavirus infection.[84] Vaccines against cholera are available; these have been used to respond

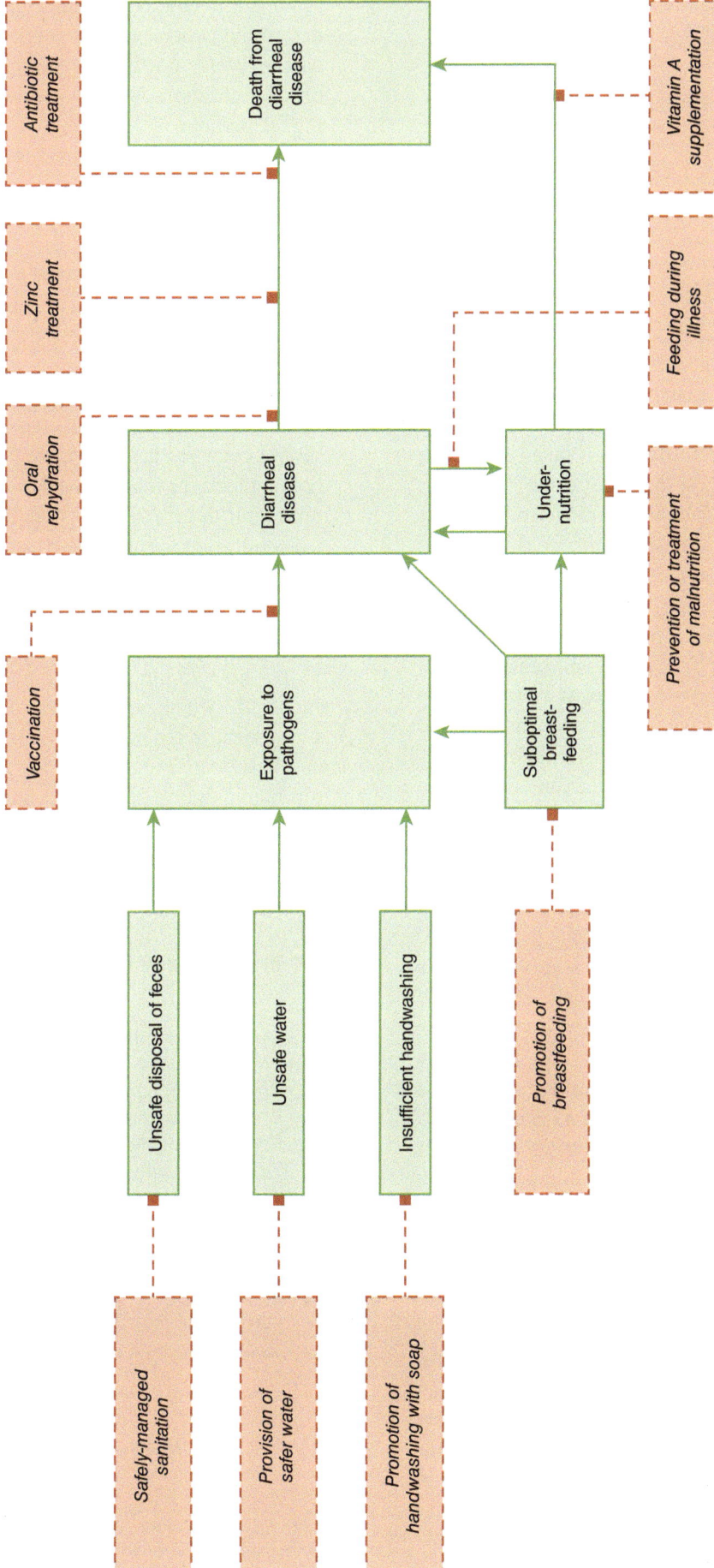

Figure 9.24 **Cause-and-Effect Diagram for Diarrheal Diseases, with Preventive Interventions.**

to outbreaks and in hot spots.[46] Vaccines against other diarrheal pathogens are being developed.

Secondary Prevention

Children with diarrheal diseases can be treated in ways that greatly reduce dehydration, undernutrition, and mortality. Some key recommendations today differ completely from how children were treated in the past. The harm caused by diarrhea can be reduced by:

- *Oral rehydration.* A discovery that has probably saved millions of lives over the past 50 years is that children with diarrhea absorb more fluid if they drink a solution that contains both sodium and glucose.[88] This combination takes advantage of the sodium glucose co-transporter 1 (SGLT1) in the small intestine. When both sodium and glucose are in the intestine, the epithelial cells absorb the two together (see Figure 9.18). Then, because of osmosis, water is also absorbed into the epithelial cells and from there into the blood. Fluid that contains the optimal concentrations of sodium and glucose is called **oral rehydration solution**. WHO distributes recommendations to countries on how to make this solution. Countries around the world manufacture packets of glucose and electrolytes meeting these specifications, which families dissolve in water and give to their children when they have diarrhea. The use of oral rehydration solutions reduces deaths from diarrheal diseases by perhaps as much as 93%.[84,89]

- *Zinc treatment.* Zinc is an essential mineral needed for several metabolic processes. Zinc helps the immune system function. People living in low-income countries with narrow diets can have zinc deficiency.[90] When children have a bout of diarrhea, they lose more zinc than normal and have a reduced ability to absorb it, which increases their zinc needs. Children with diarrhea who are given zinc supplements have less severe symptoms, recover more quickly, and are less likely to have a repeat bout of diarrhea.[90] The WHO recommends that all children in low- and middle-income countries with diarrheal diseases be given zinc supplements for 10-14 days.[91]

- *Antibiotics for children with bacterial pathogens.* When *Shigella* and certain other bacteria are the cause of diarrheal disease, taking **antibiotics** can shorten the illness and prevent many adverse consequences.[46,92] However, antibiotics are not helpful for people with diarrhea caused by other types of organisms like viruses or by cryptosporidium, and can even be harmful.[92,93] Many clinics in low-income countries cannot carry out tests that determine which organisms are causing diarrhea, so the WHO currently recommends antibiotics only for children with bloody diarrhea.[93,94] If testing for pathogens becomes more widely available, antibiotic treatment for diarrheal disease may be better targeted to children with proven bacterial infections.[46]

- *Feeding during illness.* A remarkably simple intervention to treat children with diarrhea—a recommendation that may seem so obvious that it feels unnecessary to state—is feeding. In the past, pediatricians recommended children with diarrhea be given "bowel rest"—that is, no feeding for 12–48 hours, followed by gradually restarting feeding over several days. Studies have clearly shown that withholding food during diarrheal disease just increases undernutrition.[40,53] Infants and children should be fed continuously during diarrheal disease.

By one estimate, the interventions most responsible for reducing deaths from diarrhea from 1980 to 2015 were oral rehydration, reduction of undernutrition, and Vitamin A supplementation.[95] But the World Health Organization estimates that 69% of the remaining deaths are attributable to unsafe drinking water, unsafe sanitation, or inadequate hygiene, so the ultimate solution to this problem lies in WASH facilities.[70] One of the United Nation's 17 Sustainable Development Goals is to provide safe drinking water and sanitation for everyone by 2030.[96]

Box 9.5 Strategy Summary

- ■ Primary Prevention
  - Safely-managed sanitation
  - Provision of safe water
  - Promotion of handwashing with soap
  - Breastfeeding promotion
  - Prevention or treatment of undernutrition
  - Vitamin A supplementation
  - Vaccination
- ■ Secondary Prevention
  - Oral rehydration
  - Zinc treatment
  - Antibiotics for children with bacterial pathogens
  - Feeding during illness

Box 9.6 Key Words–Diarrhea Diseases

Acute bloody diarrhea
Acute watery diarrhea
Adenovirus type 40 or 41

Antibiotic
Antibody, antibodies
Bile acids
Colon
Crypts
Dehydration
Diarrhea
Diarrheal (or diarrhoeal) diseases
Duodenum
Dysentery
Enteroaggregative E. coli
Enteroinvasive E. coli
Enteropathogenic E. coli
Enterotoxigenic E. coli
Epithelium, epithelial cells
Fecal-oral route
Fomite
Gastroenteritis
Gastrointestinal tract
Glucose
Gut microbiome
Hypochlorite
Ileum
Inflammation
Jejunum
Large intestine
Lumen
Macronutrients
Micronutrients
Microvillus (plural microvilli)
Minerals
Night blindness
Norovirus
Oral rehydration solution
Osmosis
Pathogen
Persistent diarrhea
Pit latrine
Potassium
Rectum
Rotavirus
Sanitation
Small intestine
Sodium
Sodium-glucose co-transporter 1 (SGLT1)
Stools
Stunted, stunting
Villus (plural villi)
Vitamin A
Vitamins
WASH

Resources–Diarrheal Diseases

- Platts-Mills JA, Liu J, Rogawski ET, et al. Use of quantitative molecular diagnostic methods to assess the aetiology, burden, and clinical characteristics of diarrhoea in children in low-resource settings: a reanalysis of the MAL-ED cohort study. *Lancet Glob Health*. 2018;6(12):e1309-e1318. doi: 10.1016/S2214-109X(18)30349-8. This is one of the largest studies on the different pathogens that cause diarrheal illness.
- Wolf J, Hubbard S, Brauer M, et al. Effectiveness of interventions to improve drinking water, sanitation, and handwashing with soap on risk of diarrhoeal disease in children in low-income and middle-income settings: a systematic review and meta-analysis. *The Lancet*. 2022;400(10345): 48-59. doi:10.1016/S0140-6736(22)00937-0.
- The World Health Organization has many resources on diarrheal illness. The *Safer Water, Better Health* report provides evidence for the many specific health benefits of safer water. The plan to prevent diarrhea and pneumonia is *Ending Preventable Child Deaths from Pneumonia and Diarrhoea by 2025: The Integrated Global Action Plan for Pneumonia and Diarrhoea (GAPPD)*. These are available at http://www.who.int/publications. A web page on *Water, sanitation, and hygiene (WASH)* has many other resources at https://www.who.int /health-topics/water-sanitation-and-hygiene-wash
- The WHO and UNICEF have a *Joint Monitoring Programme for Water Supply, Sanitation, and Hygiene* that tracks progress on the availability of these facilities (including the "sanitation ladder") at https://washdata.org

Lower Respiratory Infections

Introduction

In December 2019, the world learned that a new virus was infecting people in Wuhan, China. What followed was a pandemic that readers will not forget, with billions of people infected, millions dying, and extraordinary disruptions in daily life from attempts to contain the virus.

The COVID-19 pandemic was unique, but it was only the most vivid example of a major, ongoing public health problem: infections of the lung and small airways, called **lower respiratory infections** or **LRI**, and often referred to **pneumonia**. The Global Burden of Disease project estimates that COVID-19 killed 7.3 million people worldwide from 2020 through 2022.[97] But just before the pandemic, LRI killed an estimated 2.5 million people in only a single year.[98]

Lower respiratory infections (LRI) affect nearly everyone, but they kill mainly young children and older adults.[70] In young children, LRI deaths have fallen sharply over the past few decades, but LRI is still the leading cause of death after the first few weeks of life in low-income countries. In older adults, LRI are among the top killers in every country.

Many different pathogens cause LRI, and it is common for people to be infected by a combination— for example, both a virus and a bacterium. This section covers LRI as a group, with additional detail on **SARS-CoV-2** (the virus that causes COVID-19) and other important pathogens.

Physiology of the Lung and Respiratory Tract

The lungs supply oxygen to the blood and remove carbon dioxide from it. They are at the base of the **respiratory tract**, the channels (or **airways**) through which air enters and leaves the body. The respiratory tract includes the nose and throat, the **trachea** (windpipe), the large **bronchi** (singular— **bronchus**), and smaller airways called **bronchi- oles** (**Figure 9.25**). The bronchioles end in hundreds of millions of tiny, spherical sacs called **alveoli** (singular—**alveolus**).

Figure 9.26 shows a diagram of an alveolus. The respiratory tract is lined with **epithelium**, composed of a single layer of **epithelial cells**. Each alveolus is wrapped with capillaries through which blood flows.

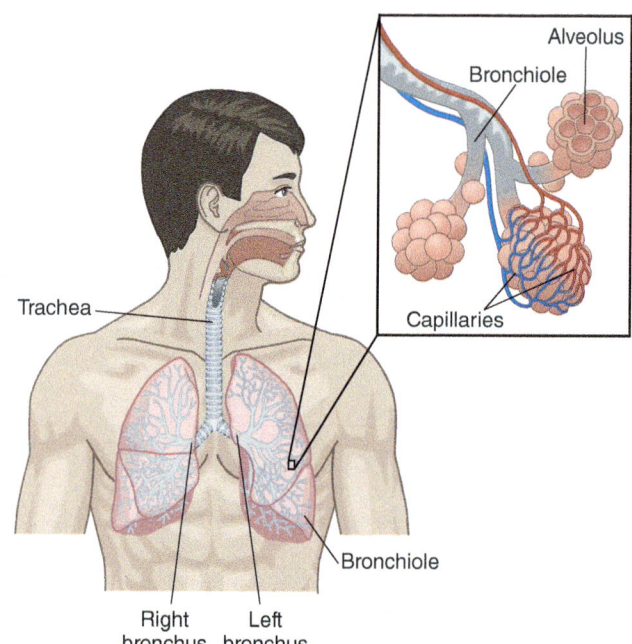

Figure 9.25 The Lung, Bronchioles, and Alveoli. The lung is composed of a branching network of large airways called bronchi and small airways called bronchioles, which end in tiny air sacs called alveoli.
© MAYO FOUNDATION FOR MEDICAL EDUCATION & RESEARCH

The capillaries themselves are lined with a single layer of cells called **endothelium**. Between the capillary endothelium and the alveolar epithelium is an extremely thin, delicate membrane. Gases like carbon

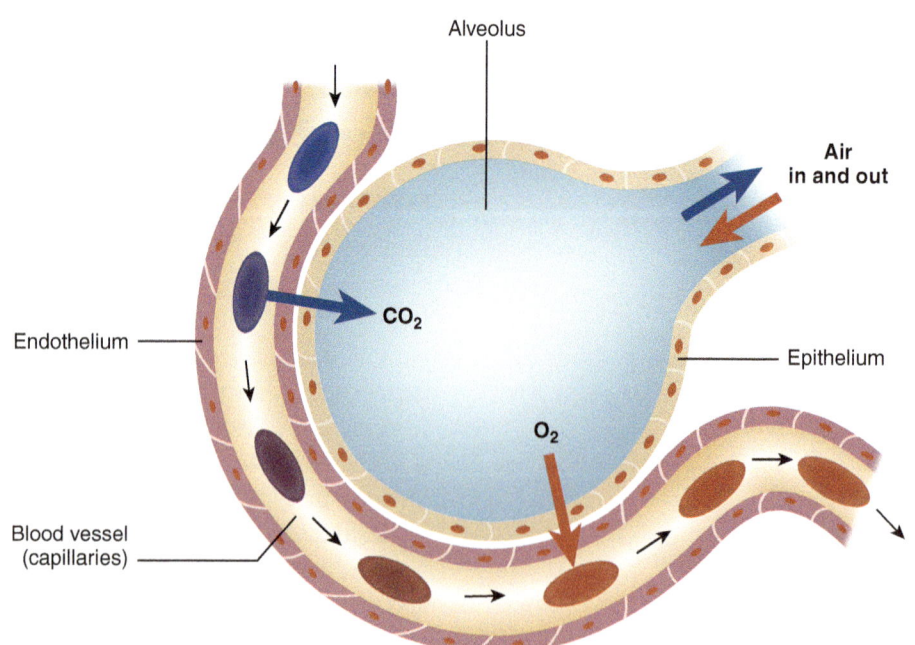

Figure 9.26 How Lung Alveoli Supply Oxygen to Blood and Remove Carbon Dioxide. The airways supply fresh air to the alveoli. Blood that is full of carbon dioxide and depleted of oxygen enters capillaries that wrap around the alveoli. As the blood passes the alveoli, carbon dioxide diffuses across the lining of the capillaries (endothelium) and the lining of the alveoli (epithelium) into the alveoli. Oxygen diffuses across the epithelium and endothelium in the opposite direction. This leaves the blood exiting the lungs full of oxygen and depleted of carbon dioxide.

dioxide and oxygen can diffuse across the endothelium, the epithelium, and the membrane between them, but fluid cannot.

The alveoli are full of air, which is constantly refreshed by breathing. Blood flows through the capillaries that wrap around the alveoli. When the blood flows in, it is full of carbon dioxide but depleted of oxygen, which makes it bluish in color. As the blood passes the alveoli, carbon dioxide diffuses out of the blood and oxygen in (Figure 9.26). The blood flowing out of the capillaries is then full of oxygen and depleted of carbon dioxide and has a deep red color.

Pathophysiology of Lower Respiratory Infections

Infections of the respiratory tract typically start when a virus reaches and infects the epithelial cells.[99] This infection prompts immune cells to travel to the area to fight the infection. It also prompts the epithelial cells to secrete mucus into the respiratory tract. If the immune response contains the infection to the nose, throat, and trachea, the person experiences only an **upper respiratory infection (URI)**—what most people call a "cold"—with just a cough and runny nose. If the infection spreads down to the bronchioles and alveoli, it becomes a lower respiratory infection (LRI) or pneumonia.[100]

LRI are more likely to develop if the immune system or the epithelial cells are weakened. Young children with undernutrition have these problems, so they are particularly susceptible to LRI. And adults who smoke, as well as persons of any age who regularly breathe in polluted air, develop damage to their epithelial cells that increases their susceptibility.

LRI are much more dangerous than URI because they can interfere with the flow of oxygen and carbon dioxide. When the epithelium of the alveoli becomes infected, the membranes between the alveoli and the capillaries can break down, causing fluid to flow from the blood into the alveoli. This fluid partially blocks the exchange of oxygen and carbon dioxide between the capillaries and the alveoli (**Figure 9.27**).[99] People with LRI can have low oxygen levels or high carbon dioxide levels in their blood, which causes them to feel short of breath.

Some viruses, like SARS-CoV-2 and **respiratory syncytial virus (RSV)**, can cause a fatal LRI by themselves. But other viruses cause life-threatening damage by interfering with the lungs' ability to fight off other infections, paving the way for a **secondary infection** with bacteria.[99] LRI caused by bacteria can be very severe and are often fatal if not treated with **antibiotics**.

Death from LRI can happen very quickly—in a matter of days or even hours—especially in children with undernutrition. Children who survive an LRI (unlike children who survive a bout of diarrheal disease) are not at high risk of dying in the month or so afterward, but they are left with some amount of

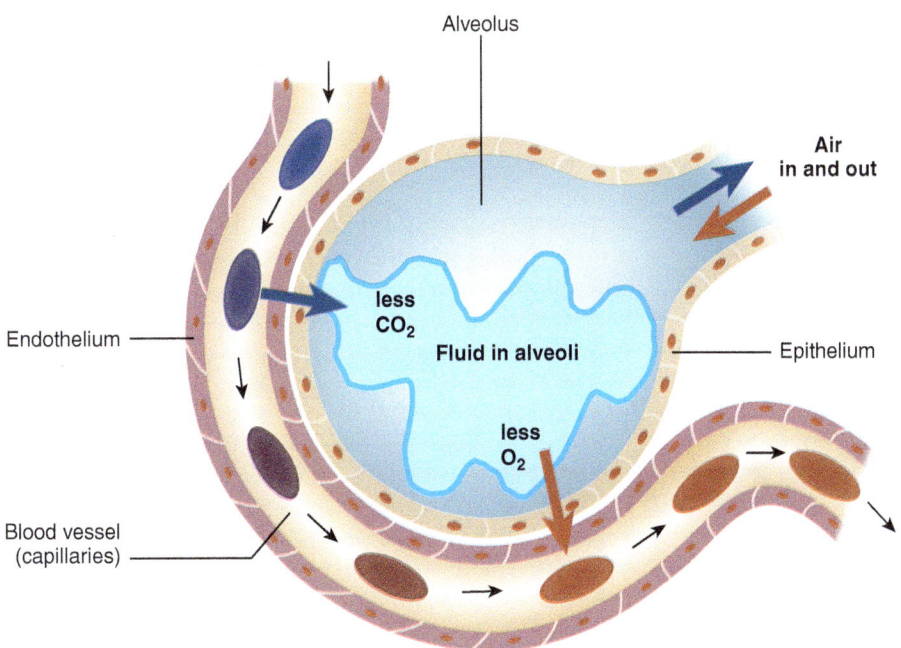

Figure 9.27 Alveolus in Person with Pneumonia. In a person with pneumonia, the epithelium is damaged and fluid flows from the blood into the alveoli. This fluid partially blocks the exchange of oxygen and carbon dioxide.

permanent damage to the lungs, which may increase their risk of chronic lung disease later in life.[101,102] In older adults, LRI can lead to other serious health problems, such as a heart attack or stroke.[103]

Pathogens That Cause LRI

A large and diverse group of viruses and bacteria can cause LRI (**Table 9.3**).[101,102,104-109] Although this list is long, in most studies a few pathogens are responsible for a large percentage of infections. Before vaccination against these pathogens was widespread, about half of deaths from LRI were caused by respiratory syncytial

Table 9.3 Pathogens Causing Lower Respiratory Infections

Most Common
Viruses
Respiratory syncytial virus (RSV)
Human rhinovirus
Human metapneumovirus
Parainfluenza virus
Influenza virus
Adenovirus
Bacteria
Streptococcus pneumoniae
Haemophilus influenzae
Staphylococcus aureus
Mycoplasma pneumoniae (older children and young adults)
Chlamydia pneumoniae
Mycobacterium tuberculosis (children in low-income countries)
Less Common
Viruses
Coronavirus
Bocavirus
Cytomegalovirus
Bacteria
Moraxella catarrhalis
Klebsiella pneumoniae
Legionella pneumophila
Enterobacteriaceae

virus (RSV), *Streptococcus pneumoniae*, *Haemophilus influenzae*, or influenza virus.[101,109] Vaccines against all four of these pathogens are now available and increasingly used around the world. With this vaccination, rates of LRI are falling and the remaining cases are more likely to be caused by the other pathogens in Table 9.3.

Viruses are more common causes of LRI than bacteria, but they tend to cause less severe infection.[110] As the COVID-19 pandemic demonstrated, though, viruses mutate much more quickly than bacteria do. With viruses, there is always a risk that a new variant will appear, causing widespread and severe infections.

Viruses that cause LRI are spread more easily in colder, drier weather. For that reason, every year there is a respiratory virus season that peaks in late fall, winter or early spring.[104-106] The pathogens causing most cases of LRI in the summer may differ from those causing LRI in the winter.

Here are notes on specific pathogens:

Streptococcus pneumoniae. *Streptococcus pneumoniae* (often called the **pneumococcus**) was once the most common and most severe cause of pneumonia.[99] Before antibiotics became available, illness from it was often rapidly fatal. Vaccines against *S. pneumonia,* called **pneumococcal conjugate vaccines or PCV**, are now given routinely to infants and older adults in many countries, making infection with this bacterium less common.

Haemophilus influenzae. *Haemophilus influenzae* is a bacterium that has several types, which are assigned different letters. Type B causes the most serious infections, including pneumonia and meningitis in young children.[99] The **Hib vaccine** protects against *Haemophilus influenzae* type B, and it is included in the routine childhood vaccination schedule in many countries. This vaccine does not protect against other types of *Haemophilus influenzae.*

Respiratory Syncytial Virus. Respiratory syncytial virus (RSV) usually causes only a cold, but sometimes it causes a much more severe infection, particularly in infants who were born preterm and in older adults. In countries that vaccinate children against *Streptococcus pneumonia* and *Haemophilus influenzae,* RSV is by far the most common cause of LRI, responsible for about one-third of cases.[102] Vaccines against RSV for older adults became available in 2023. Also, a vaccine is available to be given to pregnant women that protects their babies for the first few months of life.

Influenza Virus. The influenza virus causes a pandemic of LRI every winter or spring. Each year, influenza infects billions of people and kills tens of thousands in the United States and hundreds of thousands globally. The virus does this by constantly mutating, so that people's immunity from one year's strain of the virus gives them only partial protection against an infection with the next year's strain. This annual mutation of the influenza virus is called **antigenic drift**. Less frequently, the influenza virus undergoes a major genetic change, called **antigenic shift**. When this happens, most people have little or no immunity from previous infections, so many more become infected, and their illnesses tend to be more severe. The most severe pandemic caused by antigenic shift was the great influenza pandemic of 1918-1919, which killed tens of millions of people worldwide.

Influenza virus strains come in two types—Type A and Type B—and the Type A strains are numbered based on two proteins in their surface, one labeled H and the other N. In the early 2020s, typically one Type A(H1N1) strain and one Type A(H3N2) strain, along with one Type B strain, were circulating in humans. However, a Type A(H5N1) virus was circulating in birds (so-called "bird flu"). It is possible that this virus could evolve to infect humans, perhaps causing the next major antigenic shift and a deadly pandemic.[99]

Fortunately, vaccines against influenza are widely available. The vaccines are produced to match four specific strains of the virus. Experts update these vaccines every year to try to match the strains of virus that they expect will circulate in the coming months. Some years, the match between strains in vaccines and the strains that are circulating is excellent. When this occurs, the vaccines are highly effective in preventing influenza infection. Other years, the virus mutates in a surprising direction, so the vaccines do not match them closely, and the vaccines are less effective. However, even if they do not prevent infections, the vaccines always make the influenza illness less severe and reduce the risk of dying. Each year, about 70% of U.S. adults over age 65, 40% of adults under 65, and 60% of children are vaccinated against influenza.[111]

Also, **antiviral medications** are available for influenza. Antiviral medications interfere with viruses' ability to make copies of themselves. If people take these drugs early in the course of illness, the drugs prevent the illness from being very severe or dangerous. Whenever the next major antigenic shift occurs, the public health response will require quick development and distribution of a new vaccine, as well as widespread use of these antiviral medications while the vaccine is being developed.

Coronavirus. Many different strains of coronaviruses cause infection in animals and in humans. In humans, most coronaviruses, most of the time, cause little more than a cold. However, even before the COVID-19 pandemic, some strains of coronaviruses originating in animals caused very serious infections in people. In 2002, a strain of coronavirus that was thought to be carried by bats caused an outbreak of **Severe Acute Respiratory Syndrome (SARS)** in Asia. Then, in 2012, a different strain of coronavirus, which was also thought to originate in bats but which infected camels, caused an outbreak of **Middle East Respiratory Syndrome (MERS)** in Saudi Arabia. Although these strains killed some people, they did not spread readily from one person to another, so the outbreaks were contained. We were not so fortunate with the strain of coronavirus called SARS-CoV-2 that emerged in China in 2019 (**Box 9.7**).

Box 9.7 **SARS-CoV-2 and the COVID-19 Pandemic**

SARS-CoV-2 is unusually dangerous for a respiratory virus. It infects not just the epithelial cells lining the alveoli but also the endothelial cells lining the capillaries that wrap around the alveoli (**Figure 9.28**). The damage to these two layers allows fluid containing proteins to leak from the blood into the alveoli. This protein-filled fluid blocks the diffusion of oxygen, so the blood in the capillaries does not receive the oxygen it needs. When this happens throughout both lungs, it is called **acute respiratory distress syndrome** (or **ARDS**).[99,112,113] People with COVID-19 have a severe cough, feel short of breath, have low levels of oxygen in their blood, and can die from a lack of oxygen. Most people with COVID-19 recover fully, but some 10–30% of those who get past the initial illness have lingering symptoms (called "long COVID") like fatigue, loss of taste and/or smell, and difficulty thinking clearly ("brain fog").[114]

The pandemic caused by SARS-CoV-2 did not arrive without warning. The annual pandemics of influenza pointed out how easily and quickly a new virus can spread around the entire world. And the SARS and MERS outbreaks showed that the coronavirus had the ability to mutate, spread among humans, and cause fatal illness.

(continues)

Box 9.7 **SARS-CoV-2 and the COVID-19 Pandemic**   *(continued)*

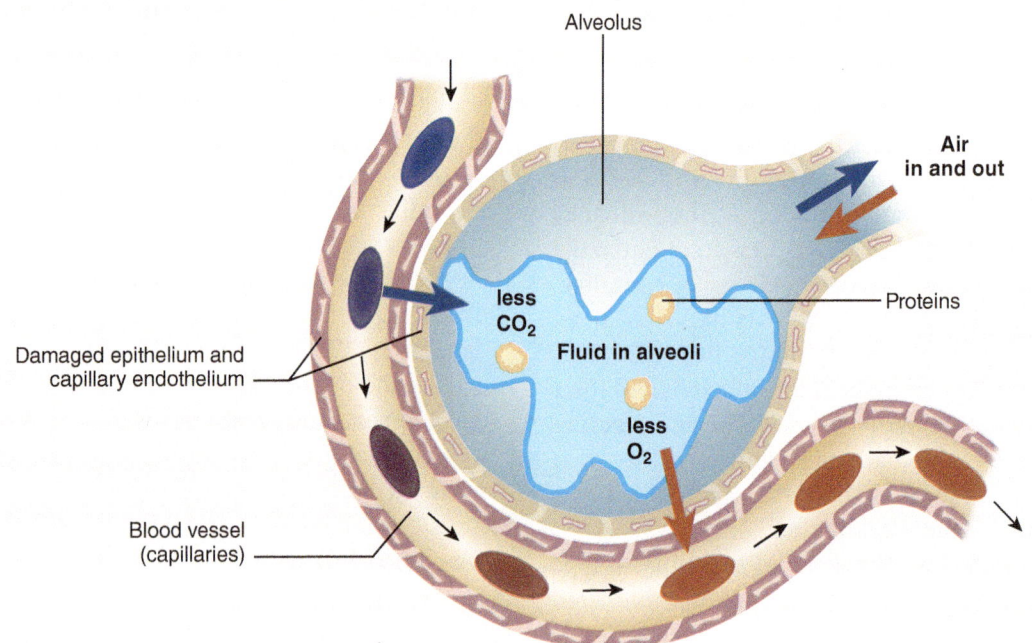

Figure 9.28 **Alveolus in Person with Acute Respiratory Distress Syndrome (ARDS) from COVID-19.** In a person with ARDS, fluid containing proteins leaks from the blood into the alveoli. This protein-filled fluid blocks the flow of oxygen into the blood.

The COVID-19 pandemic unfolded in a series of waves (**Figure 9.29**). These waves were caused by new variants of the original strain of virus as it evolved to spread more easily among humans. One pivotal event was the wave caused by the Omicron variant in the early winter of 2021–22. Omicron spread extraordinarily quickly and easily, and within months it seems to have infected nearly everyone on earth who was not already immune to the virus, as well as many who were partially immune. A CDC study showed that by the Fall of 2022, 96% of Americans had antibodies to SARS-CoV-2, indicating that they had been infected, been vaccinated, or both. Of those, 70% had evidence that they had been infected with the virus itself.[115]

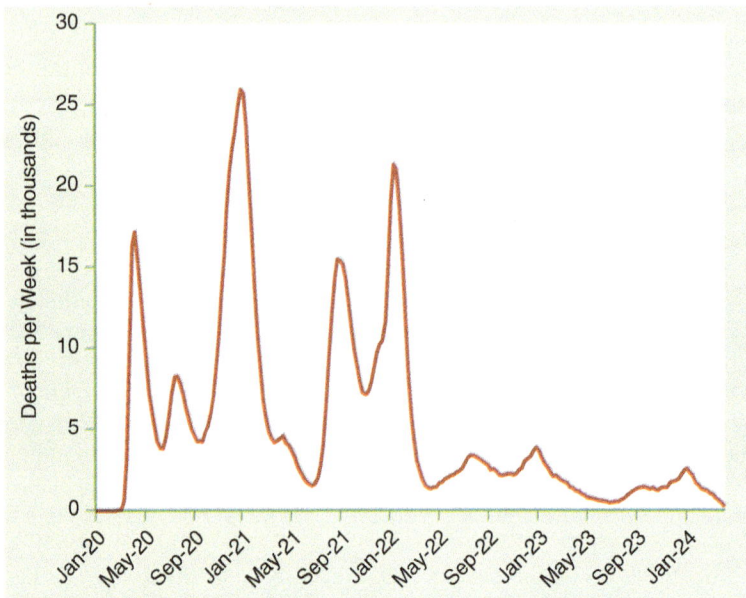

Figure 9.29 **Weekly Deaths from COVID-19 in the United States, 2020–2024.** The COVID-19 pandemic unfolded in a series of waves caused by new variants of the original virus.

Data from Centers for Disease Control and Prevention. COVID Data Tracker. Accessed July 30, 2024. https://covid.cdc.gov/

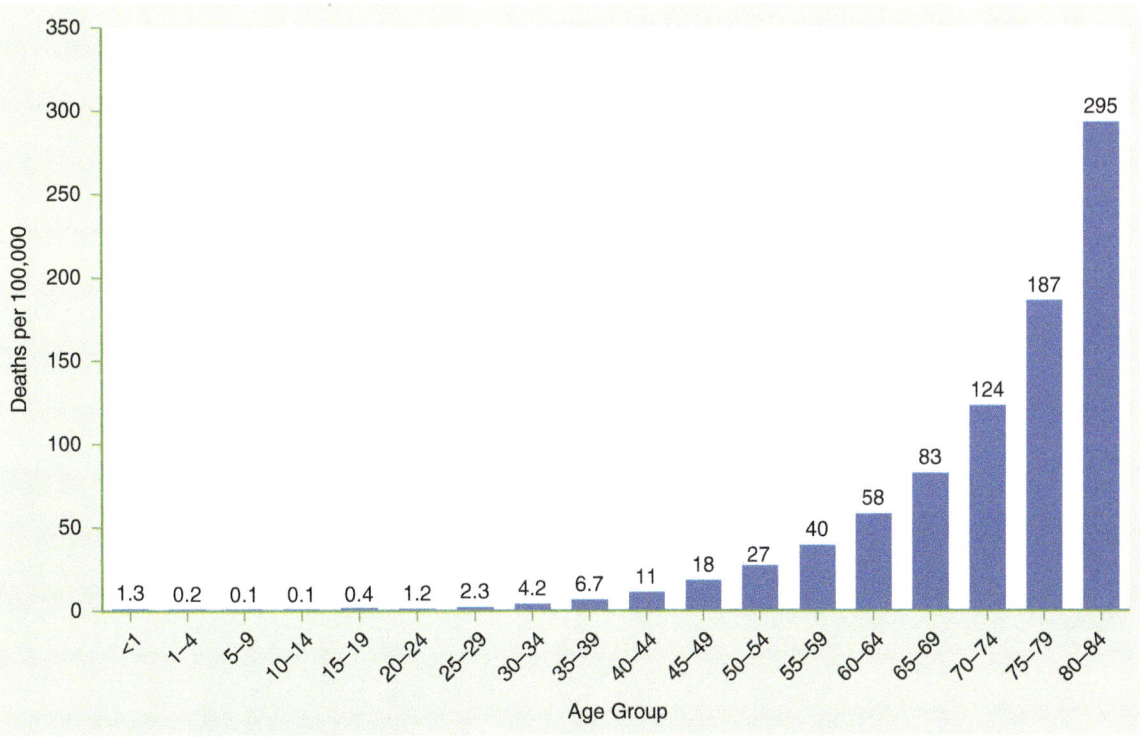

Figure 9.30 **Mortality Rates from COVID-19 in the United States through April 2024, by Age Group.**

Data from National Center for Health Statistics, Centers for Disease Control and Prevention. Underlying Cause of Death Data on CDC WONDER. Published 2023. Accessed June 12, 2024. https://wonder.cdc.gov/Deaths-by-Underlying-Cause.html

CDC estimates that, by the end of 2024, some 1.2 million Americans died from COVID-19.[116] The risk of dying was strikingly tied to age, with people over age 65 hundreds of times more likely to die than children (**Figure 9.30**).[117] Compared to this, the differences in mortality rates by race or sex were small (**Figure 9.31**).

For other viruses, it took decades to develop vaccines. In a historic achievement, vaccines against SARS-CoV-2 were developed, tested, produced, and deployed in just 12 months. By January 2022, just two years after the virus appeared, about 75% of Americans, including over 95% of those over age 65, had received two doses. After the Omicron wave passed and COVID-19 dropped out of the headlines, though, the number of people keeping up with the recommended booster doses fell sharply.

Many lessons can be drawn from this experience in planning the prevention of LRI or responding to future pandemics. Here are some:

Respiratory viruses are spread so easily that they are difficult to prevent, even in the wealthiest and most technologically-advanced societies. Efforts to contain the virus with contact tracing, isolation, and quarantine, which had been successful for SARS and MERS, were ineffective for a virus spread through airborne transmission like SARS-CoV-2. Similarly, testing for SARS-CoV-2, while much in demand, did little to nothing to prevent spread, because testing was spotty, the results arrived after spread had occurred, and many people did not isolate themselves after testing positive.

Social distancing policies can slow an epidemic wave of an airborne virus, protecting the healthcare system from being overwhelmed and buying time for the development or deployment of a vaccine.

However, people are not willing to tolerate the disruptions caused by social distancing policies for long. Even simple prevention steps like requirements to wear masks met substantial resistance over time. Travel bans were ineffective because they could never be airtight and the virus moved quickly, crossing borders long before it was recognized.

On the other hand, vaccination can be extraordinarily successful. The mRNA technology underlying the COVID-19 vaccines is a major scientific advance, allowing this and future vaccines to be developed and updated quickly. COVID-19 vaccines have been met with some skepticism, misinformation, and hostility, and far too many people died because they chose to not be vaccinated. But even with the incomplete vaccination coverage, according to estimates by researchers at the Commonwealth Fund, vaccinations in the United States prevented 3.2 million deaths through December 2022 (**Figure 9.32**).[118]

Finally, antiviral medications that are biologically effective have been somewhat disappointing in practice.[119] The drug Paxlovid was found in one study to reduce mortality from COVID-19 by 73%, but only about 10% of people with COVID-19 took it.[120] This drug has the potential to prevent tens of thousands of deaths per year, but for it to meet that potential, public health practitioners must better understand why people were hesitant to use it and make it easier for people to obtain it.[119]

(continues)

Box 9.7 **SARS-CoV-2 and the COVID-19 Pandemic** *(continued)*

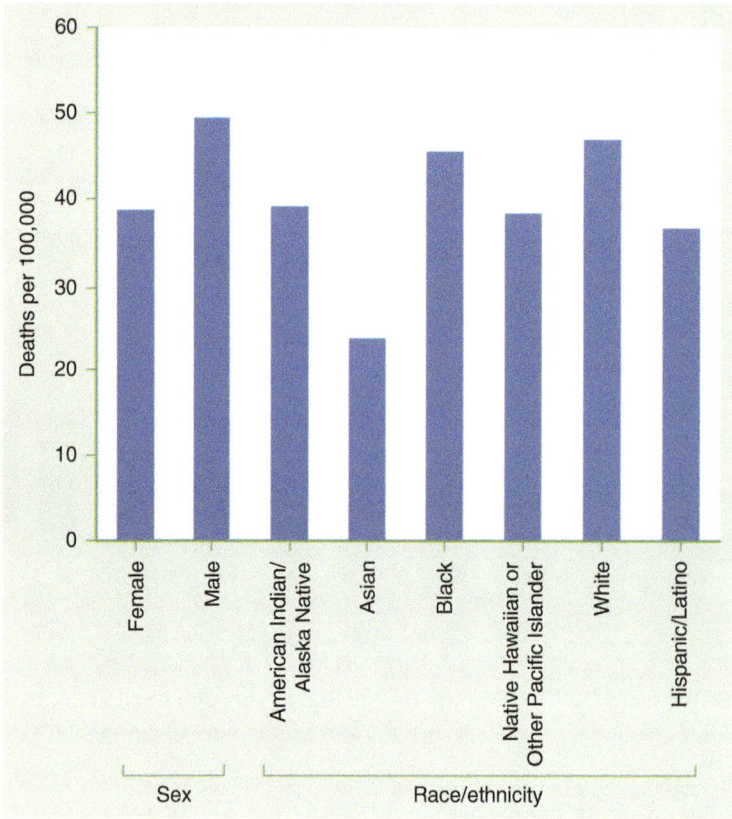

Figure 9.31 **Mortality Rates from COVID-19 in the United States through April 2024, by Race and Sex.**

Data from National Center for Health Statistics, Centers for Disease Control and Prevention. Underlying Cause of Death Data on CDC WONDER. Published 2023. Accessed June 12, 2024. https://wonder.cdc.gov/Deaths-by-Underlying-Cause.html

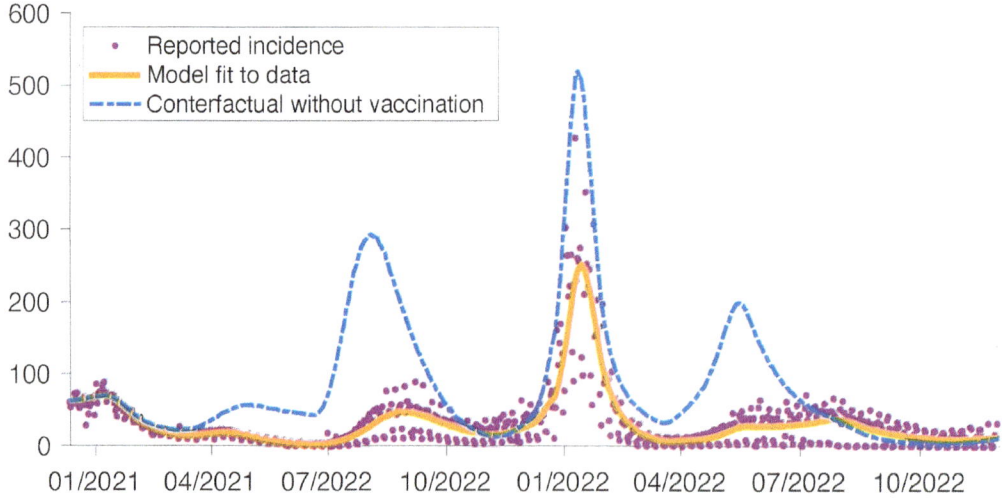

Figure 9.32 **Estimates of COVID-19 Infections Prevented in the United States by Vaccination (Through November 2022).** Model estimates of the incidence of COVID-19 infection (orange line) and what the incidence would have been (blue dashed line) if COVID-19 vaccines had not been available. The difference between the two is an estimate of the number of infections prevented by vaccination. This study estimated that between December 20, 2020 and November 30, 2022, vaccination prevented 120 million cases of COVID-19, 18.6 million COVID-related hospitalizations, and 3.3 million COVID-related deaths.

Reproduced from Meagan C. Fitzpatrick et al., "Two Years of U.S. COVID-19 Vaccines Have Prevented Millions of Hospitalizations and Deaths," To the Point (blog), Commonwealth Fund, Dec. 13, 2022. https://doi.org/10.26099/whsf-fp90

Mycobacterium tuberculosis. *Mycobacterium tuberculosis* is the bacterium that causes the disease tuberculosis. It is discussed in a separate section later in this chapter.

Transmission of Respiratory Pathogens

One way to prevent LRI is to reduce the spread of respiratory pathogens from one person to another. That requires understanding how pathogens make that jump.

Fluid in the respiratory tract of a person with a URI or LRI holds many copies of pathogens—that is, viral particles or bacterial cells. When a person coughs, sneezes, talks, or even just breathes, that person puts out droplets of this fluid into the air. The droplets come in many sizes, from microscopic (1-3 microns) to large enough to see with the naked eye.[121,122] People expel many more small droplets than large ones, and most of the pathogens are thought to be in the smaller droplets.[121] The larger droplets are heavy enough that they quickly fall onto whatever surface is below them. But the smaller droplets can dry out, leaving even smaller particles called **droplet nuclei** in the air.[122] Tiny droplets and droplet nuclei have also been called **aerosols**. The droplet nuclei are light enough that they can remain suspended in the air and travel with air currents.

Respiratory pathogens are spread when they land on an uninfected person's **mucous membranes**, which are the moist tissues lining the eyes, nose, mouth, or respiratory tract. There are theoretically four routes by which pathogens can make this trip, two involving contact and two through the air (**Figure 9.33**):[123]

- *Direct contact.* This route involves an infected person getting secretions on their hands (or on another skin surface) and then touching an uninfected person, for example by shaking hands. The uninfected person then spreads the pathogen to their mucous membranes by touching their eyes, nose, or mouth.
- *Indirect contact.* Pathogens take this route when an infected person touches or expels droplets onto an object, like a countertop or a piece of clothing, and then an infected person touches that object. Objects that are intermediate steps in scenario are called **fomites**.
- *Direct deposition.* In this route, an infected person expels large or small droplets that travel a short distance through the air and land directly on the mucous membranes of an uninfected person. This is especially likely to happen if the infected person coughs or sneezes while close to another person.
- *Airborne transmission/inhalation.* Pathogens take this route when an infected person expels smaller droplets, those droplets become droplet nuclei, and an uninfected person inhales the droplet nuclei. This route can spread the infection across large distances. It can also spread the infection between rooms within a building, with the droplet nuclei flowing through air ducts. However, as distance from the infected person increases, the concentration of droplet nuclei decreases, so spread over longer distances occurs less often.[122,123] Airborne transmission is also much less likely to happen outdoors, where there is good ventilation that dilutes the aerosols and where ultraviolet light from the sun inactivates viruses.[124,125]

In most situations, multiple routes of transmission theoretically can happen. For example, when an infected person spreads a virus to others at a party, that spread can result from direct contact (handshakes), indirect contact (people touching contaminated table tops), direct deposition (people talking with others nearby), or airborne transmission (people breathing in droplet nuclei).

Unfortunately, it is not clear how much each route contributes to the spread of each pathogen. The virus that causes measles and *Mycobacterium tuberculosis* are thought to mainly spread through airborne transmission/inhalation.[122] In the past, influenza virus was thought to spread only through direct and indirect contact. However, some researchers are now suggesting that influenza and other viruses like respiratory syncytial virus may actually be spread more often by airborne transmission/inhalation.[122]

The incomplete understanding of routes of transmission led to controversy and distrust during the COVID-19 pandemic. At first, experts assumed that SARS-CoV-2 was spread only by direct contact, indirect contact, and direct deposition, but studies later demonstrated that airborne transmission was possible.[122] Experts now agree that, although most spread seems to happen between people who are near each other, SARS-CoV-2 can be spread by airborne transmission.

Our understanding of these routes of transmission shapes how to prevent LRI. If a pathogen is spread only by indirect or direct contact, prevention depends on people avoiding touching each

Mode of transmission	Typical distance from the source	Route of transfer to another human	Respiratory tract entry mechanism	Respiratory tract entry portal	Schematic depiction
THROUGH THE AIR					
Airborne transmission/ inhalation	Any distance	Through the air (suspended in air or moving via air flows)	Inhalation	Anywhere along the respiratory tract	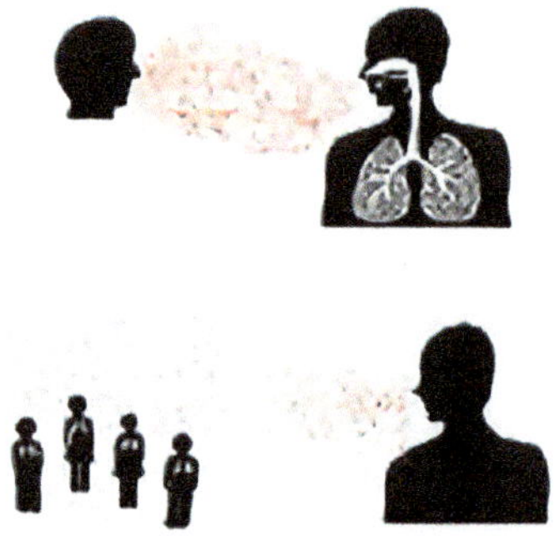
Direct deposition	Short	Through the air (semi-ballistic trajectory)	Deposition on the mucosa	Mouth, nose or eyes*	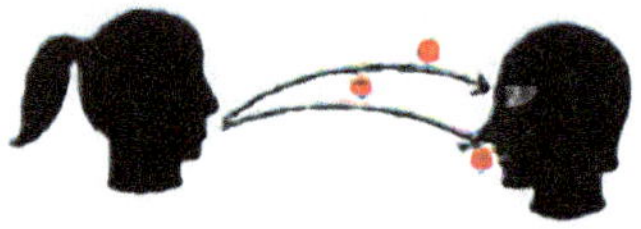
CONTACT[#]					
Direct contact	*Short*	*Not through the air*	*Direct transfer (via touch[#], usually with hands)*	*Mouth, nose or eyes**	
Indirect contact	*Any distance*	*Not through the air, although IRPs may reach an intermediate object through the air*	*Indirect transfer (via touching an intermediate object)*	*Mouth, nose or eyes**	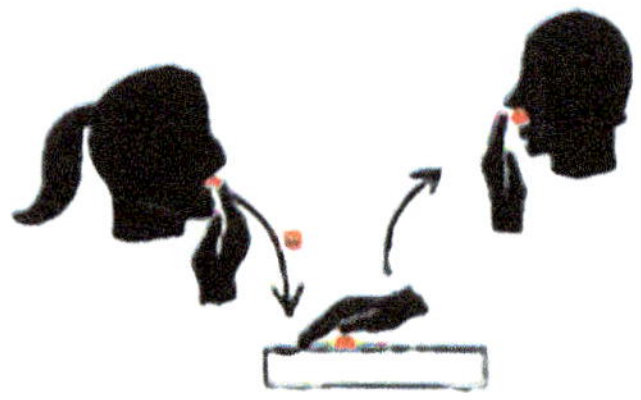

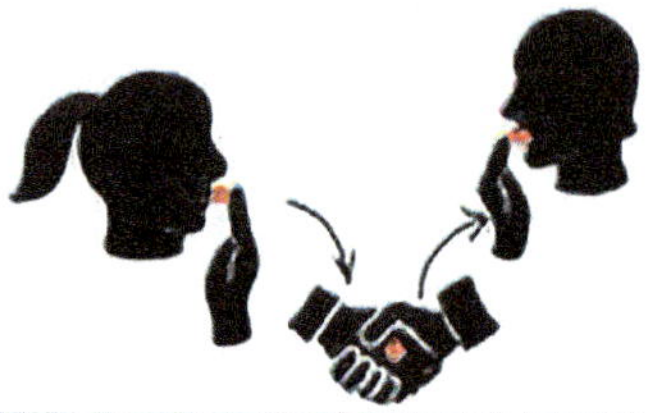

Figure 9.33 Potential Routes of Transmission of Respiratory Pathogens.

Reproduced from World Health Organization. Global Technical Consultation Report on Proposed Terminology for Pathogens That Transmit through the Air, 2024. Accessed June 27, 2024. https://www.who.int/publications/m/item/global-technical-consultation-report-on-proposed-terminology-for-pathogens-that-transmit-through-the-air

other, objects, or their own mucous membranes; this leads to recommendations for gloves, hand washing, and cleaning of surfaces. If a pathogen is spread by direct deposition, prevention depends on people maintaining a distance from each other, which leads to steps to reduce crowding. If a pathogen is spread by airborne transmission, prevention depends on tight-fitting masks, improving ventilation, directing airflow away from people, or moving activities outdoors.[122] It may be that all these actions are important.

Epidemiology: Patterns and Trends

Two groups are at high risk for lower respiratory infections: children under age five in low-income countries and adults over age 70 worldwide (**Figure 9.34**).

Among young children in low-income countries, these infections are extremely common, with about 20% of children experiencing an infection per year. Only about 1% of these infections are fatal, but in 2019 they still caused an estimated 672,000 deaths

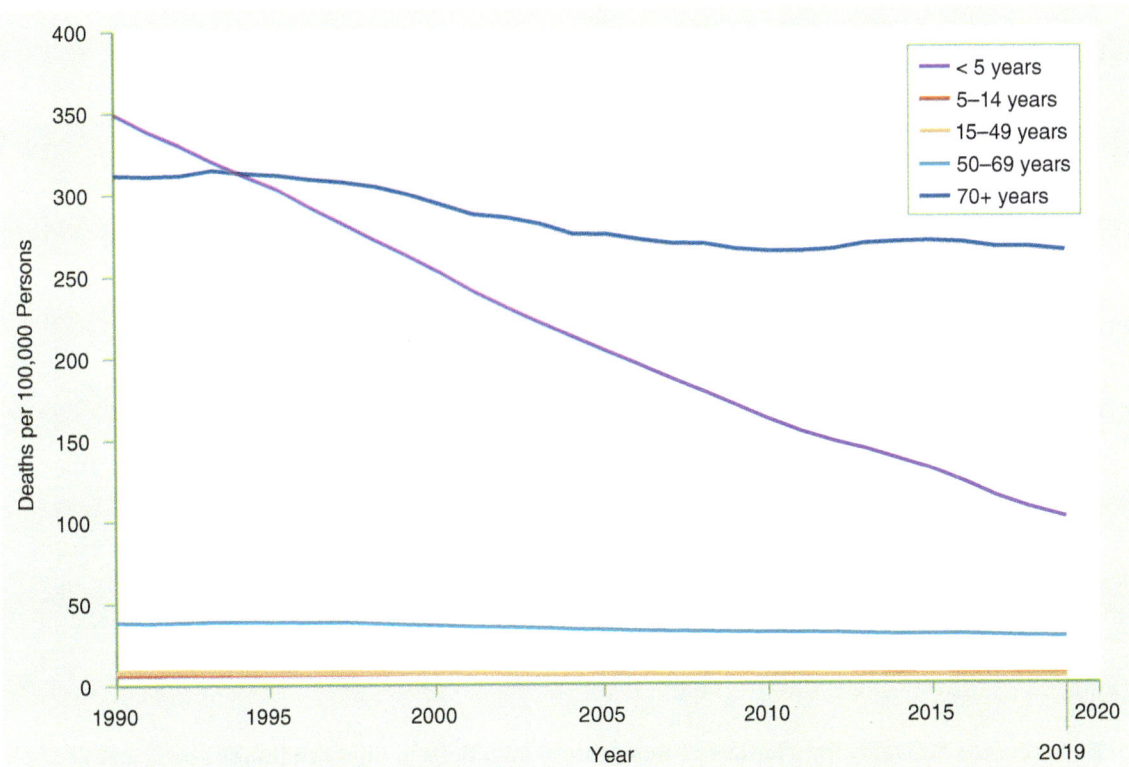

Figure 9.34 **Estimated Mortality Rates for Lower Respiratory Infections Worldwide, by Age and Year.**

Data from Global Burden of Disease Collaboration, Institute for Health Metrics and Evaluation. GBD Results Tool. Published July 12, 2023. Accessed July 11, 2023. https://vizhub.healthdata.org/gbd-results

in children under age 5.[98,101] As high as this number is, it reflects about a 70% drop from the estimated 2.2 million deaths that occurred in 1990, even with a growing global population.[98] This improvement was likely caused by a combination of vaccinations and a fall in child undernutrition. The fall in mortality from LRI has lagged in West and Central Africa and a few other low-income areas (**Figure 9.35**).

Among older adults, mortality rates from LRI are high in every country, but they are higher in sub-Saharan Africa than in high-income countries. Unlike the progress in young children, mortality rates for LRI in older adults have not fallen much in recent decades (Figure 9.34).

Risk Factors

Risk factors for LRI mostly relate either to the degree to which people are exposed to respiratory pathogens or to their susceptibility to an infection if exposed. Some risk factors are mostly important for young children, some for older adults, and some for both.

Factors that increase exposure to respiratory pathogens are:

- *Insufficient ventilation.*[126] If there is not enough ventilation, droplet nuclei linger in the air, increasing exposure to people in the area. Also, if there is little ventilation, household air pollution like smoke from indoor fires lingers, causing more harm to people's lungs.

- *Crowding.* The closer people are to each other, and the more people involved, the greater the chances that a pathogen will spread from one person to others. Studies have found that people are more likely to catch an LRI if they live with many other household members, in crowded households, or with children.[101,110,126,127]

- *Insufficient handwashing.* When people or their family members do not wash their hands regularly—most often because they do not have running water at home—they are more likely to spread respiratory pathogens by direct or indirect contact.[98,126]

Factors that increase the susceptibility of infants and young children to infections are (**Figure 9.36**):

- *Preterm birth and low birth weight.* Young children who were born early or small tend to have immature lungs and immune systems that are more vulnerable to infections.[98,110]

- *Suboptimal breastfeeding.* Breast milk is free of pathogens. Also, it contains immune cells and

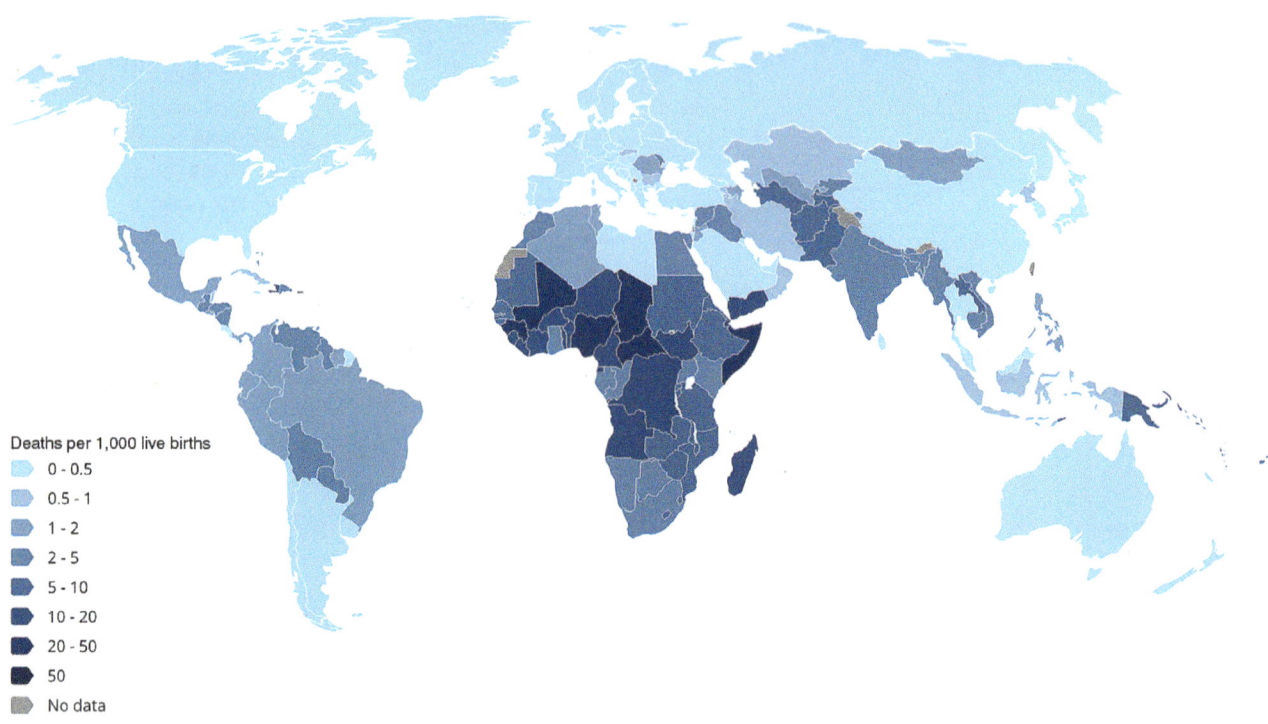

Deaths per 1,000 live births

- 0 - 0.5
- 0.5 - 1
- 1 - 2
- 2 - 5
- 5 - 10
- 10 - 20
- 20 - 50
- 50
- No data

Figure 9.35 Estimated Mortality Rate for Lower Respiratory Infections in Children Under Age 5, 2021.

Reproduced from United Nations Inter-Agency Group for Child Mortality Estimation. Accessed July 30, 2024. https://childmortality.org

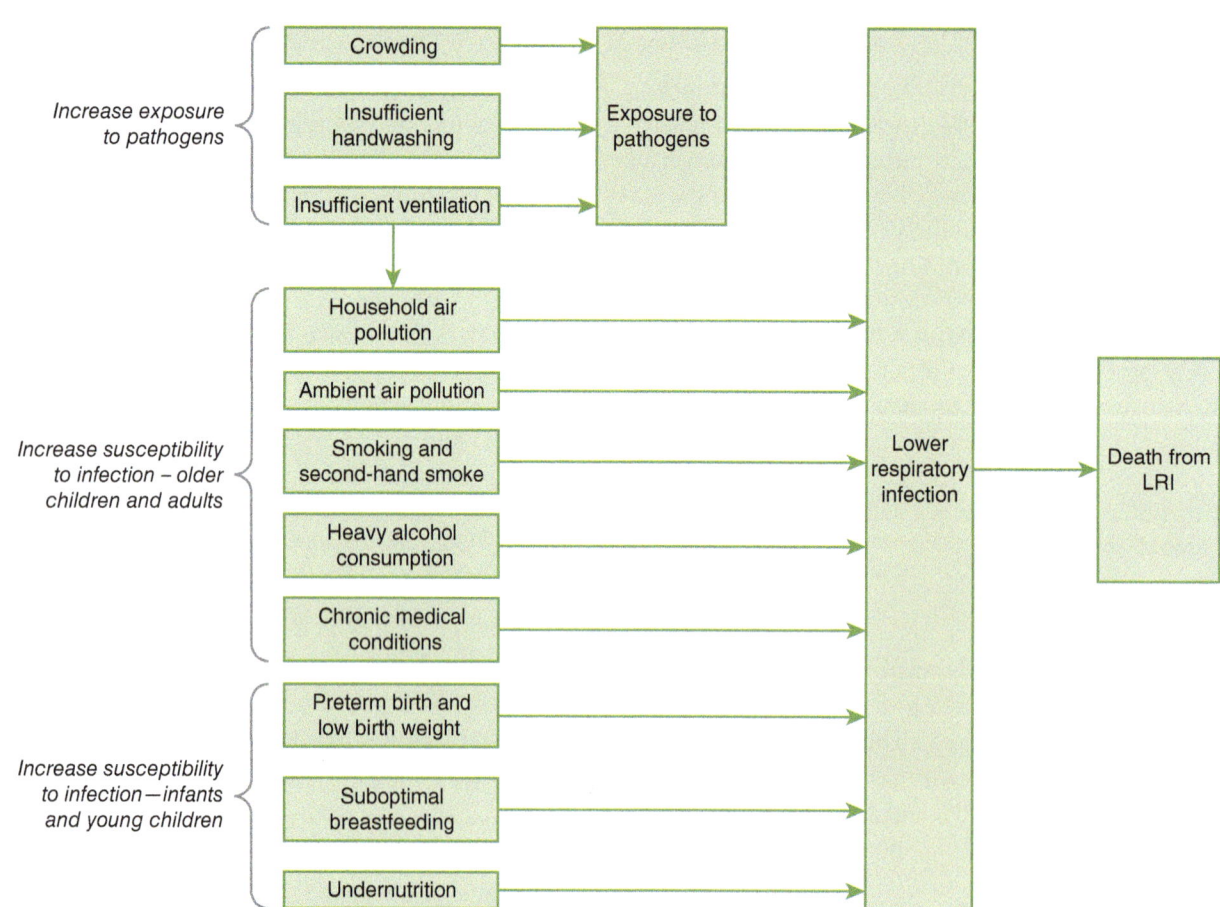

Figure 9.36 Cause-and-Effect Diagram for Lower Respiratory Infections. Risk factors for LRI can be grouped into those that increase exposure to pathogens, those that increase susceptibility to infection in infants and children, and those that increase susceptibility to infection in older children and adults.

antibodies that help protect against LRI. Children who are fed infant formula or other foods in the first six months of life are at higher risk for LRI than children who are exclusively breastfed.[98,110,126]

- *Undernutrition.*[98,101,110,126] This is the most important risk factor for young children in low-income countries with more than 50% of LRI deaths attributable to it (**Figure 9.37**).[98] Children who are malnourished have weaker immune systems and weaker epithelial barriers to infection. Different nutrients contribute to this problem, but a deficiency of zinc is particularly important.[128] More than half of children in sub-Saharan Africa have low levels of zinc.[129]

Factors that increase the susceptibility of older children and adults to infections include:

- *Household air pollution.* In low-income countries, many families burn wood, coal, crop waste, or animal dung for heat, cooking, and light. The smoke from burning these **biomass** fuels contains many pollutants that damage health, including very high concentrations of fine particles called **PM$_{2.5}$**. These tiny particles penetrate deep into the lungs, damaging the airways and making it more difficult for the lungs to fight off pathogens. Household air pollution is the second most important risk factor for young children, to which more than 30% of LRI deaths are attributable (Figure 9.35).[98] It is also an important risk factor for adult women, many of whom are heavily exposed to smoke while cooking and while indoors caring for children (Figure 9.36).[98]

- *Ambient (outdoor) particulate matter air pollution.* Air pollution that comes from outdoor sources reaches large numbers of people.[130] Like household air pollution, ambient air pollution contains many pollutants, but the most important to LRI is thought to be PM$_{2.5}$, which harm the lungs' ability to fight off infections.[98] Ambient air pollution is a risk factor for both young children and adults (Figures 9.35 and 9.36).

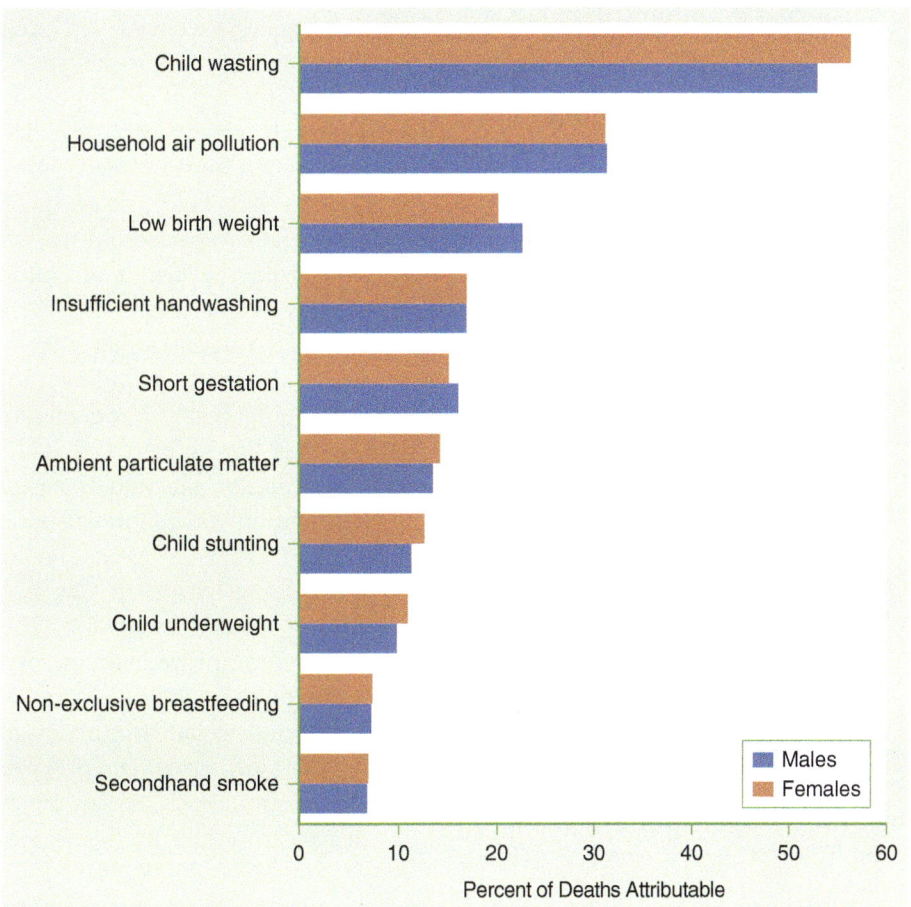

Figure 9.37 **Estimated Percentage of Fatal Lower Respiratory Infections in Children Under Age 5 Attributable to Specific Risk Factors, Worldwide.**

Data from Kyu HH, Vongpradith A, Sirota SB, et al. Age–sex differences in the global burden of lower respiratory infections and risk factors, 1990–2019: results from the Global Burden of Disease Study 2019. Lancet Infect Dis. 2022;22(11):1626-1647.

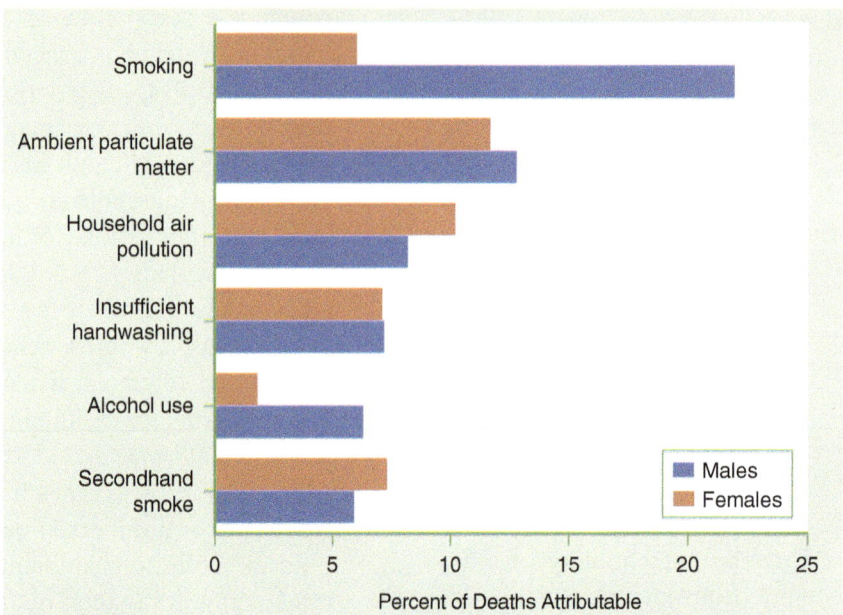

Figure 9.38 **Estimated Percentage of Fatal Lower Respiratory Infections in Adults Over Age 70 Attributable to Specific Risk Factors, Worldwide.**

Data from Kyu HH, Vongpradith A, Sirota SB, et al. Age–sex differences in the global burden of lower respiratory infections and risk factors, 1990–2019: results from the Global Burden of Disease Study 2019. *Lancet Infect Dis.* 2022;22(11):1626-1647.

Ambient and household air pollution are discussed more in Chapter 8. Chronic Respiratory Diseases.

- *Smoking and exposure to second-hand smoke.*[98,126,127,131] Even more than household and ambient air pollution, tobacco smoke harms the lungs' defenses. The greatest risk is to people who smoke, making smoking the most important risk factor for LRI in adult men globally (**Figure 9.38**). Family members exposed to second-hand smoke at home are also at increased risk.[98]

- *Heavy alcohol use.* Heavy drinking damages the immune system, and adults who are intoxicated are more likely to inhale pathogens into their airways. Between the two, people who are heavy alcohol users are at greater risk of LRI.[98,127,131]

- *Chronic medical conditions*, typically in older adults. The chronic medical conditions with the greatest impact on LRI are asthma and chronic obstructive pulmonary disease (discussed in Chapter 8. Chronic Respiratory Diseases), which harm the lungs' defenses, but people are also at greater risk for LRI if they have heart disease, chronic kidney disease, chronic liver disease, diabetes, dementia, or HIV infection.[126,127,131]

Preventive Interventions

These risk factors can be addressed with a long list of interventions, shown in **Figure 9.39**.

Core interventions are:

- *Vaccination.* Vaccines help prevent LRI in more than one way. They prevent some people from getting infected at all. They reduce the severity of illness in those people who do become infected. And by preventing infections and the spread to others, they help protect people around those who are vaccinated. Much of the progress in improving the health of children over the past century is due to vaccines. Vaccines have nearly eliminated diseases that were once dreaded killers of children, including diphtheria, pertussis (whooping cough), and measles. More recently, vaccines have greatly reduced LRI from *Streptococcus pneumoniae* and *Haemophilus influenzae*.[132] Vaccination was the most successful intervention in the COVID-19 pandemic and it continues to saves many lives each year by preventing influenza.[132] Vaccine technology keeps getting better, so new or improved vaccines will likely be central to the progress in preventing LRI in the future.

- *Antibiotic and antiviral treatment.* Antibiotics can rapidly kill bacterial pathogens and prevent deaths from LRI caused by bacteria. Antiviral drugs can reduce the severity of illness for influenza and COVID-19. In the future, antiviral drugs are likely to become available to treat infections with RSV and other viruses. While most people with pneumonia in high-income countries can visit physicians and get these medications,

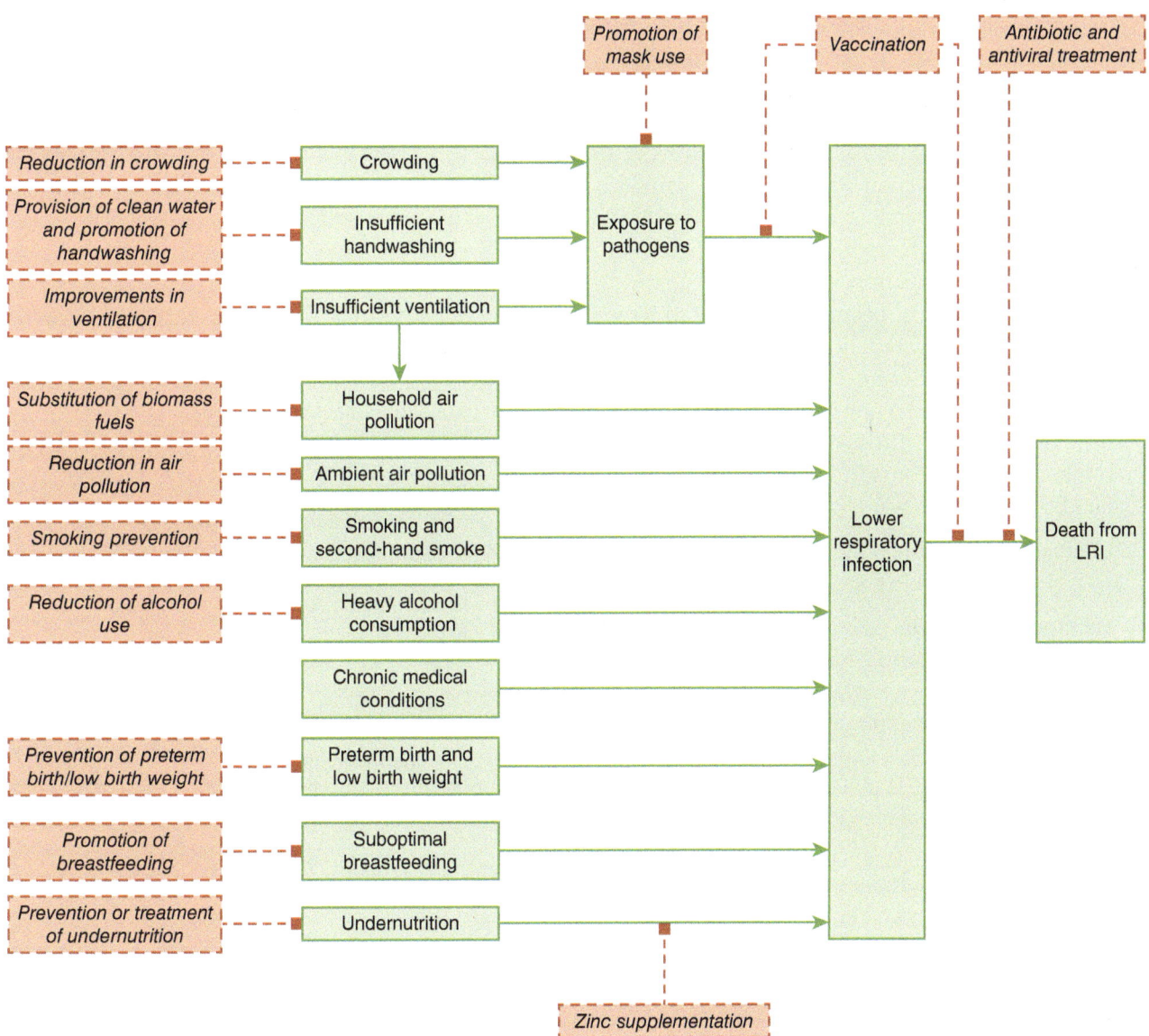

Figure 9.39 **Cause-and-Effect Diagram for Lower Respiratory Infections, with Preventive Interventions.**

this treatment is less available for people in low-income countries. In these countries, the WHO recommends antibiotics for all young children who come to health centers with rapid breathing or difficulty breathing.[94]

Interventions to help reduce people's exposure to respiratory pathogens in homes and buildings include:

- *Improvements in ventilation.* Improving ventilation can reduce infections by pathogens spread through airborne transmission and also reduce exposure to household air pollution. One way to measure the ventilation of a room is by the number of **air exchanges (or air changes) per hour**. A minimal amount of ventilation is about two air changes per hour. The CDC recommends that buildings have about 5 air changes per hour,[133] but that hospitals, where the risk of infection is greater,

have 6-15 air changes per hour.[134] In most buildings, it is possible to get high levels of ventilation by just opening windows on opposite sides (cross-ventilation), perhaps with the added help of a fan in one of the windows (forced cross-ventilation). If cold or hot outdoor temperatures make that uncomfortable, heating and air conditioning systems can be set to provide 6-12 air changes per hour and filter the air before recirculating it.[134] Systems are also available to disinfect recirculated air by treating it with ultraviolet light.[135]

- *Reduction in crowding.* In some situations, crowding can be reduced by increasing distance between people. Examples are the social distancing steps taken during the early months of the COVID-19 pandemic, such as limiting the number of people in an indoor space or enforcing a minimum distance between people. This slows the spread of respiratory pathogens and may reduce overall disease rates.

- *Promotion of mask use.* While they are difficult to study, well-designed face masks appear to reduce people's risk of infection with respiratory viruses, including influenza and COVID-19.[136-138] For them to be most effective, though, they must fit tightly on the face, which makes them uncomfortable to wear. For that reason, most people are unlikely to wear masks consistently except in special situations, such as in hospitals and during severe epidemics.
- *Provision of clean water and promotion of handwashing.* Handwashing with soap reduces rates of LRI by about 20%. Of course, for people to wash their hands, people need water in their homes.[126,139]

Interventions to reduce the susceptibility of older children and adults to LRI include:

- *Substitution of biomass fuels.* People in low-income countries burn biomass fuels like dung or crop waste because they are available and cheap. The best way to reduce exposure to indoor air pollution from these fuels is to give people inexpensive access to cleaner fuels like electricity, natural gas, and liquefied petroleum gas (LPG).[140]
- *Reduction in ambient air pollution.* Technologic improvements to reduce emissions, backed up by government policies and enforcement, can reduce ambient air pollution.
- *Smoking prevention.* See Chapter 11. Tobacco Use.
- *Reduction of alcohol use.* See Chapter 12. Alcohol Use.

Interventions to reduce the susceptibility of infants and young children to respiratory pathogens include:

- *Prevention or treatment of undernutrition.* This is discussed in the section on Maternal and Child Undernutrition in Chapter 14. Nutrition.
- *Zinc supplementation.* Giving children in low-income countries zinc supplements reduces their risk of LRI.[128]
- *Breastfeeding education and support.* See Chapter 14. Nutrition.
- *Prevention of preterm birth and low birth weight.* See Chapter 10. Diseases of the Newborn.

Many of the risk factors for LRI and interventions to prevent LRI in children overlap with those of diarrheal diseases. The WHO has adopted an integrated plan for prevention of both diarrhea and pneumonia in low-income countries. This plan includes initiatives to promote breastfeeding, handwashing, and vaccination; reduce household air pollution; and provide antibiotics for children with pneumonia.[84]

Box 9.8 Summary–Prevention of Lower Respiratory Infections

- Core interventions
  - Vaccination
  - Antibiotic and antiviral treatment
- Reduce exposure to respiratory pathogens
  - Improvements in ventilation
  - Reduction in crowding
  - Promotion of mask use
  - Provision of clean water and promotion of handwashing
- Reduce susceptibility of older children and adults
  - Substitution of biomass fuels
  - Reduction in ambient air pollution
  - Smoking prevention
  - Reduction of alcohol use
- Reduce susceptibility of young children
  - Prevention or treatment of undernutrition
  - Zinc supplementation
  - Breastfeeding education and support
  - Prevention of preterm birth and low birth weight

Box 9.9 Key Words–Lower Respiratory Infections

Acute Respiratory Distress Syndrome (ARDS)
Aerosol
Air exchanges (or air changes) per hour
Airways
Alveoli (of the lung)
Antibiotic
Antibody, antibodies
Antigenic drift
Antigenic shift
Antiviral medication
Biomass
Bronchioles
Bronchus, bronchi
Droplet nuclei
Endothelium
Epithelium, epithelial cells
Fomites
Hib vaccine
Lower respiratory infections (LRI)
Middle East Respiratory Syndrome (MERS)
Mucous membranes
$PM_{2.5}$
Pneumococcal conjugate vaccine (PCV)
Pneumococcus
Pneumonia
Respiratory syncytial virus (RSV)
Respiratory tract
SARS-CoV-2
Secondary infection
Severe Acute Respiratory Syndrome (SARS)
Trachea
Upper respiratory infection (URI)

Resources–Lower Respiratory Infections

- Aliberti S, Dela Cruz CS, Amati F, Sotgiu G, Restrepo MI. Community-acquired pneumonia. *Lancet.* 2021;398(10303):906-919. doi:10.1016/S0140-6736(21)00630-9
- Troeger C, Blacker B, Khalil IA, et al. Estimates of the global, regional, and national morbidity, mortality, and aetiologies of lower respiratory infections in 195 countries, 1990–2016: A systematic analysis for the Global Burden of Disease Study 2016. *Lancet Infect Dis.* 2018;18(11):1191-1210. doi:10.1016/S1473-3099(18)30310-4
- Kyu HH, Vongpradith A, Sirota SB, et al. Age–sex differences in the global burden of lower respiratory infections and risk factors, 1990–2019: results from the Global Burden of Disease Study 2019. *Lancet Infect Dis.* 2022;22(11):1626-1647. doi:10.1016/S1473-3099(22)00510-2
- Leung NHL. Transmissibility and transmission of respiratory viruses. *Nat Rev Microbiol.* 2021; 19(8):528-545. doi:10.1038/s41579-021-00535-6
- Leung DT, Chisti MJ, Pavia AT. Prevention and Control of Childhood Pneumonia and Diarrhea. *Pediatr Clin North Am.* 2016;63(1):67-79. doi:10.1016/j.pcl.2015.08.003
- WHO. *Ending Preventable Child Deaths from Pneumonia and Diarrhoea by 2025: The Integrated Global Action Plan for Pneumonia and Diarrhoea (GAPPD)*; 2013.

Tuberculosis

Introduction

Tuberculosis (usually abbreviated as **TB**) is an infection with a bacterium that usually involves the lungs. The bacterium is spread from one person to another through the air in crowded, poorly-ventilated settings. The infection can be cured with antibiotic drugs, and treatment of persons with active tuberculosis prevents spread to others.

Tuberculosis case rates have been falling for decades, and the disease has been nearly eliminated in the United States. But globally, tuberculosis still kills some 1.3 million persons each year, which is roughly twice the number killed by HIV.[141] The WHO has adopted a global "End TB Strategy," with a goal to reduce deaths from tuberculosis by 90% from 2015 to 2030.[142] Unfortunately, without enough funding or commitment from national leaders, this initiative will probably not meet that goal.

Pathophysiology of Tuberculosis

Mycobacterium tuberculosis

Tuberculosis is caused by *Mycobacterium tuberculosis*, a slow-growing bacterium that, under a microscope, looks like a tiny rod. Rod-shaped bacteria are called **bacilli** (**Figure 9.40**). To make bacteria visible under a microscope, microbiologists apply colorful chemical "stains" to them. *Mycobacterium tuberculosis* retains the color from these stains even after being washed with acid, so it is called an **"acid-fast" bacillus**, usually abbreviated as **AFB**.

Infection Versus Disease

In tuberculosis, there is a distinction between *TB infection* and *TB disease*.

Mycobacterium tuberculosis can live and grow in nearly any tissue in the human body, but by far the most common infection site is the lung. When *Mycobacterium tuberculosis* enters a person's lungs, the organism invades lung tissues and makes copies of itself. The person's immune system responds, sending **macrophages** and **cytotoxic T lymphocytes** to the

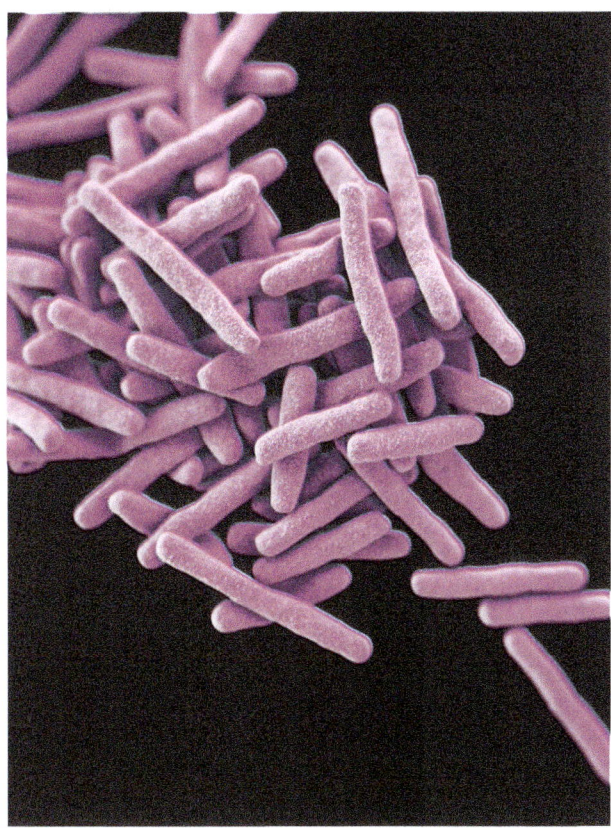

Figure 9.40 *Mycobacterium tuberculosis.* The bacteria that cause tuberculosis look like tiny rods and are called bacilli.
Courtesy of James Archer/CDC.

area. (See the HIV/AIDS section earlier in this chapter for a discussion of the immune system.) These cells try to kill the organism through **phagocytosis** and **cell-mediated immunity,** but *Mycobacterium tuberculosis* can resist these immune cell attacks.[143] Often the result is a standoff, in which small "colonies" of *M. tuberculosis* organisms remain alive but are surrounded by immune cells and encased in small pockets called **granulomas** (**Figure 9.41**). A colony of bacteria (or perhaps even a single organism) in a granuloma can remain dormant for years, during which the person is perfectly healthy. This condition is called **latent TB infection**, or often just *TB infection*.

For about 5% of people infected, the immune response fails, allowing the bacteria to spread and cause damage to other areas of the lung and other organs. This is considered **active tuberculosis**, often called just *TB disease*. When it occurs shortly after the initial infection it is called **primary active tuberculosis**.[143]

The other 95% of people who develop latent TB infection are not necessarily safe. If their immune systems later become weakened, the dormant bacteria

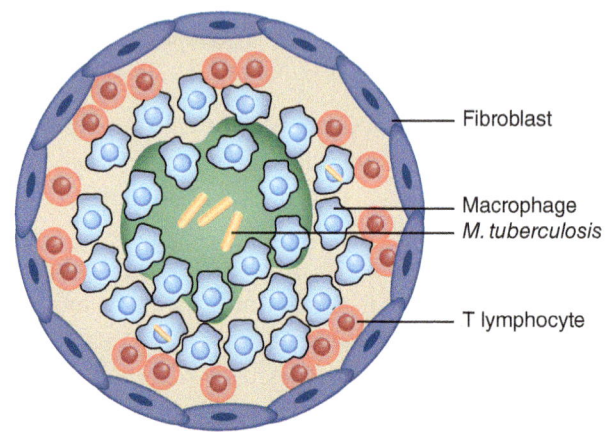

Figure 9.41 Granuloma in Person with Tuberculosis Infection. In most people, the initial infection with *Mycobacterium tuberculosis* leads to the bacteria becoming encased in granulomas. The bacteria live in the center of these granulomas, surrounded by immune cells and the remains of dead human cells, and can remain alive for many years.

can break out of the granulomas and spread to other areas of the lung or body. This is called **secondary or reactivation tuberculosis** (**Figure 9.42**), and it can occur in persons with malnutrition, chronic

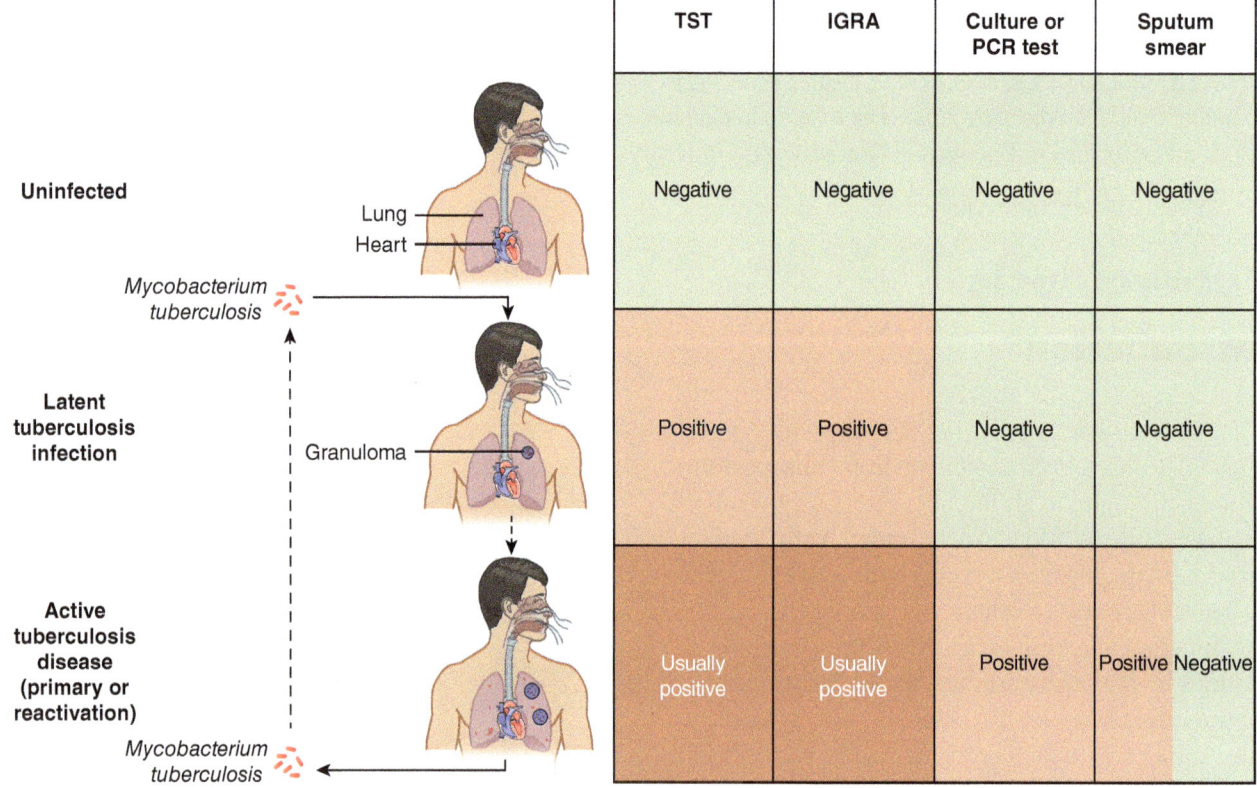

Figure 9.42 Stages of Tuberculosis Infection and Test Results. Most people infected with *Mycobacterium tuberculosis* develop latent tuberculosis infection. In this stage, they are not contagious. However, if their immune systems later become weakened, the bacteria can spread to other areas of the lung or body, which is called active tuberculosis disease. Also, a small percentage of people develop active tuberculosis disease when first infected. People with active tuberculosis disease can spread the infection to others.

diseases like diabetes, HIV infection, or just the weakness of aging. About 5-10% of people with latent TB infection will have a reactivation at some time.[144]

Symptoms and Tests

People with latent tuberculosis infection have no symptoms. However, tests of their immune system show signs that they have been infected. This most common test is the **tuberculin skin test (TST)**. In this test, a small amount of protein from *M. tuberculosis* (the **purified protein derivative or PPD**) is injected into the skin. In a person who has been infected, T lymphocytes will respond by traveling to the area, and within two days a hard bump will form at the site of the injection. Another test of the immune system is a blood test called the **interferon-gamma release assay, or IGRA** (also known by its trade name QuantiFERON).

People with either primary or secondary active tuberculosis typically have fevers, periods of intense sweating at night, a persistent cough, and weight loss.[143] X-rays of their lungs show tissue damage and inflammation. The *Mycobacterium tuberculosis* bacteria can be identified by laboratory tests of their **sputum**—that is, the mucus in their respiratory tract that they expel when coughing (Figure 9.42).

People with active tuberculosis also usually have positive TST and IGRA tests. Because the tests measure the body's immune response, not the infection itself or the disease, the tests usually remain positive even after these persons are cured.[145]

Transmission

Mycobacterium tuberculosis is spread from one person to others through airborne transmission/inhalation. When a person with active tuberculosis coughs, sings, or speaks, that person expels droplets of **respiratory secretions** into the air. After the water in these droplets evaporates, **droplet nuclei** are left. These droplet nuclei can hold a few *Mycobacterium tuberculosis* organisms. The droplet nuclei are small enough to remain suspended in the air and be blown from room to room as the air moves. They also are small enough that, if inhaled by another person, they penetrate deep into that person's lungs, where they can establish a new infection.[146]

Some people with active tuberculosis are far more likely to spread the infection than others. A simple laboratory test can identify them. A sample of their sputum is smeared on a glass slide, stained, and then viewed with a microscope. If enough acid-fast bacilli

are in the sputum for them to be visible, these people are called "**smear-positive**" and considered particularly contagious.[146]

Epidemiology: Patterns and Trends

The WHO estimates that about a quarter of the world's population is infected with *Mycobacterium tuberculosis*, and about 10 million people develop active tuberculosis every year. Some 1.3 million people die from active tuberculosis every year, of whom nearly 170,000 are HIV-positive.[141]

Between 2000 and 2019, the estimated global incidence and mortality rates of active tuberculosis fell by about 2% per year (**Figure 9.43**).[141] However, this gradual improvement was interrupted by the COVID pandemic in 2020-2021.

At a global scale, tuberculosis is strongly linked to poverty. In the least-affected regions—the United States, Canada, western Europe and Australia—there are fewer than 10 cases of active tuberculosis per 100,000 persons per year. In the most heavily affected regions—Sub-Saharan Africa, South Asia, Southeast Asia, and the Pacific islands—the TB incidence is 10 to 200 times higher, with rates between 100 and 600 cases per 100,000 per year (**Figure 9.44**).[141]

In the United States, only about 8,000 people are diagnosed with active tuberculosis each year. About 70% are immigrants from other countries. Among those born in the United States, active tuberculosis is concentrated in poor or marginalized persons. About 5% each of people with active TB in the United States are HIV positive, homeless, or incarcerated.[147]

Risk Factors

Risk factors for tuberculosis mostly fall in two categories: those that increase the risk that persons will be exposed to the bacteria and those that increase the likelihood that an initial or latent tuberculosis infection will progress to active tuberculosis (**Figure 9.45**).

People are more likely to be exposed to *M. tuberculosis* in situations with:

- *Crowding.* The increased risk from crowding stems from simple math: when more people are in an enclosed space, there is a higher chance that at least one will have active tuberculosis, and if so, there are more people who can catch the infection from him or her. An extreme example is Tibetan refugees living in India, many of whom are monks or nuns living in large group facilities. Nearly all are infected with *Mycobacterium tuberculosis*, and

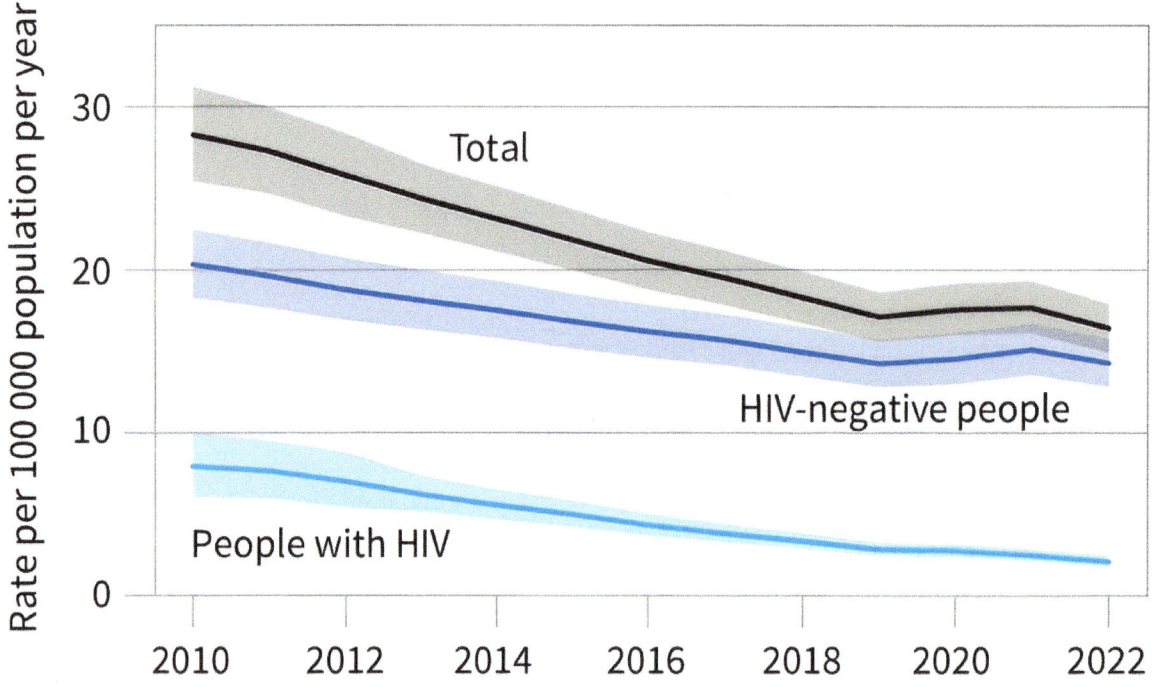

Figure 9.43 **Global Trends in the Incidence of Tuberculosis.**

Reproduced from World Health Organization. Global Tuberculosis Report 2023. World Health Organization. Published 2024. Accessed June 30, 2024. https://www.who.int/teams/global-tuberculosis-programme/tb-reports/global-tuberculosis-report-2023

their incidence rate for active tuberculosis is more than twice the rates in the countries with the highest incidence.[148] More commonly, people living in households with more than five members

are about twice as likely to develop active tuberculosis as those in smaller households.[149]

- *Poor ventilation.* In well-ventilated spaces, droplet nuclei are quickly flushed outdoors. But in spaces

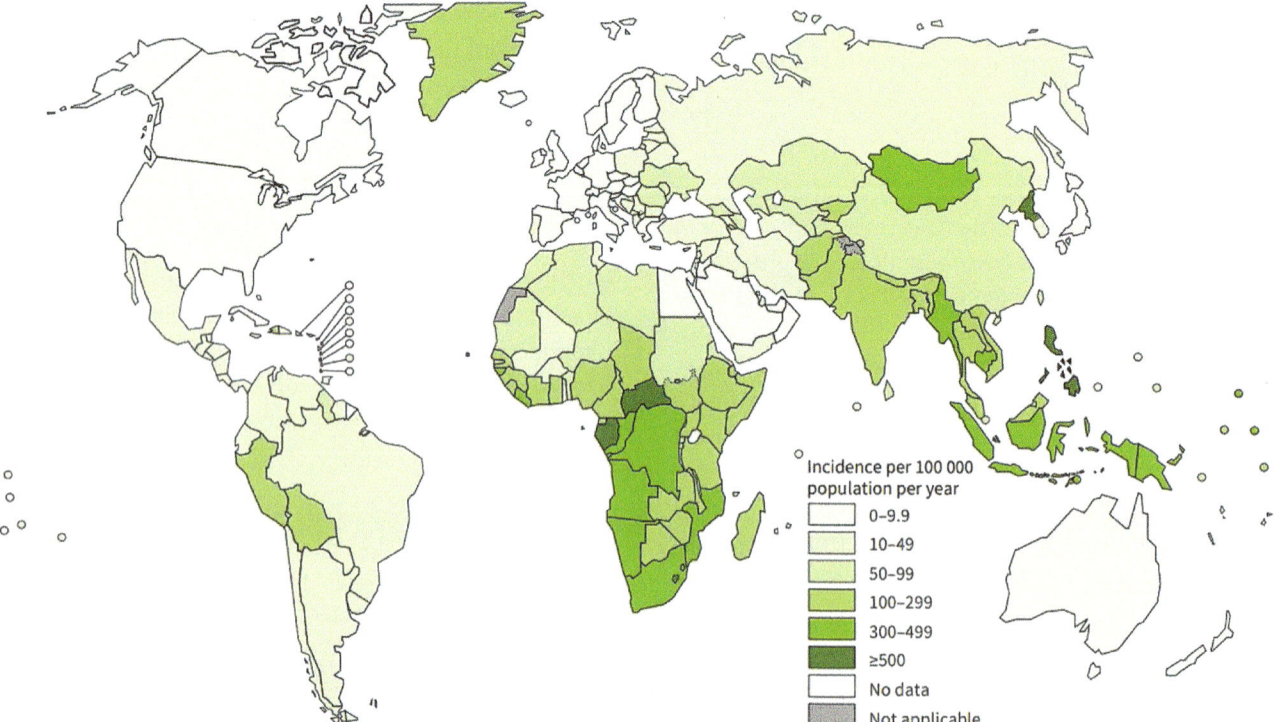

Figure 9.44 **Estimated Incidence of Tuberculosis by Country, 2021.**

Reproduced from World Health Organization. Global Tuberculosis Report 2023. World Health Organization. Published 2024. Accessed June 30, 2024. https://www.who.int/teams/global-tuberculosis-programme/tb-reports/global-tuberculosis-report-2023

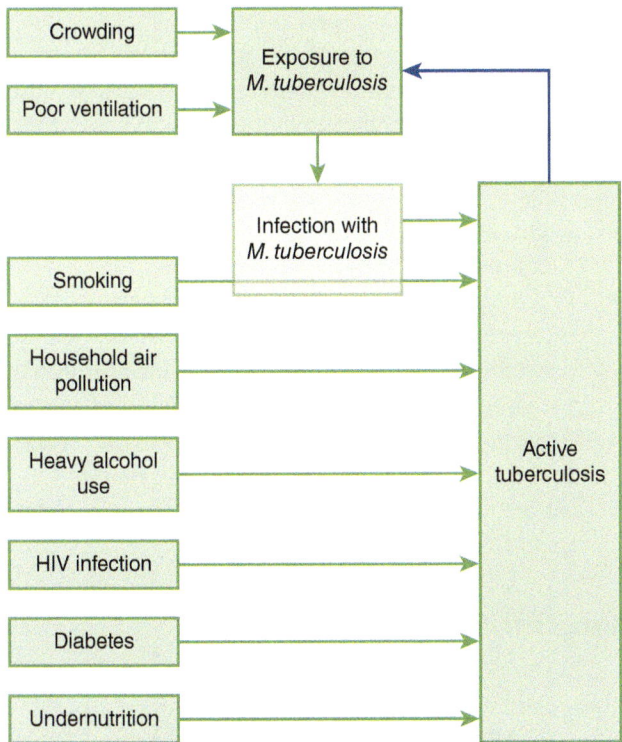

Figure 9.45 Cause-and-Effect Diagram for Tuberculosis. For a person to become infected with *Mycobacterium tuberculosis*, that person must be exposed to the organism. Among those who are exposed and infected, though, there are several risk factors that increase the likelihood that that person will develop active tuberculosis.

with poor ventilation, droplet nuclei linger where people can inhale them. Tuberculosis is rarely transmitted outdoors but is readily spread inside poorly ventilated homes and other buildings.[149-153]

People with an initial infection with *M. tuberculosis* are more likely to develop active tuberculosis if they have:

- *Undernutrition*, which weakens the immune system. For example, people with latent tuberculosis infection who are underweight are several times more likely to develop active tuberculosis.[154] The WHO estimates that about 20% of cases of TB are attributable to undernutrition.[155]
- *HIV infection*. HIV attacks the immune cells that are needed in the body's battle against the bacteria. People with HIV infection are much more likely to develop active tuberculosis, regardless of whether they are in the early stages of HIV infection or have AIDS. Taken as a group, people with HIV infection are about 20 times as likely to develop active tuberculosis as those without HIV.[156] In the 1980s, the HIV/AIDS pandemic changed tuberculosis across the globe, leading

to outbreaks and prompting experts to overhaul their tuberculosis prevention strategies.

- *Heavy alcohol consumption.* Alcohol weakens the macrophages that try to contain *Mycobacterium tuberculosis* in the lung. People who drink heavily are about three times as likely to develop active tuberculosis.[157] Experts estimate that in countries where drinking is common, about 25% of cases of active tuberculosis are attributable to alcohol use.[157]
- *Diabetes* and other chronic diseases such as chronic lung or kidney disease.[143] People with diabetes are about 50% more likely to develop active tuberculosis.[158]
- *Smoking.* Like alcohol, tobacco smoke interferes with the macrophages in the lung, weakening their ability to contain *M. tuberculosis*.[159] People who smoke are more than twice as likely as nonsmokers to develop active tuberculosis.[160,161] Smoking has also been shown to increase the risk of latent tuberculosis infection. In addition, children who are exposed to second-hand tobacco smoke at home are also more likely to acquire latent tuberculosis infection.[162]
- *Household air pollution.* In low-income countries, children in families that burn wood, charcoal, or animal dung for heat and cooking indoors are at greater risk of developing active tuberculosis, likely because of the damage from the smoke makes the lungs more susceptible to the bacteria.[140,149,163-165] Household air pollution is discussed more in Chapter 8. Chronic Respiratory Diseases.

Tuberculosis is especially likely to spread in settings with a combination of risks. For example, in the United States, outbreaks of TB occur in jails and homeless shelters because they serve persons at high risk (such as those with alcoholism or HIV infection) and they are both crowded and poorly-ventilated.[143]

The link between poverty and tuberculosis is so strong that some experts view poverty as an independent risk factor.[145] People living in poverty are more likely to have several risk factors, including malnutrition, household crowding, and inadequate ventilation at home. They are also more likely to smoke, have diabetes, and be exposed to others with tuberculosis.

Preventive Interventions

Rates of active tuberculosis in the United States and Europe fell for decades before antibiotics were discovered. This decline was due to improvements in social conditions, particularly better nutrition and housing. Today, tuberculosis rates can be reduced by likewise improving social conditions, or they can be reduced by using biomedical tools, particularly vaccination and antibiotics.

Reduction of Risk Factors

Active tuberculosis can be prevented by (**Figure 9.46**):

- *Reduction of crowding* in homes, workplaces, and public buildings like jails and homeless shelters.
- *Improvements in ventilation* in healthcare facilities, homes, workplaces, and in buildings where high-risk people are present. To help prevent the spread of TB in healthcare facilities and other high-risk settings, the WHO recommends "natural ventilation" (that is, open windows) rather than mechanical ventilation or recirculated air, even if the recirculated air is filtered.[166] CDC recommends that all buildings have at least 5 air changes per hour of ventilation, but that hospitals have 6-15 air changes per hour.[133,134] Mechanical ventilation systems should be set to increase the proportion of circulated air that comes from outdoors.
- *Reduction of undernutrition.* See Chapter 14. Nutrition.

- *Smoking prevention.* See Chapter 11. Tobacco Use.
- *Substitution of biomass fuels.* Substituting biomass fuels used in homes with cleaner fuels would help prevent tuberculosis in the same way that it helps prevent other lower respiratory infections.[140]
- *Reduction of alcohol consumption.* See Chapter 12. Alcohol Use.
- *Prevention or treatment of HIV infection.* All the interventions discussed earlier in this chapter to prevent or treat HIV infection have the additional benefit of reducing the risk of tuberculosis.
- *Prevention of diabetes.* Preventing type 2 diabetes is very difficult, but if possible, it would help reduce tuberculosis rates. See Chapter 7. Chronic Metabolic Disease.

Vaccination

Since the 1940s, many countries have used a vaccine against tuberculosis called Bacillus Calmette-Guerin (**BCG**).[167] The BCG vaccine is made from a weakened strain of a bacterium called *Mycobacterium bovis*, a close relative of *Mycobacterium tuberculosis* that infects cattle. Most countries in the world now give BCG vaccine to all babies soon after

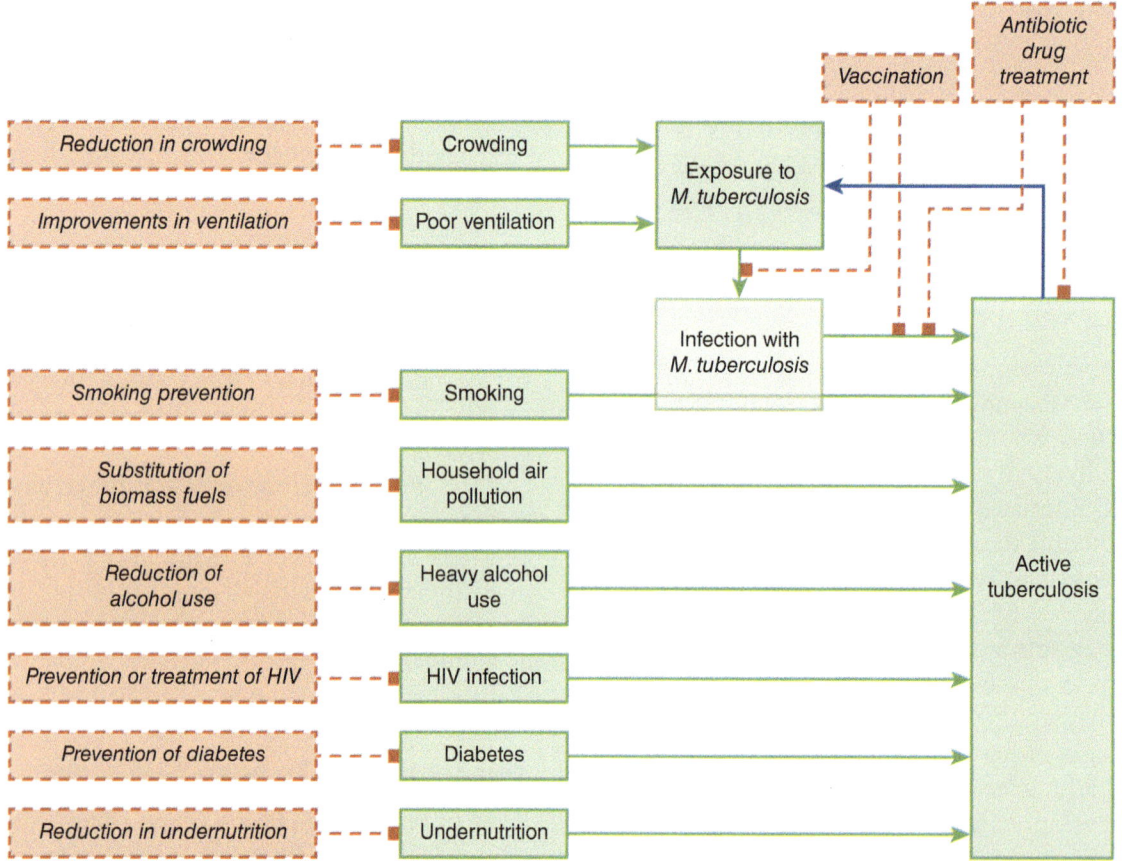

Figure 9.46 **Cause-and-Effect Diagram for Tuberculosis, with Preventive Interventions.**

birth.[168] This reduces the risk that these children will develop active tuberculosis before age 10 by about 35%, but it does not help them when they are older.[169]

The low effectiveness of BCG has prompted a push for better vaccines. As of this writing, several studies are testing newer-technology vaccines that may reduce the risk of active tuberculosis in adults by 50%.[145,170] Also, researchers are studying whether giving BCG booster doses to adolescents helps protect them as teenagers and adults.

Antibiotic Drug Treatment for Persons with Active Tuberculosis

If people with active tuberculosis take certain antibiotics, they can be cured and can no longer spread the infection to others. For that reason, antibiotic treatment of people with active tuberculosis is a cornerstone of any strategy to prevent others from developing tuberculosis and reduce TB rates in populations.

Antibiotics take longer to work against tuberculosis than they do against other bacterial infections. People with active tuberculosis stop spreading the infection after taking these drugs for just a few days, but it usually takes months of a combination of drugs for them to be cured. [151] As of this writing, experts recommend that typical adults with active tuberculosis take drugs called **isoniazid** (usually abbreviated as **INH**) and **rifampin** (also called **rifampicin**) for 6 months, combined with two other antibiotic drugs for the first two months.[145,171]

Some strains of *M. tuberculosis* have become resistant to these antibiotics. Globally, about 3% of new tuberculosis cases and 17% of previously-treated cases are caused by bacteria that are resistant to rifampin or to multiple drugs.[141] Other drugs—some newly developed, some "repurposed"—are available to treat people with drug-resistant tuberculosis, but these other drugs can be expensive and have more side effects than INH and rifampin. Treatment for drug-resistant tuberculosis may take 6 to 18 months.[172]

It can be difficult for people with tuberculosis to take these drugs consistently for 6 or more months, particularly after they feel healthy again. It is important that people with TB adhere to the full treatment course, though, because if they take these drugs intermittently or stop taking them early, they may relapse with a strain of *Mycobacterium tuberculosis* that is now resistant to antibiotics. To promote adherence to drug treatment, for many years the WHO recommended **directly-observed therapy (DOT)**, in which a medical or lay worker (or

sometimes a family member) observed the person with TB taking each dose. The WHO now recommends instead offering patients **treatment support**.[173] Like DOT, treatment support may involve a healthcare worker or trained lay worker observing a patient take pills, but the observation may be by video, or the worker may use other technological tools like digital medication monitors. Also, treatment support can include other forms of help, such as food or money.[173]

Providing medical treatment for people with tuberculosis is complicated. There are many drugs to choose from. Medical staff must offer their patients treatment support, must conduct medical tests, and must evaluate how well their patients are responding to treatment. The medical staff doing that work may not be highly trained in tuberculosis, so they will need expert guidance. With this in mind, in 1989, global experts in tuberculosis developed rules and protocols for how people with tuberculosis should be identified, tested, treated, and followed. These detailed protocols have become known as the Styblo model (named for the expert who first developed the protocols).[174] This model of highly-standardized procedures is still used today for tuberculosis control in countries worldwide. A person with tuberculosis in India is likely to be treated and supported very much like a person with tuberculosis in Zimbabwe.

Antibiotic Drug Treatment for Persons With or At Risk for Infection

WHO recommends that people with latent tuberculosis infection also take antibiotics to prevent them from developing active tuberculosis. Treatment typically involves isoniazid alone for 6–9 months, or combinations of drugs for three months.[144,145]

Finally, WHO recommends preventive drug treatment for two other groups of people who do not have active tuberculosis but who are at very high risk for infection:[144]

- *Household members of persons with active tuberculosis.* Household members of people with active TB are 10–25 times as likely as the general population to have active tuberculosis themselves.[144] Accordingly, WHO recommends that household members of people with active tuberculosis be evaluated, tested for latent tuberculosis infection if possible, and given antibiotics preventively if the TST or IGRA test is positive or the tests cannot be done.[144] **Contact tracing** is the term used to describe the process of identifying and

Box 9.10 Summary–Prevention of Tuberculosis

- Reduction in crowding
- Improvements in ventilation
- Reduction in undernutrition
- Smoking prevention
- Substitution of biomass fuels
- Reduction of alcohol consumption
- Prevention or treatment of HIV infection
- Prevention of diabetes
- Vaccination
- Antibiotic drug treatment of persons with active tuberculosis, persons with latent tuberculosis infection, persons with HIV infection, and household members of persons with active tuberculosis

Box 9.11 Key Words–Tuberculosis

Acid-fast, acid-fast bacilli (AFB)
Active tuberculosis
Bacillus, bacilli
BCG
Cell-mediated immunity
Contact tracing
Cytotoxic T lymphocytes
Directly-observed therapy (DOT)
Droplet nuclei
Granuloma
Interferon-gamma release assay (IGRA)
Isoniazid (INH)
Latent TB infection
Macrophage
Phagocytosis
Primary active tuberculosis
Purified protein derivative (PPD)
Reactivation tuberculosis
Respiratory secretions
Rifampin, rifampicin
Secondary tuberculosis
Smear-positive
Sputum
TB
Treatment support
Tuberculin skin test (TST)

finding these household members so that they can receive this treatment.

- *Persons with HIV infection.* The WHO recommends that all people with HIV infection receive antibiotic treatment for tuberculosis, regardless of whether they have known latent tuberculosis infection or know of an exposure to others with tuberculosis.[142,144] This recommendation is based on the very high risk that people with HIV will develop active tuberculosis.

Resources–Tuberculosis

- The Centers for Disease Control and Prevention provides information and guidance on prevention, diagnosis, and treatment of tuberculosis, along with data on tuberculosis cases in the United States. www.cdc.gov/tb
- Furin J, Cox H, Pai M. Tuberculosis. *Lancet.* 2019;393(10181):1642-1656. doi:10.1016/S0140-6736(19)30308-3
- Churchyard G, Kim P, Shah NS, et al. What we know about tuberculosis transmission: An overview. *J Infect Dis.* 2017;216:S629-S635. doi:10.1093/infdis/jix362
- Nardell EA. Transmission and institutional infection control of tuberculosis. *Cold Spring Harb Perspect Med.* 2016;6(2). doi:10.1101/cshperspect.a018192
- The Lancet Commission Task Force on Safe Work, Safe School, and Safe Travel, report on Proposed Non-infectious Air Delivery Rates (NADRE) for reducing exposure to airborne respiratory infectious diseases. This Provides guidance on ventilation for prevention of tuberculosis, COVID-19, and other diseases. Published November 2022.
- The World Health Organization issues "Consolidated Guidelines" for prevention and treatment of tuberculosis, as well as an annual Global Tuberculosis Report on progress of the End TB plan. Available at: https://www.who.int/health-topics/tuberculosis

Malaria

Introduction

Malaria is an infection with a **protozoan** organism that is spread by the bite of a mosquito. Every year, this disease kills hundreds of thousands of people, most of whom are young children, and sickens many times that number.[175] In the mid-20th century, the World Health Organization (WHO) tried unsuccessfully to eradicate malaria. But since 2000, public health programs have made renewed progress, which has prompted the WHO to set an ambitious goal of reducing malaria mortality by 90% by 2030.[176] This initiative is struggling, though, with the development of insecticide-resistant mosquitoes and drug-resistant protozoa, as well as a shortage of funding.

Pathophysiology of Malaria

Life Cycle of Plasmodium

The organism that causes malaria is one of several species of protozoa called **Plasmodium**. This organism is a parasite that grows inside the cells of humans and mosquitoes. *Plasmodium* has an extremely complicated life cycle, involving three different cycles, in which it reproduces itself (**Figure 9.47**), and it undergoes several transformations of its appearance (**Figure 9.48**). The reproduction cycles within the overall life cycle are:

- **Exo-erythrocytic cycle**. When a *Plasmodium*-infected mosquito bites a human, **sporozoites** are injected into the human's bloodstream. Within an hour, the sporozoites travel to the liver, where they enter liver cells (**hepatocytes**). Inside the infected hepatocytes, over several days, each sporozoite makes tens of thousands of copies of itself, turning into a **schizont**.[177] The schizont then ruptures from the hepatocyte, releasing thousands of **merozoites** into the blood.[178,179]

- **Erythrocytic cycle**. In the blood, the merozoites enter **red blood cells**, which are also called **erythrocytes**. Inside the red blood cells, the merozoites transform into ring-like **trophozoites**. Much like the sporozoites in liver cells, the trophozoites in red blood cells then make copies of themselves, turning into schizonts. These schizonts and the red blood cells around them then rupture, spilling new merozoites into the blood. These merozoites then enter other red blood cells and repeat the cycle.[178-180]

The erythrocytic cycle repeats every 24 to 72 hours, depending on the species of *Plasmodium* involved. Each time the red blood cells spill new merozoites, the organisms stimulate the human's immune system, causing the human to have a fever. Sometimes, the erythrocytic cycle is synchronized across the many infected red blood

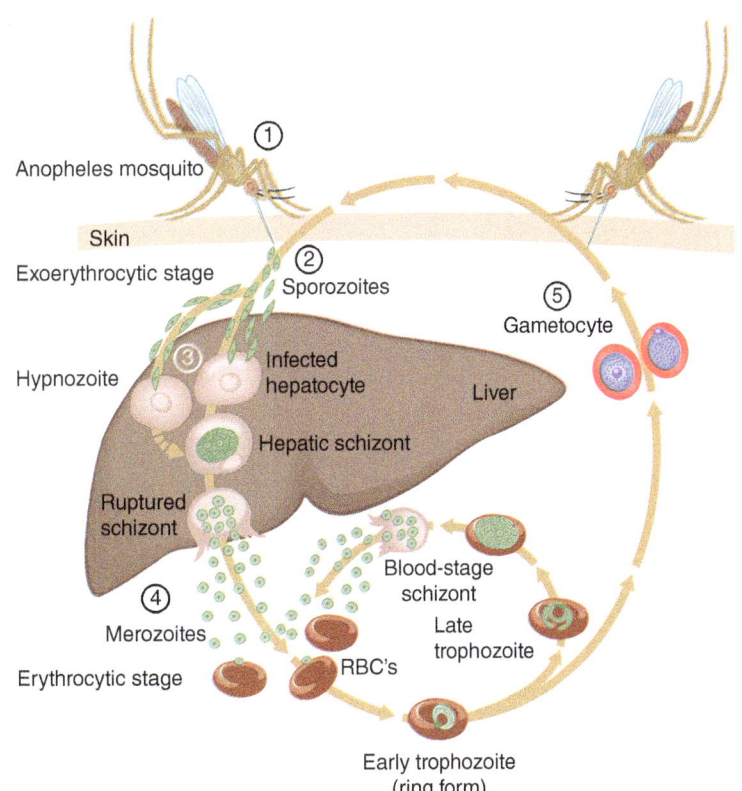

Figure 9.47 Life Cycle of the Malaria Parasite. After a bite from an infected mosquito (1), sporozoites (2) infect liver cells (hepatocytes). In the liver, the protozoa multiply to become schizonts; this is called the exo-erythrocytic cycle. These schizonts rupture and release merozoites (4) into the blood. The merozoites infect red blood cells, where they undergo repeated cycles of reproduction; this is called the erythrocytic cycle. A few take a different path, becoming gametocytes (5), which then infect another mosquito; this is called the sporogenic cycle. Also, some but not all species of malaria parasites have a stage called hypnozoites (3), which can remain dormant in the liver for many years before they become active again.

Hill AV. Vaccines against malaria. *Philos Trans R Soc Lond B Biol Sci.* 2011;366(1579):2806-2814. doi:10.1098/rstb.2011.0091.

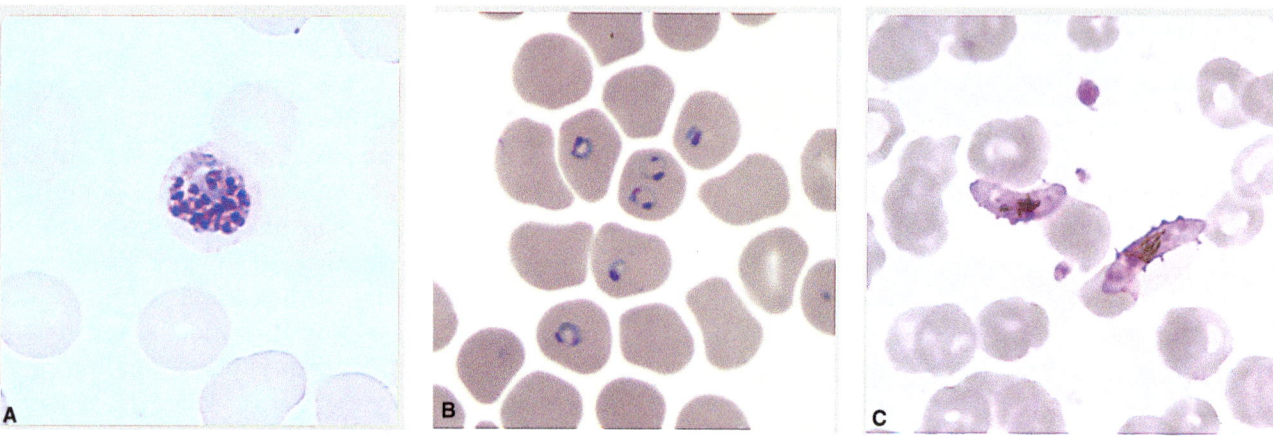

Figure 9.48 Appearance of *Plasmodium falciparum* Parasites in Blood. **A.** Schizont, **B.** Ring trophozoites, **C.** Gametocytes.
Centers for Disease Control and Prevention, Malaria. Figures B (Schizont of P. falciparum), G (Gametocytes of P. falciparum with Laveran's bibs), and H (Rings of P. falciparum) in thin blood smears. https://www.cdc.gov/dpdx/malaria/index.html

cells. When that happens, people with malaria can develop sudden, high fevers that reappear regularly every one to three days.[179,181]

- **Sporogenic cycle.** While most of the trophozoites in red blood cells become schizonts, a few take a different path, maturing into either male or female forms called **gametocytes**. Then, when mosquitoes bite humans, the mosquitoes pick up these gametocytes. Inside mosquitoes, over about one to three weeks, the male and female gametocytes join and produce new sporozoites.[178]

All the species of *Plasmodium* that infect humans undergo these same reproduction cycles, with one exception. When **Plasmodium vivax** and **Plasmodium ovale** sporozoites infect liver cells, some are transformed into **hypnozoites**.[178,181] These hypnozoites are inactive forms that can remain dormant inside liver cells for months or even years, before becoming active again. The ability of hypnozoites to hide in the liver explains why people who seem cured of malaria from *Plasmodium vivax* or *ovale* can have long-delayed relapses.[178]

Plasmodium Species

The species responsible for most malaria deaths is **Plasmodium falciparum**, which causes nearly all cases in sub-Saharan Africa and about half of the cases of malaria in other parts of the world. *Plasmodium falciparum* is particularly deadly for two reasons. First, it can infect a much higher percentage of red blood cells than other species, causing more damage to the blood. Second, it can cause the infected red blood cells to stick to walls of the body's tiniest blood vessels, which can block the flow of blood, starving organs like the brain of oxygen.[179,182]

Other than in Africa, the second most common species causing malaria is *Plasmodium vivax*, which can thrive in more varied environments than *P. falciparum* can.[175,181,182] *P. vivax* usually does not kill, but when children or adults are infected for months or years it causes **anemia** (low levels of **hemoglobin** or red blood cells), malnutrition, and low birth weight.[180] Infection with *Plasmodium vivax* is uncommon in sub-Saharan Africa because many people there are genetically resistant to it.[182] However, in other areas of the world where mosquitoes carry both *Plasmodium falciparum* and *Plasmodium vivax*, it is common for people to be infected with both organisms.[183]

Other species that can cause malaria in humans are *Plasmodium ovale*, which is similar to *Plasmodium vivax*, and **Plasmodium malariae**, which is considered the least dangerous species, but can cause a persistent infection.[180,182]

The Anopheles Mosquito

In epidemiology, a **vector** is an organism (like an insect or rodent) that carries an infectious agent (like a virus, bacterium, or protozoan) and transmits it to another organism (like a human). The vector that carries *Plasmodium* and transmits it to humans is any of about 40 species of **Anopheles** mosquitoes (**Figure 9.49**).[184] *Anopheles* species that can spread malaria are found in most of the world, including places with cool climates.[178,183]

Anopheles mosquitoes have their own complicated life cycle (**Figure 9.50**). A mature female mosquito lays eggs on the surface of standing fresh water.[184] About 2–3 days later, the eggs hatch into **larvae**.[178] On the surface of that water, over 4-10 days, the larvae eat algae or other microorganisms, grow, and then become **pupae,** like caterpillars becoming cocoons.

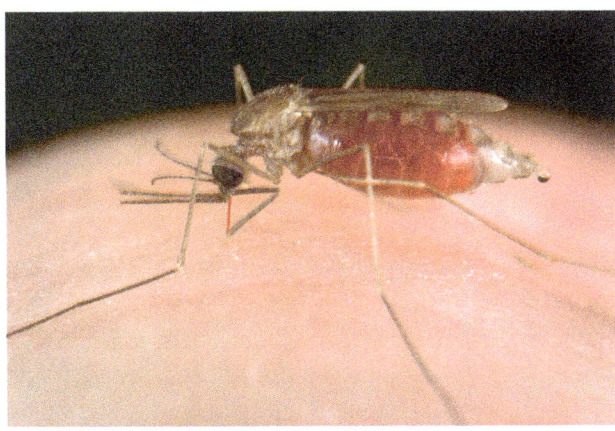

Figure 9.49 *Anopheles* **Mosquito.**

Courtesy of James Gathany/CDC.

Through metamorphosis, in another 2–3 days, adult mosquitoes emerge from the pupae.[178]

Adult male mosquitoes feed only on plant nectar, attempt to mate, and die after about a week. Adult females also feed on plant nectar but need to take in blood to develop eggs, so they bite humans or animals, drinking a **blood meal**. After blood meals, the adult females rest for a few days—they prefer dark, sheltered areas such as tree wells or the inside walls of houses—during which they develop eggs.[185] After this rest, the adult mosquitoes lay eggs on the surface of water. The females repeat this cycle of biting and laying eggs a few times before dying. For a female *Anopheles* mosquito to spread malaria, it must bite humans at least twice—once to get infected and a second time, 7–10 days later, to pass the infection to a new human.[183]

Some *Anopheles* species prefer to bite humans and some prefer to bite other animals (like cattle), but even those that prefer animals sometimes bite humans.[184] Those that prefer humans are more effective at spreading malaria.[182] Two species that strongly prefer humans and that are potent vectors for malaria in Africa are **Anopheles gambiae** and **Anopheles funestus**.[178,181]

To run successful malaria control programs, public health workers must know the habits of the *Anopheles* species that are spreading malaria in their area. For example, different *Anopheles* species have different preferences for water. Some prefer small, shallow collections of fresh water in ditches, uncovered containers, and animal hoof prints; others prefer large, open water like lakes, swamps, and rice fields.[184] Nearly all *Anopheles* mosquitoes that can transmit malaria prefer rural areas, which means that malaria is mainly a rural problem.[186] However, the species **Anopheles stephensi**, which was recently introduced to the Horn of Africa, likes urban environments, so it may cause a surge in malaria in African cities.[187] Some *Anopheles* species tend to bite humans indoors and some outdoors.[184] All *Anopheles* mosquitoes prefer to bite

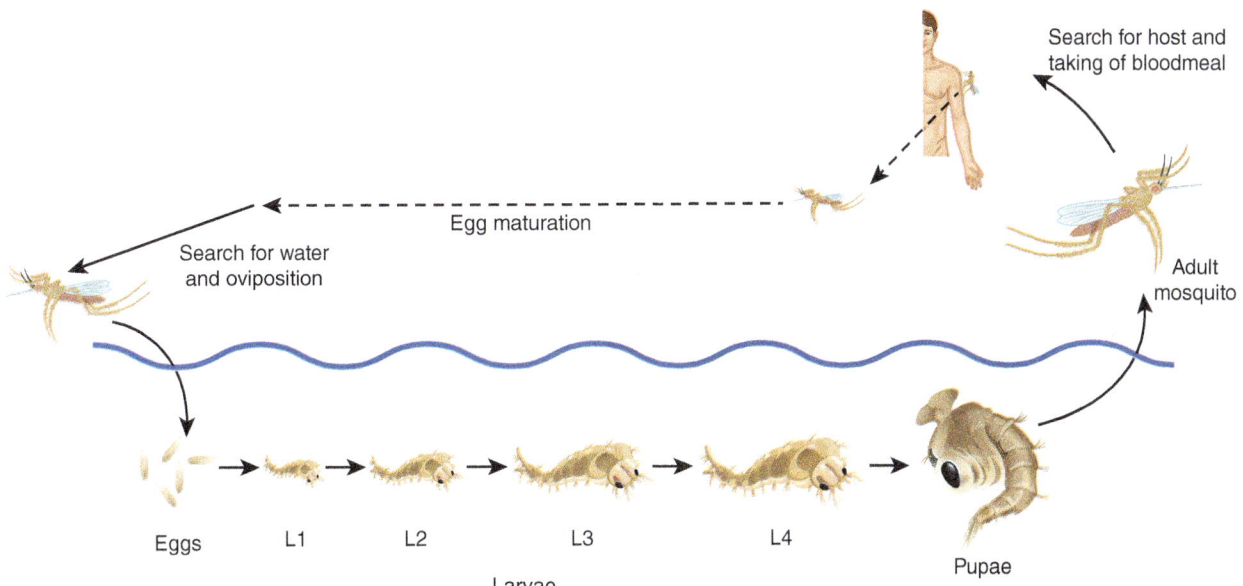

Search for host and taking of bloodmeal

Egg maturation

Search for water and oviposition

Adult mosquito

Eggs   L1   L2   L3   L4   Pupae

Larvae

Figure 9.50 **Life Cycle of Anopheles Mosquitoes.** A mature female mosquito lays eggs (called oviposition) on the surface of standing fresh water. About 2–3 days later, the eggs hatch into larvae, which grow over 4–10 days. The larvae then become pupae, like caterpillars becoming cocoons. Another 2–3 days later, adult mosquitoes emerge from the pupae. Adult females need to bite humans or animals and take in a blood meal to develop eggs. For a female mosquito to spread malaria, it must bite humans at least twice: once to get infected with malaria organisms and once to pass the organisms to a new human.

Okuneye, K., Eikenberry, S. E., & Gumel, A. B. Weather-driven malaria transmission model with gonotrophic and sporogonic cycles. Journal of biological dynamics, 2019; 13(sup1), 288-324.

humans between dusk and dawn, which is why sleeping under bed nets can protect people from malaria even if those people spend their daylight hours outdoors.[182,184]

Environmental Conditions Supporting Malaria

For malaria to spread, environmental conditions must support the *Plasmodium* protozoa, the *Anopheles* mosquitoes, and their access to humans (**Figure 9.51**). The most important factor is temperature. In cooler temperatures, the sporogenic cycle in mosquitoes takes longer. If adult female mosquitoes die before this cycle is complete, they cannot spread the infection to humans. This is the main reason that malaria does not spread in cooler climates.[181] To breed, *Anopheles* needs standing water, so malaria tends to occur on land that is wet and flat, and not in areas that are dry or hilly. Malaria typically peaks in the warm and rainy seasons, when standing water is present, and wanes in cool or dry seasons. *Anopheles* mosquitoes need access to plants so that they can feed on plant nectar. And, of course, the mosquitoes need access to humans, which depends on factors like the distance of housing from standing water, and how easily mosquitoes can enter that housing. It also matters how close humans are to other humans or animals (like farm animals) that are alternative sources of blood for mosquitoes.[181] The variations in these conditions cause malaria to be very spotty, even in hard-hit regions. Specific villages in the same region or even specific households can become "hot spots" for malaria in a single season, and those "hot spots" can change from one season to the next.[188-190]

Humans can cause surges in malaria by changing environmental conditions. For example, when people irrigate land for agriculture, it can create standing water in which *Anopheles* can breed, leading to local outbreaks.[191] And urban neighborhoods without good drainage can create puddles that support *Anopheles stephensi*.[175] Global warming is likely to change the spread of malaria, but it is very difficult to predict what those changes will be.[175]

Human Evolutionary Responses to Plasmodium

Malaria has had such a profound impact on people that evolution has stepped in to limit the damage. The main "food" that *Plasmodium* consumes inside red blood cells is hemoglobin, the protein that carries oxygen. Over thousands of years, evolution has selected genes for altered types of hemoglobin that help protect people from malaria. Examples are the **thalassemia** gene and genes for hemoglobin types S, C, and E.[179,183] When people inherit a single copy of these genes, they can still become infected with *Plasmodium*, but they are partially protected from the worst consequences.[183] For

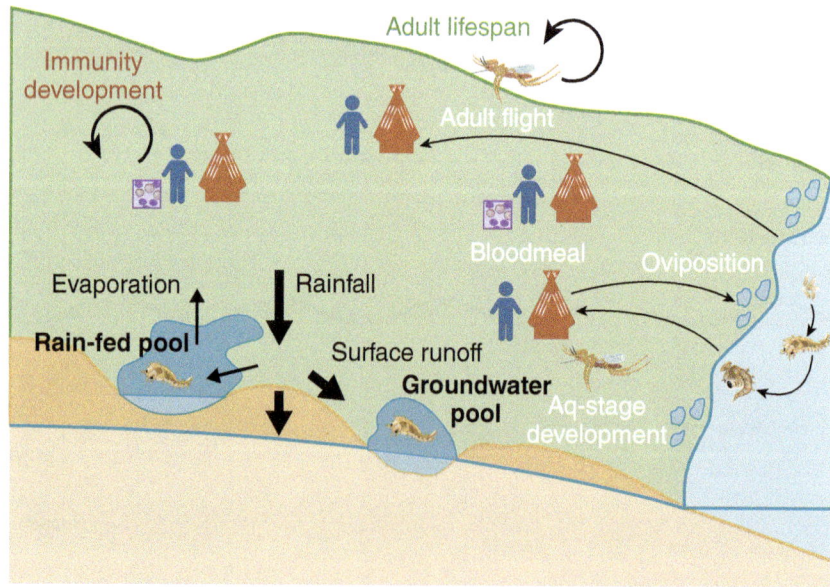

Figure 9.51 Environmental Determinants of Malaria Transmission Around the Koka Reservoir in Ethiopia. The Figure shows an example of local environmental conditions and their impact on spread of malaria. Malaria transmission requires warm temperatures, standing water, short distances between housing and that water, housing that allows mosquitoes to enter, and the availability of persons and/or farm animals as sources of blood for adult mosquitoes.

example, people with one copy of the thalassemia gene are about half as likely to die from malaria as people with two normal hemoglobin genes.[192] The altered gene with the biggest benefit is the gene for hemoglobin type S. People with one copy of this gene are 90% less likely to die from malaria.[193] This biologic advantage is so large that more than 30% of people in some parts of Africa and about 8% of African-Americans now have the "sickle cell trait"—that is, one copy of the hemoglobin S gene. Unfortunately, these genes harm people who are unlucky enough to inherit two copies, causing their red blood cells to collapse and form odd shapes. For people with two copies of hemoglobin type S, this is called **sickle cell disease**.

Impact of Malaria on Health

Malaria can cause a fatal illness, a mild illness, or no symptoms at all.

When people are infected with *Plasmodium*, their immune systems try to kill the invading organisms by producing **antibodies**.[179] The shape-shifting nature of *Plasmodium* enables it to resist these antibodies, but the immune response does limit the number of *Plasmodium* organisms that survive and the damage they cause, as well as reduce the chance of a new infection.[182] In areas where malaria is common, because of this immune response, most people with the infection have few symptoms.[180,183] Those who do experience symptoms usually have only an intermittent fever and fatigue from anemia.

However, a small percentage develops **severe malaria**, which harms many organ systems.[182] The most dangerous manifestation of severe malaria is **cerebral malaria**, caused by damage to the brain from inflammation and blockage of flow of blood through blood vessels. Cerebral malaria can kill children very quickly.[179,180,183] Malaria can also cause severe anemia, which can be fatal in infants, or fatal damage to the lungs or kidneys.[180,183] And malaria is particularly dangerous in pregnancy—both to the parent and to the developing fetus.[181-183]

In areas of Africa where malaria is very common, nearly all children become infected early in life. Those who are less than six months old are partially protected

from severe malaria by antibodies they received when they were in the womb. Most of those older than five years of age are partially protected by antibodies from their own earlier infections. Those between the ages of six months and five years, though, are often becoming infected for the first time. It is when young children have these initial infections that they are most likely to have develop severe malaria.[183]

People who grow up in areas without malaria do not develop antibodies to it. If these people as adults travel to areas with malaria and become infected, they are also more likely to develop severe malaria.[183]

Treatment of Malaria

Antimalarial drugs that can cure or prevent the disease have been available for hundreds of years. The first was **quinine**, a chemical used by Native Americans in the Andes as early as the 1600s.[194] Quinine was the main drug used to treat malaria until the 1940s, when it was mainly replaced by **chloroquine**, a chemically-related drug.[194] People relied on chloroquine and other related drugs to treat malaria until the 1970s, when *Plasmodium falciparum* in Africa started to become resistant to these drugs.

In the 1990s, the drug **artemisinin** was shown effective in curing malaria.[195] Artemisinin comes from a weed that grows in China, and it had been used as a traditional medicine for malaria for many years.[196] Artemisinin's action on *Plasmodium* is entirely different from that of quinine and chloroquine, so it can cure malaria that is caused by chloroquine-resistant organisms. Since the 1990s, researchers have developed several synthetic antimalarial drugs that are chemically related to artemisinin. Experts now recommend that malaria be routinely treated with **artemisinin-based combination therapy (ACT)**—that is, one antimalarial drug chemically related to artemisinin and an additional drug that is usually chemically related to chloroquine.[184]

Some areas of Southeast Asia now have *Plasmodium* that is partially resistant to artemisinin and the drugs related to it.[175,197] Resistance to artemisinin is not a big problem in Africa yet, but it could threaten malaria control in the future.[175]

Box 9.12 History of Malaria Control

Malaria has bedeviled humans for thousands of years, since the beginning of agriculture. The ancient Romans, who struggled with it, recognized that it was connected to stagnant water and the clearing of land for farming.[192] For most of recorded history, the risk of malaria extended far beyond the tropics, including Europe and North and South America. By one estimate, three-fourths of the world's population in 1900 lived in areas where malaria circulated.[198]

(continues)

Box 9.12 **History of Malaria Control** *(continued)*

Major breakthroughs in malaria control took place in the early 1900s during building of the Panama Canal. At first, the massive project was hindered by workers ill and dying from both malaria and yellow fever. By 1897, researchers had described the life cycle of *Plasmodium* and had shown that *Anopheles* mosquitoes were vectors. Public health experts hired by the canal project put that knowledge to use by draining swamps, eliminating or spraying oil on standing water, and installing screens around the verandas where workers slept. These steps worked, nearly eliminating yellow fever and greatly reducing malaria. The success inspired public health experts elsewhere to control malaria by disrupting mosquito breeding places and protecting people from mosquito bites at night.

The next major breakthrough was the discovery in the 1940s that a chemical known as **DDT** sprayed on interior walls of homes killed mosquitoes for months afterward. This **indoor residual spraying** eliminated malaria from some areas, with the disease not returning after spraying stopped.[199] Encouraged by that success, public health experts believed that they could **eliminate malaria** from other areas (that is, stop all local spread) and eventually **eradicate malaria** across the entire world. In 1955, the WHO approved a global malaria eradication campaign, based mostly on indoor residual spraying of DDT.[199] The campaign also used chloroquine widely for treatment. The campaign mostly abandoned efforts to disrupt mosquito breeding sites or protect humans from mosquito bites in other ways.

This campaign sharply reduced or eliminated malaria from many areas, but in sub-Saharan Africa and some parts of the Western Pacific, after initial successes, malaria rates resurged, with especially deadly consequences (**Figure 9.52**).[192] By 1969, the WHO acknowledged that the global eradication campaign had failed. The primary reason was that *Anopheles* had become resistant to DDT. More broadly, experts blame the failure on over-reliance on a single intervention, lack of research into other approaches, and a weak evaluation system.[199]

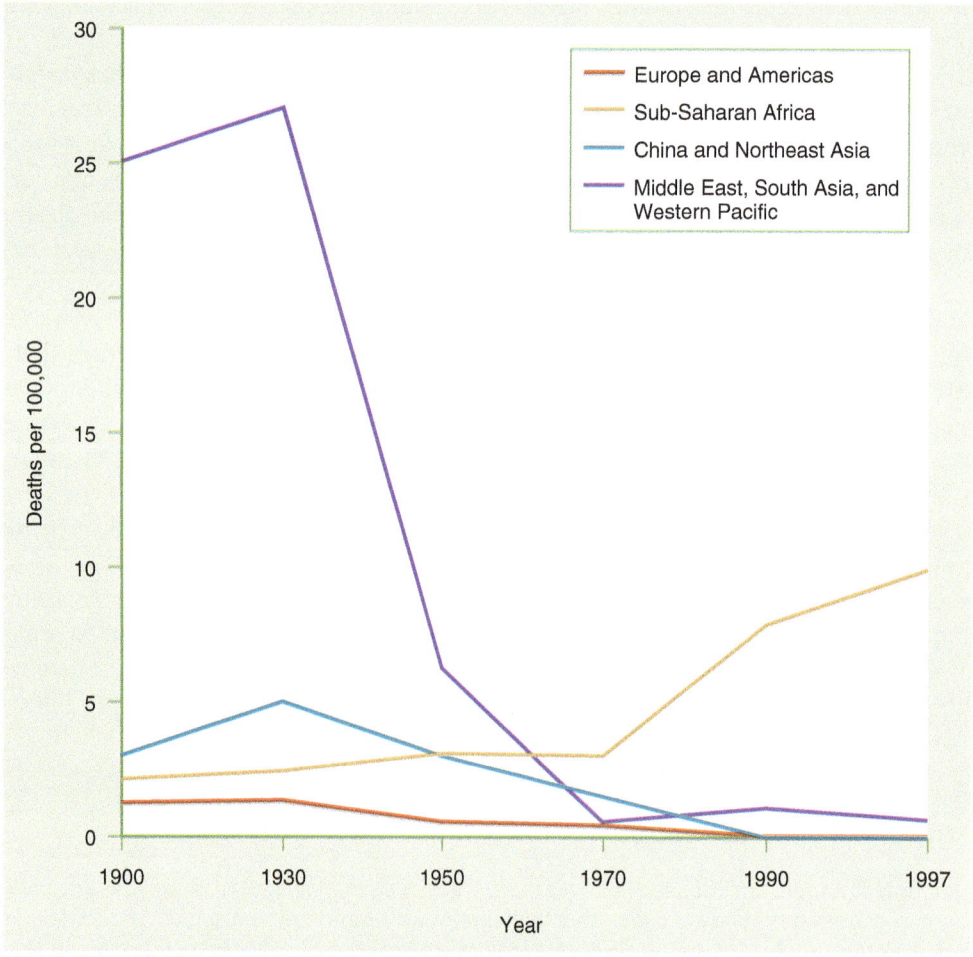

Figure 9.52 Trends in Estimated Malaria Deaths by Region, 1900–1997.

Data from Carter R, Mendis KN. Evolutionary and historical aspects of the burden of malaria. *Clin Microbiol Rev.* 2002;15(4):564-594. doi:10.1128/CMR.15.4.564-594.2002.

In the 1970s and 1980s, prospects for the control of malaria looked very grim. The two main tools—DDT and chloroquine—were becoming ineffective, and the failure of the eradication campaign made it difficult to obtain support for control programs. Between 1970 and the late 1990s, the estimated number of global deaths from malaria nearly doubled.[192]

Research continued, though. In the 1980s and 1990s, researchers showed that bed nets infused with insecticides could kill *Anopheles* mosquitoes, reduce bites, and sharply reduce malaria deaths in children.[200] In the 2000s, health organizations began to distribute these insecticide-treated nets on a huge scale in Africa, and malaria rates began to fall. When artemisinin arrived to treat chloroquine-resistant malaria in the 1990s it was another huge step forward. These breakthroughs led public health leaders to reconsider the goal of eliminating malaria from entire countries and ultimately eradicating it worldwide. The current WHO plan sets targets to eliminate malaria from 35 countries and to reduce the global mortality by 90% by 2030.[176,182]

Epidemiology: Patterns and Trends

The numbers of people affected by malaria are staggering. The WHO estimates that each year nearly 250 million people across 86 countries have malaria with symptoms severe enough that they seek medical care, and more than 600,000 die from the illness.[175]

Geographically, malaria is present in the warmer areas of every continent, but it is most heavily concentrated in sub-Saharan Africa, where nearly 95% of the global cases occur (**Figure 9.53**).[175] In fact, about 40% of the cases and deaths occur in just two countries—Nigeria and the Democratic Republic of the Congo.

Figure 9.54 shows estimates of the percentage of people in sub-Saharan Africa who are infected and the mortality rate from malaria by age group. Some 10%–20% of people in this entire region are infected with *Plasmodium*. As the graph shows, though, deaths from malaria are heavily concentrated in young children and, to a lesser extent, in older adults. About three-fourths of people who die from malaria are children under five.[175] In the hard-hit African countries, more than one-third of pregnant women are estimated to have malaria.[175]

Malaria rates were even worse a couple of decades ago. Between 2000 and 2015, renewed prevention programs cut the malaria mortality rate almost in half (**Figure 9.55**). Since 2015, rates have continued to fall in Southeast Asia and the Americas. However, in a worrisome trend, in recent years progress has slowed, stalled or gone into reverse in the African, Western Pacific, and Eastern Mediterranean regions.[175]

Risk Factors

Figure 9.56 shows the chain of cause and effect that leads to malaria. For a human to develop malaria, that person must be bitten by an *Anopheles* mosquito and that mosquito must be carrying *Plasmodium*. Also, the illness is more likely if that person is not already immune to the organism. Tracing these events backward, the underlying risk factors for infection are:

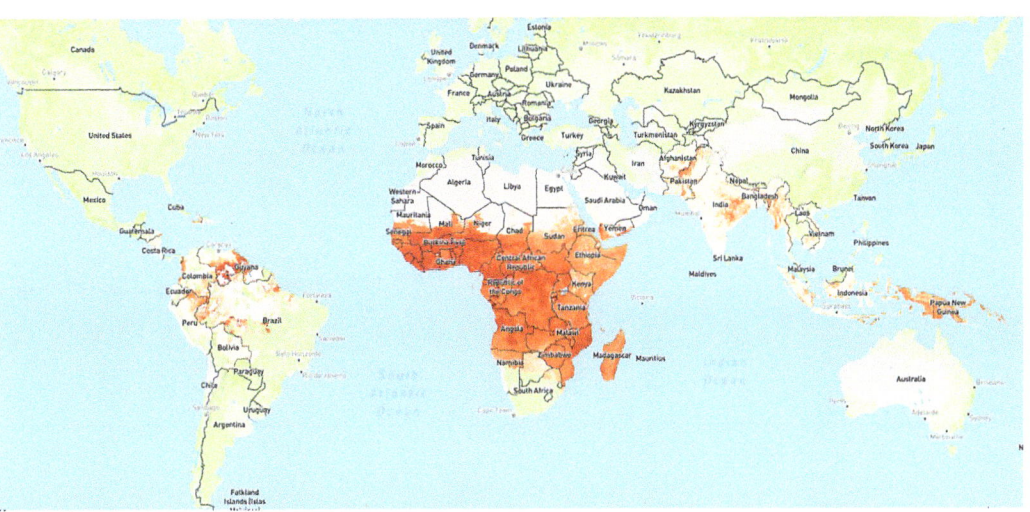

Figure 9.53 *Plasmodium falciparum* **Malaria Mortality, 2020–2022.**

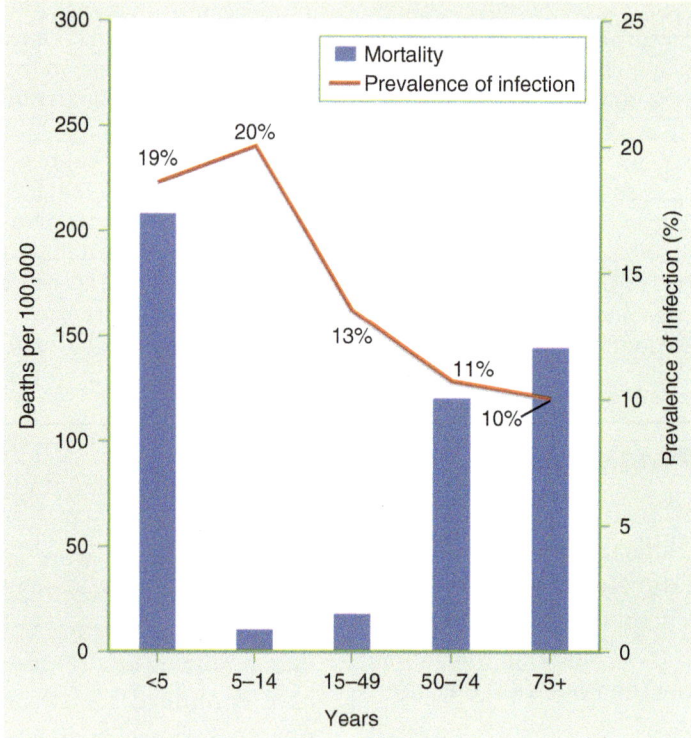

Figure 9.54 Estimated Malaria Prevalence and Mortality by Age Group in Sub-Saharan Africa, 2019. In sub-Saharan Africa, the prevalence of infection is very high in all age groups, but most deaths from malaria are in young children and older adults.

Data from Global Burden of Disease Collaboration, Institute for Health Metrics and Evaluation. GBD Results Tool. Accessed April 10, 2024. https://vizhub.healthdata.org/gbd-results

- *Unprotective housing.* People who live in huts with mud walls, thatched roofs, and open eaves (the gap between the top of the wall and the roof) are more likely to catch malaria than those living in houses with cement or brick walls, metal roofs, and closed eaves.[184,188,201-204]

The main reason that malaria does not spread in high-income countries with hot climates is that people avoid mosquitoes by staying inside closed, air-conditioned homes.

- *Outdoor activities at night.* Protective housing helps only those people who stay inside houses

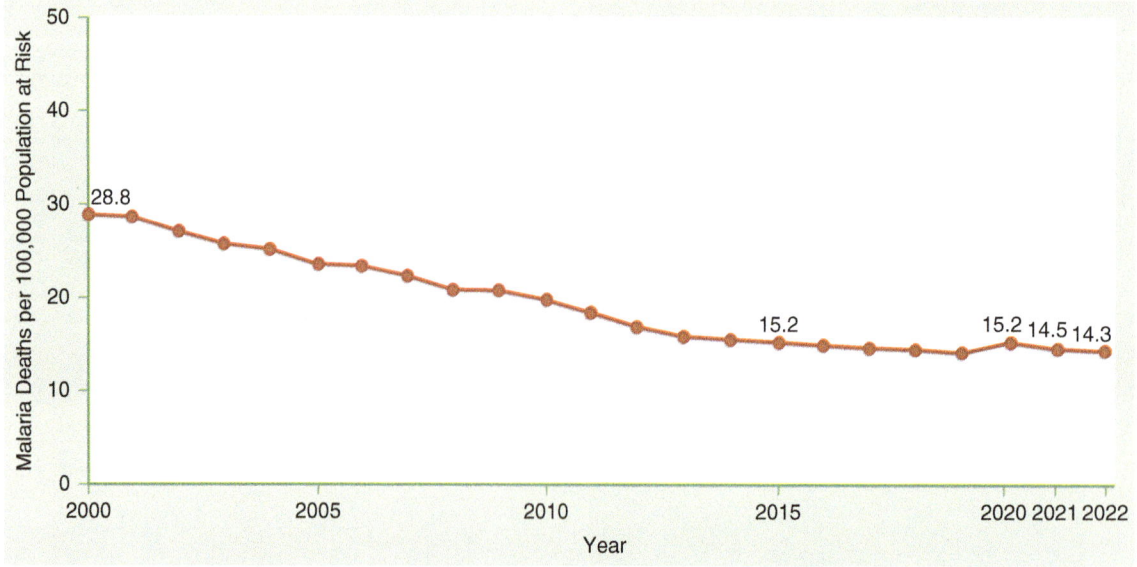

Figure 9.55 Trend in Mortality Rate from Malaria, Worldwide, 2000–2022.

Reproduced from World Health Organization. World Malaria Report 2023.; 2023. Accessed July 1, 2024. https://www.who.int/teams/global-malaria-programme/reports/world-malaria-report-2023

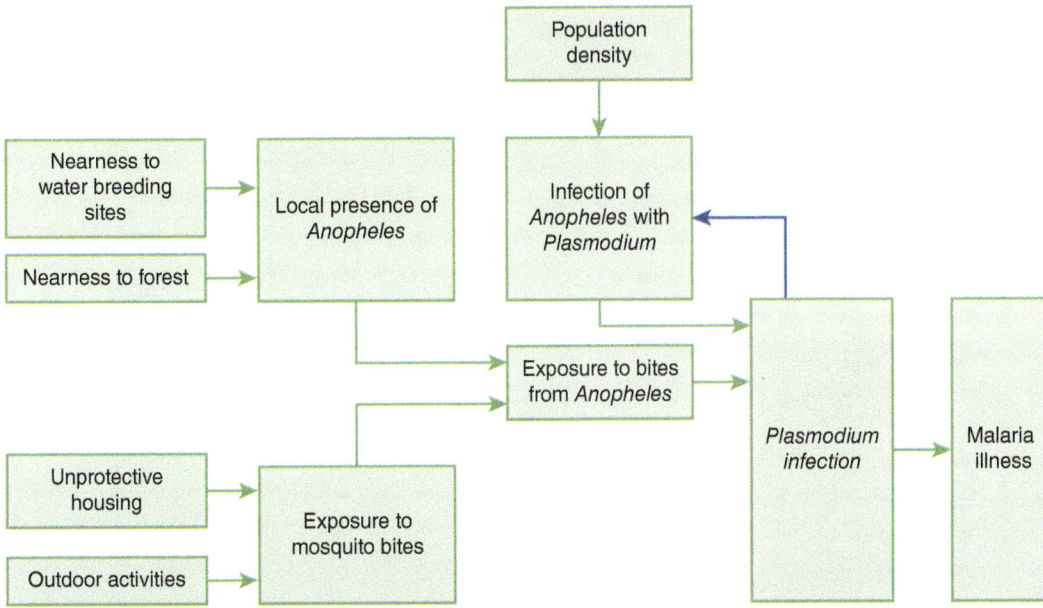

Figure 9.56 **Cause-and-Effect Diagram for Malaria.**

when *Anopheles* mosquitoes are biting. People are at greater risk of infection if they spend time outside at night for social activities, work, travel, or sleeping in the heat.[188,205]

- *Nearness to water breeding sites.* In villages with malaria, people living in houses closer to water sources like ponds, dams or irrigated fields are more likely to develop malaria.[188]
- *Nearness to forest.* Although agriculture often increases malaria risk, so does living close to a forest, probably because *Anopheles* mosquitoes prefer resting in shaded areas and because they need access to plants for the plant nectar.[188]
- *Population density.* Studies have found that people are more likely to catch malaria if they are crowded within households or their houses are close to each other. This may be simply because more humans mean more sources of blood for mosquitoes. Or it may be because crowding makes it easier for an individual *Anopheles* mosquito to bite two different humans during its life span.[188]

Preventive Interventions

The chain of events that leads to people getting sick with malaria offers several opportunities for prevention (**Figure 9.57**). Experience says that no single intervention can eradicate this disease, though; a combination is needed. The WHO malaria plan has three elements to it—vector control, chemoprevention, and diagnostic testing and treatment—but there are additional options.

Primary Prevention

Vector Control. Where there are fewer mosquitoes, humans are less likely to catch malaria. For that reason, public health experts have always used **vector control** (that is, reducing *Anopheles* populations) as the main way to prevent the disease. Insecticides are one—but not the only—method for vector control. Options include:

- *Insecticide-treated bed nets.* Maybe the most important development in malaria control in the past 50 years has been nets that are infused with insecticides, which people sleep under at night. The main insecticides recommended by the WHO for these nets are called **pyrethroids**.[176] These nets protect people from *Anopheles* in two ways: they physically block mosquitoes, and they kill those mosquitoes that rest on the nets. Insecticide-treated nets reduce the incidence of malaria by about half and reduce mortality rates from all causes in young children by 18%.[182] Malaria control programs have embraced these to the point that, by WHO estimates, in 2022, 70% of households in sub-Saharan Africa had at least one insecticide-treated net and about half of people slept under them.[175] However, the impact of these nets is limited by two factors. First, of course, they do not protect people who sleep outdoors or are active outdoors at night.[205] Second, in some areas *Anopheles* mosquitoes are becoming resistant to pyrethroid insecticides. In those areas, the WHO recommends that bed net manufacturers use combinations of insecticides.[175,182,183]

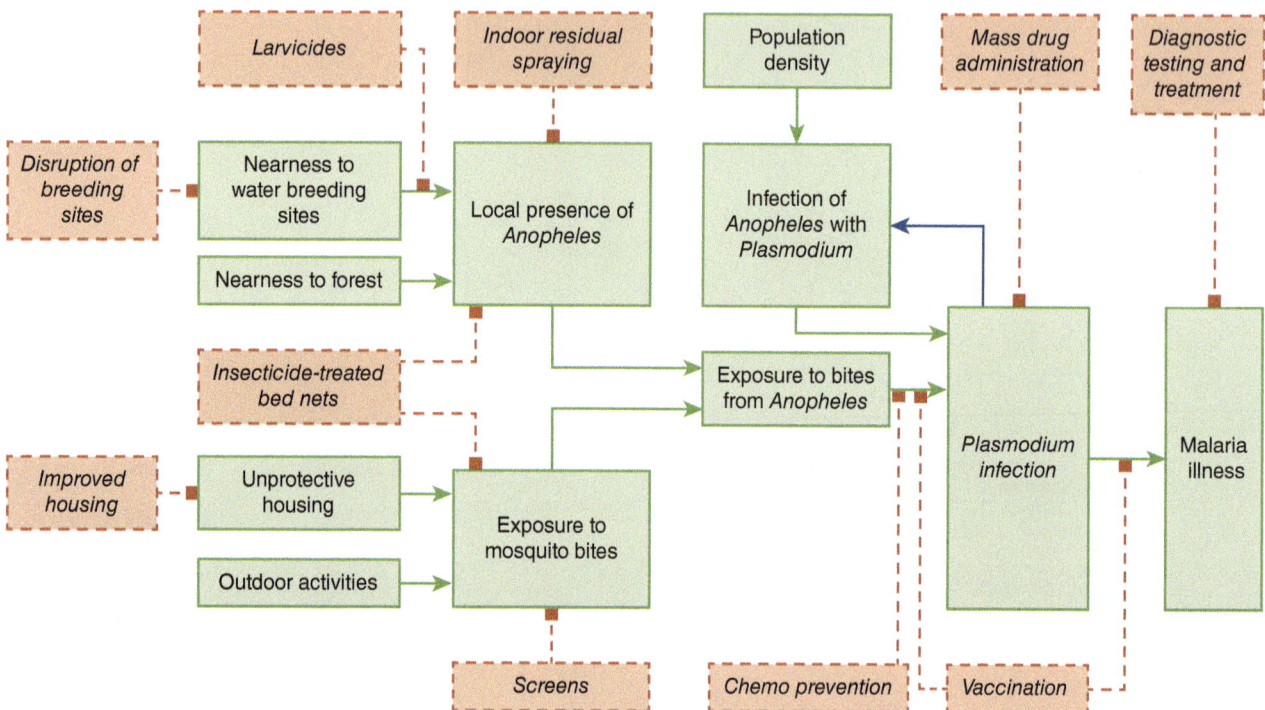

Figure 9.57 **Cause-and-Effect Diagram for Malaria, with Preventive Interventions.**

- *Indoor residual spraying of insecticides.* Public health teams can kill *Anopheles* mosquitoes and protect humans by spraying long-lasting insecticides on the internal surfaces of homes— walls, ceilings, and eaves.[182,184] But despite its endorsement by the WHO, indoor residual spraying is used in only a small (and shrinking) proportion of homes in malaria-prone areas of Africa.[175,184] Families often dislike the disruption of the spraying and the appearance of walls that have been treated.

- *Larvicide use in breeding sites.* **Larvicides** are chemicals or biologic agents that kill mosquito larvae in water breeding sites. Larvicides have been very effective in reducing *Anopheles* levels and controlling malaria in the past.[206-208] The WHO recommends using larvicides where breeding sites are "few, fixed, and findable," typically in urban areas, but not where water breeding sites are "abundant, scattered, and variable," typically in rural areas.[184] Chemical larvicides have somewhat fallen out of favor in recent years because they can harm species other than *Anopheles*. However, they may be replaced by biologic larvicides, which are bacteria that kill *Anopheles* larvae but have little effect on fish or other species.[206]

- *Disruption of Anopheles breeding sites.* Throughout recorded history, people have reduced the spread of malaria by draining swamps, irrigating fields intermittently instead of continuously, and eliminating other collections of standing water.[192]

Today, where it is practical, disrupting water sites where *Anopheles* breed can still help prevent malaria.[207,208]

Protection of Humans from Mosquito Bites

- *Improved housing.* People can be protected from *Anopheles* mosquitoes at night with housing that is sealed—that is, with cement or brick walls without gaps, metal roofs, and closed eaves.[184]

- *Screens.* At a much lower cost, people can cut the number of *Anopheles* mosquitoes inside houses and lower malaria risk if they install screens on windows, open doorways, and eaves.[184,209]

Where it is practical, malaria risk can also be reduced by locating or relocating houses further from water sources or forests.

Chemoprevention. **Chemoprevention** means using antimalarial medications not to cure infection but to prevent it. The WHO endorses several approaches:

- ***Intermittent preventive treatment of malaria in pregnancy*** involves women taking three or more doses of antimalarial drugs during the second and third trimester, regardless of whether they are infected with *Plasmodium*.[183,184,197] This treatment cures those who are already infected and prevents others from becoming infected. It has been shown to reduce miscarriage and low birth weight.[193] Today, just under half of pregnant women in areas with high malaria rates are receiving three doses of antimalarials.[175] The WHO estimates that treating all pregnant women in areas where malaria is common would prevent low birth weight in 500,000 infants every year.[175]

- *Perennial malaria chemoprevention* (formerly called **intermittent preventive treatment of malaria in infants**) is a similar approach, involving giving infants and young children three to 12 doses of antimalarial drugs, usually when the children receive their routine vaccines.[184] This reduces malaria and also anemia in children.[193]
- *Intermittent preventive treatment of malaria in school-aged children* (5–15 years) extends this idea to older children, with doses of medicines given at schools.[197]
- *Seasonal malaria chemoprevention* involves giving all children in age groups at high risk for severe malaria antimalarial drugs during the rainy season, when malaria rates rise.[175,184,197] It has been shown to greatly reduce deaths from malaria in young children.[193]
- *Mass drug administration* involves trying to give antimalarials to every child and every adult in a defined geographic area over a short period of time.[183,184,197,210] In theory, this helps more than just those people who receive the treatment. By reducing the number of humans carrying the organism, it may lower *Plasmodium* infection rates in mosquitoes, which prevents spread even to people who are not treated with antimalarials.[184] But studies have not proven that it is effective in this way, and experts worry that it may increase the parasite's resistance to antimalarials, so this intervention is not recommended routinely.[184]

Vaccination. After many years of research and development, two vaccines are now available and recommended by the WHO for children in areas with high malaria rates.

A vaccine called **RTS,S/AS01** and sold under the brand name **Mosquirix**, provokes an immune response that can prevent sporozoites from infecting liver cells.[211,212] It is given to infants in four doses starting at when an infant is five months old.[175] In studies in Africa, it reduced infections in children under age 5 by about one-third and mortality by about one-fourth.[182] As of 2024, only limited supplies of this vaccine were available, but it was included in the routine infant immunization schedule in Ghana, Kenya, and Malawi, and several other countries were scaling up its use.[175,213]

In 2023, the WHO endorsed a second malaria vaccine, called **R21/Matrix-M**. Like the RTS,S/AS01 vaccine, this second vaccine induces immunity to sporozoites and is meant for infants and young children. In studies in Africa, a three-dose series of this vaccine reduced malaria by 75%.[197]

Secondary Prevention–Diagnostic Testing and Treatment with ACT

If people with fever or other symptoms of malaria take antimalarial drugs early in their illness, their risk of dying from malaria is very low.[180,182,184] That requires that the diagnosis of malaria be confirmed by a laboratory test. Rapid diagnostic tests—like the rapid tests used to diagnose COVID-19—now make this possible. In the past, people in hard-hit areas of Africa who had fever often simply took ant malarial drugs, without first getting tested. WHO recommends instead that all adults in areas with malaria who have a fever first be tested for malaria, and only those who are found infected be treated with antimalarials.[184]

Box 9.13 Summary–Prevention of Malaria

- Vector control
  - Insecticide-treated bed nets
  - Indoor residual spraying of insecticides
  - Larvicide use in breeding sites
  - Disruption of *Anopheles* breeding sites
- Protection of humans from mosquito bites
  - Improved housing
  - Screens
- Chemoprevention
  - Intermittent preventive treatment in pregnancy
  - Perennial malaria chemoprevention
  - Intermittent preventive treatment of malaria in school-aged children
  - Seasonal malarial chemoprevention
  - Mass drug administration
- Vaccination
- Diagnostic testing and treatment with antimalarials

Box 9.14 Key Words–Malaria

Anemia
Anopheles
Anopheles funestus
Anopheles gambiae

(continues)

Box 9.14 **Key Words–Malaria** *(continued)*

Anopheles stephensi
Antibodies
Antimalarial drug
Artemisinin
Artemisinin-based combination therapy (ACT)
Blood meal
Cerebral malaria
Chemoprevention
Chloroquine
DDT
Elimination of malaria
Eradiation of malaria
Erythrocytes
Erythrocytic cycle
Exo-erythrocytic cycle
Gametocyte
Hemoglobin
Hepatocyte
Hypnozoites
Indoor residual spraying
Intermittent preventive treatment of malaria in
    infants
Intermittent preventive treatment of malaria in
    pregnancy
Intermittent preventive treatment of malaria in
    school-aged-children
Larva, larvae
Larvicides
Mass drug administration
Merozoite
Mosquirix
Perennial malaria chemoprevention
Plasmodium
Plasmodium falciparum
Plasmodium malariae
Plasmodium ovale
Plasmodium vivax
Protozoa
Pupa, pupae
Pyrethroid
Quinine
R21/Matrix-M

Red blood cells
RTS,S/AS01
Schizont
Seasonal malarial chemoprevention
Severe malaria
Sickle cell disease
Sporogenic cycle
Sporozoite
Thalassemia
Trophozoite
Vector
Vector control

Resources–Malaria

- The CDC has a series of web pages that provide plain-language descriptions of the biology of *Plasmodium* and *Anopheles* at www.cdc.gov/dpdx/malaria

- Poespoprodjo JR, Douglas NM, Ansong D, Kho S, Anstey NM. Malaria. *Lancet*. 2023;402(10419):2328-2345. doi:10.1016/S0140-6736(23)01249-7. This is an excellent state-of-the-art review of malaria biology, prevention, and treatment.

- Ippolito MM, Moser KA, Cunningham C, Kabuya JB, Juliano JJ. Antimalarial drug resistance and implications for the WHO Global Technical Strategy. *Curr Epidemiol Rep*. 2021;8:46-62. doi: 10.1007/s40471-021-00266-5

- The World Health Organization publishes extensive resources on malaria. Their high-level strategy is summarized in the *Global Technical Strategy for Malaria 2016–2030 (2021 Update)*. Detailed recommendations for prevention and control are in the *WHO Guidelines for Malaria*. And each year the WHO publishes a *World Malaria Report* that summarizes the state of disease prevention programs around the world. All are available at www.who.int/publications

References

1. Bureau of the Census. *1850 Census: Mortality Statistics of the Seventh Census of the United States, 1850.*; 1855. Available at: https://www.census.gov/library/publications/1855/dec/1850b.html

2. McGinnis M, Tyring S. Introduction to Mycology. In: Baron S, ed. *Medical Microbiology*. 4th ed. University of Texas Medical Branch at Galveston; 1996. Accessed May 1, 2024. Available at: https://www.ncbi.nlm.nih.gov/books/NBK8125/

3. Yaeger RG. Protozoa: Structure, Classification, Growth, and Development. In: Baron S, ed. *Medical Microbiology*. 4th ed.

University of Texas Medical Branch at Galveston; 1996. Accessed May 1, 2024. Available at: https://www.ncbi.nlm.nih.gov/books/NBK8325/

4. UNAIDS. *The Path That Ends AIDS: 2023 UNAIDS Global AIDS Update*. 2023. Accessed June 26, 2024. Available at: https://thepath.unaids.org/

5. Kumar V, Abbas AK, Aster JC, Turner JR. Acquired Immunodeficiency Syndrome (AIDS). In: Kumar V, Abbas AK, Aster JC, Turner JR, eds. *Robbins & Cotran Pathologic Basis of Disease*. 10th ed. Elsevier; 2021:247-258.

6. Chatzileontiadou DSM, Sloane H, Nguyen AT, Gras S, Grant EJ. The Many Faces of CD4+ T Cells: Immunological and Structural Characteristics. *Int J Mol Sci.* 2020;22(1):73. Published 2020 Dec 23. doi:10.3390/ijms22010073

7. Hall JE, Hall ME. Resistance of the body to infection: II. Immunity and allergy. In: *Guyton and Hall Textbook of Medical Physiology.* 14th ed. Elsevier; 2021:459-470.

8. Kumar V, Abbas AK, Aster JC, Turner JR. The normal immune response. In: *Robbins & Cotran Pathologic Basis of Disease.* 10th ed. Elsevier; 2021:190-203.

9. Ronen K, Sharma A, Overbaugh J. HIV transmission biology: Translation for HIV prevention. *AIDS.* 2015;29(17):2219-2227. doi:10.1097/QAD.0000000000000845.

10. Shaw GM, Hunter E. HIV transmission. *Cold Spring Harb Perspect Med.* 2012;2(11):a006965.doi:10.1101/cshperspect.a006965.

11. Patel P, Borkowf CB, Brooks JT, Lasry A, Lansky A, Mermin J. Estimating per-act HIV transmission risk: A systematic review. *AIDS.* 2014;28(10):1509-1519. doi:10.1097/QAD.0000000000000298

12. Weiss HA, Dickson KE, Agot K, Hankins CA. Male circumcision for HIV prevention: Current research and programmatic issues. *AIDS.* 2010;24(Suppl 4):S61-S69. doi:10.1097/01.aids.0000390708.66136.f4

13. Rouzioux C, Costagliola D, Burgard M, et al. Estimated timing of mother-to-child human immunodeficiency virus type 1 (HIV-1) transmission by use of a Markov model. *Am J Epidemiol.* 1995;142(12):1330-1337. doi:10.1093/oxfordjournals.aje.a117601

14. Centers for Disease Control and Prevention. *HIV Surveillance Report, 2022.* 2024. Accessed November 19, 2024. Available at: http://www.cdc.gov/hiv-data/nhss/hiv-diagnoses-deaths-prevalence.html

15. Centers for Disease Control and Prevention. Atlas Plus. CDC. 2024. Accessed May 5, 2024. Available at: https://www.cdc.gov/nchhstp/atlas/index.htm

16. UNAIDS. AIDSinfo. UNAIDS.org. 2024. Accessed May 5, 2024. Available at: https://aidsinfo.unaids.org/

17. Bearman PS, Moody J, Stovel K. Chains of affection: The structure of adolescent romantic and sexual networks. *Am J Sociol.* 2004;110(1):44-91. doi:10.1086/386272

18. Sauter SR, Ratnayake A, Campbell MB, Kissinger PJ. Sexual networks and STI infection among young black men who have sex with women in a Southern U.S. City. *J Adolesc Health.* 2023;72(5):730-736. doi:10.1016/j.jadohealth.2022.11.248

19. El-Bassel N, Shaw SA, Dasgupta A, Strathdee SA. Drug use as a driver of HIV risks: Re-emerging and emerging issues. *Curr Opin HIV AIDS.* 2014;9(2):150-155. doi:10.1097/COH.0000000000000035

20. Probst C, Simbayi LC, Parry CDH, Shuper PA, Rehm J. Alcohol use, socioeconomic status and risk of HIV infections. *AIDS Behav.* 2017;21(7):1926-1937. doi:10.1007/s10461-017-1758-x

21. Morojele NK, Shenoi S V., Shuper PA, Braithwaite RS, Rehm J. Alcohol use and the risk of communicable diseases. *Nutrients.* 2021;13(10):3317. doi:10.3390/nu13103317

22. Centers for Disease Control and Prevention. Alcohol Use and Your Health. CDC. April 14, 2022. Accessed August 8, 2023. Available at: https://www.cdc.gov/alcohol/fact-sheets/alcohol-use.htm

23. Bagby G, Amedee A, Siggins R, Molina P, Nelson S, Veazey R. Alcohol and HIV Effects on the Immune System. *Alcohol Research.* 2015;37(2):287-297.

24. Baggaley RF, White RG, Boily MC. HIV transmission risk through anal intercourse: Systematic review, meta-analysis and implications for HIV prevention. *Int J Epidemiol.* 2010;39(4):1048-1063. doi:10.1093/ije/dyq057

25. Weiss HA, Quigley MA, Hayes RJ. Male circumcision and risk of HIV infection in sub-Saharan Africa: a systematic review and meta-analysis. *AIDS.* 2000;14(15):2361-2370. doi:10.1097/00002030-200010200-00018

26. Morris BJ, Wamai RG, Henebeng EB, et al. Estimation of country-specific and global prevalence of male circumcision. *Popul Health Metr.* 2016;14:4. doi:10.1186/s12963-016-0073-5

27. Hughes JP, Baeten JM, Lingappa JR, et al. Determinants of per-coital-act HIV-1 infectivity among African HIV-1-serodiscordant couples. *J Infect Dis.* 2012;205(3):358-365. doi:10.1093/infdis/jir747

28. John GC, Nduati RW, Mbori-Ngacha DA, et al. Correlates of mother-to-child human immunodeficiency virus type 1 (HIV-1) transmission: Association with maternal plasma HIV-1 RNA load, genital HIV-1 DNA shedding, and breast infections. *J Infect Dis.* 2001;183(2):206-212. doi:10.1086/317918

29. Prendergast AJ, Goga AE, Waitt C, et al. Transmission of CMV, HTLV-1, and HIV through breastmilk. *Lancet Child Adolesc Health.* 2019;3(4):264-273. doi:10.1016/S2352-4642(19)30024-0

30. Garnett GP, Anderson RM. Sexually transmitted diseases and dexual behavior: Insights from mathematical models. *J Infect Dis.* 1996;174(Suppl 2):S150-S161. doi:10.1093/infdis/174.Supplement_2.S150

31. Centers for Disease Control and Prevention. Effectiveness of prevention strategies to reduce the risk of acquiring or transmitting HIV. CDC. Published 2022. Accessed May 7, 2024. Available at: https://www.cdc.gov/hiv/risk/estimates/preventionstrategies.html

32. Awad SF, Sgaier SK, Lau FK, et al. Could circumcision of HIV-positive males benefit voluntary medical male circumcision programs in Africa? Mathematical modeling analysis. *PLoS One.* 2017;12(1):e0170641. doi:10.1371/journal.pone.0170641

33. Aspinall EJ, Nambiar D, Goldberg DJ, et al. Are needle and syringe programmes associated with a reduction in hiv transmission among people who inject drugs: A systematic review and meta-analysis. *Int J Epidemiol.* 2014;43(1):235-248. doi:10.1093/ije/dyt243

34. Ghosn J, Taiwo B, Seedat S, Autran B, Katlama C. HIV. *Lancet.* 2018;392(10148):685-697. doi:10.1016/S0140-6736(18)31311-4

35. Nolen S. New drug provides total protection from HIV in trial of young African women. *The New York Times.* June 21, 2024. Accessed June 26, 2024. Available at: https://www.nytimes.com/2024/06/21/health/lenacapavir-hiv-prevention-africa.html

36. Lee JH, Crotty S. HIV vaccinology: 2021 update. *Semin Immunol.* 2021;51:101470. doi:10.1016/j.smim.2021.101470

37. Rodger AJ, Cambiano V, Phillips AN, et al. Risk of HIV transmission through condomless sex in serodifferent gay couples with the HIV-positive partner taking suppressive antiretroviral therapy (PARTNER): Final results of a multicentre, prospective, observational study. *Lancet.* 2019;393(10189):2428-2438. doi:10.1016/S0140-6736(19)30418-0

38. Hall JE, Hall ME. Gastrointestinal physiology. In: *Guyton and Hall Textbook of Medical Physiology.* 14th ed. Elsevier; 2021:787-839.

39. Field M. Intestinal ion transport and the pathophysiology of diarrhea. *J Clin Invest.* 2003;111(7):931-943. doi:10.1172/JCI18326

40. WHO. Diarrhoeal disease. WHO. March 7, 2024. Accessed April 11, 2024. Available at: https://www.who.int/news-room/fact-sheets/detail/diarrhoeal-disease

41. Liu J, Platts-Mills JA, Juma J, et al. Use of quantitative molecular diagnostic methods to identify causes of diarrhoea in children: a reanalysis of the GEMS case-control study. *Lancet.* 2016;388(10051):1291-1301. doi:10.1016/S0140-6736(16)31529-X

42. Ballard SB, Requena D, Mayta H, et al. Enteropathogen changes after rotavirus vaccine scale-up. *Pediatrics.* 2022;149(1):e2020049884. doi:10.1542/peds.2020-049884

43. Platts-Mills JA, Liu J, Rogawski ET, et al. Use of quantitative molecular diagnostic methods to assess the aetiology, burden, and clinical characteristics of diarrhoea in children in low-resource settings: A reanalysis of the MAL-ED cohort study. *Lancet Glob Health.* 2018;6(12):e1309-e1318. doi:10.1016/S2214-109X(18)30349-8

44. Kotloff KL, Nataro JP, Blackwelder WC, et al. Burden and aetiology of diarrhoeal disease in infants and young children in developing countries (the Global Enteric Multicenter Study, GEMS): A prospective, case-control study. *Lancet.* 2013;382(9888):209-222. doi:10.1016/S0140-6736(13)60844-2

45. Keusch GT, Walker CF, Das JK, Horton S, Habte D. Diarrheal diseases. In: *Disease Control Priorities, Third Edition (Volume 2): Reproductive, Maternal, Newborn, and Child Health.* The World Bank; 2016:163-185. doi:10.1596/978-1-4648-0348-2_ch9

46. Mokomane M, Kasvosve I, Melo E de, Pernica JM, Goldfarb DM. The global problem of childhood diarrhoeal diseases: Emerging strategies in prevention and management. *Ther Adv Infect Dis.* 2018;5(1):29-43. doi:10.1177/2049936117744429

47. Kumar V, Abbas AK, Aster JC, Turner JR. Infectious enterocolitis. In: *Robbins & Cotran Pathologic Basis of Disease.* 10th ed.; 2021:787-798.

48. Anderson EJ, Weber SG. Rotavirus infection in adults. *Lancet Infect Dis.* 2004;4(2):91-99. doi:10.1016/S1473-3099(04)00928-4

49. Barzilay EJ, Schaad N, Magloire R, et al. Cholera surveillance during the Haiti epidemic—The first 2 years. *N Engl J Med.* 2013;368(7):599-609. doi:10.1056/nejmoa1204927

50. Mac Kenzie WR, Hoxie NJ, Proctor ME, et al. A massive outbreak in Milwaukee of Cryptosporidium infection transmitted through the public water supply. *N Engl J Med.* 1994;331(3):161-167. doi:10.1056/NEJM199407213310304

51. Pinto DJ, Vinayak S. Cryptosporidium: Host-parasite interactions and pathogenesis. *Curr Clin Microbiol Rep.* 2021;8(2):62-67. doi:10.1007/s40588-021-00159-7

52. Acosta AM, De Burga RR, Chavez CB, et al. Relationship between growth and illness, enteropathogens and dietary intakes in the first 2 years of life: Findings from the MAL-ED birth cohort study. *BMJ Glob Health.* 2017;2(4). doi:10.1136/bmjgh-2017-000370

53. Brown KH. Diarrhea and malnutrition. *J Nutr.* 2003;133(1):328S-332S. doi:10.1093/jn/133.1.328S

54. Checkley W, Buckley G, Gilman RH, et al. Multi-country analysis of the effects of diarrhoea on childhood stunting. *Int J Epidemiol.* 2008;37(4):816-830. doi:10.1093/ije/dyn099

55. Rogawski ET, Liu J, Platts-Mills JA, et al. Use of quantitative molecular diagnostic methods to investigate the effect of enteropathogen infections on linear growth in children in low-resource settings: longitudinal analysis of results from the MAL-ED cohort study. *Lancet Glob Health.* 2018;6(12):e1319-e1328. doi:10.1016/S2214-109X(18)30351-6

56. Nasrin D, Blackwelder WC, Sommerfelt H, et al. Pathogens associated with linear growth faltering in children with diarrhea and impact of antibiotic treatment: The Global Enteric Multicenter Study. *J Infect Dis.* 2021;224:S848-S855. doi:10.1093/infdis/jiab434

57. Kandrait D, Vasudeo N, Zodpey S, Kumbhalkar D. Brief report. Risk factors for subclinical vitamin A deficiency in children under the age of 6 years. *J Trop Pediatr.* 2000;46(4):239-241. doi:10.1093/tropej/46.4.239

58. Sommer A, Djunaedi E, Loeden AA, et al. Impact of vitamin A supplementation on childhood mortality. *Lancet.* 1986;327(8491):1169-1173. doi:10.1016/S0140-6736(86)91157-8

59. Mason J, Greiner T, Shrimpton R, Sanders D, Yukich J. Vitamin A policies need rethinking. *Int J Epidemiol.* 2015;44(1):283-292. doi:10.1093/ije/dyu194

60. World Health Organization. Vitamin A deficiency. World Health Organization. 2020. Accessed April 14, 2024. Available at: https://www.who.int/data/nutrition/nlis/info/vitamin-a-deficiency

61. Mason J, Greiner T, Shrimpton R, Sanders D, Yukich J. Vitamin A policies need rethinking. *Int J Epidemiol.* 2015;44(1):283-292. doi:10.1093/ije/dyu194

62. Sommer A, Katz J, Tarwotjo I. Increased risk of respiratory disease and diarrhea in children with preexisting mild vitamin A deficiency. *Am J Clin Nutr.* 1984;40(5):1090-1095. doi:10.1093/ajcn/40.5.1090

63. Thornton KA, Mora-Plazas M, Marín C, Villamor E. Vitamin A deficiency is associated with gastrointestinal and respiratory morbidity in school-age children. *J Nutr.* 2014;144(4):496-503. doi:10.3945/jn.113.185876

64. Fawzi WW, Herrera MG, Willett WC, Nestel P, el Amin A, Mohamed KA. Dietary vitamin A intake and the incidence of diarrhea and respiratory infection among Sudanese children. *J Nutr.* 1995;125(5):1211-1221. doi:10.1093/jn/125.5.1211

65. Han X, Ding S, Lu J, Li Y. Global, regional, and national burdens of common micronutrient deficiencies from 1990 to 2019: A secondary trend analysis based on the Global Burden of Disease 2019 study. *EClinicalMedicine.* 2022;44:101299. doi:10.1016/j

66. Song P, Adeloye D, Li S, et al. The prevalence of vitamin A deficiency and its public health significance in children in low and middle-income countries: A systematic review and modelling analysis. *J Glob Health.* 2023;13:04084. doi:10.7189/JOGH.13.04084

67. UNICEF. Vitamin A: Nearly two in three children in need were protected with the requisite two annual high-dose vitamin A supplements in 2022. UNICEF. March 2023. Accessed April 14, 2024. Available at: https://data.unicef.org/topic/nutrition/vitamin-a-deficiency/

68. Eisenberg JNS, Trostle J, Sorensen RJD, Shields KF. Toward a systems approach to enteric pathogen transmission: from individual independence to community interdependence. *Annu Rev Public Health.* 2012;33(1):239-257. doi:10.1146/annurev-publhealth-031811-124530

69. UN Inter-agency Group for Child Mortality Estimation. Child mortality stillbirth, and cause of death estimates.

Childmortality.org. March 13, 2024. Accessed April 13, 2024. Available at: https://childmortality.org

70. Global Burden of Disease Collaboration, Institute for Health Metrics and Evaluation. *GBD Results Tool.* July 12, 2023. Accessed July 11, 2023. Available at: https://vizhub.healthdata.org/gbd-results/

71. Johansen ØH, Abdissa A, Zangenberg M, et al. A comparison of risk factors for cryptosporidiosis and non-cryptosporidiosis diarrhoea: A case-case-control study in Ethiopian children. *PLoS Negl Trop Dis.* 2022;16(6):0010508. doi:10.1371/JOURNAL.PNTD.0010508

72. Mengistie B, Berhane Y, Worku A. Prevalence of diarrhea and associated risk factors among children under-five years of age in Eastern Ethiopia: A cross-sectional study. *Open J Prev Med.* 2013;03(07):446-453. doi:10.4236/ojpm.2013.37060

73. Getachew B, Mengistie B, Mesfin F, Argaw R. Factors associated with acute diarrhea among children aged 0-59 months in Harar Town, Eastern Ethiopia. *East Afr J Health Biomed Sci.* 2018;2(1):26-35.

74. Arvelo W, Kim A, Creek T, et al. Case-control study to determine risk factors for diarrhea among children during a large outbreak in a country with a high prevalence of HIV infection. Int *J Infect Dis.* 2010;14(11):e1002-e1007. doi:10.1016/j.ijid.2010.06.014

75. Wolf J, Hubbard S, Brauer M, et al. Effectiveness of interventions to improve drinking water, sanitation, and handwashing with soap on risk of diarrhoeal disease in children in low-income and middle-income settings: a systematic review and meta-analysis. *Lancet.* 2022;400(10345):48-59. doi:10.1016/S0140-6736(22)00937-0

76. Otsuka Y, Agestika L, Widyarani, Sintawardani N, Yamauchi T. Risk factors for undernutrition and diarrhea prevalence in an urban slum in Indonesia: Focus on water, sanitation, and hygiene. *Am J Trop Med Hyg.* 2019;100(3):727-732. doi:10.4269/ajtmh.18-0063

77. Berendes DM, Fagerli K, Kim S, et al. Survey-Based assessment of water, sanitation, and animal-associated risk factors for moderate-to-severe iarrhea in the Vaccine Impact on Diarrhea in Africa (VIDA) study: The Gambia, Mali, and Kenya, 2015-2018. *Clin Infect Dis.* 2023;76:S132-S139. doi:10.1093/cid/ciac911

78. Gebru T, Taha M, Kassahun W. Risk factors of diarrhoeal disease in under-five children among health extension model and non-model families in Sheko district rural community, Southwest Ethiopia: Comparative cross-sectional study. *BMC Public Health.* 2014;14(1):395. doi:10.1186/1471-2458-14-395

79. Wolf J, Prüss-Ustün A, Cumming O, et al. Systematic review: Assessing the impact of drinking water and sanitation on diarrhoeal disease in low-and middle-income settings: Systematic review and meta-regression. *Trop Med Int Health.* 2014;19(8):928-942. doi:10.1111/tmi.12331

80. Ganguly E, Sharma PK, Bunker CH. Prevalence and risk factors of diarrhea morbidity among under-five children in India: A systematic review and meta-analysis. *Indian J Child Health (Bhopal).* 2015;2(4):152-160.

81. Acácio S, Mandomando I, Nhampossa T, et al. Risk factors for death among children 0-59 months of age with moderate-to-severe diarrhea in Manhiça district, southern Mozambique. *BMC Infect Dis.* 2019;19(1). doi:10.1186/s12879-019-3948-9

82. Turin CG, Ochoa TJ. The role of maternal breast milk in preventing infantile diarrhea in the developing world. *Curr Trop Med Rep.* 2014;1(2):97-105. doi:10.1007/s40475-014-0015-x

83. Victora CG, Bahl R, Barros AJD, et al. Breastfeeding in the 21st century: Epidemiology, mechanisms, and lifelong effect. *The Lancet.* 2016;387:475-490. http://mics

84. World Health Organization. *Ending Preventable Child Deaths from Pneumonia and Diarrhoea by 2025: The Integrated Global Action Plan for Pneumonia and Diarrhoea (GAPPD).* 2013. Accessed June 26, 2024. Available at: https://www.who.int/publications/i/item/9789241505239

85. WHO and UNICEF Joint Monitoring Program. *Sanitation.* 2023. Accessed November 18, 2024. Available at: https://washdata.org/monitoring/sanitation

86. Meki CD, Ncube EJ, Voyi K. Frameworks for mitigating the risk of waterborne diarrheal diseases: A scoping review. *PLoS One.* 2022;17:e0278184. doi:10.1371/journal.pone.0278184

87. Ngari MM, Mwalekwa L, Timbwa M, et al. Changes in susceptibility to life-threatening infections after treatment for complicated severe malnutrition in Kenya. *Am J Clin Nutr.* 2018;107(4):626-634. doi:10.1093/ajcn/nqy007

88. Binder HJ, Brown I, Ramakrishna BS, Young GP. Oral rehydration therapy in the second decade of the twenty-first century. *Curr Gastroenterol Rep.* 2014;16(3). doi:10.1007/s11894-014-0376-2

89. Munos MK, Walker CLF, Black RE. The effect of oral rehydration solution and recommended home fluids on diarrhoea mortality. *Int J Epidemiol.* 2010;39(Suppl 1):i75-i87. doi:10.1093/ije/dyq025

90. Gupta S, Brazier AKM, Lowe NM. Zinc deficiency in low- and middle-income countries: prevalence and approaches for mitigation. *J Hum Nutr Diet.* 2020;33(5):624-643. doi:10.1111/jhn.12791

91. Dhingra U, Kisenge R, Sudfeld CR, et al. Lower-Dose Zinc for Childhood Diarrhea—A Randomized, Multicenter Trial. *N Engl J Med.* 2020;383(13):1231-1241. doi:10.1056/nejmoa1915905

92. Pavlinac PB, Platts-Mills JA, Liu J, et al. Azithromycin for bacterial watery diarrhea: A reanalysis of the AntiBiotics for Children with Severe Diarrhea (ABCD) trial incorporating molecular diagnostics. *J Infect Dis.* 2024;229(4):988-998. doi:10.1093/infdis/jiad252

93. Ahmed T, Chisti MJ, Rahman MW, et al. Effect of 3 days of oral azithromycin on young children with acute diarrhea in low-resource settings: A randomized clinical trial. *JAMA Netw Open.* 2021;4(12). doi:10.1001/jamanetworkopen.2021.36726

94. World Health Organization, UNICEF. *Integrated Management of Childhood Illness.* 2014. Accessed June 26, 2024. Available at: https://www.who.int/publications/m/item/integrated-management-of-childhood-illness---chart-booklet-(march-2014)

95. Black R, Fontaine O, Lamberti L, et al. Drivers of the reduction in childhood diarrhea mortality 1980-2015 and interventions to eliminate preventable diarrhea deaths by 2030. *J Glob Health.* 2019;9(2). doi:10.7189/jogh.09.020801

96. United Nations (UN). UN Sustainable Development Goal 6. 2015. Accessed April 17, 2024. Available at: https://sdgs.un.org/goals/goal6

97. Institute for Health Metrics and Evaluation. COVID-19 Projections. Global Burden of Disease. April 1, 2023. Accessed April 24, 2024. Available at: https://covid19.healthdata.org/global

98. Kyu HH, Vongpradith A, Sirota SB, et al. Age–sex differences in the global burden of lower respiratory infections and risk factors, 1990–2019: results from the Global Burden of Disease Study 2019. *Lancet Infect Dis.* 2022;22(11):1626-1647. doi:10.1016/S1473-3099(22)00510-2

99. Husain A. Pulmonary infections. In: Kumar V, Abbas AK, Aster JC, Turner JR, eds. *Robbins & Cotran Pathologic Basis of Disease.* 10th ed. Elsevier; 2021:705-714.

100. Aliberti S, Dela Cruz CS, Amati F, Sotgiu G, Restrepo MI. Community-acquired pneumonia. *Lancet.* 2021;398(10303):906-919. doi:10.1016/S0140-6736(21)00630-9

101. Fischer Walker CL, Rudan I, Liu L, et al. Global burden of childhood pneumonia and diarrhoea. *Lancet.* 2013;381(9875):1405-1416. doi:10.1016/S0140-6736(13)60222-6

102. O'Brien KL, Baggett HC, Brooks WA, et al. Causes of severe pneumonia requiring hospital admission in children without HIV infection from Africa and Asia: the PERCH multi-country case-control study. *Lancet.* 2019;394(10200):757-779. doi:10.1016/S0140-6736(19)30721-4

103. Conrad A, Valour F, Vanhems P. Burden of influenza in the elderly: A narrative review. *Curr Opin Infect Dis.* 2023;36(4):296-302. doi:10.1097/QCO.0000000000000931

104. Jain S, Williams DJ, Arnold SR, et al. Community-acquired pneumonia requiring hospitalization among U.S. children. *N Engl J Med.* 2015;372(9):835-845. doi:10.1056/nejmoa1405870

105. Zar HJ, Barnett W, Stadler A, Gardner-Lubbe S, Myer L, Nicol MP. Aetiology of childhood pneumonia in a well vaccinated South African birth cohort: A nested case-control study of the Drakenstein Child Health Study. *Lancet Respir Med.* 2016;4(6):463-472. doi:10.1016/S2213-2600(16)00096-5

106. Jain S, Self WH, Wunderink RG, et al. Community-acquired pneumonia requiring hospitalization among U.S. adults. *N Engl J Med.* 2015;373(5):415-427. doi:10.1056/nejmoa1500245

107. Prina E, Ranzani OT, Torres A. Community-acquired pneumonia. In: *Lancet.* 2015;386(9998):1097-1108. doi:10.1016/S0140-6736(15)60733-4

108. Arnold FW, Summersgill JT, Lajoie AS, et al. A worldwide perspective of atypical pathogens in community-acquired pneumonia. *Am J Respir Crit Care Med.* 2007;175(10):1086-1093. doi:10.1164/rccm.200603-350OC

109. Troeger C, Blacker B, Khalil IA, et al. Estimates of the global, regional, and national morbidity, mortality, and aetiologies of lower respiratory infections in 195 countries, 1990–2016: A systematic analysis for the Global Burden of Disease Study 2016. *Lancet Infect Dis.* 2018;18(11):1191-1210. doi:10.1016/S1473-3099(18)30310-4

110. Rudan I, O'Brien KL, Nair H, et al. Epidemiology and etiology of childhood pneumonia in 2010: Estimates of incidence, severe morbidity, mortality, underlying risk factors and causative pathogens for 192 countries. *J Glob Health.* 2013;3(1). doi:10.7189/jogh.03.010401

111. Centers for Disease Control and Prevention. Influenza Vaccination Coverage for Persons 6 Months and Older. CDC; 2024. Accessed April 25, 2024. Available at: https://www.cdc.gov/flu/fluvaxview/interactive-general-population.htm

112. Swenson KE, Hardin CC. Pathophysiology of Hypoxemia in COVID-19 Lung Disease. *Clin Chest Med.* 2023;44(2):239-248. doi:10.1016/j.ccm.2022.11.007

113. Hariri LP, North CM, Shih AR, et al. Lung histopathology in coronavirus disease 2019 as compared with severe acute respiratory sydrome and H1N1 influenza: A systematic review. *Chest.* 2021;159(1):73-84. doi:10.1016/j.chest.2020.09.259

114. Greenhalgh T, Sivan M, Perlowski A, Nikolich J. Long COVID: A clinical update. *Lancet.* 2024;404(10453):707-724. doi:10.1016/S0140-6736(24)01136-X

115. Jones JM, Manrique IM, Mars, et al. Estimates of SARS-CoV-2 Seroprevalence and Incidence of primary SARS-CoV-2 infections among blood donors, by COVID-19 vaccinationstatus-United States, April 2021-September 2022. *MMWR Morb Mortal Wkly Rep.* 2023;72(22):601-605. Available at: https://www.fda.gov/media/151027/download

116. Centers for Disease Control and Prevention. COVID Data Tracker. Accessed April 25, 2024. Available at: https://covid.cdc.gov/covid-data-tracker

117. Centers for Disease Control and Prevention. Provisional Multiple Cause of Death Data. CDC WONDER. April 14, 2024. Accessed April 24, 2024. Available at: https://wonder.cdc.gov/mcd-icd10-provisional.html

118. Fitzpatrick M, Moghadas S, Pandey A, Galvani A. Two years of U.S. COVID-19 vaccines have prevented millions of hospitalizations and deaths The Commonwealth Fund. 2022. Accessed April 21, 2024. Available at: https://www.commonwealthfund.org/blog/2022/two-years-covid-vaccines-prevented-millions-deaths-hospitalizations

119. Bai Y, Du Z, Wang L, et al. Public health impact of Paxlovid as treatment for COVID-19, United States. *Emerg Infect Dis.* 2024;30(2):262-269. doi:10.3201/eid3002.230835

120. Hansen K, Makkar SR, Sahner D, Fessel J, Hotaling N, Sidky H. Paxlovid (nirmatrelvir/ritonavir) effectiveness against hospitalization and death in N3C: A target trial emulation study Key points. *Medrxiv.* Published online 2023. doi:10.1101/2023.05.26.23290602

121. Marr LC, Tang JW. A paradigm shift to align transmission routes with mechanisms. *Clin Infect Dis.* 2021;73(10):1747-1749. doi:10.1093/cid/ciab722

122. Leung NHL. Transmissibility and transmission of respiratory viruses. *Nat Rev Microbiol.* 2021;19(8):528-545. doi:10.1038/s41579-021-00535-6

123. World Health Organization. Global technical consultation report on proposed terminology for pathogens that transmit through the air. 2024. Accessed June 27, 2024. Available at: https://www.who.int/publications/m/item/global-technical-consultation-report-on-proposed-terminology-for-pathogens-that-transmit-through-the-air

124. Bulfone TC, Malekinejad M, Rutherford GW, Razani N. Outdoor transmission of SARS-CoV-2 and other respiratory viruses: A systematic review. *J Infect Dis.* 2021;223(4):550-561. doi:10.1093/infdis/jiaa742

125. Wang CC, Prather KA, Sznitman J, et al. Airborne transmission of respiratory viruses. *Science.* 2021;373(6558). doi:10.1126/science.abd9149

126. Sarfo JO, Amoadu M, Gyan TB, et al. Acute lower respiratory infections among children under five in Sub-Saharan Africa: A scoping review of prevalence and risk factors. *BMC Pediatr.* 2023;23(1). doi:10.1186/s12887-023-04033-x

127. Torres A, Peetermans WE, Viegi G, Blasi F. Risk factors for community-acquired pneumonia in adults in Europe: A literature review. *Thorax.* 2013;68(11):1057-1065. doi:10.1136/thoraxjnl-2013-204282

128. Lassi ZS, Moin A, Bhutta ZA. Zinc supplementation for the prevention of pneumonia in children aged 2 months to 59

months. *Cochrane Database Syst Rev.* 2016;12(12):CD005978. doi:10.1002/14651858.CD005978.pub3

129. Victora CG, Christian P, Vidaletti LP, Gatica-Domínguez G, Menon P, Black RE. Revisiting maternal and child undernutrition in low-income and middle-income countries: Variable progress towards an unfinished agenda. *Lancet.* 2021;397(10282):1388-1399. doi:10.1016/S0140 -6736(21)00394-9

130. World Health Organization. *Compendium of WHO and Other UN Guidance on Health and Environment: 2024 Update.* 2024.

131. Rivero-Calle I, Cebey-López M, Pardo-Seco J, et al. Lifestyle and comorbid conditions as risk factors for community-acquired pneumonia in outpatient adults (NEUMO-ES-RISK project). *BMJ Open Respir Res.* 2019;6(1). doi:10.1136/bmjresp-2018-000359

132. Leung DT, Chisti MJ, Pavia AT. Prevention and control of childhood pneumonia and diarrhea. *Pediatr Clin North Am.* 2016;63(1):67-79. doi:10.1016/j.pcl.2015.08.003

133. Centers for Disease Control and Prevention. Ventilation in buildings. May 12, 2023. Accessed July 18, 2023. Available at: https://www.cdc.gov/coronavirus/2019-ncov /community/ventilation.html

134. Centers for Disease Control and Prevention. Guidelines for environmental infection control in health-care facilities: Recommendations of the CDC and the Healthcare Infection Control Practices Advisory Committee (HICPAC). 2019. Accessed June 27, 2024. Available at: https://www.cdc.gov /infectioncontrol/guidelines/environmental/index.html

135. Centers for Disease Control and Prevention. Upper-room ultraviolet germicidal irradiation. April 9, 2021. Accessed April 24, 2024. Available at: https://www.cdc.gov /coronavirus/2019-ncov/community/ventilation/UVGI.html

136. bin-Reza F, Lopez Chavarrias V, Nicoll A, Chamberland ME. The use of masks and respirators to prevent transmission of influenza: A systematic review of the scientific evidence. *Influenza Other Respir Viruses.* 2012;6(4):257-267. doi:10 .1111/j.1750-2659.2011.00307.x

137. Sleator RD, Smith N. COVID-19: did the masks work? *Future Microbiol.* 2024;19(11):997-1002. doi:10.1080/174 60913.2024.2343558

138. Andrejko KL, Pry JM, Myers JF, et al. Effectiveness of face mask or respirator use in indoor public settings for prevention of SARS-CoV-2 infection—California, February—December 2021. *MMWR Morb Mortal Wkly Rep.* 2022;71(6):212-216. doi:10.15585/mmwr.mm7106e1

139. Ross I, Bick S, Ayieko P, et al. Effectiveness of handwashing with soap for preventing acute respiratory infections in low-income and middle-income countries: A systematic review and meta-analysis. *Lancet.* 2023;401(10389):1681-1690. doi:10.1016/S0140-6736(23)00021-1

140. Gordon SB, Bruce NG, Grigg J, et al. Respiratory risks from household air pollution in low-and middle-income countries. *Lancet Respir Med.* 2014;2(10):823-860. doi:10 .1016/S2213-2600(14)70168-7

141. World Health Organization. *Global Tuberculosis Report 2023.* World Health Organization; 2024. Accessed June 30, 2024. Available at: https://www.who.int/teams/global -tuberculosis-programme/tb-reports/global-tuberculosis -report-2023

142. World Health Organization. *Implementing the End TB Strategy: The Essentials, 2022 Update.* 2022. Accessed January 6, 2024. Available at: https://www.who.int/publications/i /item/9789240065093

143. Frank KM, McAdam AJ. Mycobacterial infections. In: Kumar V, Abbas AK, Aster JC, Turner JR, eds. *Robbins & Contran Pathologic Basis of Disease.* 10th Edition. Elsevier; 2022:367-373.

144. World Health Organization. *WHO Consolidated Guidelines on Tuberculosis. Module 1, Prevention: Tuberculosis Preventive Treatment.* 2022. Accessed July 1, 2024. Available at: https://www.who.int/publications/i/item/9789240001503

145. Furin J, Cox H, Pai M. Tuberculosis. *Lancet.* 2019;393 (10181):1642-1656. doi:10.1016/S0140-6736(19)30308-3

146. Churchyard G, Kim P, Shah NS, et al. What we know about tuberculosis transmission: An Overview. *J Infec Dis.* 2017;216:S629-S635. doi:10.1093/infdis/jix362

147. Schildknecht KR, Pratt RH, Feng PJI, Price SF, Self JL. Tuberculosis-United States, 2022. *MMWR Morb Mortal Wkly Rep.* 2022;72(12):297-303.

148. Dierberg KL, Dorjee K, Salvo F, et al. Improved detection of tuberculosis and multidrug-resistant tuberculosis among Tibetan refugees, India. *Emerg Infect Dis.* 2016;22(3):463-468. doi:10.3201/eid2203.140732

149. Khaliq A, Khan. I.H., Akhtar MW, Chaudhry MN. Environmental risk factors and social determinants of pulmonary tuberculosis in Pakistan. *Epidemiology: Open Access.* 2015;5(3):1-9. doi:10.4172/2161-1165.1000201

150. Wardani DWSR, Wahono EP. Housing condition as tuberculosis infection risk factor. *Indian J Public Health Res Dev.* 2019;10(3). doi:10.5958/0976-5506.2019.00577.1

151. Nardell EA. Transmission and institutional infection control of tuberculosis. *Cold Spring Harb Perspect Med.* 2016;6(2). doi:10.1101/cshperspect.a018192

152. Yates TA, Khan PY, Knight GM, et al. The transmission of Mycobacterium tuberculosis in high burden settings. *Lancet Infect Dis.* 2016;16:227-238.

153. Deol AK, Shaikh N, Middelkoop K, Mohlamonyane M, White RG, McCreesh N. Importance of ventilation and occupancy to Mycobacterium tuberculosis transmission rates in congregate settings. *BMC Public Health.* 2022;22(1). doi:10.1186/s12889-022-14133-5

154. Koethe JR, Von Reyn CF. Protein-calorie malnutrition, macronutrient supplements, and tuberculosis. *Int J Tuberc Lung Dis.* 2016;20(7):857-863. doi:10.5588/ijtld.15.0936

155. World Health Organization. *Global Tuberculosis Report 2023.* 2023. Accessed June 30, 2024. Available at: https:// www.who.int/publications/i/item/9789240083851

156. Kwan C, Ernst JD. HIV and tuberculosis: A deadly human syndemic. *Clin Microbiol Rev.* 2011;24(2):351-376. doi:10 .1128/CMR.00042-10

157. Rehm J, Samokhvalov A V., Neuman MG, et al. The association between alcohol use, alcohol use disorders and tuberculosis (TB). A systematic review. *BMC Public Health.* 2009;9(450). doi:10.1186/1471-2458-9-450

158. Hayashi S, Chandramohan D. Risk of active tuberculosis among people with diabetes mellitus: systematic review and meta-analysis. Trop Med Int Health. 2018;23(10):1058-1070. doi:10.1111/tmi.13133

159. Lugg ST, Scott A, Parekh D, Naidu B, Thickett DR. Cigarette smoke exposure and alveolar macrophages: mechanisms for lung disease. *Thorax.* 2022;77(1):94-101. doi:10.1136/thoraxjnl-2020-216296

160. Feldman C, Theron AJ, Cholo MC, Anderson R. Cigarette smoking as a risk factor for tuberculosis in adults: Epidemiology and aspects of disease pathogenesis. *Pathogens.* 2024;13(2). doi:10.3390/pathogens13020151

161. Chiang CY, Slama K, Enarson DA. Associations between tobacco and tuberculosis. *Int J Tuberc Lung Dis.* 2007;11(3):258-262.

162. du Preez K, Mandalakas AM, Kirchner HL, et al. Environmental tobacco smoke exposure increases Mycobacterium tuberculosis infection risk in children. *Int J Tuberc Lung Dis.* 2011;15(11):1490-1497. doi:10.5588/ijtld.10.0759

163. Jafta N, Jeena PM, Barregard L, Naidoo RN. Association of childhood pulmonary tuberculosis with exposure to indoor air pollution: A case control study. *BMC Public Health.* 2019;19(1). doi:10.1186/s12889-019-6604-9

164. Obore N, Kawuki J, Guan J, Papabathini SS, Wang L. Association between indoor air pollution, tobacco smoke and tuberculosis: An updated systematic review and meta-analysis. *Public Health.* 2020;187. doi:10.1016/j.puhe.2020.07.031

165. Kurmi OP, Sadhra CS, Ayres JG, Sadhra SS. Tuberculosis risk from exposure to solid fuel smoke: a systematic review and meta-analysis. *J Epidemiol Community Health.* 2014;68(12):1112-1118. doi:10.1136/jech-2014-204120

166. World Health Organization. *WHO Consolidated Guidelines on Tuberculosis Module 1: Prevention Infection Prevention and Control.*; 2020. Accessed July 1, 2024. Available at: https://www.who.int/publications/i/item/9789240055889

167. Abubakar I, Pimpin L, Ariti C, et al. Systematic review and meta-analysis of the current evidence on the duration of protection by bacillus Calmette—Guérin vaccination against tuberculosis. *Health Technol Assess.* 2013;17(37). doi:10.3310/hta17370

168. Zwerling A, Behr MA, Verma A, Brewer TF, Menzies D, Pai M. The BCG world atlas: A database of global BCG vaccination policies and practices. *PLoS Med.* 2011;8(3). doi:10.1371/journal.pmed.1001012

169. Martinez L, Cords O, Liu Q, et al. Infant BCG vaccination and risk of pulmonary and extrapulmonary tuberculosis throughout the life course: a systematic review and individual participant data meta-analysis. *Lancet Glob Health.* 2022;10(9):e1307-e1316. doi:10.1016/S2214-109X(22)00283-2

170. Tait DR, Hatherill M, Van Der Meeren O, et al. Final analysis of a trial of M72/AS01 E vaccine to prevent tuberculosis. *N Engl J Med.* 2019;381(25):2429-2439. doi:10.1056/nejmoa1909953

171. World Health Organization. *WHO Consolidated Guidelines on Tuberculosis Module 4: Treatment Drug-Susceptible Tuberculosis Treatment.* 2022. Accessed June 20, 2024. Available at: https://www.who.int/publications/i/item/9789240048126

172. World Health Organization. *WHO Consolidated Guidelines on Tuberculosis Module 4: Treatment Drug-Resistant Tuberculosis Treatment (2022 Update).* 2022. Accessed June 20, 2024. Available at: https://www.who.int/publications/i/item/9789240063129

173. World Health Organization. *WHO Consolidated Guidelines on Tuberculosis Module 4: Treatment Tuberculosis Care and Support.* 2022. Accessed July 1, 2024. Available at: https://www.who.int/publications/i/item/9789240047716

174. Arnadottir T. The Styblo model 20 years later: What holds true? *Int J Tuberc Lung Dis.* 2009;13(6):672-690.

175. World Health Organization. *World Malaria Report 2023.* 2023. Accessed July 1, 2024. Available at: https://www.who.int/teams/global-malaria-programme/reports/world-malaria-report-2023

176. World Health Organization. *Global Technical Strategy for Malaria: 2016–2030. 2021 Update.* 2021. Accessed July 1, 2024. Available at: https://www.who.int/publications/i/item/9789240031357

177. Roques M, Bindschedler A, Beyeler R, Heussler VT. Same, same but different: Exploring Plasmodium cell division during liver stage development. *PLoS Pathog.* 2023;19(3). doi:10.1371/JOURNAL.PPAT.1011210

178. Centers for Disease Control and Prevention. Malaria. CDC. March 19, 2024. Accessed April 2, 2024. Available at: https://www.cdc.gov/dpdx/malaria/index.html

179. Frank K, McAdam A. Parasitic Infections. In: Kumar V, Abbas AK, Aster JC, Turner JR, eds. *Robbins & Cotran Pathologic Basis of Disease.* 10th ed. Elsevier; 2021:388-390.

180. Milner DA. Malaria pathogenesis. *Cold Spring Harb Perspect Med.* 2018;8(1). doi:10.1101/cshperspect.a025569

181. World Health Organization. *Epidemiological Approach for Malaria Control: Guide for Tutors.* 2013. Accessed July 1, 2024. Available at: https://iris.who.int/bitstream/handle/10665/96351/9789241506014_tutors_guide_eng.pdf

182. Tedioisi F, Lengeler C, Castro M, et al. Malaria control. In: Holmes K, Bertozzi S, Bloom B, eds. *Major Infectious Diseases.* 3rd ed. International Bank for Reconstruction and Development/The World Bank; 2017. Accessed March 31, 2024. Available at: https://www.ncbi.nlm.nih.gov/books/NBK525176/

183. Phillips MA, Burrows JN, Manyando C, Van Huijsduijnen RH, Van Voorhis WC, Wells TNC. Malaria. *Nat Rev Dis Primers.* 2017;3. doi:10.1038/nrdp.2017.50

184. World Health Organization. *WHO Guidelines for Malaria.* 2023. Accessed July 1, 2024. Available at: https://www.who.int/publications/i/item/guidelines-for-malaria

185. Centers for Disease Control and Prevention. *Life Cycle of Anopheles Species Mosquitos.* CDC. August 24, 2023. Accessed April 2, 2024. Available at: https://www.cdc.gov/mosquitoes/about/life-cycles/anopheles.html

186. Doumbe-Belisse P, Kopya E, Ngadjeu CS, et al. Urban malaria in sub-Saharan Africa: Dynamic of the vectorial system and the entomological inoculation rate. *Malar J.* 2021;20(1). doi:10.1186/s12936-021-03891-z

187. Takken W, Lindsay S. Increased threat of urban malaria from *Anopheles stephensi* mosquitoes, Africa. *Emerg Infect Dis.* 2019;25(7):1431-1433. doi:10.3201/eid2507.190301

188. Bannister-Tyrrell M, Verdonck K, Hausmann-Muela S, Gryseels C, Muela Ribera J, Peeters Grietens K. Defining micro-epidemiology for malaria elimination: systematic review and meta-analysis. *Malar J.* 2017;16(1). doi:10.1186/s12936-017-1792-1

189. Dieng S, Ba EH, Cissé B, et al. Spatio-temporal variation of malaria hotspots in Central Senegal, 2008–2012. *BMC Infect Dis.* 2020;20(1). doi:10.1186/s12879-020-05145-w

190. Endo N, Eltahir EAB. Environmental determinants of malaria transmission around the koka reservoir in Ethiopia. *Geohealth.* 2018;2(3):104-115. doi:10.1002/2017GH000108

191. Stresman GH. Beyond temperature and precipitation: Ecological risk factors that modify malaria transmission. *Acta Trop.* 2010;116(3):167-172. doi:10.1016/j.actatropica.2010.08.005

192. Carter R, Mendis KN. Evolutionary and historical aspects of the burden of malaria. *Clin Microbiol Rev.* 2002;15(4):564-594. doi:10.1128/CMR.15.4.564-594.2002

193. Poespoprodjo JR, Douglas NM, Ansong D, Kho S, Anstey NM. Malaria. *Lancet.* 2023;402(10419):2328-2345. doi:10.1016/S0140-6736(23)01249-7

194. Achan J, Talisuna AO, Erhart A, et al. Quinine, an old antimalarial drug in a modern world: Role in the treatment of malaria. *Malar J.* 2011;10. doi:10.1186/1475-2875-10-144

195. Faurant C. From bark to weed: The history of artemisinin. *Parasite.* 2011;18(3):215-218. doi:10.1051/parasite/2011183215

196. White NJ, Hien TT, Nosten FH. A Brief History of Qinghaosu. *Trends Parasitol.* 2015;31(12):607-610. doi:10.1016/j.pt.2015.10.010

197. González-Sanz M, Berzosa P, Norman FF. Updates on malaria epidemiology and prevention strategies. *Curr Infect Dis Rep.* 2023;25(7):131-139. doi:10.1007/s11908-023-00805-9

198. Hay SI, Guerra CA, Tatem AJ, Noor AM, Snow RW. The global distribution and population at risk of malaria: past, present, and future. *Lancet Infect Dis.* 2004;4(6):327-336. doi:10.1016/S1473-3099(04)01043-6

199. Nájera JA, González-Silva M, Alonso PL. Some lessons for the future from the global malaria eradication programme (1955-1969). *PLoS Med.* 2011;8(1). doi:10.1371/journal.pmed.1000412

200. Lengeler C, Snow RW. From efficacy to effectiveness: insecticide-treated bednets in Africa. *Bull World Health Organ.* 1996;74(3):325-332.

201. Leandro-Reguillo P, Thomson-Luque R, Monteiro WM, De Lacerda MVG. Urban and architectural risk factors for malaria in indigenous Amazonian settlements in Brazil: A typological analysis. *Malar J.* 2015;14(1). doi:10.1186/s12936-015-0806-0

202. Nguela RL, Bigoga JD, Armel TN, et al. The effect of improved housing on indoor mosquito density and exposure to malaria in the rural community of Minkoameyos, Centre Region of Cameroon. *Malar J.* 2020;19(1). doi:10.1186/s12936-020-03232-6

203. Tusting LS, Ippolito MM, Willey BA, et al. The evidence for improving housing to reduce malaria: A systematic review and meta-analysis. *Malar J.* 2015;14(1). doi:10.1186/s12936-015-0724-1

204. Rek JC, Alegana V, Arinaitwe E, et al. Rapid improvements to rural Ugandan housing and their association with malaria from intense to reduced transmission: a cohort study. *Lancet Planet Health.* 2018;2:e83-e94.

205. Monroe A, Asamoah O, Lam Y, et al. Outdoor-sleeping and other night-time activities in northern Ghana: Implications for residual transmission and malaria prevention. *Malar J.* 2015;14(1). doi:10.1186/s12936-015-0543-4

206. Derua YA, Kweka EJ, Kisinza WN, Githeko AK, Mosha FW. Bacterial larvicides used for malaria vector control in sub-Saharan Africa: Review of their effectiveness and operational feasibility. *Parasit Vectors.* 2019;12(1). doi:10.1186/s13071-019-3683-5

207. Tusting LS, Thwing J, Sinclair D, et al. Mosquito larval source management for controlling malaria. *Cochrane Database of Syst Rev.* 2013;2013(8). doi:10.1002/14651858.D008923.pub2

208. Fillinger U, Lindsay SW. Larval source management for malaria control in Africa: Myths and reality. *Malar J.* 2011;10(353):1-10.

209. Saili K, de Jager C, Masaninga F, et al. House screening reduces exposure to indoor host-seeking and biting malaria vectors: Evidence from rural South-East Zambia. *Trop Med Infect Dis.* 2024;9(1). doi:10.3390/tropicalmed9010020

210. Shah MP, Hwang J, Choi L, Lindblade KA, Kachur SP, Desai M. Mass drug administration for malaria. *Cochrane Database of Syst Rev.* 2021;2021(9). doi:10.1002/14651858.CD008846.pub3

211. Laurens MB. RTS,S/AS01 vaccine (Mosquirix™): An overview. *Hum Vaccin Immunother.* 2019;15(4):757-765. doi:10.1080/21645515.2019.1669415

212. Zavala F. RTS,S: the first malaria vaccine. *J Clin Invest.* 2022;132(1). doi:10.1172/JCI156588

213. Asante KP, Mathanga DP, Milligan P, et al. Feasibility, safety, and impact of the RTS,S/AS01E malaria vaccine when implemented through national immunisation programmes: evaluation of cluster-randomised introduction of the vaccine in Ghana, Kenya, and Malawi. *Lancet.* 2024;504(10437):1660-1670. doi:10.1016/S0140-6736(24)00004-7

CHAPTER 10

Diseases of the Newborn

The health of newborn infants is a key measure of the health of an entire society. It mostly reflects the health of women during and before pregnancy, but it has consequences for the infants' entire lives.

In United States health statistics, the two leading listed causes of deaths for infants are actually clusters of causes: 1) disorders related to preterm birth and low birth weight and 2) congenital malformations. This chapter defines these terms and discusses the biologic causes and prevention of those two clusters. Many risk factors are involved, and the risk factors for these two clusters overlap.

Preterm Birth and Low Birth Weight

Introduction

A newborn's chances of survival are closely tied to that newborn's weight at birth (**Figure 10.1**).[1] In the United States, babies born weighing 2,200 grams (just under 5 pounds) are about seven times more likely to die in the first year as babies born weighing 3,600 grams (8 pounds). An infant with a weight at birth below 2,500 grams is said to have **low birth weight**.

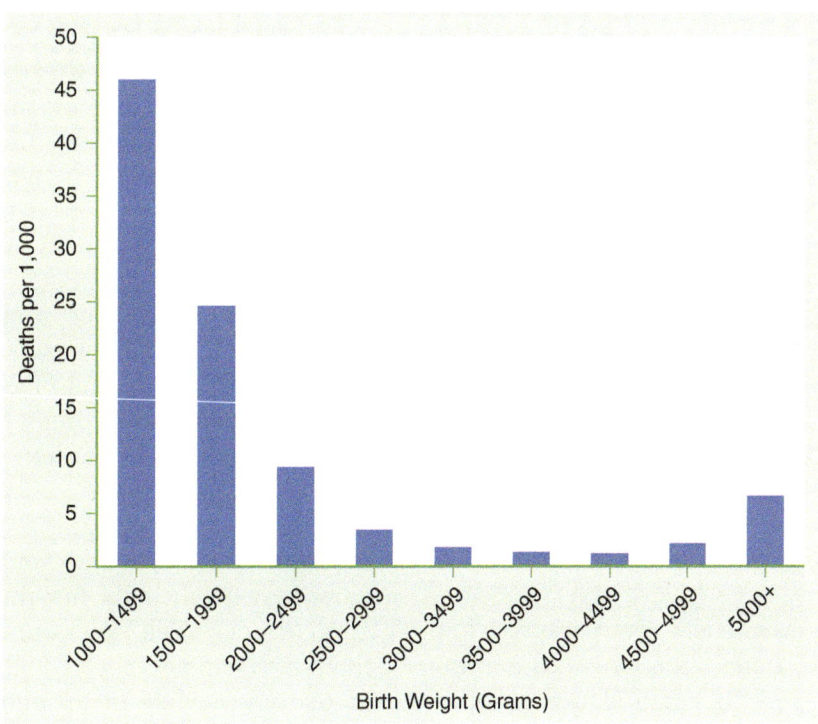

Figure 10.1 **Infant Mortality by Birth Weight in the United States, 2007–2021.**

Data from Centers for Disease Control and Prevention. WONDER Natality Files. CDC. Published 2024. Accessed May 14, 2024. https://wonder.cdc.gov/natality.html

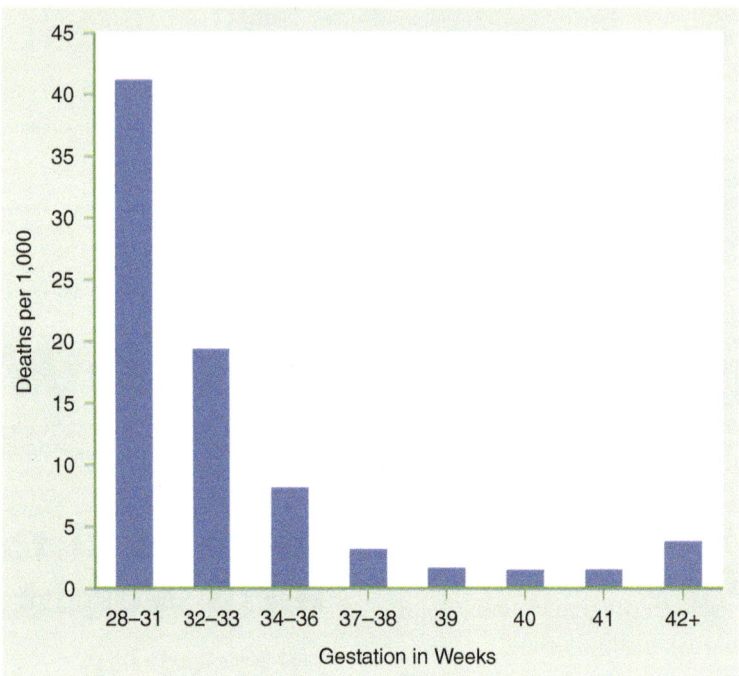

Figure 10.2 Infant Mortality by Length of Gestation in the United States, 2007–2021.

Data from Centers for Disease Control and Prevention. WONDER Natality Files. CDC. Published 2024. Accessed May 14, 2024. https://wonder.cdc.gov/natality.html

Likewise, the duration of the pregnancy has a large impact on the chances that an infant will survive (**Figure 10.2**).[1] The **gestation**, or gestational period, is counted as the time from the mother's last menstrual period to the infant's birth. The healthiest infants are born after a gestation of 40 weeks. A **preterm birth** is a birth that occurs before 37 weeks gestation; these infants are called **premature**. Infants born before 35 weeks gestation are more than five times as likely to die in the first year as infants born after 40 weeks, despite high-technology medical care for premature babies. Preventing infant mortality today depends less on the quality of medical care for infants than on prevention of low birth weight and preterm birth.

The health risks of low birth weight and preterm birth do not end with an infant surviving to the first birthday. Infants born small or early are more likely to have long-term health problems, such as chronic lung disease and developmental problems from a lack of oxygen to the brain. Even adults who were born small or early are more likely to die of heart disease and diabetes.[2]

There are many causes and contributors to low birth weight and to preterm birth, some tied to pregnancy and some tied to the health of women when they become pregnant. At a global scale, the largest driver is **undernutrition** in women. In the United States, major contributors include infections, use of drugs during pregnancy, and a condition called **pre-eclampsia**, which is discussed in Box 10.1. However, many of the causes of low birth weight and of preterm birth in high-income countries are not well understood. And there are important racial and socioeconomic differences that are likewise not fully explained.

Physiology of Fetal Growth

A fetus grows inside the **uterus**, within a fluid-filled space that is covered by an inner membrane called the **amnion** and an outer membrane called the **chorion** (**Figure 10.3**). The fluid inside this space is called **amniotic fluid**. The fetus obtains oxygen and nutrients needed for growth and disposes of carbon dioxide and metabolic waste products through the **umbilical cord** and the **placenta**. The placenta serves as the interface between the fetus and the parent. It is implanted into the lining of the uterus. Fluids, chemicals, most drugs, and gases like oxygen flow freely across the placenta, but the mother's and fetus' cells usually do not.

The 40-week gestation is divided into three **trimesters** of about three months each. The fetus grows very slowly in the first trimester (gaining about 10 grams per week), picks up speed in the second trimester (gaining about 65 grams per week), and grows very quickly in the third trimester (gaining nearly 200 grams per week **Figure 10.4**).[3] Many organs are still being developed in the third trimester. A gestation that is shortened by even a week or two leads to a birth weight that is hundreds of grams below optimal and organs that are not fully mature.

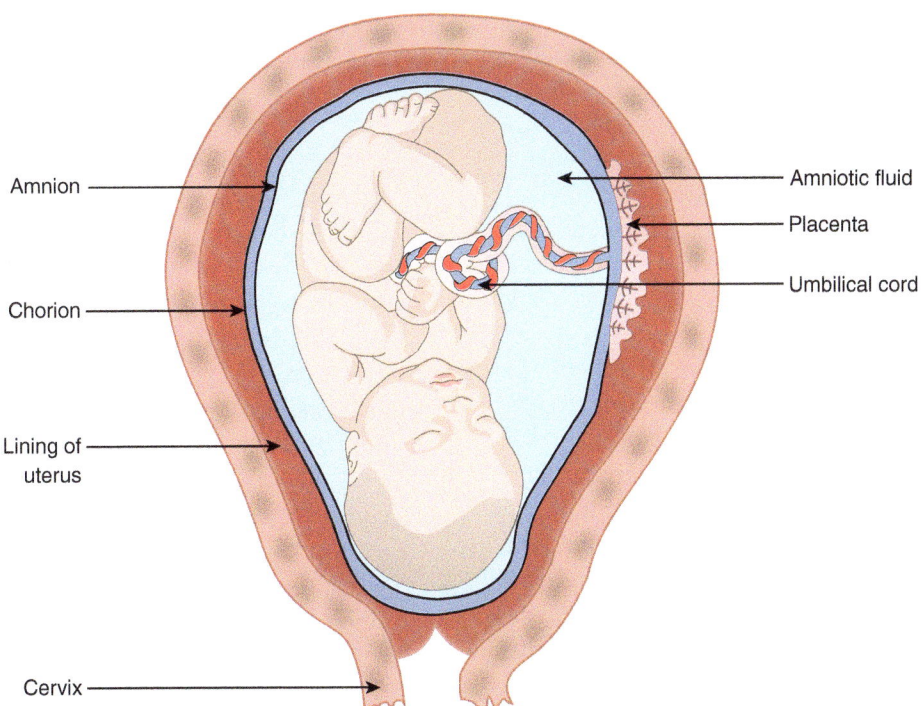

Figure 10.3 The Fetus, Placenta, and Uterus. A fetus grows inside the mother's uterus, within a space filled with amniotic fluid. That space is covered by an inner membrane called the amnion and an outer membrane called the chorion. The fetus obtains oxygen and nutrients and disposes of carbon dioxide and metabolic waste products through the umbilical cord and the placenta.

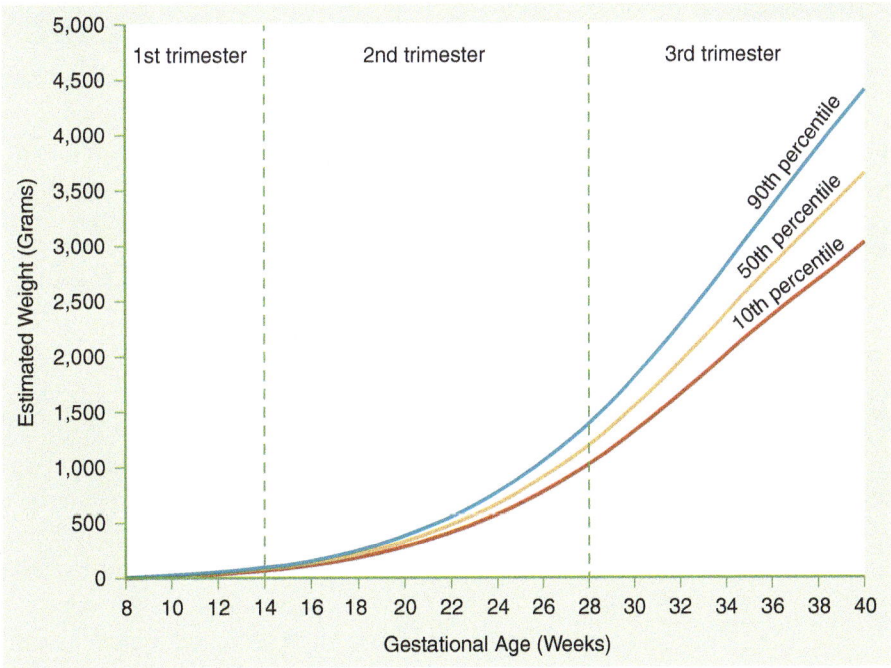

Figure 10.4 Fetal Growth During Pregnancy. A fetus grows very slowly in the first trimester, picks up speed in the 2nd trimester, and grows very quickly in the third trimester.

Data from Grantz KL, Grewal J, Kim S, et al. Unified standard for fetal growth: the Eunice Kennedy Shriver National Institute of Child Health and Human Development Fetal Growth Studies. Am J Obstet Gynecol. 2022;226(4):576-587.e2. doi:10.1016/j.ajog.2021.12.006

Physiology of Labor

When a fetus is fully grown and developed, three changes happen that begin labor and end in birth. The opening of the uterus (called the **cervix**) expands (**dilates**). The amnion and chorion membranes break, causing the amniotic fluid to leak out. And the uterus begins to contract, pushing the fetus out through the cervix and vagina.

Because it is so unhealthy for a baby to be born early, there is much interest in what exactly initiates these three changes. **Inflammation** plays a key role.[4] Inflammation is ordinarily a response of the body's immune system to foreign invading organisms. It involves recruitment and activation of many different types of immune cells. Among those cells are **regulatory T lymphocytes** that suppress other immune cells to prevent an overreaction that would hurt the body's own tissues.

Pregnancy poses a risk that the mother's immune system will attack the fetus as a foreign invader. To avoid this, adult women regulatory T lymphocytes are activated during pregnancy, suppressing the inflammatory response (**Figure 10.5**).[4] This immune suppression may be why women are especially susceptible to infections like influenza and COVID-19 when they are pregnant. After a full gestation, though, this suppression ends, and the immune system becomes activated again, provoking inflammation. The inflammatory response generates chemical messengers that cause the uterus to contract, the cervix to soften, and the membranes to rupture.[5]

The female hormone **progesterone** also plays an important role in initiation of labor. Throughout pregnancy, levels of progesterone are very high, and these high levels seem to help delay the onset of labor. In a healthy pregnancy, progesterone levels fall just before labor starts.[4] This is why there is much research recently on giving pregnant women progesterone to try to prevent early labor.

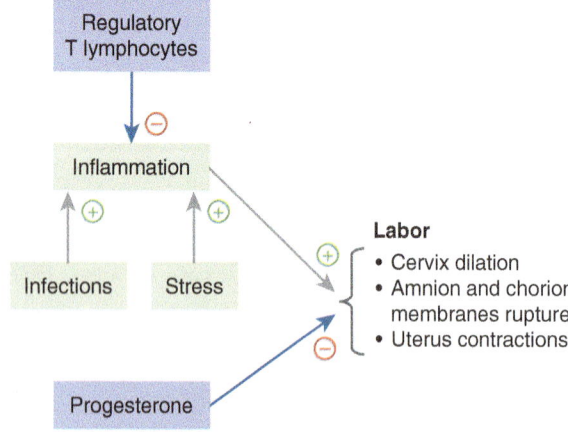

Figure 10.5 Role of Inflammation in Initiation of Labor. Inflammation triggers the onset of labor, including cervical dilation, rupture of membranes, and contractions of the uterus. In a healthy pregnancy, regulatory T lymphocytes suppress inflammation until the pregnancy reaches term. However, infections or stress during pregnancy can overcome this suppression, causing inflammation and triggering early labor. Also, throughout pregnancy, levels of the female hormone progesterone are high, which helps delay labor. In a healthy pregnancy, progesterone levels fall just before labor starts.

Pathophysiology of Preterm Birth and Low Birth Weight

There are three possible reasons why an infant would have a low birth weight:

- **Spontaneous preterm birth**. Labor spontaneously begins early.
- **Fetal growth restriction** (also called **intrauterine growth restriction** or small for gestational age). The fetus grows slower than is normal during gestation.
- **Iatrogenic** or **medically-indicated preterm birth**. A medical provider deliberately gives a pregnant woman medications to initiate labor or conducts a cesarean section before the end of the pregnancy, usually to protect the mother or the fetus from a dangerous condition.

The frequency of these reasons varies across settings, but in the United States, about 1/3 of low birth weight is due to fetal growth restriction and 2/3 to preterm birth.[1] Of babies born preterm in the United States, about one-third of the early deliveries are iatrogenic.[5]

The causes and risk factors for these three reasons for low birth weight overlap.

Spontaneous Preterm Birth

It is not well understood why some women spontaneously go into labor early, but a common thread is early or abnormally high levels of inflammation.[4-6] Inflammation, even occurring long before 40 weeks of gestation, can inappropriately start labor (Figure 10.5).

Most important, infections of the amnion and chorion membranes (**intrauterine infections**) can induce inflammation that triggers early labor.[6] Intrauterine infections with bacteria are found in 25%–40% of spontaneous preterm births, with a higher percentage in the especially early births.[5,7] The bacteria causing these infections are thought to enter the uterus mainly from the vagina through the cervix.[5]

It is normal for bacteria to live in the vagina. For most women, the dominant bacteria are various species of *Lactobacillus*, which appear to be healthful.[7,8] However, in some the vagina instead is colonized with bacteria that are unhealthy and **anaerobic**—that is, they do not need oxygen to survive. This condition is called **bacterial vaginosis**. In the past, the bacterium *Gardnerella vaginalis* was thought to be the only anaerobic organism involved, but now experts believe the condition instead reflects a shift in the entire **microbiome** of the vagina from *Lactobacillus* to many species of anaerobic bacteria.[7] There are degrees of severity of bacterial vaginosis; while many with it have no symptoms, some have a vaginal discharge, itching, and burning.[9] Pregnant women with bacterial vaginosis are much more likely to have a preterm birth.[5] This suggests that the unusual bacteria in the vagina can ascend into the uterus, causing an intrauterine infection and triggering labor.

Bacterial vaginosis is not generally considered a sexually transmitted disease, but it is linked to sexual activity. Young women rarely develop the condition until they start having sex, and women are more likely to have bacterial vaginosis if they have more sex partners.[10-13]

Other **genital infections** (infections of the vagina or cervix) that are clearly sexually transmitted also can trigger preterm labor. For example, women are more likely to have preterm birth if they have gonorrhea (infection with the bacterium *Neisseria gonorrheae*), infection with *Chlamydia trachomatis*, syphilis, or infection with the protozoa *Trichomonas vaginali*.[5,14,15] Other organisms that can infect the membranes and that have been associated with preterm birth are species of *Mycoplasma* and *Ureaplasma*, which are very small, simple bacteria that cause few if any symptoms and are thought to spread sexually.[5,16]

Infections in other areas of the body have also been linked to preterm labor. For example, pregnant women with malaria, pneumonia, or urinary tract infections are more likely to go into labor early.[6,17] It may be that these infections increase inflammation throughout the body, which is enough to trigger early labor.

Finally, pregnant women who under high levels of psychological or social stress are more likely to go into preterm labor. Inflammation may be the connection. Stress can prompt the release of hormones that increase inflammation or promote contractions of the uterus.[4-6,18]

Fetal growth restriction

There are several reasons why an infant may not grow as much as others. Some fetuses are just genetically programmed to be small, inheriting genes from small parents. Others do not reach their full genetic potential because they do not get enough nutrients, for example, if their mothers are malnourished or their placentas are inadequate (see section on pre-eclampsia). And still other fetuses fail to grow because they are exposed to toxic chemicals (from parents' smoking or other drug use) or infections during the pregnancy.[17,19-21]

Iatrogenic Preterm Birth

For many women delivering a baby preterm, the cause was a deliberate decision by a medical provider.[5] These iatrogenic preterm deliveries are rising worldwide. In some countries, as many as half of preterm births are iatrogenic.[22,23]

The most common reason for iatrogenic preterm delivery—between half and three-fourth of cases—is **pre-eclampsia** (**Box 10.1**), and the medical provider is concerned that allowing the pregnancy to continue is too risky for the mother or the fetus.[24-26] This is sometimes the wisest decision. However, one study from the United States found that the medical reason for the iatrogenic preterm delivery was "not evidence-based" more than half the time.[27]

Box 10.1 Pre-eclampsia

Pre-eclampsia is a condition of pregnancy in which the placenta creates serious risks to both the mother and the fetus. Pregnant women with pre-eclampsia have **hypertension** (high blood pressure) and **proteinuria** (protein appearing in the urine) and often have damage to one or more organs. The condition is called pre-eclampsia because, left untreated, it may lead to **eclampsia**, which is characterized by seizures or coma.[28]

Epidemiology

About 4% of pregnant women develop pre-eclampsia.[25,29,30] For unknown reasons, the condition is much more common in women of African and South Asian descent (including African-Americans in the United States), as well as those who live in lower-income neighborhoods.[29,31] Particularly disturbing, rates of pre-eclampsia in the United States have been gradually rising over the past quarter century.[32,33] The cause of this increase is not clear.

Pathophysiology

The origins of pre-eclampsia can be traced to the two weeks after an egg is fertilized. The early embryo implants itself in the lining of the uterus, with some of its cells "invading" the lining to build a bridge to the mother's arteries—a bridge that is to become the placenta. During a healthy pregnancy, this bridge grows to allow for high-volume flow of oxygen and nutrients to the fetus. In pre-eclampsia, the embryo's cells do not invade the lining of the uterus deeply enough.[29] This restricts the flow of oxygen and nutrients to the placenta. The placenta, under stress from lack of oxygen, then secretes a variety of harmful compounds that enter the mother's circulation.[25] These compounds damage the **endothelium** that lines the small blood vessels throughout the body.

(continues)

Box 10.1 **Pre-eclampsia** *(continued)*

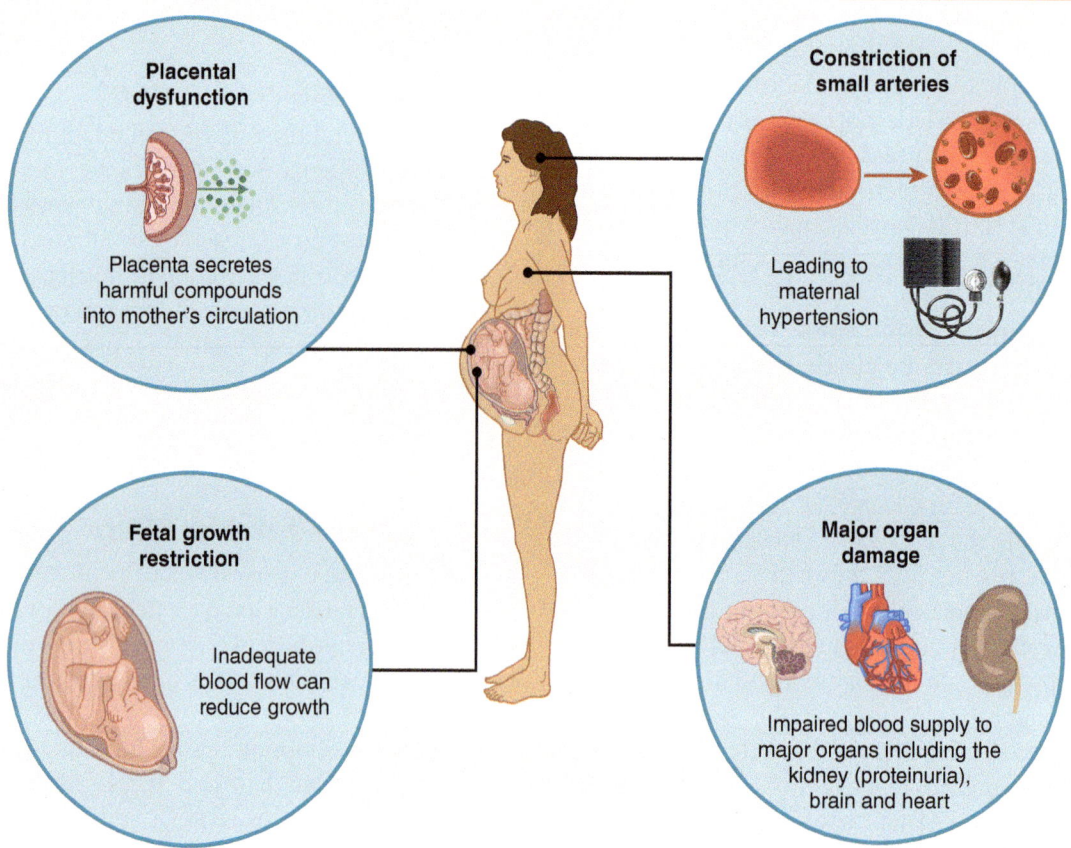

Figure 10.6 **Pre-eclampsia.** In pre-eclampsia, the placenta releases harmful compounds into the mother's circulation, causing damage to the lining of arteries, constriction of small arteries, and damage to many organ systems. The two key signs of pre-eclampsia are high blood pressure and the presence of protein in the urine.

Although the groundwork for pre-eclampsia is laid in the early weeks of a pregnancy, the signs of it do not appear until late in gestation—usually after the 34th week. At that point, damage to the **endothelial cells** causes widespread problems for the pregnant woman (**Figure 10.6**). The small arteries **constrict** (become narrower), which raises the blood pressure. The blood vessels also "leak" protein through the kidneys into the urine, causing proteinuria, and the resulting shortage of protein in the blood causes fluid swelling in the legs. And the damaged blood vessels do not supply enough blood to the mother's major organs, like the brain, heart, liver, and kidneys—or to the fetus.[28] Inadequate blood flow to the fetus can slow its growth and the damage to the mother's organs can lead to seizures or other very serious health problems.

Fortunately, pre-eclampsia disappears within days after the placenta is delivered. But when a woman develops pre-eclampsia in the 34th week, the medical provider must make the difficult decision about whether the pregnancy can safely continue. A delivery may save the parent's life but cause the child to be born preterm.

Risk Factors

Women are more likely to develop pre-eclampsia if they are relatively older (30s or beyond) and if it is their first pregnancy. They are also more likely to develop pre-eclampsia if before pregnancy they have risk factors for cardiovascular disease, specifically, obesity, diabetes, hypertension, or high blood **triglycerides**.[25,29,34] In this way, pregnancy acts as a kind of test that identifies women who are more likely to develop heart disease or stroke later in life.[25]

Primary Prevention

Primary prevention of pre-eclampsia involves reducing its risk factors, not just in pregnancy but also in women of childbearing age who might become pregnant. That points to the population-based interventions to prevent heart disease and stroke, particularly *promotion of exercise and healthy eating*.[29] Studies have shown that exercise during pregnancy reduces the risk of pre-eclampsia by a strikingly high 40%.[35]

Secondary Prevention

Two other interventions during pregnancy can reduce the risk of pre-eclampsia:

- If women at high risk take *low-dose aspirin* every day beginning near the end of the first trimester, it reduces their risk of pre-eclampsia, fetal growth restriction, and the need for iatrogenic delivery by about 15%–20%.[30] The benefits of aspirin are even greater in preventing pre-eclampsia that starts early in pregnancy.[29]
- If women who ordinarily have a low intake of the mineral calcium take *calcium supplements* during the second half of pregnancy, their risk of pre-eclampsia falls by about half, and their risk of preterm birth falls by about 25%. Calcium supplements are generally unnecessary in the United States, where most women get enough calcium, but they are very important for low-income women in some countries who have limited diets.

Epidemiology: Patterns and Trends

In the United States, about 8% of infants are born with low birth weight and about 10% are born preterm. These percentages were falling slowly from the early 2000s until about 2014 but have been rising slowly since.[1] Both conditions are more common in infants born of women who are either under 25 or over 35, Black, or with less education (**Figure 10.7**).[1] These demographic differences are larger for especially early preterm births. For example, Black women are more than twice as likely as White women to deliver before 32 weeks gestation.[1] The high rates of low birth weight and preterm birth in Black women may be because they are more likely to have pre-eclampsia or bacterial vaginosis (see below), and/or because they are more likely to experience psychosocial stress. For many immigrant groups, the more time they spend in the United States, the higher the preterm birth rate.[5]

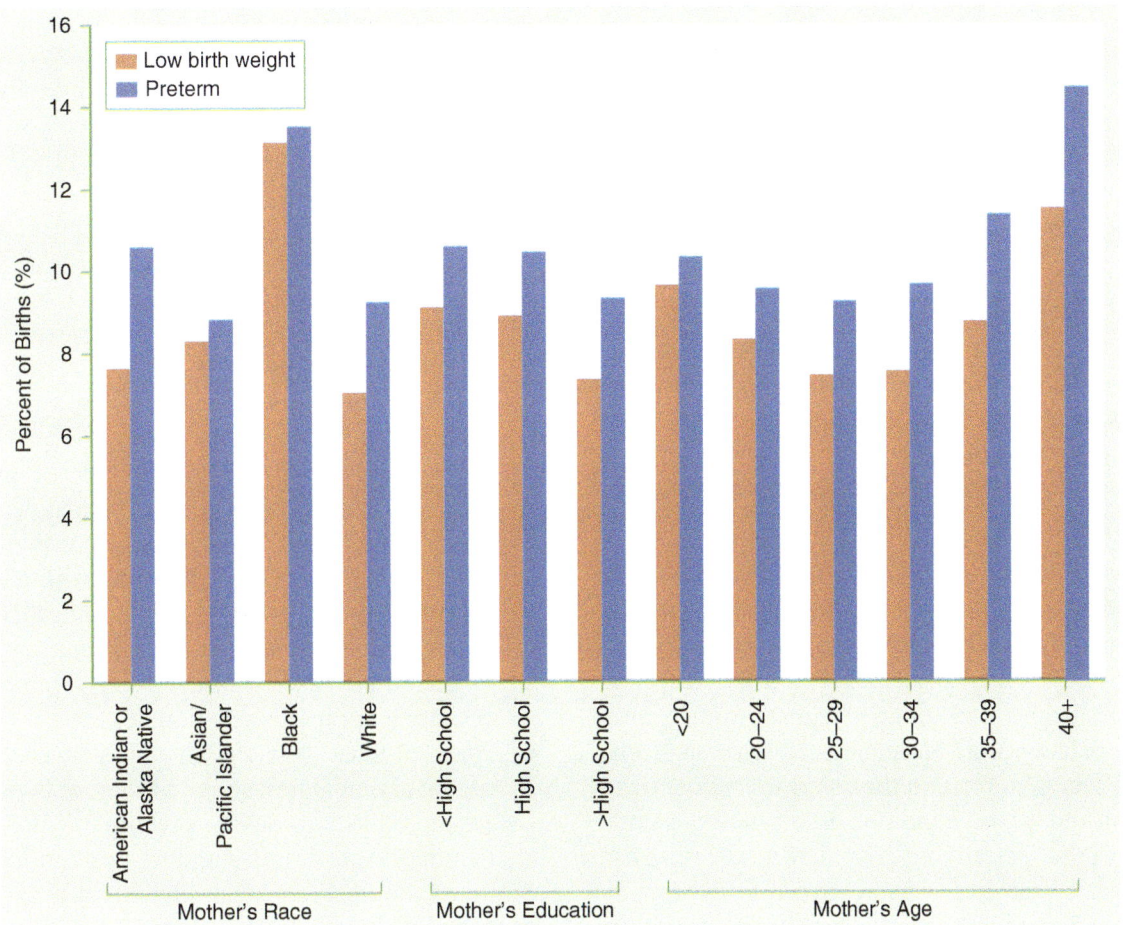

Figure 10.7 **Low Birth Weight and Preterm Birth in the United States by Mothers' Age, Race, and Education, 2007–2019.**

Data from Centers for Disease Control and Prevention. WONDER Natality Files. CDC. Published 2024. Accessed May 14, 2024. https://wonder.cdc.gov/natality.html

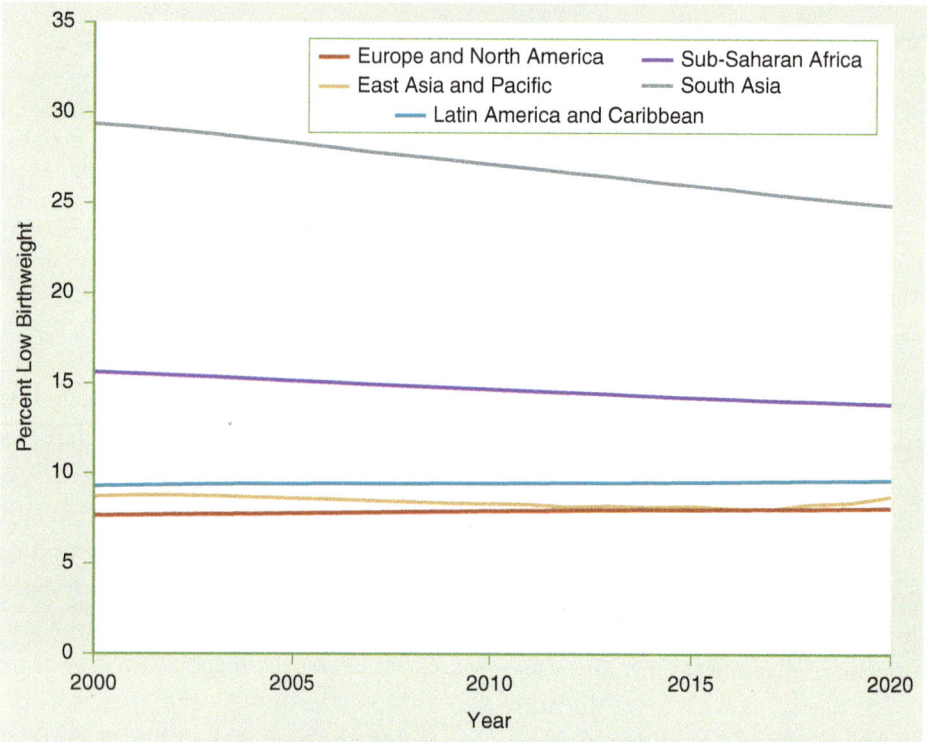

Figure 10.8 Estimates of Low Birth Weight by Global Region, 2000–2020.

Data from UNICEF. Low Birth Weight. Published July 2, 2023. Accessed May 14, 2024. https://data.unicef.org/topic/nutrition/low-birthweight/

Globally, the rates of low birth weight are highest in South Asia, followed by Sub-Saharan Africa. In both regions, the rates of low birth weight are falling slowly, probably because of economic development and improved nutrition (**Figure 10.8**).[36,37]

Risk Factors

The multiple causes of low birth weight lead to a long list of risk factors, some of which operate by more than one mechanism, and a complicated cause-and-effect diagram (**Figure 10.9**).

Potentially modifiable risk factors for spontaneous preterm birth include:

- *Bacterial vaginosis.* This condition is extremely common and strongly linked to preterm birth.[7] In one national study of adult women in the United States, 29% had bacterial vaginosis, most of whom had no symptoms.[11] Pregnant women with bacterial vaginosis are more than twice as likely to deliver preterm, and the risk rises to more than seven-fold if the condition is diagnosed before 16 weeks gestation.[38] For unknown reasons, bacterial vaginosis is more common in women of Sub-Saharan African descent, including those raised in Africa and those raised on other continents.[7] In the same national study of U.S. women, those who were Black were more than twice as

likely as those who were White to have bacterial vaginosis.[11] The higher rates of bacterial vaginosis in Black women may explain half of their excess preterm birth rates.[5]

- *Genital and intrauterine infections.* Pregnant women are more likely to deliver preterm if they have infections of the cervix with bacteria like *Neisseria gonorrhea*, *Chlamydia*, and *Mycoplasma*, some of which may spread to the amnion and chorion. Most of these infections are transmitted through sex.

- *Other maternal infections.* The risk of preterm birth also is higher in pregnant women who have infections at other sites, including urinary tract infections, pneumonia, **periodontal disease** (infection of the gums), malaria, and HIV.[5,6,39,40] At a global level, malaria is a major contributor to preterm birth because it is so common and because it approximately doubles the risk.[6,39]

- *Stress.* Studies have shown that women experiencing psychological stress, anxiety, or depression are more likely to deliver preterm.[6,41] Also, those required to work in a standing position for more than 6 hours a day are at higher risk for preterm birth; this may be the result of psychological stress, because physical activity itself during pregnancy does not increase the risk, and recreational exercise seems beneficial.[5,6]

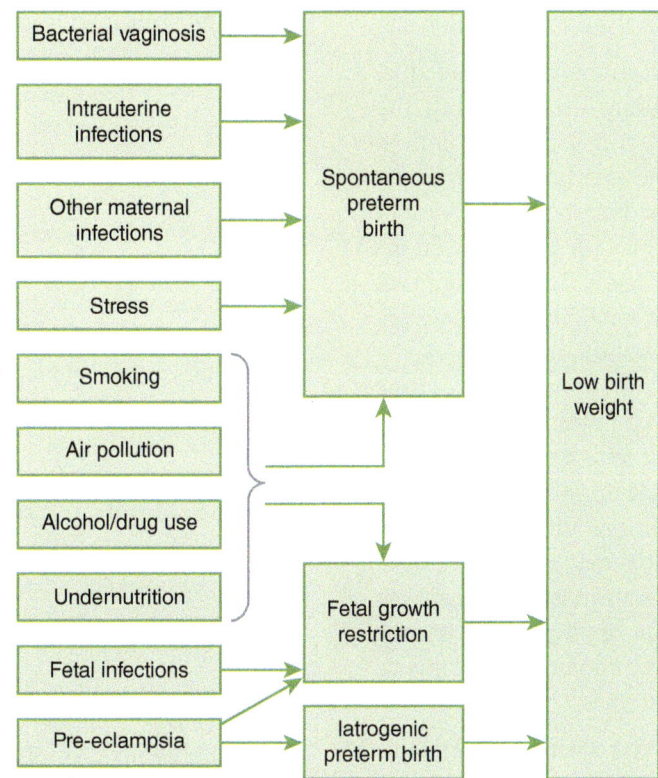

Figure 10.9 Cause-and-Effect Diagram for Low Birth Weight. Risk factors for low birth weight can exert their effects through spontaneous preterm birth, fetal growth restriction, or iatrogenic preterm birth. Some risk factors (such as smoking) have an effect through more than one of these routes.

Several factors related to nutrition and exposure to toxic chemicals are harmful in two ways, increasing the risk of both preterm birth and fetal growth restriction:

- *Smoking.* Smoking during pregnancy increases the risk of preterm birth by about 50%, and it has an even larger impact on fetal growth restriction, approximately doubling the risk.[42,43] While smoking rates have fallen over the years, about 4% of women still admit to smoking during their pregnancies.[1]

- *Air pollution.* For adverse outcomes of pregnancy, as for many other health problems, the risk of air pollution parallels the risk of smoking. The increase in risk of preterm birth and low birth weight from **ambient** (outdoor) **air pollution** is only about 10%, but the population impact can be large because so many people are exposed to it.[44] In low-income countries, a larger increase in risk (about 30%) has been found from **household** (indoor) **air pollution** from burning solid fuels like coal, wood, dung, or crop waste for heat and cooking.[45,46] Ambient and household air pollution are discussed more in Chapter 8. Chronic Respiratory Diseases.

- *Heavy alcohol consumption* and *drug use.* Pregnant women drinking three or more alcoholic drinks per day are much more likely to have an infant with fetal growth restriction and to have an infant born preterm.[47] Use of cocaine during pregnancy more than triples the risk of preterm birth and fetal growth restriction, and use of opioids and other street drugs has similar effects.[5,48-50]

- *Undernutrition.* Women who are undernourished are more likely to have an infant born preterm or with fetal growth restriction.[51,52] This is particularly important in some low-income countries. Shortages of both **macronutrients** (carbohydrate, fats, and proteins) and **micronutrients** (vitamins and minerals) appear to be important. For example, in a study in rural Bangladesh, underweight women were about 50% more likely than overweight women to have an infant with fetal growth restriction and twice as likely to have an infant born preterm.[53] Separately, pregnant women with low levels of iron, folic acid, and zinc are more likely to deliver preterm.[5] Pregnancy tends to deplete the body of nutrients, so those who become pregnant again soon after a delivery are more likely to be undernourished. Women who have an interval of less than 6 months between pregnancies have more than double the risk of preterm birth.[5]

Two other risk factors for fetal growth restriction are:

- *Fetal infections.* Some infections involve not just the membranes surrounding the fetus, but the fetus itself. These fetal infections are less common causes of low birth weight, but they can cause the most harm to the fetus, leading to stillbirth or life-long disabilities. Children with these infections tend to have "symmetric" growth restriction, that is, small heads along with small bodies, which is a sign of poor development of the brain.

- *Pre-eclampsia.* Women who have pre-eclampsia have an inadequate flow of nutrients through the placenta to the fetus, so the fetus tends to grow less. At the same time, pre-eclampsia puts women at risk for the potentially fatal condition of eclampsia. Facing that risk, medical providers often induce delivery or conduct a cesarean section early, so that the child may have an **iatrogenic preterm birth**. The causes and prevention of pre-eclampsia are discussed more in Box 10.1.

There are other known risk factors for preterm birth that are not included in Figure 10.9 because they are not modifiable. In particular, women are more likely to deliver preterm if they have had a previous preterm birth, if they are carrying twins (or more), or if they have structural problems with the uterus.[17]

Finally, women with less income or education are more likely to have a preterm birth.[54] It is not difficult to understand how a combination of the proven risk factors in Figure 10.9 could cause this. For example, people with less income or education are more likely to live or work in stressful conditions, to smoke, to use drugs, and to be exposed to air pollution.[55] This explanation is consistent with the theory that social disadvantage harms health by multiple risks "piling on" to each other.

Preventive Interventions

Many diverse interventions can contribute to reducing low birth weight (**Figure 10.10**):

Primary Prevention

- *Sexual risk reduction and condom promotion.* Because the organisms that cause most intrauterine infections are thought to be spread by sex, these infections should occur less often in populations with lower-risk sexual behavior, that is, with people having fewer partners, in less-connected sexual networks, and/or using condoms more often. The risk is at the population level; even a person who has only one partner is at relatively high risk of sexually transmitted diseases if that partner is in a highly-connected sexual network. That means the preventive intervention is—if possible—to reduce the risky sexual behavior of the entire network.

- *Social and financial support* during pregnancy. Some experts have recommended policies to support people during pregnancy to reduce their stress.[56] While there is no proof that this approach reduces preterm birth, some European countries have adopted policies along these lines. Examples are requiring that employers exempt pregnant workers from night shifts and offer paid pregnancy work leave.[56] The Province of Manitoba, Canada, provides an unrestricted income supplement of about $60 per month to low-income pregnant women during the second and third trimesters. While the evaluations of this policy are limited, those who received this income supplement had lower rates of preterm birth and low birth weight than others who did not.[57,58]

- *Smoking prevention.* Smoking prevention should reduce rates of preterm birth and low birth weight. Ideally, women should not be smoking at the time that they become pregnant, so smoking prevention efforts should be directed at entire populations, not just to those who are pregnant. But even when women quit smoking during pregnancy, they are about 15% less likely to have a child preterm or with low birth weight.[59] Smoking prevention is discussed in Chapter 11. Tobacco Use.

- *Reduction in air pollution.* The consistent link between low birth weight and both ambient and household air pollution suggests that reducing air pollution should reduce rates of low birth weight. See Chapter 8. Chronic Respiratory Diseases.

- *Reduction of alcohol and drug use.* Similarly, the strong links between low birth weight and both heavy alcohol use and other drug use suggest that reducing use of alcohol and drugs should reduce low birth weight. For more, see Chapter 12. Alcohol Use and Chapter 13. Use of Addictive Drugs.

- *Improvements in nutrition and supplementation* for women of childbearing age in developing countries. In countries with high rates of undernutrition, improving the nutritional status of those who become pregnant reduces the rates of low birth weight. Even changes during pregnancy can help. In many low-income countries, pregnant women are given dietary supplements of macronutrients (protein and energy) and/or micronutrients (vitamins and minerals).[60] Studies generally show that macronutrient supplements reduce rates of low birth weight, and micronutrient supplements reduce rates of both low birth weight and preterm

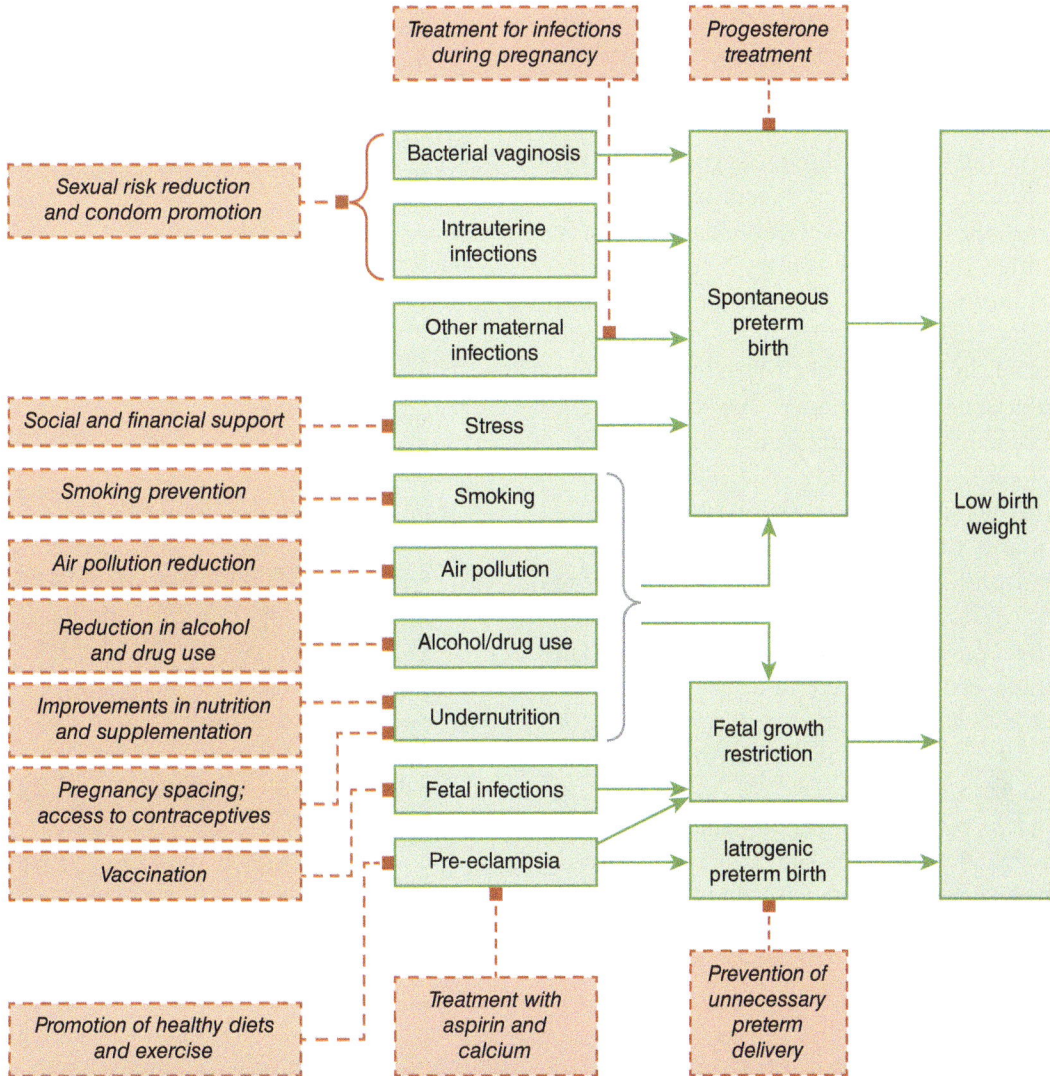

Figure 10.10 Cause-and-Effect Diagram for Low Birth Weight, with Preventive Interventions.

birth.[60-64] Separately, studies in many high-income countries have found that giving pregnant women supplements containing omega-3 fatty acids reduces the risk of preterm birth.[65] Chapter 14. Nutrition discusses undernutrition in mothers and children in more depth.

- *Pregnancy spacing and access to contraceptives.* Because a short time interval between pregnancies can lead to low birth weight and preterm birth, increasing this interval can help prevent these problems. Spacing of pregnancies requires that women have ready access to contraceptives.

- *Vaccination.* Vaccination against **rubella** prevents fetal infection caused by this virus. The most effective approach is to vaccinate the general population, which prevents the spread of the virus, even to those who are not vaccinated.

- *Promotion of healthy diets and exercise* to prevent pre-eclampsia. Pre-eclampsia is less likely to

occur in women who are at lower risk for cardiovascular disease (see Box 10.1), so it should be partially preventable by promoting healthy eating and exercise. This promotion should be directed at all women, not just those who are pregnant.[35]

Secondary Prevention

- *Treatment with aspirin and calcium.* As discussed in Box 10.1, pre-eclampsia can be partially prevented by women at high risk taking low-dose aspirin or calcium supplements during pregnancy.[56,66-68]

- *Prevention of unnecessary preterm delivery.* Medical providers are often faced with hard choices about whether to induce labor in a woman who has pre-eclampsia or whose fetus is showing signs of problems. Nonetheless, the high rate of non-medically indicated deliveries suggests that standards should be put in place to avoid delivering infants preterm unnecessarily. An international group of obstetricians has called for "action plans" to reduce these unnecessary iatrogenic preterm deliveries.[22]

- *Treatment for infections during pregnancy.* It certainly makes sense for pregnant women who have treatable infections such as malaria, sexually transmitted diseases, or urinary tract infections to take antimalarials or antibiotics to cure those infections. Unfortunately, this treatment may not reliably reduce low birth weight. Treatment for malaria definitely reduces low birth weight and probably reduces preterm birth, and antibiotic treatment of urinary tract infections may have this benefit.[40,69,70] But, surprisingly, studies have found that antibiotic treatment of sexually transmitted diseases during or even before pregnancy does not reduce preterm birth.[56,71] Likewise, despite bacterial vaginosis being an important cause of preterm birth, studies of antibiotic treatment of this condition during or before pregnancy have not shown reductions in preterm birth.[38,56,71]

- *Progesterone treatment during pregnancy for women with a short cervix.* Some women have a cervix that is shorter than others. Studies suggest that if these women take progesterone in the second trimester it may delay labor and help prevent preterm birth.[72,73]

Box 10.2 Summary–Prevention of Prematurity and Low Birth Weight

- Primary prevention
  - Sexual risk reduction and condom promotion
  - Social and financial support during pregnancy
  - Smoking prevention
  - Reduction in air pollution
  - Reduction of alcohol and drug use
  - Improvements in nutrition and supplementation for women of childbearing age in developing countries.
  - Pregnancy spacing and access to contraceptives.
  - Vaccination
  - Promotion of healthy diets and exercise
- Secondary Prevention
  - Treatment with aspirin and calcium
  - Prevention of unnecessary preterm delivery
  - Treatment for infections during pregnancy
  - Progesterone treatment during pregnancy for women with a short cervix

---

Box 10.3 Key Words–Prematurity and Low Birth Weight

Ambient air pollution
Amnion
Amniotic fluid
Anaerobic
Bacterial vaginosis
Birth defects
Cervix
Chorion
Congenital anomalies
Congenital malformations
Constrict
Dilate
Eclampsia
Endothelium, endothelial cells
Fetal growth restriction
Genital infections
Gestation
Household air pollution
Hypertension
Iatrogenic preterm birth
Inflammation
Intrauterine growth restriction
Intrauterine infection
Low birth weight
Macronutrients
Medically-indicated preterm birth
Microbiome
Micronutrients
Periodontal disease
Placenta
Pre-eclampsia
Premature (in an infant)
Preterm birth
Progesterone
Proteinuria
Regulatory T lymphocytes
Rubella
Spontaneous preterm birth
Triglycerides
Trimester
Umbilical cord
Undernutrition
Uterus

Resources–Prematurity and Low Birth Weight

- CDC WONDER, at https://wonder.cdc.gov/, is an interactive website that allows analysis of U.S. data on birth weight, the length of gestation, and their determinants, linked to infant mortality.
- Blencowe H, Krasevec J, de Onis M, et al. National, regional, and worldwide estimates of low birthweight

in 2015, with trends from 2000: a systematic analysis. *Lancet Glob Health.* 2019;7(7):e849-e860. doi:10.1016/S2214-109X(18)30565-5. This is the most comprehensive analysis of the rates of low birth weight globally.

- https://data.unicef.org/topic/nutrition/low-birth weight/ This interactive website by UNICEF has extensive data on estimates of low birth weight and its determinants worldwide.

- Goldenberg RL, Culhane JF, Iams JD, Romero R. Epidemiology and causes of preterm birth. *Lancet.* 2008;371(9606):75-84. doi:10.1016/S0140-6736 (08)60074-4. This review article is not recent, but it is the clearest and most comprehensive review available on the causes of preterm birth.

- Iams JD, Romero R, Culhane JF, Goldenberg RL. Primary, secondary, and tertiary interventions to reduce the morbidity and mortality of preterm birth. *Lancet.* 2008;371(9607):164-175. doi:10.1016/S0140-6736(08)60108-7. This review article (paired with the one above) is the clearest and most comprehensive review of the prevention of spontaneous preterm birth.

- Romero R, Dey SK, Fisher SJ. Preterm labor: One syndrome, many causes. *Science (1979).* 2014;345(6198):760-765. doi:10.1126/science .1251816

Congenital Malformations

Introduction

Some babies are born with abnormally-structured arms, legs, or internal organs. Among the more common problems are **congenital heart defects**, **spina bifida** (a malformation of the spine and spinal cord), **clubfoot**, and **cleft lip**. This chapter will call these **congenital malformations** and define them as structural abnormalities in an infant that are present at birth.

The terminology for this health problem is confusing, because even organizations of experts use different labels and different definitions.[74] Other terms used for congenital malformations are **birth defects**, **congenital anomalies**, **congenital abnormalities**, or just **congenital disorders**. When many organizations use these terms, they mean to include not just *structural* abnormalities but also *functional* abnormalities present at birth, such as sickle cell anemia and the metabolic disease phenylketonuria (PKU). However, the Global Burden of Disease project (which refers to these as "congenital

birth defects") limits the term to structural abnormalities.[74] Because this book uses the Global Burden of Disease analyses to guide which diseases are covered, this chapter will limit its focus to structural abnormalities. And it will use the term congenital malformations to emphasize that the abnormalities are in structure, not just function.

Congenital malformations are often categorized as **major** or **minor**, with the major ones defined as those that have significant medical, social or cosmetic consequences;[75] examples include heart defects and clubfoot. Minor congenital malformations pose little or no problems;[75] examples are wide-set eyes and a tiny sixth finger.

Congenital malformations can be caused by defective chromosomes (like Down syndrome), individual defective genes, toxic chemicals and drugs, nutritional deficiencies, or infections. Like all diseases, congenital malformations are often caused by multiple factors operating together. The causes of most congenital malformations are not known. However, several modifiable factors have been identified.

Normal Development of the Embryo and Fetus

Human development begins when a sperm cell from the father fertilizes an **ovum** (egg cell) from the mother. Normally, when each sperm cell or ovum is formed, the 23 pairs of chromosomes found in human cells split into 23 individual chromosomes. Then when a sperm cell fertilizes an ovum, their chromosomes pair up, with one of each pair from each parent. The **zygote** that is formed by this combination then divides repeatedly, becoming an embryo of about 100 cells over 7 days. The embryo then implants itself in the lining of the uterus, its cells differentiate into groups of specialized cells, and those specialized cells develop into organs.

The basic structure of most key organs in the embryo and fetus is built in the first trimester of pregnancy (**Figure 10.11**). Much of that development takes place in the first few weeks.

In the first four weeks after conception (six weeks after the mother's last menstrual period), a flat disc in the embryo folds over onto itself, creating the **neural tube** that will become the brain and spinal cord.[76] In about the same time period, the heart's four chambers and large blood vessels are formed. The heart is mostly developed by the end of the first trimester, but the brain continues to grow in number of cells and the connections among them throughout the pregnancy.

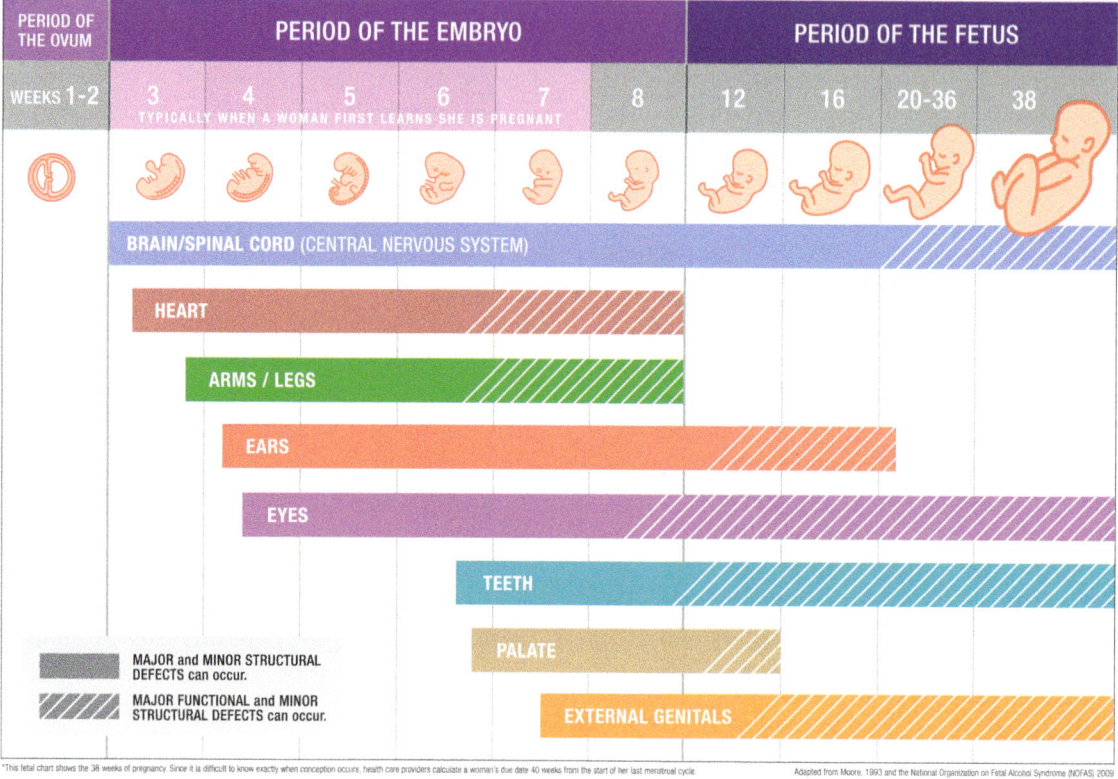

PERIOD OF THE OVUM	PERIOD OF THE EMBRYO							PERIOD OF THE FETUS			
WEEKS 1-2	3	4	5	6	7		8	12	16	20-36	38
	TYPICALLY WHEN A WOMAN FIRST LEARNS SHE IS PREGNANT										

BRAIN/SPINAL CORD (CENTRAL NERVOUS SYSTEM)

HEART

ARMS / LEGS

EARS

EYES

TEETH

PALATE

EXTERNAL GENITALS

- MAJOR and MINOR STRUCTURAL DEFECTS can occur.
- MAJOR FUNCTIONAL and MINOR STRUCTURAL DEFECTS can occur.

*This fetal chart shows the 38 weeks of pregnancy. Since it is difficult to know exactly when conception occurs, health care providers calculate a woman's due date 40 weeks from the start of her last menstrual cycle.

Adapted from Moore, 1993 and the National Organization on Fetal Alcohol Syndrome (NOFAS) 2009

Figure 10.11 Vulnerable Periods of Development for Organ Systems in the Embryo and Fetus. The basic structure of most key organs in the embryo and fetus is built in the first trimester of pregnancy. Much of that development takes place in the first few weeks, before many women know that they are pregnant.

Chart adapted from Moore 1993 and the National Organization of Fetal Alcohol Syndrome 2009 and designed by MotherToBaby, 2025.

The limbs, eyes, and ears start to develop soon after the brain and heart begin; their basic structures are in place by six weeks after conception (eight weeks after the last menstrual period).

Pathophysiology of Malformations

In this multi-step process, much can go wrong.

Errors can start even before fertilization. For example, sometimes an ovum (or less often, a sperm cell) contains a pair of chromosomes instead of only individual chromosomes. When that cell joins the cell from the other parent, it creates a triplet of chromosomes called a **trisomy**. If this happens with the 21st chromosome, the zygote has **Trisomy 21** and the child at birth has **Down syndrome**. This can also happen with other chromosomes, such as the 13th and the 18th. Many trisomies end in miscarriage, but some infants with these problems complete a normal gestation and are born alive. Other errors can occur as chromosomes are copied from parents to zygotes, involving not full chromosomes but parts of them; depending on the chromosomes involved, these errors can also lead to Down syndrome or to

other congenital malformations. Trisomies and these related problems are called **chromosomal defects**, and they are more common in mothers who are older because the chromosomes in their **ova** are more likely to split abnormally.[77-79] About 12%–15% of congenital malformations are the result of these chromosomal defects.[80,81]

Defects in individual genes happen if errors (**mutations**) occur when a gene is copied. Some of these single-gene mutations can cause congenital malformations if they are present in the genes from just one parent, while others will cause congenital malformations only if they are present in the genes of both parents. About 2%–4% of congenital malformations are the result of single-gene mutations.[80,81]

Most children with congenital malformations are not believed to have genetic problems, though. For these children, other errors occur during the development of organs.

Genes are often called "blueprints" for an organism, but a better analogy is that genes are "recipes"— instructions on how to build an organism. A human is built based on the instructions in human genes from the ingredients that are present in the uterus. These ingredients are the fluids, proteins, chemicals,

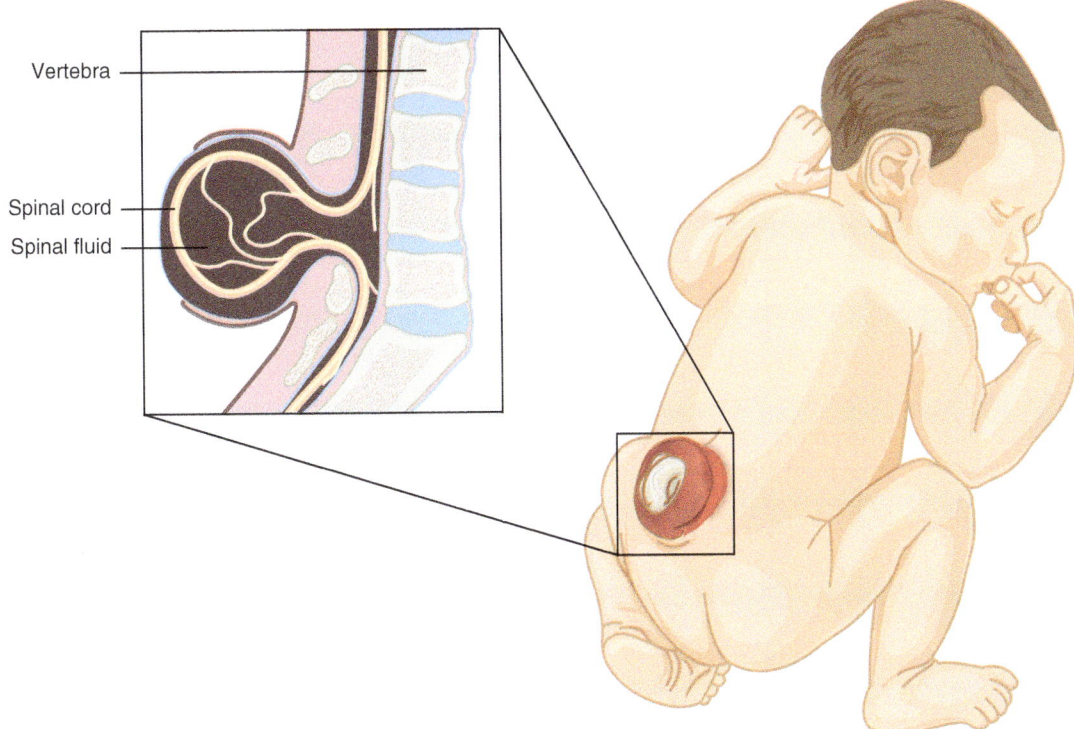

Figure 10.12 Spina Bifida. Neural tube defects result when the neural tube does not fully close. Spina bifida, in which the defect is on the lower end, is the most common neural tube defect.

Coutersy of Centers for Disease Control and Prevention.

and gases in the mother's blood in the early weeks of a pregnancy. As with a recipe one might use in the kitchen, if the ingredients available are not exactly what the recipe calls for, the end product might not be as the recipe intends. Malformations in humans can arise from a deficiency of certain ingredients (such as the vitamin **folate**), the presence of harmful compounds (such as alcohol or the drug thalidomide), or disease conditions of the mother (such as the high blood sugar of diabetes). Malformations can also arise if an infectious agent (such as a virus or bacterium) interferes with cells that are developing into organs. And malformations can even occur from an inappropriately high temperature during development, for example, if the woman has a fever during pregnancy.

Neural tube defects are particularly important because they have such a profound impact on children and families, and because they are largely preventable. Neural tube defects result when the neural tube created in the third or fourth week after conception does not fully close. The most common neural tube defects are an opening at the lower end of the spinal cord called spina bifida (**Figure 10.12**), an opening at the back of the brain called an **encephalocele**, and the near-complete failure of the brain to develop called **anencephaly** (**Figure 10.13**). Neural tube defects are much more common when the woman does not have

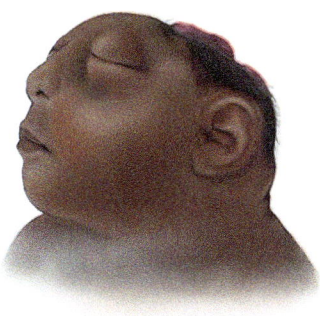

Figure 10.13 Anencephaly. The most severe form of neural tube defect is anencephaly, which is the near-complete failure of the brain to develop.

Coutersy of Centers for Disease Control and Prevention.

enough folate during the first four weeks of a pregnancy (**Box 10.4**).

Epidemiology: Patterns and Trends

Prevalence of Major Malformations

In the United States, about 3% of infants have major congenital malformations.[7,80] Estimates of the frequency of the most common major congenital malformations are shown in **Figure 10.14**.[78] They include:

Box 10.4 Folate and Congenital Malformations

In 1944–1945, World War II caused the people in Western Netherlands to suffer through a disaster that became known as the Dutch Hunger Winter. Over a few months, an estimated 20,000 people died of starvation, and those who survived consumed an average of only about 600 calories a day.[82] Since then, the Hunger Winter has been used extensively by epidemiologists to study the effects of malnutrition on health. One key observation they made was that babies who were conceived during this winter were about twice as likely to be born with neural tube defects.[83] That left many to wonder if neural tube defects were caused by a nutritional deficiency.

Twenty years after the war ended, a pediatrician who ran a birth defects clinic in Liverpool, England pursued this idea. Working with two obstetricians, he developed tests to measure vitamin levels in blood and began testing women who had affected infants. In 1965, the team published a paper showing that those who had given birth to children with neural tube defects had lower levels of folate than those who had had healthy children.[84,85]

Folate (also called **folic acid**) is a vitamin found in green leafy vegetables that is essential for DNA synthesis and cell growth. When not enough folate is available to growing cells, DNA breaks down and cells die.[76] This damages rapidly-growing cell lines, like those in the fetus that are developing into the brain and spinal cord. The idea that a folate deficiency could cause the brain or spinal cord to develop abnormally made biologic sense.

Even in the 1960s, folic acid was widely available as a vitamin supplement, so it was natural for the pediatrician to follow up his study by giving women folic acid and seeing if it prevented neural tube defects in their babies. Hampered by practical obstacles and ethical objections, though, that study was not completed for another quarter century.[84] But in 1991, researchers announced the results: among women who had previously had children with a neural tube defect, those who took high-dose folic acid supplements before and during pregnancy were 72% less likely to have a child with a neural tube defect.[76,86] In the next few years, two other studies of lower-dose folic acid supplements were done in women without histories of infants with neural tube defects. Both also found large reductions in neural tube defects.[87,88]

That left public health experts to consider how to give folic acid to all pregnant women. They were unlikely to get the amount of folate they needed to prevent neural tube defects from food. By one estimate, that would require eating 12 cups of raw spinach a day. They were not likely to get it from a vitamin pill either, because less than one-fourth of women of reproductive age took a daily multivitamin pill. And by the time they knew they were pregnant, it was mostly too late; women need high levels of folate in their systems in the first 28 days after conception.[76] The only option left was to add folic acid to the ordinary food supply—that is, to fortify foods with folic acid.

Based on this thinking, in 1996 the U.S. Food and Drug Administration required that any flour and other grain products labeled as "enriched" must be fortified with folic acid.[76] Afterwards, the number of children born annually with neural tube defects in the United States dropped by about 35% and the severity of spina bifida cases that did occur dropped 70%.[89,90] Other countries also required food fortification, and an analysis of eight such countries found that afterwards rates of neural tube defects fell by an average of 46%.[76] While more needs to be done to protect babies globally, folic acid fortification is now considered one of the great public health achievements of the past few decades.[76]

- *Chromosomal abnormalities*, such as Down syndrome, Trisomy 13, and Trisomy 18,
- *Musculoskeletal abnormalities*, such as clubfoot (**Figure 10.15**), other defects of the arms of legs, and **gastroschisis** (an opening in the abdominal wall),
- *Congenital heart defects*, of which there are many types (**Figure 10.16**),
- **Orofacial clefts**, including cleft lip and **cleft palate** (roof of the mouth), and
- *Neural tube defects*, including spina bifida, encephalocele, and anencephaly.

These congenital malformations individually occur at a rate between 2 and 20 per 10,000 births.[78] When individual congenital malformations are grouped by the organ involved, congenital heart defects may be the most common. One study estimated that 120 children per 10,000 in the United States (1.2%) had any type of congenital heart defect, and that rates of congenital heart defects in low-income countries were about twice that.[91]

Another common congenital malformation is **fetal alcohol syndrome** (**Figure 10.17**). This problem does not appear in Figure 10.14 because it is often not recognized at birth. Alcohol use during pregnancy directly damages the developing fetus in several ways, with the brain particularly affected.[92] Fetal alcohol syndrome is a combination of a thin upper lip, a smooth ridge between the nose and upper lip, a small head size (called **microcephaly**), and shorter-than-average height.[93] Studies in which school-aged children have been assessed in person

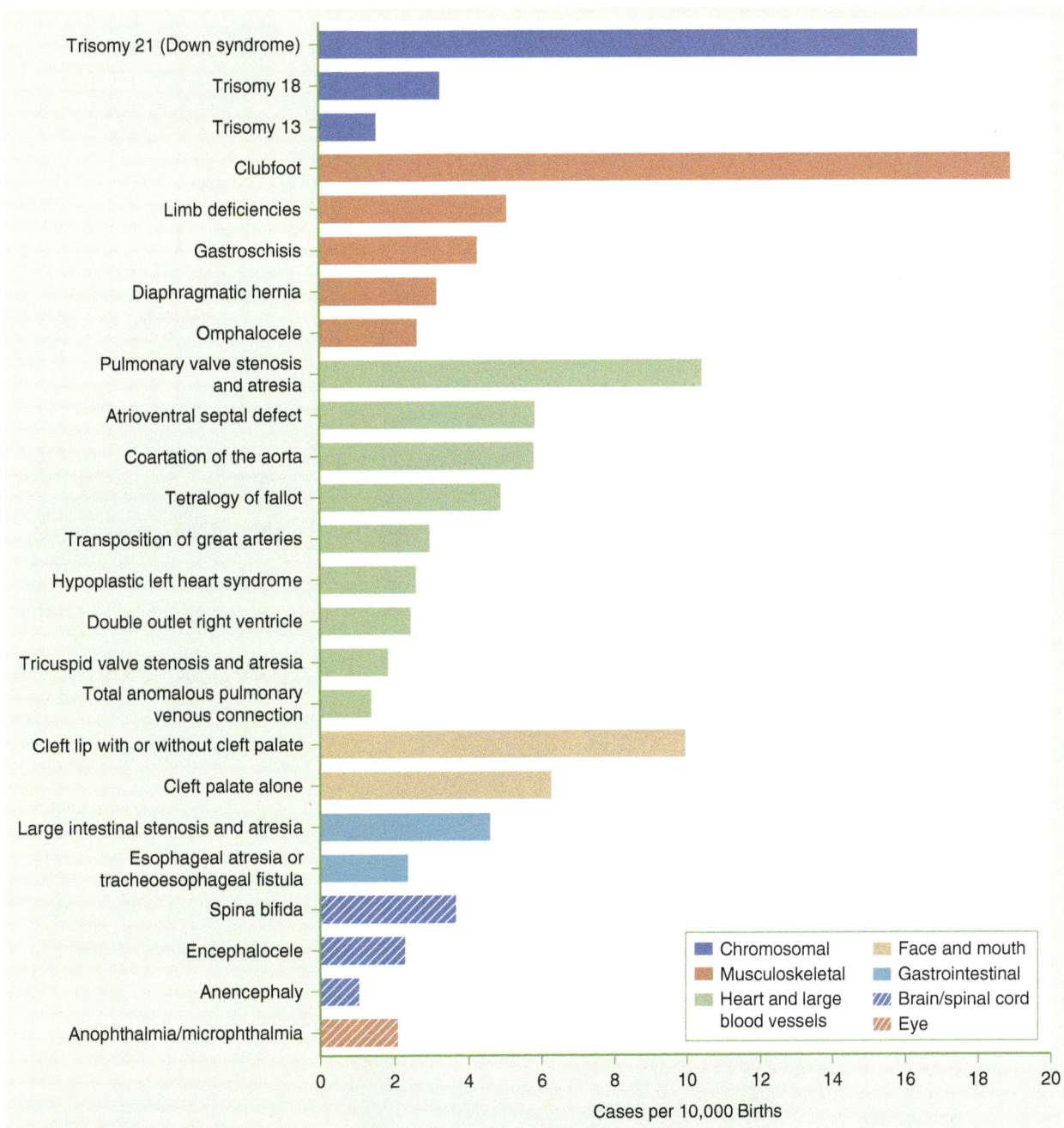

Figure 10.14 **Prevalence of Major Birth Defects in the United States, 2016–2020.**

Data from Stallings EB, Isenburg JL, Rutkowski RE, et al. National population-based estimates for major birth defects, 2016–2020. Birth Defects Res. 2024;116(1). doi:10.1002/bdr2.2301

have estimated that about 7 children per 1,000 in the United States have fetal alcohol syndrome.[94] That would make fetal alcohol syndrome several times more common than any malformation in Figure 10.14. And many more infants have brain damage from exposure to alcohol called **fetal alcohol spectrum disorders (FASD)**. FASD includes fetal alcohol syndrome, but also includes more subtle developmental, intellectual or behavioral problems in children. One study of four communities estimated conservatively that 1%–5% of school-aged children have FASD.[95]

Differences by Age and Race/Ethnicity

Congenital malformations caused by chromosomal defects are more common when mothers are older than 35 years of age. Older age may also increase the risk of congenital malformations that are not caused by abnormal chromosomes, but to a smaller degree.[78] There also appears to be a slight increase in risk of some congenital malformations in infants of older fathers.[96]

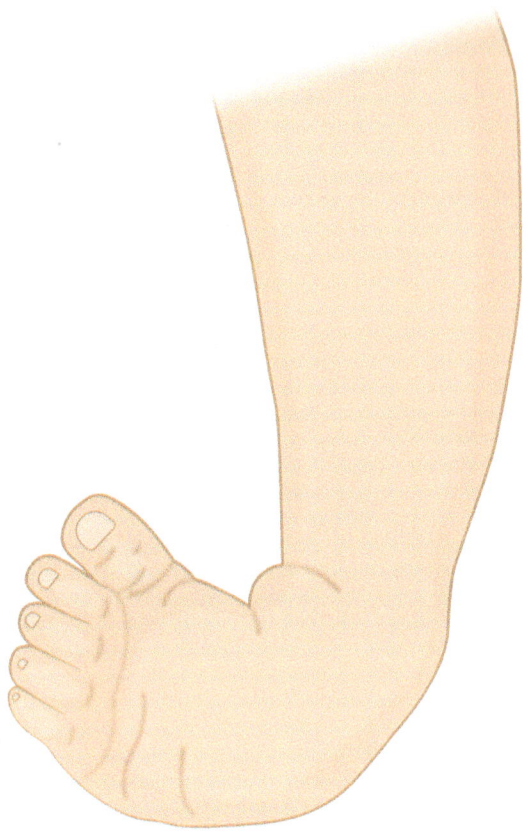

Figure 10.15 Clubfoot.

Coutersy of Centers for Disease Control and Prevention.

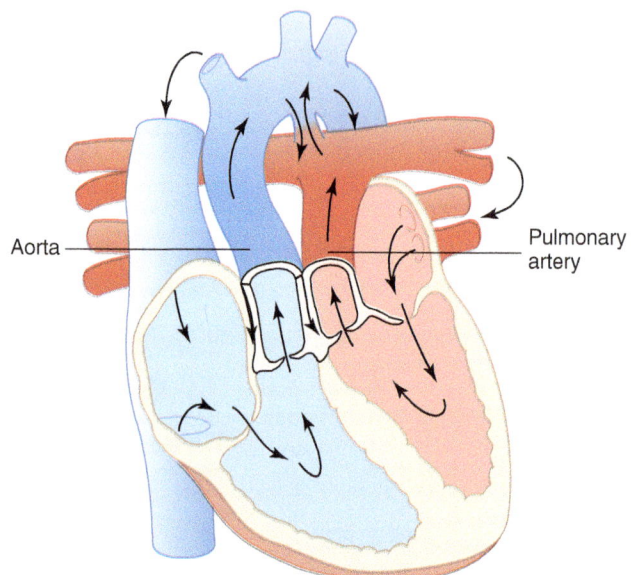

Aorta

Pulmonary artery

Figure 10.16 Transposition of the great arteries.
There are many types of congenital heart defects, in which the heart does not develop normally. This is one example: a defect in which the large arteries are switched, that is, the aorta arises from the right ventricle and the pulmonary artery arises from the left ventricle. .

Coutersy of Centers for Disease Control and Prevention.

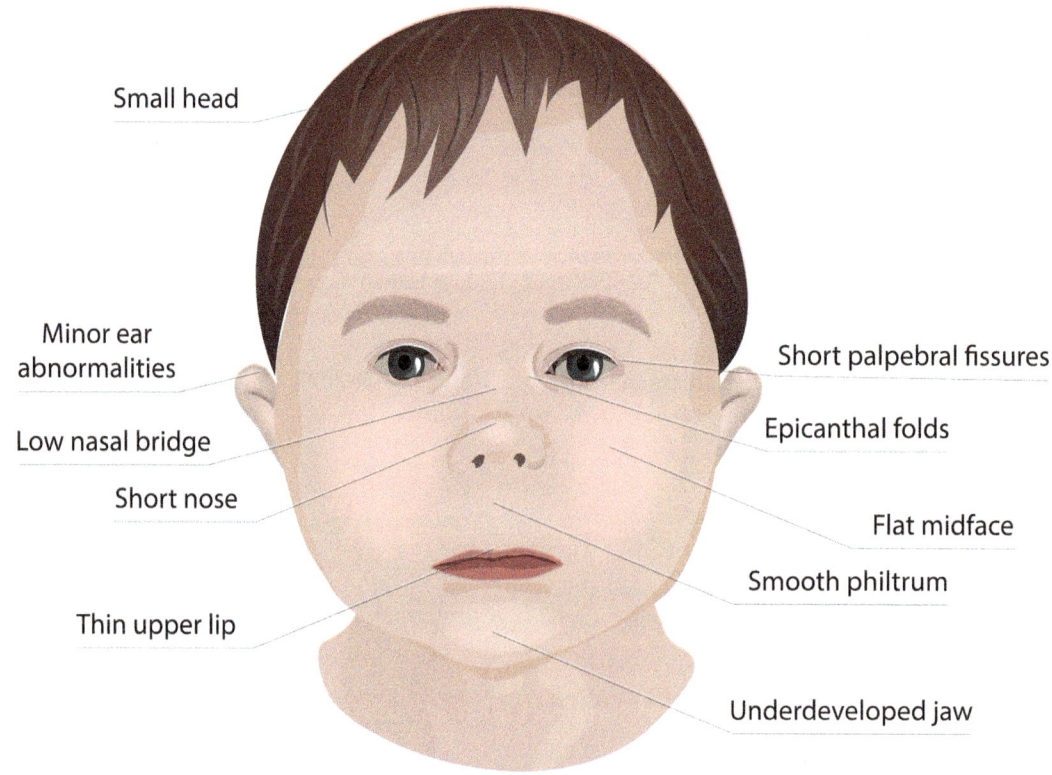

Small head

Minor ear abnormalities

Low nasal bridge

Short nose

Thin upper lip

Short palpebral fissures

Epicanthal folds

Flat midface

Smooth philtrum

Underdeveloped jaw

Figure 10.17 Facial Features of Fetal Alcohol Syndrome. Children with fetal alcohol syndrome may have these subtle patterns to their facial features.

© Maniki_rus/Shutterstoc

In the United States, the rates of some congenital malformations such as cleft lip, heart defects, and limb defects are more common in American Indian/Alaska Natives, for reasons that are not known.[97]

Risk Factors

The established modifiable risk factors for congenital malformations relate to the health conditions and exposures early in pregnancy (**Figure 10.18**):

- *Alcohol consumption.* Even low levels of alcohol consumption during pregnancy are associated with brain damage in children.[98] Experts estimate that about 1 in 67 women who drink alcohol during pregnancy will give birth to a child with fetal alcohol syndrome,[99] and about 1 in 13 will have a child with fetal alcohol spectrum disorder.[98] This risk factor is extremely important because it is so common: on surveys, 14% of women in the United States admit to drinking and 5% to binge drinking during pregnancy.[100] Drinking during pregnancy is even more common in Europe and the countries of the former Soviet Union.[98,99]

- *Other drug use.* More than one hundred drugs are known and dozens more are suspected to increase the risk of congenital malformations when taken during pregnancy.[101,102] Drugs for which the connection to congenital malformations is particularly strong are labelled **teratogens** or **teratogenic drugs**. The list of teratogens includes drugs to treat infections, high blood pressure, epilepsy, and rheumatoid arthritis. For example, about 1 in 10 of those who take the antiepileptic drug valproate during pregnancy will have a child with a major malformation.[103] Unfortunately, use of prescription medications during pregnancy is high and increasing.[104] Nine in ten American women use at least one prescription medication during pregnancy and 2% take at least one teratogenic drug.[101] The list of teratogenic drugs also includes some over-the-counter drugs and recreational drugs like cocaine.[105]

- *Smoking.* While the major risk of smoking during pregnancy is fetal growth restriction (see the previous section in this chapter), smoking also increases by about 10–20% the risk of several congenital malformations, including heart defects, cleft lip, and limb defects.[106-108]

- *Exposure to teratogenic chemicals.* While there is reason to worry that exposure to chemicals in the environment or workplace may cause congenital malformations, there are few chemicals for which there is strong evidence.[104] One exception is **polychlorinated biphenyls (PCBs)**, chemicals that can be present in fish. In one study, children of women who ate moderate amounts of fish contaminated with PCBs before and during pregnancy had smaller head sizes and intellectual problems.[109] Another is the metal **mercury**. If mercury is discharged into bodies of water, the chemical methylmercury can accumulate in fish, and if pregnant women eat those fish, it can lead to brain damage to their infants.[110]

- *Deficiency of folate and other micronutrients.* Folate deficiency in pregnancy increases the risk of neural tube defects and maybe also congenital heart defects and orofacial clefts (see Box 10.1).[76] Deficiencies of other micronutrients may also increase the risk of congenital malformations. For example, a deficiency of Vitamin B12 has also been linked to neural tube defects.[76] In some areas of the world where salt is not fortified with iodine, a deficiency in iodine in pregnancy

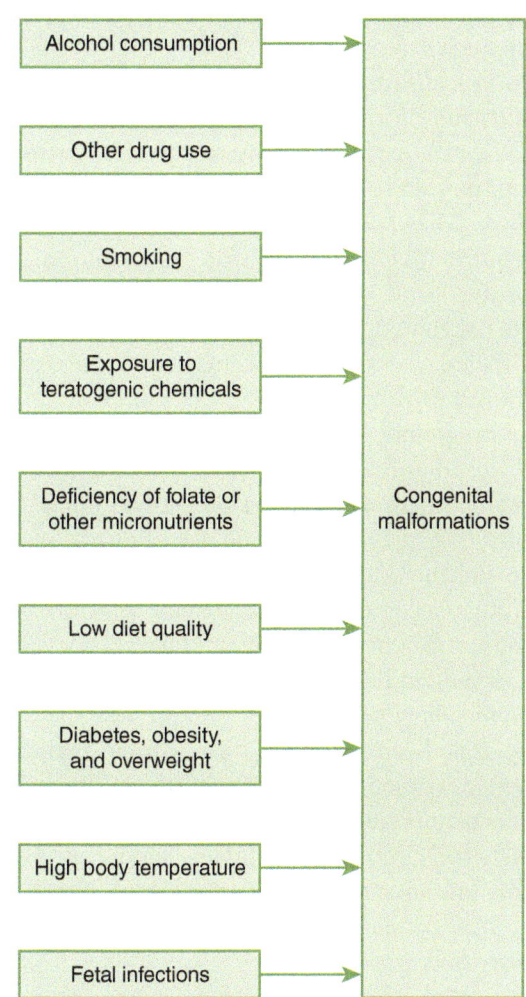

Figure 10.18 **Cause-and-Effect Diagram for Congenital Malformations.**

can cause infants to have intellectual deficits and hearing loss.[111]

- *Low diet quality.* The healthfulness of the food that people eat can be summarized in a "Diet Quality Index," which measures how closely a person's diet matches the U.S. Dietary Guidelines. The Diet Quality Index gives positive points for fruits, vegetables, whole grains, and minerals, and negative points for foods high in fats and sugar. Women who have low scores on this index are more likely to have children with neural tube defects, orofacial clefts, congenital heart defects, and other congenital malformations.[112-114] This risk of low diet quality has been found even in those who take vitamin supplements during pregnancy.[114]

- *Diabetes, obesity, and overweight.* Women with either type 1 or type 2 diabetes are more likely to have children with a variety of malformations, including neural tube defects.[76] The high blood sugar in diabetes damages fetal cells, including those in the neural tube.[76] Overweight and obesity also increase the risk of several types of congenital malformations, with higher risk as body mass index increases.[76,114,115]

- *Fetal infections.* Some viruses, bacteria, and other infectious agents cross the placenta and affect the fetus. When they do, they harm many developing organs, leading to problems such as brain damage, deafness, eye abnormalities, and congenital heart defects.[116] The list of agents that cause fetal infections includes: the viruses **rubella**, **cytomegalovirus**, **Zika** (which is spread by mosquitoes), and herpes; the bacteria *Treponema pallidum* (a sexually-transmitted infection that causes congenital **syphilis**); and the protozoan *Toxoplasma gondii* (which causes a disease called **toxoplasmosis**).[17]

- *High body temperature.* High body temperature during the first trimester is associated with having a child with malformations, including neural tube defects. High temperature has this effect regardless of whether it is from a fever or from the pregnant women spending time in a hot tub or spa.[117,118]

Preventive Interventions

These risk factors can be addressed by (**Figure 10.19**):

- *Reduction of alcohol consumption* by pregnant women and women of reproductive age. Those who are pregnant should be strongly discouraged from drinking any alcohol. But the damage from alcohol begins very early in pregnancy—as early

as the third week after conception—before most women know they are pregnant.[98] That means that prevention of fetal alcohol syndrome and fetal alcohol spectrum disorder depends in large part on preventing alcohol use among those *who might become* pregnant. Pregnancies are very difficult to predict: nearly half of pregnancies are unplanned, and nearly 5% of women of reproductive age have an unintended pregnancy each year.[119] The only reliable way to reduce alcohol use in early pregnancy for entire populations is to discourage alcohol use in all women in their reproductive years. That requires a population-based approach, as discussed in Chapter 12. Alcohol Use.

- *Reduction in the prescribing of teratogenic drugs.* Healthcare providers should prescribe drugs that can cause congenital malformations less often to patients who are pregnant and women of reproductive age.

- *Smoking prevention.* See Chapter 11. Tobacco Use.

- *Reduction in exposure to teratogenic chemicals.* women who are or who may become pregnant should be protected from potentially teratogenic chemicals in workplaces.

- Food *fortification with folic acid and other micronutrients.* Fortification of foods with folic acid has been extraordinarily successful in reducing neural tube defects in the United States (Box 10.2).[76] While some other countries also require folic acid fortification, many cases of neural tube defects across the world could be prevented if foods in every country were fortified.[116] Similarly, iodine fortification of salt should be universal to prevent iodine deficiency in pregnancy (as well as iodine deficiency in children and adults).[116]

- *Micronutrient supplementation.* Not all micronutrients that prevent congenital malformations can be delivered through food fortification. Expert groups recommend that women who are pregnant or may become pregnant take a daily vitamin supplement that contains folic acid.[64,120]

- *Promotion of healthy diets.* Because low diet quality has been linked to congenital malformations, women of reproductive age (regardless of whether they take multivitamins) should eat diets high in fruits, vegetables, and whole grains, and low in saturated fats and sugar. Promotion of healthy eating is discussed in Chapter 14. Nutrition.

- *Prevention of obesity and diabetes.* Prevention of obesity, which would also reduce rates of diabetes, should help reduce congenital malformations.

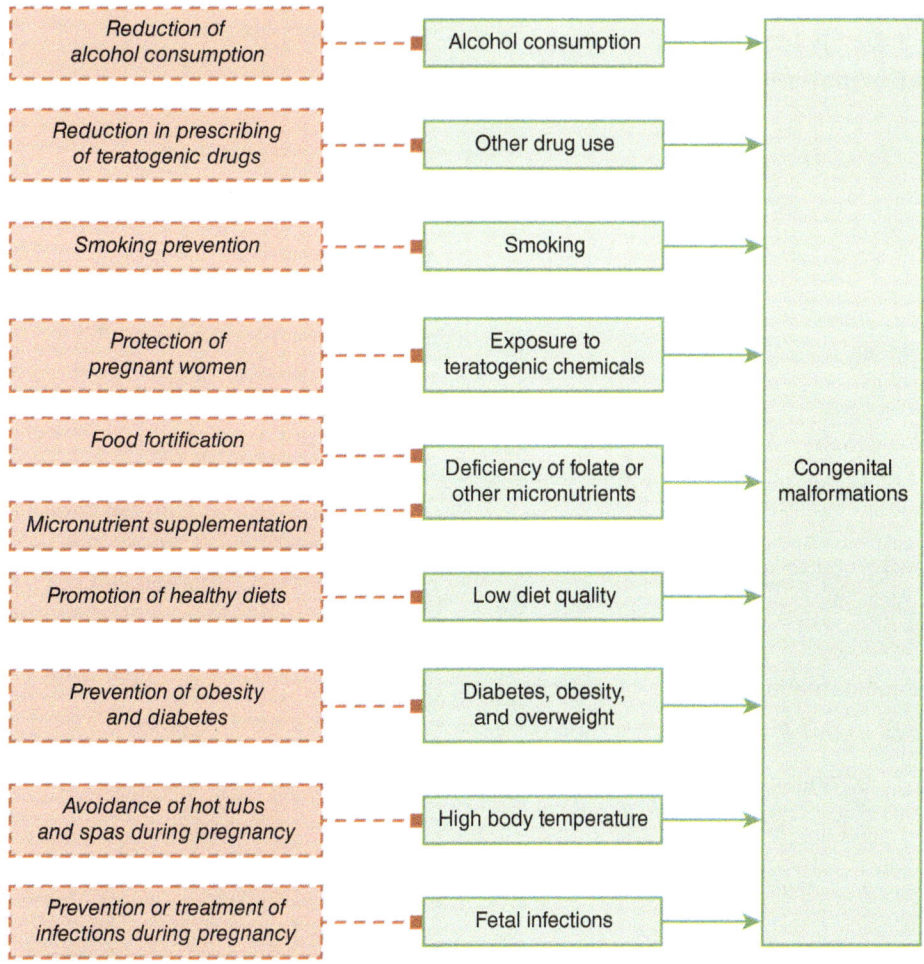

Figure 10.19 **Cause-and-Effect Diagram for Congenital Malformations, with Preventive Interventions.**

Prevention of obesity and diabetes is discussed in Chapter 8. Chronic Metabolic Diseases.

- *Avoidance of high temperatures during pregnancy.* While it would not prevent many congenital malformations, women should be advised to avoid hot tubs or spas during pregnancy or when they might become pregnant.

- *Prevention or treatment of infections during pregnancy.* There are different ways to prevent or treat each of the infections that can involve the fetus. For example, rubella can be prevented by vaccination. Cytomegalovirus infection can be treated with antiviral medications.[121] Zika virus infection can be prevented by mosquito control. Toxoplasmosis, caused by an organism carried by cats that can sometimes get into farm animals, can be prevented by those who might become pregnant by avoiding cat feces and not eating undercooked meat.[122] And congenital syphilis can be prevented by testing women for syphilis during pregnancy and treating those found to be infected with antibiotics.

Today, major congenital malformations can often be detected in the first or second trimester of pregnancy with a combination of tests of the mother's blood, tests of amniotic fluid, tests of the fetus' chromosomes, and ultrasound images of the fetus.[116]

Box 10.5 **Summary–Prevention of Congenital Malformations**

- Reduction of alcohol consumption by pregnant women and women of reproductive age
- Reduction in prescribing of teratogenic drugs
- Smoking prevention
- Reduction in exposure to teratogenic chemicals
- Food fortification with folic acid and other micronutrients
- Micronutrient supplementation
- Promotion of healthy diets
- Prevention of obesity and diabetes
- Avoidance of high temperatures during pregnancy
- Prevention or treatment of infections during pregnancy

Box 10.6 Key Words–Congenital Malformations

Anencephaly
Birth defects
Chromosomal defects
Cleft lip
Cleft palate
Clubfoot
Congenital abnormalities
Congenital anomalies
Congenital disorders
Congenital heart defects
Congenital malformations
Cytomegalovirus
Down syndrome
Encephalocele
Fetal alcohol spectrum disorder (FASD)
Fetal alcohol syndrome
Folate, folic acid
Gastroschisis
Major congenital malformations (major birth defects)
Mercury
Microcephaly
Minor congenital malformations (minor birth defects)
Mutation
Neural tube
Neural tube defects
Orofacial clefts
Ovum, Ova
Polychlorinated biphenyls (PCBs)
Rubella
Spina bifida
Syphilis
Toxoplasmosis
Trisomy
Trisomy 21
Zika
Zygote

Resources–Congenital Malformations

- Stallings EB, Isenburg JL, Rutkowski RE, et al. National population-based estimates for major birth defects, 2016–2020. *Birth Defects Res.* 2024; 116(1). doi:10.1002/bdr2.2301
- Zimmerman MS, Smith AGC, Sable CA, et al. Global, regional, and national burden of congenital heart disease, 1990–2017: A systematic analysis for the Global Burden of Disease Study 2017. *Lancet Child Adolesc Health.* 2020;4(3):185-200. doi:10.1016/S2352-4642(19)30402-X
- Popova S, Charness ME, Burd L, et al. Fetal alcohol spectrum disorders. *Nat Rev Dis Primers.* 2023;9(1). doi:10.1038/s41572-023-00420-x
- Crider KS, Qi YP, Yeung LF, et al. Folic acid and the prevention of birth defects: 30 years of opportunity and controversies. *Annu Rev Nutr* 2022;42:423-452. doi:10.1146/annurev-nutr-043 020-091647
- Wang Y, Smolinski NE, Thai TN, et al. Common teratogenic medication exposures—a population-based study of pregnancies in the United States. *Am J Obstet Gynecol MFM.* 2024;6(1):1-11. doi:10.1016/j.ajogmf .2023.101245

References

1. Centers for Disease Control and Prevention (CDC). *WONDER Natality Files.* Published 2024. Accessed May 14, 2024. Available at: https://wonder.cdc.gov/natality .html
2. Risnes K, Bilsteen JF, Brown P, et al. Mortality among young adults born preterm and early term in 4 Nordic nations. *JAMA Netw Open.* 2021;4(1). doi:10.1001/jamanetworkopen .2020.32779
3. Grantz KL, Grewal J, Kim S, et al. Unified standard for fetal growth: The Eunice Kennedy Shriver National Institute of Child Health and Human Development Fetal Growth Studies. *Am J Obstet Gynecol.* 2022;226(4):576-587.e2. doi:10.1016/j.ajog.2021.12.006
4. Green ES, Arck PC. Pathogenesis of preterm birth: Bidirectional inflammation in mother and fetus. *Semin Immunopathol.* 2020;42(4):413-429. doi:10.1007/s00281 -020-00807-y
5. Goldenberg RL, Culhane JF, Iams JD, Romero R. Epidemiology and causes of preterm birth. *Lancet.* 2008;371(9606): 75-84. doi:10.1016/S0140-6736(08)60074-4
6. Romero R, Dey SK, Fisher SJ. Preterm labor: One syndrome, many causes. *Science.* 2014;345(6198):760-765. doi:10.1126/science.1251816
7. van de Wijgert JHHM, Jespers V. The global health impact of vaginal dysbiosis. *Res Microbiol.* 2017;168(9-10): 859-864. doi:10.1016/j.resmic.2017.02.003
8. Rampersaud R, Randis TM, Ratner AJ. Microbiota of the upper and lower genital tract. *Semin Fetal Neonatal Med.* 2012;17(1):51-57. doi:10.1016/j.siny.2011.08.006
9. Onderdonk AB, Delaney ML, Fichorova RN. The human microbiome during bacterial vaginosis. *Clin Microbiol Rev.* 2016;29(2):223-238. doi:10.1128/CMR.00075-15
10. Bautista CT, Wurapa E, Sateren WB, Morris S, Hollingsworth B, Sanchez JL. Bacterial vaginosis: A synthesis of the literature on etiology, prevalence, risk factors, and relationship with chlamydia and gonorrhea infections. *Mil Med Res.* 2016;3(1). doi:10.1186/s40779-016-0074-5
11. Koumans EH, Sternberg M, Bruce C, et al. The prevalence of bacterial vaginosis in the United States, 2001–2004; Associations with symptoms, sexual behaviors, and

reproductive health. *Sex Transm Dis*. 2007;34(11):864-869. doi:10.1097/OLQ.0b013e318074e565

12. Roxby AC, Mugo NR, Oluoch LM, et al. Low prevalence of bacterial vaginosis in Kenyan adolescent girls and rapid incidence after first sex. *Am J Obstet Gynecol*. 2023;229(3):282. e1-282. doi:10.1016/j.ajog.2023.06.044

13. Verstraelen H, Verhelst R, Vaneechoutte M, Temmerman M. The epidemiology of bacterial vaginosis in relation to sexual behaviour. *BMC Infect Dis*. 2010;10(81):1-11. doi:10.1186/1471-2334-10-81

14. Van Gerwen OT, Craig-Kuhn MC, Jones AT, et al. Trichomoniasis and adverse birth outcomes: A systematic review and meta-analysis. *BJOG*. 2021;128(12):1907-1915. doi:10.1111/1471-0528.16774

15. Gao R, Liu B, Yang W, et al. Association of maternal sexually transmitted infections with risk of preterm birth in the United States. *JAMA Netw Open*. 2021;4(11):E2133413. doi:10.1001/jamanetworkopen.2021.33413

16. Jonduo ME, Vallely LM, Wand H, et al. Adverse pregnancy and birth outcomes associated with Mycoplasma hominis, Ureaplasma urealyticum, and Ureaplasma parvum: A systematic review and meta-analysis. *BMJ Open*. 2022; 12(8). doi:10.1136/bmjopen-2022-062990

17. Husain AN, Koo SC. Prematurity and fetal growth restriction. In: Kumar V, Abbas AK, Aster JC, Turner JR, eds. *Robbins & Cotran Pathologic Basis of Disease*. 10th ed. Elsevier; 2021:457-459.

18. Olson DM, Severson EM, Verstraeten BSE, Ng JWY, McCreary JK, Metz GAS. Allostatic load and preterm birth. *Int J Mol Sci*. 2015;16(12):29856-29874. doi:10.3390 /ijms161226209

19. Dall'Asta A, Brunelli V, Prefumo F, Frusca T, Lees CC. Early onset fetal growth restriction. *Matern Health Neonatol Perinatol*. 2017;3(1). doi:10.1186/s40748-016-0041-x

20. McCowan L, Horgan RP. Risk factors for small for gestational age infants. *Best Pract Res Clin Obstet Gynaecol*. 2009;23(6):779-793. doi:10.1016/j.bpobgyn.2009.06.003

21. Burton GJ, Jauniaux E. Pathophysiology of placental-derived fetal growth restriction. *Am J Obstet Gynecol*. 2018;218(2):S745-S761. doi:10.1016/j.ajog.2017.11 .577

22. Valencia CM, Mol BW, Jacobsson B, et al. FIGO good practice recommendations on modifiable causes of iatrogenic preterm birth. *Int J Gynaecol Obstet*. 2021;155(1):8-12. doi:10.1002/ijgo.13857

23. Chen C, Zhang JW, Xia HW, et al. Preterm birth in China between 2015 and 2016. *Am J Public Health*. 2019;109(11):1597-1604. doi:10.2105/AJPH.2019.305287

24. Wang MJ, Kuper SG, Steele R, Sievert RA, Tita AT, Harper LM. Outcomes of medically indicated preterm births differ by indication. *Am J Perinatol*. 2018;35(8):758-763. doi:10.1055/s-0037-1615792

25. Poon LC, Shennan A, Hyett JA, et al. The International Federation of Gynecology and Obstetrics (FIGO) initiative on pre-eclampsia: A pragmatic guide for first-trimester screening and prevention. *Int J Gynaecol Obstet*. 2019;145(S1):1-33. doi:10.1002/ijgo.12802

26. Ananth CV, Vintzileos AM. Maternal-fetal conditions necessitating a medical intervention resulting in preterm birth. *Am J Obstet Gynecol*. 2006;195(6):1557-1563. doi:10.1016/j.ajog.2006.05.021

27. Gyamfi-Bannerman C, Fuchs KM, Young OM, Hoffman MK. Nonspontaneous late preterm birth: Etiology and outcomes. *Am J Obstet Gynecol*. 2011;205(5):456.e1-456. e6. doi:10.1016/j.ajog.2011.08.007

28. Ellenson LH, Pirog EC. Disorders of late pregnancy. In: Kumar V, Abbas AK, Aster JC, Turner JR, eds. *Robbins & Cotran Pathologic Basis of Disease*. 10th ed. Elsevier; 2021:1030-1032.

29. Dimitriadis E, Rolnik DL, Zhou W, et al. Pre-eclampsia. *Nat Rev Dis Primers*. 2023;9(1). doi:10.1038/s41572-023 -00417-6

30. Henderson JT, Vesco KK, Senger CA, Thomas RG, Redmond N. Aspirin use to prevent preeclampsia and related morbidity and mortality: Updated evidence report and systematic review for the US Preventive Services Task Force. *JAMA*. 2021;326(12):1192-1206. doi:10.1001/jama .2021.8551

31. Thompson J, Onyenaka C, Oduguwa E, et al. Trends and racial/ethnic disparities in the rates of pre-eclampsia by HIV status in the US. *J Racial Ethn Health Disparities*. 2021;8(3):670-677. doi:10.1007/s40615-020-00826-3

32. Wen T, Schmidt CN, Sobhani NC, et al. Trends and outcomes for deliveries with hypertensive disorders of pregnancy from 2000 to 2018: A repeated cross-sectional study. *BJOG*. 2022;129(7):1050-1060. doi:10.1111/1471 -0528.17038

33. Fingar KR, Mabry-Hernandez I, Ngo-Metzger Q, Wolff T, Steiner CA, Elixhauser A. Delivery hospitalizations involving preeclampsia and eclampsia, 2005–2014. *AHRQ Statistical Brief*. 2017;(222):1-28.

34. Wiznitzer A, Mayer A, Novack V, et al. Association of lipid levels during gestation with preeclampsia and gestational diabetes mellitus: A population-based study. *Am J Obstet Gynecol*. 2009;201(5):482.e1-482.e8. doi:10.1016/j.ajog .2009.05.032

35. Davenport MH, Ruchat SM, Poitras VJ, et al. Prenatal exercise for the prevention of gestational diabetes mellitus and hypertensive disorders of pregnancy: A systematic review and meta-analysis. *Br J Sports Med*. 2018;52(21):1367-1375. doi:10.1136/bjsports-2018-099355

36. Blencowe H, Krasevec J, de Onis M, et al. National, regional, and worldwide estimates of low birthweight in 2015, with trends from 2000: A systematic analysis. *Lancet Glob Health*. 2019;7(7):e849-e860. doi:10.1016/S2214 -109X(18)30565-5

37. UNICEF. Low birthweight. UNICEF. Published July 2023. Accessed May 20, 2024. Available at: https://data.unicef .org/topic/nutrition/low-birthweight

38. Klebanoff MA, Schuit E, Lamont RF, et al. Antibiotic treatment of bacterial vaginosis to prevent preterm delivery: Systematic review and individual participant data meta-analysis. *Paediatr Perinat Epidemiol*. 2023;37(3):239-251. doi:10.1111/ppe.12947

39. Hussein H, Shamsipour M, Yunesian M, et al. Prenatal malaria exposure and risk of adverse birth outcomes: a prospective cohort study of pregnant women in the Northern Region of Ghana. *BMJ Open*. 2022;12(8). doi:10 .1136/bmjopen-2021-058343

40. Poespoprodjo JR, Douglas NM, Ansong D, Kho S, Anstey NM. Malaria. *Lancet*. 2023;402(10419):2328-2345. doi:10.1016/S0140-6736(23)01249-7

41. Becker M, Mayo JA, Phogat NK, et al. Deleterious and protective psychosocial and stress-related factors predict risk of spontaneous preterm birth. *Am J Perinatol*. 2023;40(1):74-88. doi:10.1055/s-0041-1729162

42. Cnattingius S. The epidemiology of smoking during pregnancy: Smoking prevalence, maternal characteristics, and pregnancy outcomes. *Nicotine Tob Res.* 2004;6(Suppl 2):s125-s140. doi:10.1080/14622200410001669187

43. Iñiguez C, Ballester F, Costa O, et al. Maternal smoking during pregnancy and fetal biometry. *Am J Epidemiol.* 2013;178(7):1067-1075. doi:10.1093/aje/kwt085

44. Bekkar B, Pacheco S, Basu R, Basu R, Denicola N. Association of air pollution and heat exposure with preterm birth, low birth weight, and stillbirth in the US: A systematic review. *JAMA Netw Open.* 2020;3(6). doi:10.1001/jamanetworkopen.2020.8243

45. Amegah AK, Quansah R, Jaakkola JJK. Household air pollution from solid fuel use and risk of adverse pregnancy outcomes: A systematic review and meta-analysis of the empirical evidence. *PLoS One.* 2014;9(12). doi:10.1371/journal.pone.0113920

46. Younger A, Alkon A, Harknett K, Jean Louis R, Thompson LM. Adverse birth outcomes associated with household air pollution from unclean cooking fuels in low-and middle-income countries: A systematic review. *Environ Res.* 2022;204:112274. doi:10.1016/j.envres.2021.112274

47. Patra J, Bakker R, Irving H, Jaddoe VWV, Malini S, Rehm J. Dose-response relationship between alcohol consumption before and during pregnancy and the risks of low birthweight, preterm birth and small for gestational age (SGA): A systematic review and meta-analyses. *BJOG.* 2011;118(12):1411-1421. doi:10.1111/j.1471-0528.2011.03050.x

48. Bosworth OM, Padilla-Azain MC, Adgent MA, et al. Prescription opioid exposure during pregnancy and risk of spontaneous preterm delivery. *JAMA Netw Open.* 2024;7(2):E2355990. doi:10.1001/jamanetworkopen.2023.55990

49. Kennare R, Heard A, Chan A. Substance use during pregnancy: Risk factors and obstetric and perinatal outcomes in South Australia. *Aust N Z J Obstet Gynaecol.* 2005;45(3):220-225. doi:10.1111/j.1479-828X.2005.00379.x

50. Gouin K, Murphy K, Shah PS. Effects of cocaine use during pregnancy on low birthweight and preterm birth: systematic review and metaanalyses. *Am J Obstet Gynecol.* 2011;204(4):340.e1-340.e12. doi:10.1016/j.ajog.2010.11.013

51. Bryce E, Gurung S, Tong H, et al. Population attributable fractions for risk factors for spontaneous preterm births in 81 low-and middle-income countries: A systematic analysis. *J Glob Health.* 2022;12:04013. doi:10.7189/jogh.12.04013

52. Ramakrishnan U, Grant F, Goldenberg T, Zongrone A, Martorell R. Effect of women's nutrition before and during early pregnancy on maternal and infant outcomes: A systematic review. *Paediatr Perinat Epidemiol.* 2012;26(Suppl 1):285-301. doi:10.1111/j.1365-3016.2012.01281.x

53. Khanam R, Lee AC, Mitra DK, et al. Maternal short stature and under-weight status are independent risk factors for preterm birth and small for gestational age in rural Bangladesh. *Eur J Clin Nutr.* 2019;73(5):733-742. doi:10.1038/s41430-018-0237-4

54. McHale P, Maudsley G, Pennington A, et al. Mediators of socioeconomic inequalities in preterm birth: a systematic review. *BMC Public Health.* 2022;22(1). doi:10.1186/s12889-022-13438-9

55. Mikati I, Benson AF, Luben TJ, Sacks JD, Richmond-Bryant J. Disparities in distribution of particulate matter emission sources by race and poverty status. *Am J Public Health.* 2018;108(4):480-485. doi:10.2105/AJPH.2017.304297

56. Iams JD, Romero R, Culhane JF, Goldenberg RL. Primary, secondary, and tertiary interventions to reduce the morbidity and mortality of preterm birth. *Lancet.* 2008;371(9607):164-175. doi:10.1016/S0140-6736(08)60108-7

57. Brownell M, Nickel NC, Chartier M, et al. An unconditional prenatal income supplement reduces population inequities in birth outcomes. *Health Aff.* 2018;37(3):447-455. doi:10.1377/hlthaff.2017.1290

58. Brownell MD, Chartier MJ, Nickel NC, et al. Unconditional prenatal income supplement and birth outcomes. *Pediatrics.* 2016;137(6):e20152992.

59. Lumley J, Chamberlain C, Dowswell T, Oliver S, Oakley L, Watson L. Interventions for promoting smoking cessation during pregnancy. In: Chamberlain C, ed. *Cochrane Database Syst Rev.* 2009;(3):CD001055. doi:10.1002/14651858.CD001055.pub3

60. Keats EC, Haider BA, Tam E, Bhutta ZA. Multiple-micronutrient supplementation for women during pregnancy. *Cochrane Database Syst Rev.* 2019;(3):CD004905. doi:10.1002/14651858.CD004905.pub6

61. Da Silva Lopes K, Ota E, Shakya P, et al. Effects of nutrition interventions during pregnancy on low birth weight: An overview of systematic reviews. *BMJ Glob Health.* 2017;2(3). doi:10.1136/bmjgh-2017-000389

62. Bhutta ZA, Das JK, Rizvi A, et al. Evidence-based interventions for improvement of maternal and child nutrition: What can be done and at what cost? *Lancet.* 2013;382(9890):452-477. doi:10.1016/S0140-6736(13)60996-4

63. Ota E, Hori H, Mori R, Tobe-Gai R, Farrar D. Antenatal dietary education and supplementation to increase energy and protein intake. *Cochrane Database Syst Rev.* 2015;(6):CD000032. doi:10.1002/14651858.CD000032.pub3

64. Keats EC, Das JK, Salam RA, et al. Effective interventions to address maternal and child malnutrition: an update of the evidence. *Lancet Child Adolesc Health.* 2021;5(5):367-384. doi:10.1016/S2352-4642(20)30274-1

65. Middleton P, Gomersall JC, Gould JF, Shepherd E, Olsen SF, Makrides M. Omega-3 fatty acid addition during pregnancy. *Cochrane Database Syst Rev.* 2018;(11):CD003402. doi:10.1002/14651858.CD003402.pub3

66. Henderson J, Vesko K, Senger C. Aspirin use to prevent pre-eclampsia and related morbidity and mortality. *AHRQ Evid Synth.* 2021;(205). Accessed May 14, 2024. Available at: https://www.ncbi.nlm.nih.gov/books/NBK574449/

67. Hofmeyr GJ, Lawrie TA, Atallah ÁN, Torloni MR. Calcium supplementation during pregnancy for preventing hypertensive disorders and related problems. *Cochrane Database Syst Rev.* 2018;10(10). doi:10.1002/14651858.CD001059.pub5

68. Hofmeyr GJ, Belizán JM, Von Dadelszen P. Low-dose calcium supplementation for preventing pre-eclampsia: A systematic review and commentary. *BJOG.* 2014;121(8):951-957. doi:10.1111/1471-0528.12613

69. Smaill FM, Vazquez JC. Antibiotics for asymptomatic bacteriuria in pregnancy. *Cochrane Database Syst Rev.* 2019;(11):CD000490. doi:10.1002/14651858.CD000490.pub4

70. Ansaldi Y, Martinez de Tejada Weber B. Urinary tract infections in pregnancy. *Clin Microbiol Infect.* 2023;29(10):1249-1253. doi:10.1016/j.cmi.2022.08.015

71. Andrews WW, Goldenberg RL, Hauth JC, Cliver SP, Copper R, Conner M. Interconceptional antibiotics to prevent spontaneous preterm birth: A randomized clinical trial. *Am J Obstet Gynecol.* 2006;194(3):617-623. doi:10.1016/j.ajog.2005.11.049

72. Conde-Agudelo A, Romero R. Vaginal progesterone for the prevention of preterm birth: Who can benefit and who cannot? Evidence-based recommendations for clinical use. *J Perinat Med.* 2023;51(1):125-134. doi:10.1515/jpm-2022-0462

73. Care A, Nevitt SJ, Medley N, et al. Interventions to prevent spontaneous preterm birth in women with singleton pregnancy who are at high risk: Systematic review and network meta-analysis. *BMJ.* 2022;376:e064547. doi:10.1136/bmj-2021-064547

74. Malherbe H, Modell B, Blencowe H, Strong K, Aldous C. A review of key terminology and definitions used for birth defects globally. *J Community Genet.* 2023;14(3):241-262. doi:10.1007/s12687-023-00642-2

75. World Health Organization, Centers for Disease Control and Prevention (CDC), International Clearinghouse for Birth Defects. *Birth Defects Surveillance: A Manual for Program Managers.* World Health Organization; 2020. Accessed October 22, 2024. https://www.who.int/publications/i/item/9789240015395

76. Crider KS, Qi YP, Yeung LF, et al. Folic acid and the prevention of birth defects: 30 years of opportunity and controversies. *Annu Rev Nutr.* 2022;42:423-452. doi:10.1146/annurev-nutr-043020

77. Centers for Disease Control and Prevention (CDC). Update on overall prevalence of major birth defects—Atlanta, Georgia, 1978-2005. *MMWR Morb Mortal Wkly Rep.* 2008;57(1):1-5.

78. Stallings EB, Isenburg JL, Rutkowski RE, et al. National population-based estimates for major birth defects, 2016–2020. *Birth Defects Res.* 2024;116(1):e2301. doi:10.1002/bdr2.2301

79. Harris BS, Bishop KC, Kemeny HR, Walker JS, Rhee E, Kuller JA. Risk factors for birth defects. *Obstet Gynecol Surv.* 2017;72(2):123-135. www.obgynsurvey.com|123

80. Feldkamp ML, Carey JC, Byrne JLB, Krikov S, Botto LD. Etiology and clinical presentation of birth defects: Population based study. *BMJ (Online).* 2017;357:j2249. doi:10.1136/bmj.j2249

81. Toufaily MH, Westgate MN, Lin AE, Holmes LB. Causes of congenital malformations. *Birth Defects Res.* 2018;110(2):87-91. doi:10.1002/bdr2.1105

82. Lumey LH, Van Poppel FWA. The Dutch famine of 1944–1945: Mortality and morbidity in past and present generations. *Soc Hist Med.* 1994;7(2):229-246. doi:10.1093/shm/7.2.229

83. Brown AS, Susser ES. Sex differences in prevalence of congenital neural defects after periconceptional famine exposure. *Epidemiology.* 1997;8(1):55-58. doi:10.1097/00001648-199701000-00009

84. Schorah C. Dick Smithells, folic acid, and the prevention of neural tube defects. *Birth Defects Res A Clin Mol Teratol.* 2009;85(4):254-259. doi:10.1002/bdra.20544

85. Wald NJ. Commentary: A brief history of folic acid in the prevention of neural tube defects. *Int J Epidemiol.* 2011;40(5):1154-1156. doi:10.1093/ije/dyr131

86. MRC Vitamin Study Research Group. Prevention of neural tube defects: Results of the Medical Research Council Vitamin Study. *Lancet.* 1991;338(8760):131-137.

87. Czeizel AE, Dudás I. Prevention of the first occurrence of neural-tube defects by periconceptional vitamin supplementation. *N Engl J Med.* 1992;327(26):1832-1835. doi:10.1056/NEJM199212243272602

88. Berry RJ, Li Z, Erickson JD, et al. Prevention of neural-tube defects with folic acid in China. *N Engl J Med.* 1999;341(20):1485-1490. doi:10.1056/NEJM199911113412001

89. Williams J, Mai CT, Mulinare J, et al. Updated estimates of neural tube defects prevented by mandatory folic acid fortification—United States, 1995–2011. *MMWR Morb Mortal Wkly Rep.* 2015;64(1):1-5.

90. Mai CT, Evans J, Alverson CJ, et al. Changes in spina bifida lesion level after folic acid fortification in the US. *J Pediatr.* 2022;249:59-66.e1. doi:10.1016/j.jpeds.2022.06.023

91. Zimmerman MS, Smith AGC, Sable CA, et al. Global, regional, and national burden of congenital heart disease, 1990–2017: A systematic analysis for the Global Burden of Disease Study 2017. *Lancet Child Adolesc Health.* 2020;4(3):185-200. doi:10.1016/S2352-4642(19)30402-X

92. Riley EP, Infante MA, Warren KR. Fetal alcohol spectrum disorders: An overview. *Neuropsychol Rev.* 2011;21(2):73-80. doi:10.1007/s11065-011-9166-x

93. Williams JF, Smith VC. Fetal alcohol spectrum disorders. *Pediatrics.* 2015;136(5):e1395-e1406. doi:10.1542/peds.2015-3113

94. May PA, Baete A, Russo J, et al. Prevalence and characteristics of fetal alcohol spectrum disorders. *Pediatrics.* 2014;134(5):855-866. doi:10.1542/peds.2013-3319

95. May PA, Chambers CD, Kalberg WO, et al. Prevalence of fetal alcohol spectrum disorders in 4 US communities. *JAMA.* 2018;319(5):474-482. doi:10.1001/jama.2017.21896

96. Yang Q, Wen SW, Leader A, Chen XK, Lipson J, Walker M. Paternal age and birth defects: How strong is the association? *Human Reproduction.* 2007;22(3):696-701. doi:10.1093/humrep/del453

97. Canfield MA, Mai CT, Wang Y, et al. The association between race/ethnicity and major birth defects in the United States, 1999–2007. *Am J Public Health.* 2014;104(9):e14-e23. doi:10.2105/AJPH.2014.302098

98. Popova S, Charness ME, Burd L, et al. Fetal alcohol spectrum disorders. *Nat Rev Dis Primers.* 2023;9(1):11. doi:10.1038/s41572-023-00420-x

99. Popova S, Lange S, Probst C, Gmel G, Rehm J. Estimation of national, regional, and global prevalence of alcohol use during pregnancy and fetal alcohol syndrome: a systematic review and meta-analysis. *Lancet Glob Health.* 2017;5(3):e290-e299. doi:10.1016/S2214-109X(17)30021-9

100. Gosdin LK, Deputy NP, Kim SY, Dang EP, Denny CH. Alcohol consumption and binge drinking during pregnancy among adults aged 18-49 years—United States, 2018–2020. *MMWR Morb Mortal Wkly Rep.* Accessed May 27, 2024. Available at: https://www.cdc.gov/mmwr

101. Wang Y, Smolinski NE, Thai TN, et al. Common teratogenic medication exposures—a population-based study of pregnancies in the United States. *Am J Obstet Gynecol MFM.* 2024;6(1):1-11. doi:10.1016/j.ajogmf.2023.101245

102. Eltonsy S, Martin B, Ferreira E, Blais L. Systematic procedure for the classification of proven and potential teratogens for use in research. *Birth Defects Res A Clin Mol Teratol.* 2016;106(4):285-297. doi:10.1002/bdra.23491

103. Tomson T, Battino D, Bonizzoni E, et al. Comparative risk of major congenital malformations with eight different antiepileptic drugs: A prospective cohort study of the EURAP registry. *Lancet Neurol.* 2018;17(6):530-538. doi:10.1016/S1474-4422(18)30107-8

104. Feldkamp ML, Botto LD, Carey JC. Reflections on the etiology of structural birth defects: Established teratogens and risk factors. *Birth Defects Res A Clin Mol Teratol.* 2015;103(8):652-655. doi:10.1002/bdra.23392

105. Cleveland Clinic. Teratogens. October 21, 2022. Accessed May 27, 2024. https://my.clevelandclinic.org/health/articles/24325-teratogens

106. Leite M, Albieri V, Kjaer SK, Jensen A. Maternal smoking in pregnancy and risk for congenital malformations: Results of a Danish register-based cohort study. *Acta Obstet Gynecol Scand.* 2014;93(8):825-834. doi:10.1111/aogs.12433

107. Hackshaw A, Rodeck C, Boniface S. Maternal smoking in pregnancy and birth defects: A systematic review based on 173,687 malformed cases and 11.7 million controls. *Hum Reprod Update.* 2011;17(5):589-604. doi:10.1093/humupd/dmr022

108. Sullivan PM, Dervan LA, Reiger S, Buddhe S, Schwartz SM. Risk of congenital heart defects in the offspring of smoking mothers: A population-based study. *J Pediatr.* 2015;166(4):978-984.e2. doi:10.1016/j.jpeds.2014.11.042

109. Agency for Toxic Substances and Disease Registry. Polychlorinated biphenyls (PCBs) toxicity. Centers for Disease Control and Prevention. May 24, 2023. Accessed May 27, 2024. https://www.atsdr.cdc.gov/csem/polychlorinated-biphenyls/adverse_health.html

110. Harada M. Congenital minamata disease: Intrauterine methylmercury poisoning. *Birth Defects Res A Clin Mol Teratol.* 2010;88(10):906-909. doi:10.1002/bdra.20756

111. Lisco G, De Tullio A, Triggiani D, et al. Iodine deficiency and iodine prophylaxis: An overview and update. *Nutrients.* 2023;15(4):1004. doi:10.3390/nu15041004

112. Botto LD, Krikov S, Carmichae SL, Munger RG, Shaw GM, Feldkamp ML. Lower rate of selected congenital heart defects with better maternal diet quality: A population-based study. *Arch Dis Child Fetal Neonatal Ed.* 2016;101(1):F43-F49. doi:10.1136/archdischild-2014-308013

113. Carmichael SL, Yang W, Feldkamp ML, et al. Reduced risks of neural tube defects and orofacial clefts with higher diet quality. *Arch Pediatr Adolesc Med.* 2012;166(2):121-126. doi:10.1001/archpediatrics.2011.185

114. Carmichael SL, Yang W, Gilboa S, et al. Elevated body mass index and decreased diet quality among women and risk of birth defects in their offspring. *Birth Defects Res A Clin Mol Teratol.* 2016;106(3):164-171. doi:10.1002/bdra.23471

115. Stothard KJ, Tennant PWG, Bell R, Rankin J. Maternal overweight and obesity and the risk of congenital anomalies: A systematic review and meta-analysis. *JAMA.* 2009;301(6):636-650.

116. Kancherla V, Oakley GP, Brent RL. Urgent global opportunities to prevent birth defects. *Semin Fetal Neonatal Med.* 2014;19(3):153-160. doi:10.1016/j.siny.2013.11.008

117. Duong HT, Shahrukh Hashmi S, Ramadhani T, Canfield MA, Scheuerle A, Kim Waller D. Maternal use of hot tub and major structural birth defects. *Birth Defects Res A Clin Mol Teratol.* 2011;91(9):836-841. doi:10.1002/bdra.20831

118. Waller DK, Hashmi SS, Hoyt AT, et al. Maternal report of fever from cold or flu during early pregnancy and the risk for noncardiac birth defects, National Birth Defects Prevention Study, 1997–2011. *Birth Defects Res.* 2018;110(4):342-351. doi:10.1002/bdr2.1147

119. Guttmacher Institute. Unintended Pregnancy in the United States. Guttmacher.org. January 2019. Accessed May 28, 2024. Available at: https://www.guttmacher.org/fact-sheet/unintended-pregnancy-united-states

120. Tuncalp Ö, Rogers LM, Lawrie TA, et al. WHO recommendations on antenatal nutrition: An update on multiple micronutrient supplements. *BMJ Glob Health.* 2022;5(7):e003375. doi:10.1136/BMJGH-2020-003375

121. Khalil A, Heath PT, Jones CE, Soe A, Ville YG. Congenital cytomegalovirus infection: Update on screening, diagnosis and treatment. *BJOG.* Published online October 21, 2024. doi:10.1111/1471-0528.17966

122. Ahmed M, Sood A, Gupta J. Toxoplasmosis in pregnancy. *Eur J Obstet Gynecol Reprod Biol.* 2020;255:44-50. doi:10.1016/j.ejogrb.2020.10.003

PART III

Behavioral and Social Risks

CHAPTER 11

Tobacco Use

No behavior or exposure kills more people than the use of tobacco. That statement is true both in the United States and on a global scale.[1] The Global Burden of Disease project estimates that each year tobacco use underlies more than 300,000 deaths in the United States and more than 8 million deaths worldwide.[1] That is like having a COVID-19 pandemic every year.

It could be far worse. While about 20% of adults in the world smoke, that percentage has fallen by about a third over the past 30 years.[2] The decrease in smoking rates did not happen on its own. It happened because public health advocates put in place anti-smoking policies at the local, national, and global level, including the world's first health-oriented global treaty, the United Nation's **Framework Convention on Tobacco Control.**

The public health battle against tobacco is far from won, though. Much more work needs to be done to implement this treaty, to enact key policies at the national, state, and local levels, and to discourage tobacco use in every country.

Tobacco use is addictive because it delivers the drug **nicotine** to users. Nearly all the damage from tobacco, though, comes not from nicotine (which by itself is not very harmful) but instead from the other chemicals in the leaf or its smoke. As discussed below, many products available today—from nicotine patches to e-cigarettes—try to reduce the health risks by separating the drug from these other chemicals and delivering only nicotine to users. Because nicotine will always be popular, there are important policy questions to answer about these newer nicotine-delivery products.

Tobacco Use and Health

Tobacco and Nicotine

Tobacco is a flowering plant that grows to a few feet tall and has large, broad leaves (**Figure 11.1**). The leaves contain nicotine, which protects the plant as a natural insecticide. The tobacco plant is native to

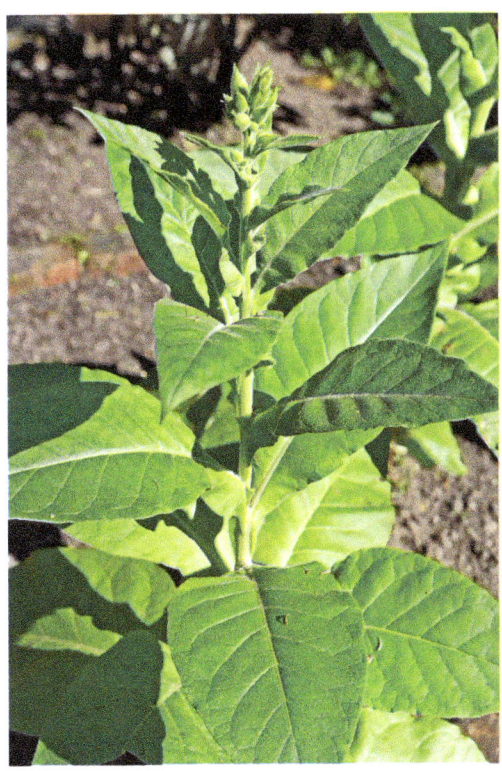

Figure 11.1 Tobacco Plant (*Nicotiana tabacum*).

the Caribbean, where it was used as a medicinal by Indigenous people. Christopher Columbus brought the plant to Europe and people around the world have cultivated it for nicotine since then.

Effects of Nicotine

When people light tobacco leaves on fire and inhale the smoke, nicotine flows into the lungs. Nicotine is then absorbed into the blood and delivered to the brain within seconds. That immediate effect allows people who smoke to unconsciously fine-tune how much nicotine is in their brains by how frequently and deeply they puff.

When nicotine first hits the brain, users experience a "rush" in which they feel both more relaxed and more alert. They also feel less anxious and are better able to concentrate and perform mental tasks.[3] The rush is caused by nicotine indirectly stimulating the release of several **neurotransmitters**, the most important of which is **dopamine**, in the brain's **reward circuit**, through which people feel pleasure.[3] This is the same reward circuit that experts believe is involved in use of all popular recreational drugs, including alcohol, cocaine, and heroin.[4] The reward circuit is discussed more in Chapter 13. Use of Addictive Drugs.

When people smoke regularly, though, their **neurons** (brain cells) adapt to high levels of nicotine. They require higher doses to experience the same pleasant effect, a pattern that is called **tolerance**. Over time, if people who smoke regularly do not get a dose of nicotine, their neurons respond as they would to a stressful situation, making the smoker irritable, anxious, and depressed—that is, feeling the symptoms of **withdrawal**. To ease or prevent those unpleasant symptoms, they light up again.[3] Together, the effects of tolerance and withdrawal are what makes smoking addictive.

Nicotine has effects on the body, too. It increases the heart rate and blood pressure. Usually this is not dangerous—it is like the effect of caffeine—but it can cause heart problems in some people.[5]

Nicotine Delivery

The more nicotine a product delivers to the user, the more pleasurable and the more addictive it is. Tobacco companies have an incentive, then, to increase the amount of nicotine that their products deliver to users. One way that they do that is through their selection and handling of the leaves. Nicotine levels vary according to the strain, which leaves on the plant are used, and how the leaves are dried and "cured."

Tobacco companies also manipulate the chemical form of nicotine. In the tobacco plant, nicotine is

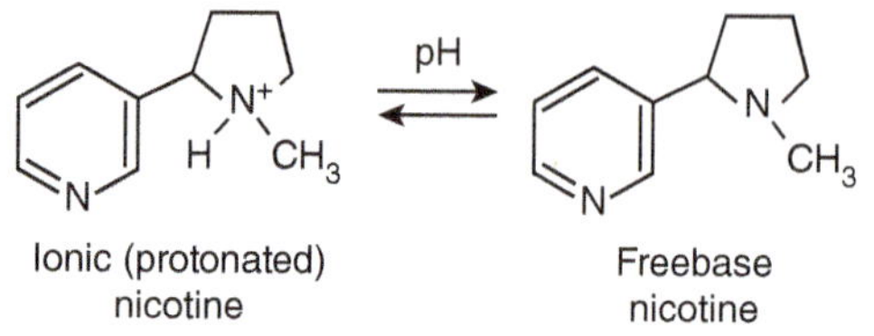

Figure 11.2 Two Forms of Nicotine. Nicotine is present in tobacco leaves in two forms, an ionic (protonated) form and a freebase form. In a more acidic environment, the ionic form predominates, and in a more basic environment, the freebase form predominates. The free base form is more easily absorbed through the lungs but feels harsh to smokers.

present in two forms (**Figure 11.2**). The "**free base**" form is easily absorbed through the lungs but feels harsh to users. The "**ionic**" or "**protonated**" form, which is more present in acidic fluids, is not well absorbed through the lungs but is less irritating.[6] The goal of tobacco manufacturers is to deliver as much "free base" nicotine as possible while minimizing the irritation.[6,7] They do this by adjusting both the total nicotine content and the pH of the tobacco leaves.

In the early 1960s, Philip Morris began treating tobacco leaves for the Marlboro brand cigarettes with ammonia, which raised the pH and increased the proportion of nicotine that was in the free base form.[8] This change delivered more nicotine to users, helping Marlboro become the nation's biggest-selling cigarette brand. More than 50 years later, JUUL used a similar combination of pH and nicotine concentration in its pod-type e-cigarettes, which led millions of teenagers to vape.[7]

Nicotine-delivery Products

Hundreds of products are available today to deliver nicotine to a user's bloodstream (**Figure 11.3**). Cigarettes emit smoke containing nicotine, which is absorbed through the lungs. This efficient delivery system has made cigarettes the most popular tobacco product and by far the biggest public health problem. Cigar and pipe smoke is mostly absorbed through the lining of the mouth. Chewing tobacco and packets of tobacco held in the mouth called **snus** likewise deliver nicotine through the mouth.[5] **Dry snuff** is a powder made from tobacco leaves that delivers nicotine through the lining of the nose. (Together, chewing tobacco, snus, and dry snuff are called **smokeless tobacco**.) All these products cause quick spikes of nicotine in the brain.

In the early 2000s, start-up companies began selling **electronic nicotine delivery systems (ENDS)**, which are more often called **e-cigarettes**.

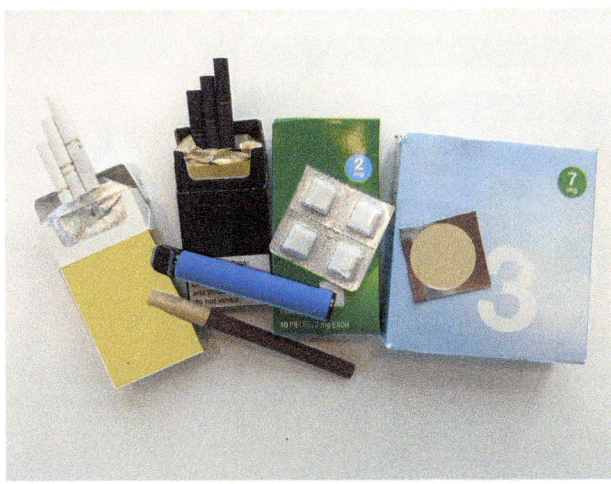

Figure 11.3 Products that Deliver Nicotine. Many different products are designed to deliver nicotine to users, including cigarettes, cigars, e-cigarettes (in blue), nicotine gum, and nicotine patches.

These devices typically contain nicotine in a liquid that is mostly **propylene glycol** or **vegetable glycerine**, with added chemicals that create flavors. When a user draws on an e-cigarette, a coil heats the liquid, creating a vapor that delivers nicotine to the "vaper's" lungs.[5,9] The vapor does not contain the toxic chemicals of cigarette smoke, but it is not just water vapor, either. The health risks and benefits of e-cigarettes are discussed further below.

In the 2010s, major tobacco corporations started selling products that deliver nicotine by heating (but not burning) tobacco leaves, under brand names IQOS, Glo, Ploom, and others. These contain toxic chemicals found in cigarette smoke, but at substantially lower levels.[10] The tobacco companies hope that consumers will see these as safer than cigarettes. It is too early to know the health effects of these products to users, but they cannot be considered safe. At this point, these heat-not-burn are mostly used by people who also continue to smoke and by young people who have never smoked.[11,12]

Pharmaceutical companies have developed many products, called **nicotine replacement therapy**, that are designed to safely deliver nicotine to people who smoke but want to quit. These products include tablets, lozenges, nasal sprays, mouth sprays, and patches that deliver nicotine through the skin.[13] The nicotine that these products deliver is the same drug that is in cigarettes and e-cigarettes, but the products do not expose users to the toxic chemicals in tobacco. These products are evaluated for their safety and approved by the FDA. Most are designed to keep nicotine at steady levels in the blood, avoiding a quick drop that would prompt people to crave tobacco.[14]

Other Constituents of Tobacco and Smoke

Tobacco smoke carries a plume of tiny particles containing thousands of chemicals, which is called "tar." As a group, these chemicals are toxic to cells, especially those lining the lungs, and dozens of them are linked to cancer. Among those chemicals are **nitrosamines** and **polycyclic aromatic hydrocarbons**, which are proven to cause cancer, and trace amounts of metals like lead, cadmium, and arsenic. Tobacco smoke also includes gases, such as those found in polluted air, and carbon monoxide, the gas that makes automobile exhaust deadly.[6]

Tobacco companies add various chemicals to leaves as they turn them into tobacco products. To attract users, they add flavorings. The U.S. government has prohibited most flavorings in cigarettes, but it still allows them in cigars.

The additive used most is **menthol**, a chemical extracted from peppermint leaves, which is arguably a flavoring, but is also very biologically active, so it might be more accurate to call it a drug.[6] Cough drops contain menthol because it numbs the back of the throat. People smoking menthol-infused cigarettes feel less irritation, making it easier for teens to start smoking and harder for adults who smoke to stop.[15] Despite the FDA's 2021 recommendation that menthol be prohibited in cigarettes, under the heavy lobbying by tobacco companies, menthol was still allowed as of 2025.

Pathophysiology of Tobacco Use

Although people smoke or chew tobacco for the nicotine, nearly all the damage to cells, tissues, and organs is caused by the other chemicals in tobacco. These chemicals directly kill many cells and transform many other cells into potential cancers.[6] When cells are killed by these chemicals, the cells' spilled contents activate the body's immune system, which responds by causing **inflammation**. That inflammation itself causes additional damage to other cells and tissues.

The cells that receive the heaviest dose of smoke's chemicals are those lining the mouth, throat, larynx (voice box), large airways, and lungs. But these chemicals also are carried by the blood to the rest of the body, causing damage to every organ.

People who do not smoke are frequently exposed to trace amounts of toxic chemicals. But people who smoke get a heavy dose of these chemicals with every puff. And when they puff for hours a day, every day,

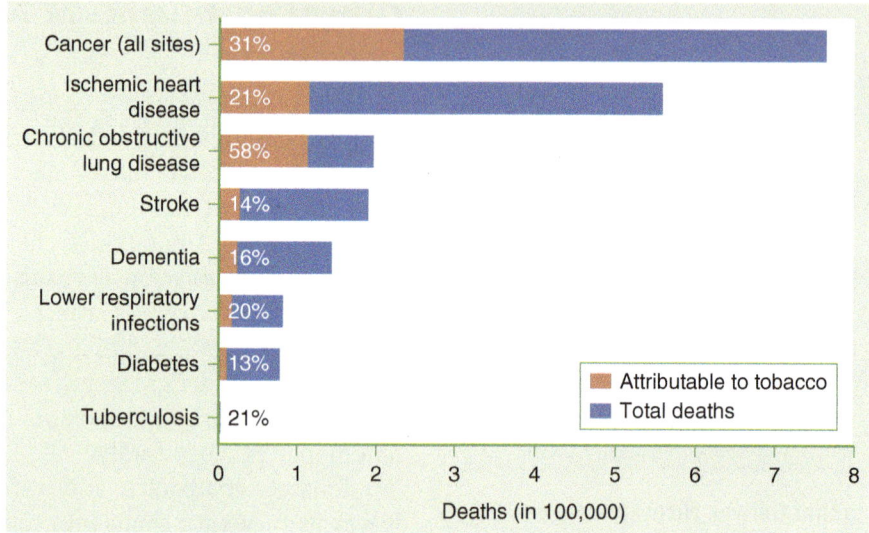

Figure 11.4 Estimated Deaths Attributable to Tobacco in the United States, by Major Causes, 2019.

Data from Global Burden of Disease Collaboration, Institute for Health Metrics and Evaluation. GBD Results Tool. Published July 12, 2023. Accessed October 27, 2023. https://vizhub.healthdata.org/gbd-results/

for years or decades, they get cumulative doses of these chemicals that are orders of magnitude higher than those of nonsmokers, causing damage that is far worse and far more widespread. That explains why smoking is a risk factor for most of the diseases covered in this book.

The other chapters describe these diseases in detail, but they are also summarized below. The diseases with the greatest impact on populations are **chronic obstructive pulmonary disease**, **cardiovascular disease** (that is, ischemic heart disease and ischemic stroke), and cancer. **Figure 11.4** shows estimates of the number and proportion of deaths attributable to tobacco use each year in the United States.

Chronic Lung Diseases and Lung Infections

The chemicals in smoke damage the cells lining the large and small airways, as well as the other lung tissues. This damage creates inflammation, causing people who smoke to cough and produce **sputum**. This inflammation also makes it more difficult for the lungs to exchange oxygen and carbon dioxide with the blood, and ultimately destroys the lung tissues. This causes chronic obstructive pulmonary disease, including its two types **chronic bronchitis** and **emphysema** (**Figure 11.5**). People who smoke are about 30 times as likely as nonsmokers to develop chronic obstructive pulmonary disease.[14] The smoke's

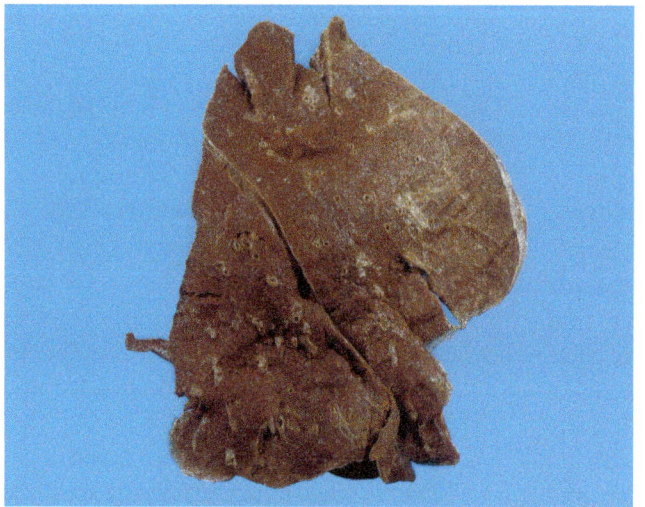
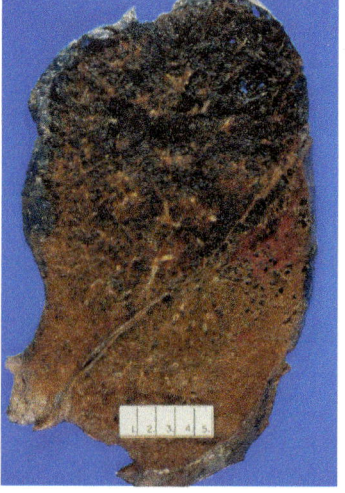

Figure 11.5 Normal Lung and Lung from Smoker with Emphysema.

© Arthur Glauberman/Science Source; © Dr. E. Walker/Science Source damage also hurts the lung's ability to fight off infections, which makes people who smoke more likely to get **tuberculosis** and other **lower respiratory infections**.[1,16,17]

Heart Disease and Stroke

The chemicals from tobacco smoke circulate in the blood, injuring the lining of the large and medium-sized arteries throughout the body. This injury to arteries is a key contributor to **atherosclerosis** (narrowing of arteries), which is a cause of heart attacks (**ischemic heart disease**) and **ischemic strokes**.[5]

Cancer

Not surprisingly, tobacco has its greatest impact on cancers arising from tissues directly touched by smoke. The Global Burden of Disease project estimates that smoking causes about three-fourths of cancers of the lung and larynx and nearly half of cancers of the mouth and **esophagus** (**Figure 11.6**). The impact on lung cancer is especially strong: people who smoke are about 20 times as likely as nonsmokers to die from this disease.[14]

But the chemicals in tobacco increase the risk of cancer throughout the body. For example, about one-third of cancers of the **cervix**, one-fourth of cancers of the **pancreas**, and one-seventh of cancers of the **colon and rectum** are attributable to tobacco (Figure 11.6). Smoking also increases the risk of breast cancer, although the relationship is much weaker than it is for other cancers.[18,19] Across all sites, nearly one-third of cancer deaths are attributable to tobacco.[1]

Diabetes and Chronic Kidney Disease

Smoking increases the risk of Type 2 diabetes by about 40%.[20] It is not clear why, but the body-wide inflammation caused by the chemicals in smoke may contribute to insulin resistance. Smoking also is associated with a small increase in the risk of chronic kidney disease.[21]

Adverse Pregnancy Outcomes

Tobacco use during pregnancy is linked to an extraordinary number and range of serious health problems for the parent and fetus. It increases the risk of an **ectopic pregnancy**. The fetus is vulnerable

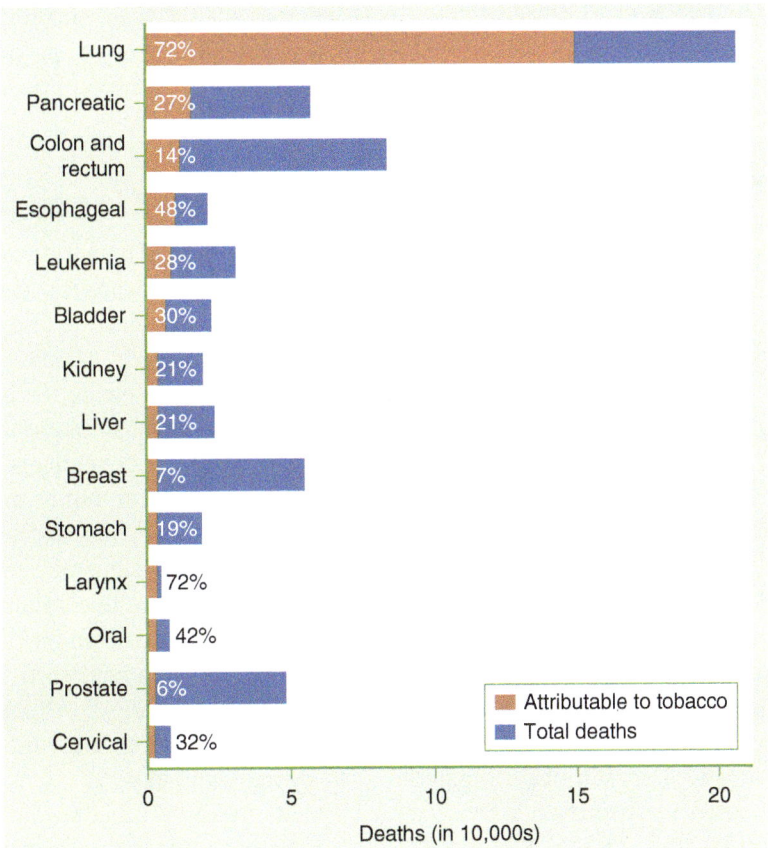

Figure 11.6 **Estimated Cancer Deaths in the United States Attributable to Tobacco, by Site, 2019.**

Data from Global Burden of Disease Collaboration, Institute for Health Metrics and Evaluation. GBD Results Tool. Published July 12, 2023. Accessed October 27, 2023. https://vizhub.healthdata.org/gbd-results/

to both nicotine and the toxic chemicals in tobacco because these chemicals are present when organs are being formed.[22,23] The fetus is likely to be born prematurely, with a low birth weight, or stillborn, and is more likely to have a **congenital malformation**. Children of women who smoke during pregnancy are more likely to die of **sudden infant death syndrome (SIDS)**. When they reach school age, they have lower average IQs.[23]

Low Back Pain

People who smoke are about 60% more likely than non-smokers to have low back pain.[24] In the United States, an estimated 20% of low back pain is attributable to smoking.[1] The mechanism for this link is not clear, but it may be that chemicals in tobacco smoke cause the cartilage in intervertebral discs to deteriorate.[25,26]

Mental Illnesses

Smoking is linked to mental illnesses. People who smoke are more likely to develop **dementia** because atherosclerosis causes narrowing of the arteries that supply blood to the brain. The chemicals in tobacco smoke lead to atherosclerosis in these arteries just as they do to arteries supplying the heart muscle.[27,28]

Also, smoking is statistically associated with **schizophrenia**, **depression**, and **anxiety disorders**.[29-31] It is difficult to be certain whether smoking causes these diseases or vice versa. However, some studies show that people who quit smoking are less likely to have anxiety, suggesting that smoking may in fact cause this illness.[32] The biologic reason for this link to smoking is not understood. It may be related to nicotine's effect on levels of dopamine and other neurotransmitters in the brain.

Health Risks of Environmental Tobacco Smoke

Nonsmokers who live with people who smoke—or who otherwise regularly breathe secondhand smoke—are more likely to develop cardiovascular disease, chronic obstructive pulmonary disease, and cancer, including cancer of the lung and breast.[33-35] Although the dose of smoke they receive is only about 1% of what people who smoke receive, the health effects are much larger than that would suggest. For example, compared to nonsmokers not exposed to environmental tobacco smoke, people who smoke have an 80% higher risk of cardiovascular disease, but nonsmokers exposed to environmental tobacco smoke have a 30% higher

risk.[34] Tobacco smoke in the air causes cardiovascular disease the same way as tobacco smoke inhaled from a cigarette does, with chemicals damaging the lining of arteries. Environmental tobacco smoke is also a risk factor for lower respiratory infections, and for asthma and tuberculosis in children.[36-38]

Health Risks of Smokeless Tobacco

People who use smokeless tobacco (chewing tobacco, snus, or dry snuff) are heavily exposed to the chemicals in tobacco leaves in the lining of the mouth or nose. This increases users' risk of developing cancer of the mouth and throat.[39] These chemicals are also absorbed into the blood, so smokeless tobacco users are also more likely to die from heart disease, stroke, and cancer in other body sites.[5,40] Use of chewing tobacco is particularly popular in India and Bangladesh, where about one on four adults use it, making this a significant public health problem in those countries.[40,41]

Overall Health Effects of Tobacco

People who smoke die younger and are much sicker when they are alive. People who start before age 25 and continue to smoke have an average life expectancy about 11 years shorter than that of nonsmokers.[14,42] In all, across the globe an astonishing 20% of deaths in men and 6% of deaths in women are attributable to smoking.[2]

Biologic Effects of E-cigarettes

Public health experts are divided over the health risks and benefits of e-cigarettes. The difference of opinion is in part because so little is known about their medium- and long-term effects. Here's what is known so far:

Vapor from e-cigarettes is nowhere near as dangerous as tobacco smoke. However, it is not harmless. It contains chemicals like **formaldehyde**, which causes cancer, but in much lower levels than in tobacco smoke.[9,43] Mice exposed to e-cigarette vapor for months show signs of damage to lung tissue, and teen users are more likely than non-users to develop a persistent cough or asthma.[44] Vapor from e-cigarettes *may* also cause damage to the cells lining arteries, as tobacco smoke does.[43] And nicotine increases heart rate and blood pressure, and may harm babies born to women who vape.[43]

At the same time, studies show that e-cigarettes can help people quit. In fact, e-cigarettes are more effective at helping people quit than nicotine patches and nicotine gum.[45]

The public health problem of e-cigarettes is not so much the products themselves but instead the lack of regulation and the way they are marketed. With no regulation, manufacturers can put any chemicals in e-cigarettes. In 2019, one or more manufacturers put Vitamin E acetate into vape liquids, causing severe lung damage in more than 2,800 users and killing more than 60.[46]

And e-cigarette manufacturers, instead of marketing these products to help adults who smoke, are marketing them to teenagers and young adults who have never smoked. They are succeeding. Teenagers in the United States are about five times as likely to vape as they are to smoke cigarettes or cigars.[47] Even assuming e-cigarettes are much safer than combustion cigarettes, if in practice they just turn nonsmokers into "vapers" and if they are rarely used by people to quit smoking, they will cause much more disease than they prevent.

Epidemiology: Patterns and Trends of Tobacco Use

The long-term trend of smoking in the United States shows remarkable progress. In 1965, more than 40% of adults smoked cigarettes; by the early 2020s, the smoking prevalence had dropped to just above 10% (**Figure 11.7**).[48] A key lesson from this is that, over time, public policies can have a big impact on drug use—even if those drugs are widely available and highly addictive.

Smoking is associated with social disadvantage. In the United States, cigarette smoking rates are nearly three times as high in people with low incomes as in those with high incomes (**Figure 11.8**). Cigarette smoking rates are similar in non-Hispanic Blacks and Whites (16%) but are far higher in either group than in Hispanics (10%) or Asians (5%).[49]

In a hopeful sign for the future, smoking rates are lower in young adults than middle-aged adults, and in 2023 only 2% of American high school students smoked cigarettes.[47,49]

Globally, smoking rates are about twice as high as they are in the United States, with large gender differences. An estimated 33% of adult men and 7% of adult women smoke.[2] Smoking rates are highest in Asia, North Africa, and Eastern Europe. The country with the world's largest number of people who smoke is China, where 50% of adult men and 4% of adult women smoke.[2] The percentage of adults who smoke is falling slowly in all regions (**Figure 11.9**).[50]

Risk Factors for Tobacco Use

The determinants of smoking are best understood through the framework of marketing.

Global sales of tobacco products are dominated by only 10 multinational conglomerates, including Philip Morris International, Altria (which includes Philip Morris USA), and British American Tobacco.[51] The business is highly profitable, with Philip Morris and British American Tobacco generating $82 billion and $35 billion in sales in 2021, respectively.[52] Because these are publicly-traded companies, they are obligated to their shareholders to maximize profits.

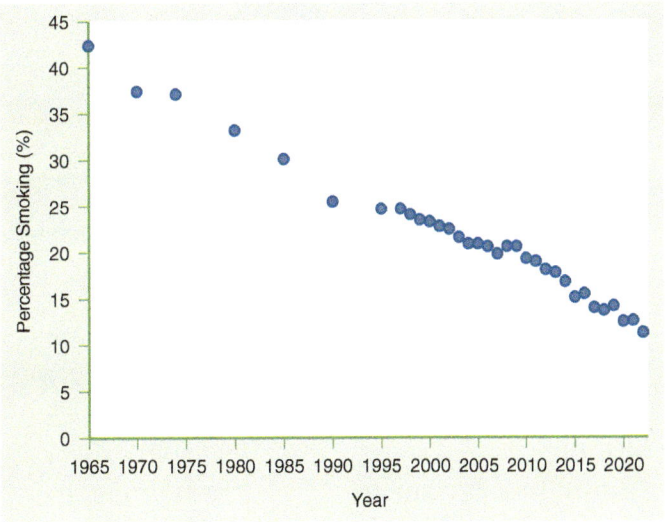

Figure 11.7 Trends in Cigarette Smoking Among Adults in the United States, 1965–2022.

Data from American Lung Association. Trends in Cigarette Smoking Rates. Published May 30, 2024. Accessed July 31, 2024. (Data from National Health Interview Survey) https://www.lung.org/research/trends-in-lung-disease/tobacco-trends-brief/overall-smoking-trends

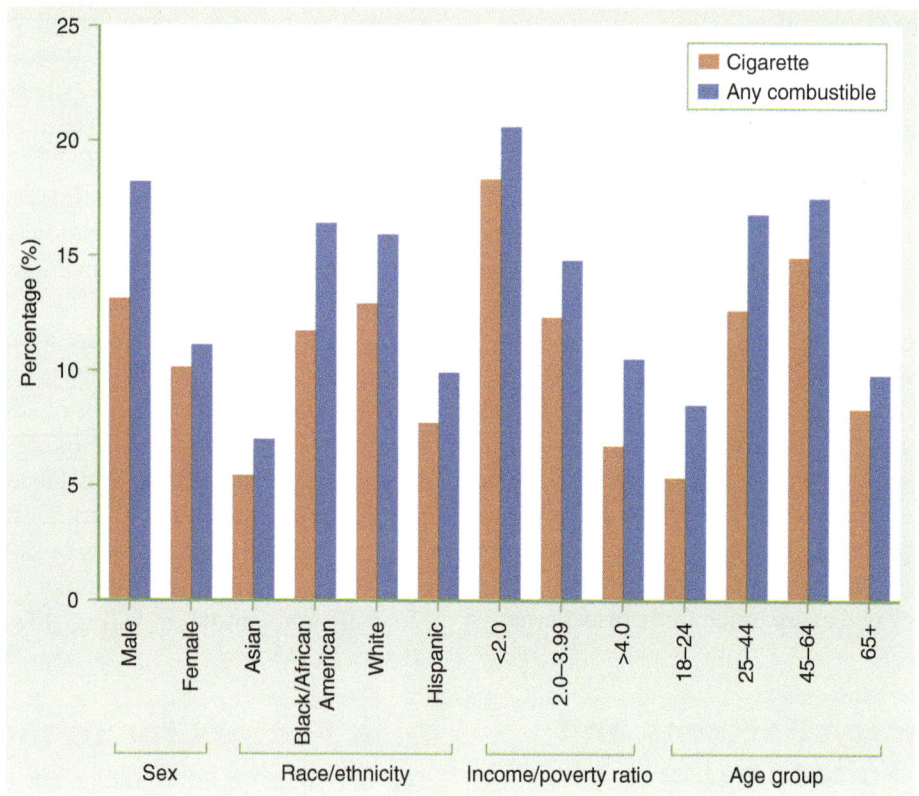

Figure 11.8 Smoking Among Adults in the United States by Demographic Group, 2021.

Data from Cornelius ME, Loretan CG, Jamal A, et al. Tobacco Product Use Among Adults-United States, 2021. *Morbidity and Mortality Weekly Report.* 2023;72(18):475-483.

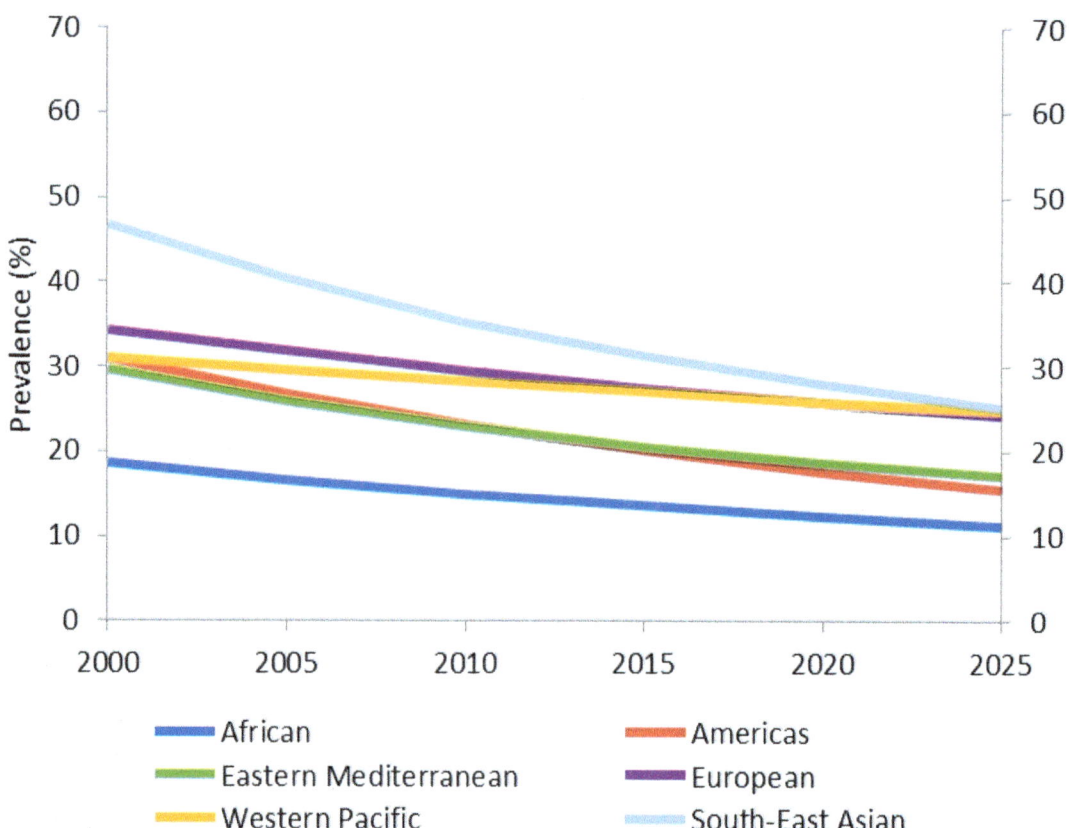

Figure 11.9 Estimated Trends in Tobacco Use and Projections by Global Region.

That means they must retain their current customers and attract new ones. Their profits enable them to spend billions to maintain and grow their customer base, so they market their products in every way that they legally can.

Although humans are attracted to nicotine, it is not natural or easy to light dried tobacco leaves on fire and breathe in the smoke. This behavior happens because the companies facilitate it and encourage it. Tobacco companies grow the plants, harvest the leaves, turn the leaves into smokable products, distribute them widely, and persuade people to start and continue smoking. All of the steps after the harvesting of the leaves can be considered marketing.

The tobacco companies design products to maximize their appeal to consumers. Then they sell those products through retailers (mostly grocery stores and convenience stores), giving those retailers large financial incentives based on the amount sold. At the same time, they give consumers discount coupons to purchase the products.[51,53] The companies encourage people to smoke by buying advertising, sponsorships, point-of-sale displays, and other forms of promotion.[53] And they employ lobbyists and public relations firms to maintain the legal and social acceptability of smoking.

With that in mind, the risk factors for smoking are (**Figure 11.10**):

- *The design of tobacco products* that makes them addictive and attractive. For example, tobacco products that deliver more nicotine cause people to smoke more and are more addictive.[54,55] Flavorings tempt teenagers and young adults to start smoking.[56,57] Menthol makes it easier for people to start smoking and harder for them to quit.[15] Features that make a tobacco product appear safer increase use.[58,59]
- *Tobacco product availability and accessibility.* The easier it is for people to obtain tobacco products, the more they will buy and use them. For example, one study showed that people who smoke who live just a little closer to the nearest store selling cigarettes were less likely to quit.[60] This risk factor includes not only the number and location of stores that sell tobacco products but also the price, whether price discounts are available, and whether teenagers can legally buy them.[60-64]
- *Tobacco promotion.* Promotion of tobacco products causes young people to experiment with smoking and to smoke regularly.[65,66] This promotion includes not just traditional advertising but also ads mailed directly to people, sponsorships of organizations and events, endorsements by social media influencers, point-of-sale displays, product placements in movies, and sales of tobacco-branded merchandise like hats and T-shirts. The United States has restricted advertising on television and radio, but many other channels for promotion of tobacco are still open. Many countries have no restrictions on tobacco advertising or promotion.
- *Social norms.* Individuals are more likely to pick up and maintain a behavior that others around them consider normal and acceptable than a behavior that others consider strange. That is the effect of "social norms," and it is particularly powerful for smoking.[67] In the United States 30 years ago, smoking indoors was considered perfectly acceptable, so much so that nonsmokers would be ashamed to ask people who smoke to stop. That norm has changed dramatically. Now smokers do not light up indoors because they are ashamed to do so.[68] Social norms are themselves influenced by tobacco product promotion; in fact, much of tobacco advertising is designed to persuade viewers that other people are smoking and are popular for it. Social norms are also influenced by the availability and accessibility of tobacco products, and by policies allowing or prohibiting smoking.

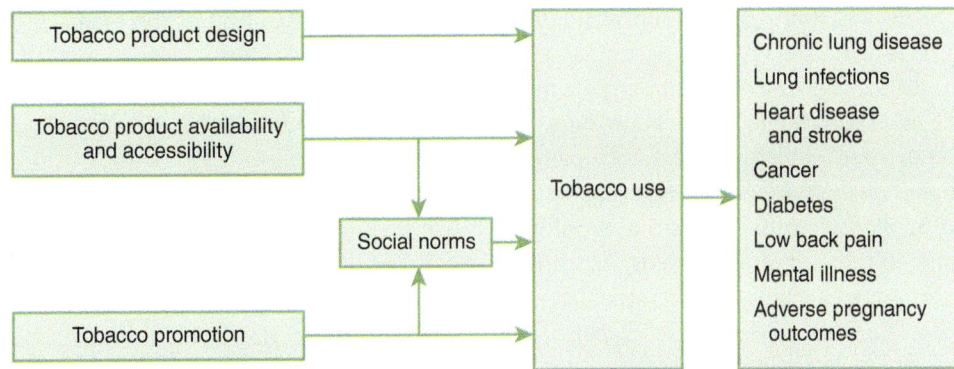

Figure 11.10 **Cause-and-Effect Diagram for Smoking and Other Forms of Tobacco Use.**

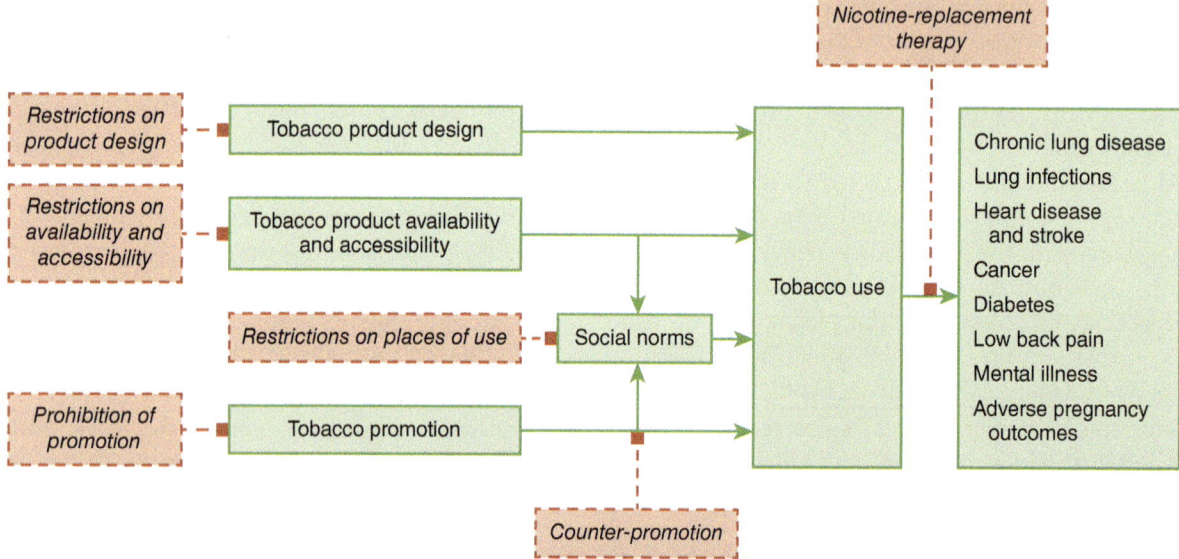

Figure 11.11 **Cause-and-Effect Diagram for Smoking and Other Forms of Tobacco Use, with Preventive Interventions.**

Preventive Interventions

Fortunately, interventions have been developed and shown to counter these risk factors (**Figure 11.11**).

Primary Prevention

- *Restrictions on product design.* Tobacco products are already regulated to make them less attractive, for example, with the U.S. prohibition on flavorings other than menthol in cigarettes. Other regulations can be put in place to reduce attractiveness or addictiveness, for example, prohibiting menthol and reducing nicotine levels.
- *Restrictions on availability and accessibility.* Many regulations on availability and accessibility are already in place in the United States, and they are effective. For example, *taxes on tobacco products* increase the product prices, reduce sales, and reduce smoking rates.[61] *Prohibitions on sales to persons under a certain age* (for example, 21) reduce smoking in underage persons.[63] More can be done to enforce these prohibitions, though. In the United States and many other countries, retail stores must have special licenses or permits to sell tobacco products. This provides an opportunity to *restrict the number, location, hours of operation, or sales practices* of these retailers. These can be paired with *prohibitions on price discounting and coupons.*
- *Prohibition of promotion.* Studies show that prohibiting advertising of tobacco products reduces smoking.[69] Governments can also restrict other forms of promotion, such as point-of-sale displays or sponsorships of concerts. In fact, the Framework Convention on Tobacco Control includes a pledge

for a comprehensive ban on tobacco advertising, sponsorships, and promotion.[70]
- *Counter-promotion. Counter-advertising* campaigns like the CDC's *Tips from Former Smokers* prompt people to quit and nudge the social norm away from smoking.[71,72] Requirements for *graphic warnings on cigarette packs* about the health risks of smoking reinforces the message from counter-advertising campaigns. These packaging requirements also prevent tobacco companies from using the space to promote smoking.
- *Restrictions on places of use.* Today, many cities and states in the United States prohibit smoking in most places where people gather, such as workplaces, bars, restaurants, school and university campuses, parks, and beaches. These restrictions have two benefits: they protect people from second-hand smoke and they make smoking less socially acceptable.[68,73]

Secondary Prevention

Helping people quit smoking can be thought of as secondary prevention of the many diseases caused by smoking. The interventions listed above as primary prevention also cause many to quit. Most who quit do it without medical help. However, some people need additional support.

People who smoke are addicted to nicotine, so substituting safer forms of nicotine can help. Those who try to quit using FDA-approved *nicotine replacement therapy* are nearly twice as likely to succeed.[13,74] And a medication called varenicline (trade name Chantix), which mimics nicotine in the brain, may be even more effective.[13,75] In the United States, states and cities provide free nicotine replacement therapy through cost-free services accessed over the telephone or the internet called **quitlines**.

E-cigarettes

Even as people gradually stop using combustion cigarettes, many people are starting or continuing to use electronic cigarettes. These devices present both an opportunity and a risk. They can help people quit, but they can also harm the health of nonsmokers. These risks and opportunities can be balanced by *regulation of e-cigarette design* to make them as safe as possible (for example, prohibiting flavorings and reducing nicotine levels) and *restrictions on e-cigarette marketing* so that it is directed only to people who already smoke regularly. That might include, for example, prohibiting sales to persons under age 25 or requiring a prescription for them to be sold.

Resources–Tobacco Use

- Benowitz NL. Nicotine addiction. *N Engl J Med.* 2010;362:2295-2303. This is an excellent review of the effects of nicotine on the brain.
- The reports of the U.S. Surgeon General on smoking and tobacco use, from the 1960s to the 2020s, are comprehensive and detailed compilations of the scientific evidence about nicotine, tobacco products, tobacco smoke, their biologic effects risks, and preventive interventions. They are available at: https://www.cdc.gov/tobacco/sgr/historical-reports/index.htm.
- CDC's *Best Practices for Comprehensive Tobacco Control Programs*, available at https://www.cdc.gov/tobacco/stateandcommunity/guides/index.htm, provides evidence-based guidance to state and local health departments on how to combat smoking and the use of other tobacco products.
- The World Health Organization's *WHO Report on the Global Tobacco Epidemic, 2023*, available at www.who.int, discusses the Framework Convention on Tobacco Control, and gives country-by-country reports on tobacco policies.

Box 11.2 **Key Words–Tobacco Use**

Anxiety disorder
Atherosclerosis
Cardiovascular disease
Cervix
Chronic bronchitis
Chronic obstructive pulmonary disease
Colon and rectum
Congenital malformations
Dementia
Depression
Dopamine
Dry snuff
E-cigarette
Ectopic pregnancy
Electronic nicotine delivery system (ENDS)
Emphysema
Esophagus
Formaldehyde
Framework Convention on Tobacco Control
Free base form of nicotine
Inflammation
Ionic form of nicotine
Ischemic heart disease
Ischemic stroke
Lower respiratory infection
Menthol
Neuron
Neurotransmitter
Nicotine
Nicotine-replacement therapy
Nitrosamines
Pancreas
Polycyclic aromatic hydrocarbons
Propylene glycol
Quitline
Reward circuit
Schizophrenia
Smokeless tobacco
Snus
Sputum
Sudden infant death syndrome (SIDS)
Tolerance
Tuberculosis
Vegetable glycerine
Withdrawal

Box 11.1 **Summary–Prevention of Tobacco Use**

- Restrictions on product design to reduce attractiveness and addictiveness
- Restrictions on availability and accessibility, including restrictions on the number and sales practices of retailers, taxes, age restrictions, and prohibitions on price discounting
- Prohibition of promotion
- Counter-promotion, including counter-advertising and graphic pack warnings
- Restrictions on places of use, such as worksites, bars, and restaurants
- Provision of nicotine replacement therapy
- Regulation of electronic cigarettes to make them safer
- Restrictions on e-cigarette marketing

References

1. Global Burden of Disease Collaboration, Institute for Health Metrics and Evaluation. GBD Results. July 12, 2023. Accessed July 11, 2023. Available at: https://vizhub.healthdata.org/gbd-results/

2. Reitsma MB, Kendrick PJ, Ababneh E, et al. Spatial, temporal, and demographic patterns in prevalence of smoking tobacco use and attributable disease burden in 204 countries and territories, 1990–2019: A systematic analysis from the Global Burden of Disease Study 2019. *Lancet.* 2021;397(10292):2337-2360. doi:10.1016/S0140-6736(21)01169-7

3. Benowitz NL. Nicotine addiction. *N Engl J Med.* 2010; 362:2295-2303.

4. Volkow ND, Blanco C. Substance use disorders: a comprehensive update of classification, epidemiology, neurobiology, clinical aspects, treatment, and prevention. *World Psychiatry.* 2023;22(2):203-229. doi:10.1002/wps.21073

5. Benowitz NL, Liakoni E. Tobacco use disorder and cardiovascular health. *Addiction.* 2022;117(4):1128-1138. doi:10.1111/add.15703

6. Office of the Surgeon General. *How Tobacco Smoke Causes Disease: The Biology and Behavioral Basis for Smoking-Attributable Disease: A Report of the Surgeon General.* Department of Health and Human Services; 2010. Accessed December 11, 2024. Available at: https://www.ncbi.nlm.nih.gov/books/NBK53017/

7. Duell AK, Pankow JF, Peyton DH. Nicotine in tobacco product aerosols: "It's déjà vu all over again." *Tob Control.* 2020;29(6):656-662. doi:10.1136/tobaccocontrol-2019-055275

8. Stevenson T, Proctor RN. The secret and soul of Marlboro. *Am J Public Health.* 2008;98(7):1184-1194. doi:10.2105/AJPH.2007.121657

9. Dinakar C, O'Connor GT. The health effects of electronic cigarettes. *N Engl J Med.* 2016;375(14):1372-1381. doi:10.1056/nejmra1502466

10. Znyk M, Jurewicz J, Kaleta D. Exposure to heated tobacco products and adverse health effects, a systematic review. *Int J Environ Res Public Health.* 2021;18(12). doi:10.3390/ijerph18126651

11. Panagiotakos DB, Georgoulis M, Kapetanstrataki M, Behrakis P. Prevalence, patterns, and determinants of electronic cigarette and heated tobacco product use in Greece: A cross-sectional survey. *Hellenic J Cardiol.* 2023;70:10-18. doi:10.1016/j.hjc.2023.01.002

12. Odani S, Tsuno K, Agaku IT, Tabuchi T. Heated tobacco products do not help smokers quit or prevent relapse: A longitudinal study in Japan. *Tob Control.* Published online 2023. doi:10.1136/tc-2022-057613

13. Thomas KH, Dalili MN, López-López JA, et al. Comparative clinical effectiveness and safety of tobacco cessation pharmacotherapies and electronic cigarettes: a systematic review and network meta-analysis of randomized controlled trials. *Addiction.* 2022;117(4):861-876. doi:10.1111/add.15675

14. Office of the Surgeon General. *The Health Consequences of Smoking—50 Years of Progress: A Report of the Surgeon General.* Department of Health and Human Services; 2014. Accessed December 11, 2024. Available at: https://www.ncbi.nlm.nih.gov/books/NBK179276/

15. Food and Drug Administration. *Preliminary Scientific Evaluation of the Possible Public Health Effects of Menthol Versus Nonmenthol Cigarettes of Menthol.* Published 2013. Accessed July 4, 2024. https://www.fda.gov/media/86497/download

16. Feldman C, Theron AJ, Cholo MC, Anderson R. Cigarette Smoking as a Risk Factor for Tuberculosis in Adults: Epidemiology and Aspects of Disease Pathogenesis. *Pathogens.* 2024;13(2). doi:10.3390/pathogens13020151

17. Kyu HH, Vongpradith A, Sirota SB, et al. Age–sex differences in the global burden of lower respiratory infections and risk factors, 1990–2019: Results from the Global Burden of Disease Study 2019. *Lancet Infect Dis.* 2022;22(11):1626-1647. doi:10.1016/S1473-3099(22)00510-2

18. Terry MB, Colditz GA. Epidemiology and risk factors for breast cancer: 21st century advances, gaps to address through interdisciplinary science. *Cold Spring Harb Perspect Med.* 2023;13(9). doi:10.1101/cshperspect.a041317

19. Luo J, Margolis KL, Wactawski-Wende J, et al. Association of active and passive smoking with risk of breast cancer among postmenopausal women: A prospective cohort study. *BMJ.* 2011;342(7796):536. doi:10.1136/bmj.d1016

20. Ley SH, Schulze MB, Hivert MF, Meigs JB, Hu FB. Risk factors for type 2 diabetes. In: Cowie CC, Casagrande SS, Menke A, Cissell MA, eds. *Diabetes in America.* 3rd ed. National Institute of Diabetes and Digestive and Kidney Diseases; 2018.

21. Xia J, Wang L, Ma Z, et al. Cigarette smoking and chronic kidney disease in the general population: A systematic review and meta-analysis of prospective cohort studies. *Nephrol Dial Transplant.* 2017;32(3):475-487. doi:10.1093/ndt/gfw452

22. Morales-Suárez-Varela M, Puig BM, Kaerlev L, Peraita-Costa I, Perales-Marín A. Safety of nicotine replacement therapy during pregnancy: A narrative review. *Int J Environ Res Public Health.* 2023;20(1). doi:10.3390/ijerph20010250

23. Havard A, Chandran JJ, Oei JL. Tobacco use during pregnancy. *Addiction.* 2022;117(6):1801-1810. doi:10.1111/add.15792

24. Shiri R, Falah-Hassani K, Heliövaara M, et al. Risk factors for low back pain: A population-based longitudinal study. *Arthritis Care Res (Hoboken).* 2019;71(2):290-299. doi:10.1002/acr.23710

25. Nasto LA, Ngo K, Leme AS, et al. Investigating the role of DNA damage in tobacco smoking-induced spine degeneration. *Spine J.* 2014;14(3):416-423. doi:10.1016/j.spinee.2013.08.034

26. Battié MC, Videman T, Kaprio J, et al. The Twin Spine Study: Contributions to a changing view of disc degeneration. *Spine J.* 2009;9(1):47-59. doi:10.1016/j.spinee.2008.11.011

27. Kalaria RN. The pathology and pathophysiology of vascular dementia. *Neuropharmacology.* 2018;134:226-239. doi:10.1016/j.neuropharm.2017.12.030

28. Wong EC, Chui HC. Vascular cognitive impairment and dementia. *Continuum (NY).* 2022;28(3):750-780.

29. Wootton RE, Richmond RC, Stuijfzand BG, et al. Evidence for causal effects of lifetime smoking on risk for depression and schizophrenia: A Mendelian randomisation study. *Psychol Med.* 2020;50(14):2435-2443. doi:10.1017/S003329171900 2678

30. Moreno-Peral P, Conejo-Cerón S, Motrico E, et al. Risk factors for the onset of panic and generalised anxiety disorders in the general adult population: A systematic

review of cohort studies. *J Affect Disord.* 2014;168:337-348. doi:10.1016/j.jad.2014.06.021

31. Zimmermann M, Chong AK, Vechiu C, Papa A. Modifiable risk and protective factors for anxiety disorders among adults: A systematic review. *Psychiatry Res.* 2020;285. doi:10.1016/j.psychres.2019.112705

32. Taylor GMJ, Lindson N, Farley A, et al. Smoking cessation for improving mental health. *Cochrane Database Syst Rev.* 2021;3(3):CD013522. Published 2021 Mar 9. doi:10.1002/14651858.CD013522.pub2

33. Kim AS, Ko HJ, Kwon JH, Lee JM. Exposure to secondhand smoke and risk of cancer in never smokers: A meta-analysis of epidemiologic studies. *Int J Environ Res Public Health.* 2018;15(9):1981. doi:10.3390/ijerph15091981

34. Digiacomo SI, Jazayeri MA, Barua RS, Ambrose JA. Environmental tobacco smoke and cardiovascular disease. *Int J Environ Res Public Health.* 2019;16(1). doi:10.3390/ijerph16010096

35. Yin P, Jiang CQ, Cheng KK, et al. Passive smoking exposure and risk of COPD among adults in China: the Guangzhou Biobank Cohort Study. *Lancet.* 2007;370:751-757. doi:10.1016/S0140-6736(07)61378-6.

36. Strzelak A, Ratajczak A, Adamiec A, Feleszko W. Tobacco smoke induces and alters immune responses in the lung triggering inflammation, allergy, asthma, and other lung diseases: A mechanistic review. *Int J Environ Res Public Health.* 2018;15(5):1033. doi:10.3390/ijerph15051033

37. Akinbami LJ, Kit BK, Simon AE. Impact of environmental tobacco smoke on children with asthma. *Acad Pediatr.* 2013;13:508-516.

38. du Preez K, Mandalakas AM, Kirchner HL, et al. Environmental tobacco smoke exposure increases Mycobacterium tuberculosis infection risk in children. *Int J Tuberc Lung Dis.* 2011;15(11):1490-1497. doi:10.5588/ijtld.10.0759

39. Wyss AB, Hashibe M, Lee YCA, et al. Smokeless tobacco use and the risk of head and neck cancer: Pooled analysis of US studies in the INHANCE consortium. *Am J Epidemiol.* 2016;184(10):703-716. doi:10.1093/aje/kww075

40. Sinha DN, Suliankatchi RA, Gupta PC, et al. Global burden of all-cause and cause-specific mortality due to smokeless tobacco use: Systematic review and meta-analysis. *Tob Control.* 2018;27(1):35-42. doi:10.1136/tobaccocontrol-2016-053302

41. Sinha DN, Gupta PC, Kumar A, et al. The poorest of poor suffer the greatest burden from smokeless tobacco use: A study from 140 countries. *Nicotine Tob Res.* 2018;20(12):1529-1532. doi:10.1093/ntr/ntx276

42. Jha P, Ramasundarahettige C, Landsman V, et al. 21st-Century hazards of smoking and benefits of cessation in the United States. *N Engl J Med.* 2013;368(4):341c350. doi:10.1056/nejmsa1211128

43. Buchanan ND, Grimmer JA, Tanwar V, Schwieterman N, Mohler PJ, Wold LE. Cardiovascular risk of electronic cigarettes: A review of preclinical and clinical studies. *Cardiovasc Res.* 2020;116(1):40-50. doi:10.1093/cvr/cvz256

44. Gotts JE, Jordt SE, McConnell R, Tarran R. What are the respiratory effects of e-cigarettes? *BMJ.* 2019;366. doi:10.1136/bmj.l5275

45. Lindson N, Butler AR, McRobbie H, et al. Electronic cigarettes for smoking cessation. *Cochrane Database Syst Rev.* 2024;2024(1):CD010216. doi:10.1002/14651858.CD010216.pub8

46. Krishnasamy VP, Hallowell BD, Ko JY, et al. Update: Characteristics of a nationwide outbreak of e-cigarette, or vaping, product use-associated lung injury—United States. *MMWR Morb Mortal Wkly Rep.* 2020;69(3):90-94.

47. Birdsey J, Cornelius M, Jamal A, et al. Tobacco product use among U.S. middle and high school students—National Youth Tobacco Survey, 2023. *MMWR Morb Mortal Wkly Rep.* 2023;72(44):1-10.

48. American Lung Association. *Trends in Cigarette Smoking Rates.* American Lung Association. May 30, 2024. Accessed July 31, 2024. Available at: https://www.lung.org/research/trends-in-lung-disease/tobacco-trends-brief/overall-smoking-trends

49. Cornelius ME, Loretan CG, Jamal A, et al. Tobacco product use among adults—United States, 2021. *MMWR Morb Mortal Wkly Rep.* 2023;72(18):475-483.

50. World Health Organization. *WHO Global Report on Trends in Prevalence of Tobacco Use 2000–2025,* 4th ed. World Health Organization; 2021. Accessed July 5, 2024. Available at: https://www.who.int/publications/i/item/9789240039322

51. Mordor Intelligence. Tobacco market size & share analysis—growth trends & forecasts (2023–2028). 2023. Accessed October 30, 2023. Available at: https://www.mordorintelligence.com/industry-reports/global-tobacco-market-industry

52. Grand View Research. Tobacco market size, share & trends analysis report. 2023. Accessed October 30, 2023. Available at: https://www.grandviewresearch.com/industry-analysis/tobacco-market

53. Federal Trade Commission. *Federal Trade Commission Cigarette Report for 2022.* 2023. Accessed July 5, 2024. Available at: https://www.ftc.gov/reports/federal-trade-commission-cigarette-report-2022-smokeless-tobacco-report-2022

54. Donny EC, Denlinger RL, Tidey JW, et al. Randomized trial of reduced-nicotine standards for cigarettes. *NEJ M.* 2015;373(14):1340-1349. doi:10.1056/nejmsa1502403

55. Staal Y, Havermans A, van Nierop L, et al. Conceptual model for the evaluation of attractiveness, addictiveness and toxicity of tobacco and related products: The example of JUUL e-cigarettes. *Regul Toxicol Pharmacol.* 2021;127. doi:10.1016/j.yrtph.2021.105077

56. Rossheim ME, Livingston MD, Krall JR, et al. Cigarette use before and after the 2009 flavored cigarette ban. *J Adolesc Health.* 2020;67(3):432-437. doi:10.1016/j.jadohealth.2020.06.022

57. Courtemanche CJ, Palmer MK, Pesko MF. Influence of the flavored cigarette ban on adolescent tobacco use. *Am J Prev Med.* 2017;52(5):e139-e146. doi:10.1016/j.amepre.2016.11.019

58. Parker MA, Villanti AC, Quisenberry AJ, et al. Tobacco product harm perceptions and new use. *Pediatrics.* 2018;142(6):e20181505. doi:10.1542/peds.2018-1505

59. Song AV, Morrell HER, Cornell JL, et al. Perceptions of smoking-related risks and benefits as predictors of adolescent smoking initiation. *Am J Public Health.* 2009;99(3):487-492. doi:10.2105/AJPH.2008.137679

60. Pulakka A, Halonen JI, Kawachi I, et al. Association between distance from home to tobacco outlet and smoking cessation and relapse. *JAMA Intern Med.* 2016;176(10):1512-1519. doi:10.1001/jamainternmed.2016.4535

61. Chaloupka FJ, Straif K, Leon ME. Effectiveness of tax and price policies in tobacco control. *Tob Control.* 2011;20(3):235-238. doi:10.1136/tc.2010.039982

62. Choi K, Hennrikus DJ, Forster JL, Moilanen M. Receipt and redemption of cigarette coupons, perceptions of cigarette companies and smoking cessation. *Tob Control.* 2013;22(6):418-422. doi:10.1136/tobaccocontrol-2012-050539

63. Friedman AS, Buckell J, Sindelar JL. Tobacco-21 laws and young adult smoking: quasi-experimental evidence. *Addiction.* 2019;114(10):1816-1823. doi:10.1111/add.14653

64. Licht AS, Hyland AJ, O'Connor RJ, et al. How do price minimizing behaviors impact smoking cessation? Findings from the international tobacco control (ITC) four country survey. *Int J Environ Res Public Health.* 2011;8(5):1671-1691. doi:10.3390/ijerph8051671

65. Office of the Surgeon General. *Preventing Tobacco Use Among Youth and Young Adults: A Report of the Surgeon General.* 2012. Accessed July 4, 2024. Available at: https://www.hhs.gov/sites/default/files/preventing-youth-tobacco-use-exec-summary.pdf

66. Robertson L, Cameron C, McGee R, Marsh L, Hoek J. Point-of-sale tobacco promotion and youth smoking: A meta-analysis. *Tob Control.* 2016;25(e2):e83-e89. doi:10.1136/tobaccocontrol-2015-052586

67. Yong HH, Chow R, East K, et al. Do social norms for cigarette smoking and nicotine vaping product use predict trying nicotine vaping products and attempts to quit cigarette smoking amongst adult smokers? Findings from the 2016–2020 International Tobacco Control Four Country Smoking and Vaping Surveys. *Nicotine Tob Res.* 2023;25(3):505-513. doi:10.1093/ntr/ntac212

68. Hoek J, Edwards R, Waa A. From social accessory to societal disapproval: Smoking, social norms and tobacco endgames. *Tob Control.* 2022;31(2):358-364. doi:10.1136/tobaccocontrol-2021-056574

69. Saffer H, Chaloupka F. The effect of tobacco advertising bans on tobacco consumption. *J Health Econ.* 2000;19(6):1117-1137. doi:10.1016/S0167-6296(00)00054-0

70. World Health Organization. *WHO Report on the Global Tobacco Epidemic, 2023 Protect People from Tobacco Smoke.* 2023. Accesed December 11, 2024. Available at: https://www.who.int/publications/i/item/9789240077164

71. McAfee T, Davis KC, Alexander RL, Pechacek TF, Bunnell R. Effect of the first federally funded US antismoking national media campaign. *Lancet.* 2013;382(9909):2003–2011. doi:10.1016/S0140-6736(13)61686-4

72. Bala MM, Strzeszynski L, Topor-Madry R. Mass media interventions for smoking cessation in adults. *Cochrane Database Syst Rev.* 2017;11(11). doi:10.1002/14651858.CD004704.pub4

73. Semple S, Dobson R, O'Donnell R, et al. Smoke-free spaces: A decade of progress, a need for more? *Tob Control.* 2022;31(2):250-256. doi:10.1136/tobaccocontrol-2021-056556

74. Hartmann-Boyce J, Chepkin SC, Ye W, Bullen C, Lancaster T. Nicotine replacement therapy versus control for smoking cessation. *Cochrane Database Syst Rev.* 2018;5(5):CD000146. Published 2018 May 31. doi:10.1002/14651858.CD000146.pub5

75. Livingstone-Banks J, Fanshawe TR, Thomas KH, et al. Nicotine receptor partial agonists for smoking cessation. *Cochrane Database Syst Rev.* 2023;5(5):CD006103. Published 2023 May 5. doi:10.1002/14651858.CD006103.pub8

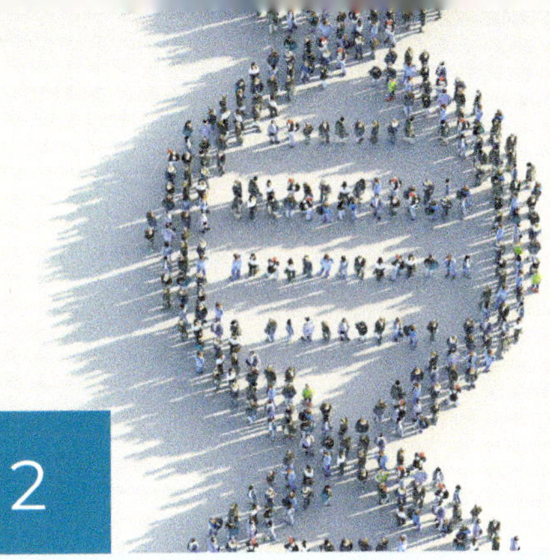

CHAPTER 12

Alcohol Use

Alcohol, or more precisely, **ethyl alcohol** or **ethanol**, is the world's most used drug. It has wide-ranging biologic effects, damaging nearly every organ system. Alcohol can kill by causing intentional or unintentional injuries, liver disease, heart disease, stroke, and cancer. Some health risks (for example, cancer) are found in all persons who drink, some (for example, injuries) are found more in people who occasionally "binge" drink, and some (for example, severe alcohol withdrawal) are found only in people who are addicted to alcohol. Globally, alcohol is responsible for some 2.6 million deaths per year, which is far less than the number killed by tobacco, but far more than the number killed by all illicit drugs combined.[1]

While humans will probably always drink alcohol, many deaths could be prevented if people were to drink less than they do today. There are big differences in drinking levels between populations, which suggests that reducing alcohol consumption at the population level is possible.

Alcohol and Alcoholic Beverages

Ethanol is a very small, simple molecule with the chemical formula CH_3—CH_2—OH (**Figure 12.1**). It is produced by micro-organisms from sugars through **fermentation**. Fermentation naturally takes place in food that is stored at warm temperatures and low oxygen levels, so alcohol has been known and used by humans for thousands of years.

U.S. government regulations classify alcoholic beverages into three types: beer, wine, and **distilled spirits**. Beer is fermented from grains and wine is fermented from grapes or other fruits. Distilled spirits are produced by distillation of fermented products, which greatly concentrates the ethanol. The final products contain very different concentrations of ethanol. Beer is about 5% ethanol and wine about 12%—although fortified wine like sherry or port is about

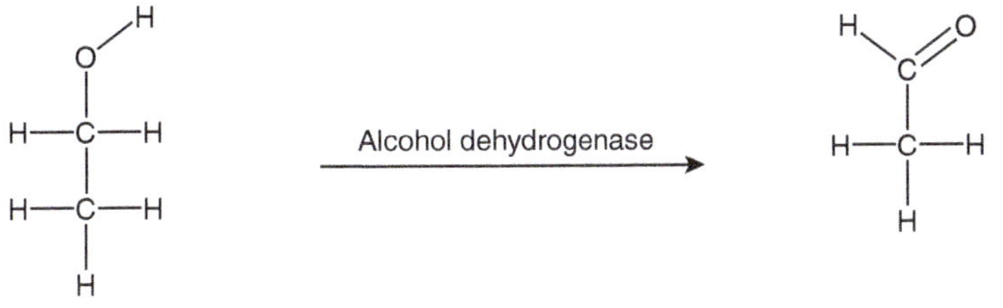

Alcohol dehydrogenase

Ethanol
Ethyl alcohol

Acetaldehyde

Figure 12.1 Ethanol and the Main Product of Its Metabolism, Acetaldehyde.

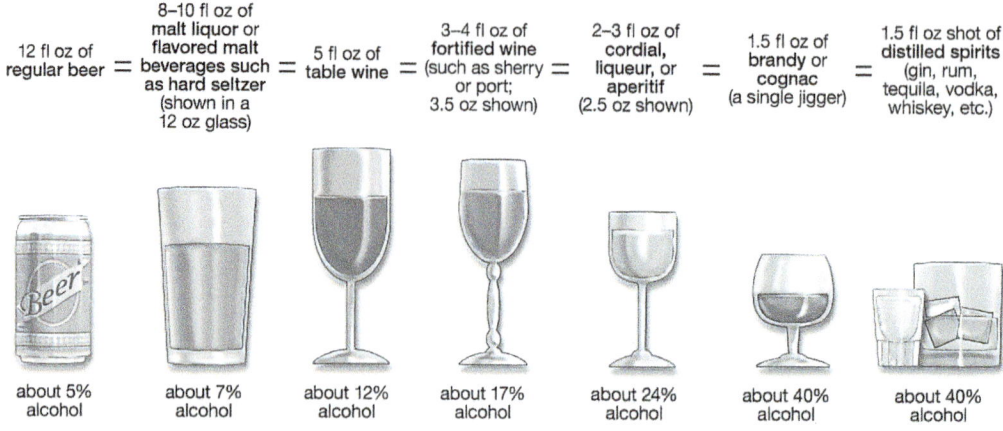

12 fl oz of regular beer = 8–10 fl oz of malt liquor or flavored malt beverages such as hard seltzer (shown in a 12 oz glass) = 5 fl oz of table wine = 3–4 fl oz of fortified wine (such as sherry or port; 3.5 oz shown) = 2–3 fl oz of cordial, liqueur, or aperitif (2.5 oz shown) = 1.5 fl oz of brandy or cognac (a single jigger) = 1.5 fl oz shot of distilled spirits (gin, rum, tequila, vodka, whiskey, etc.)

about 5% alcohol | about 7% alcohol | about 12% alcohol | about 17% alcohol | about 24% alcohol | about 40% alcohol | about 40% alcohol

Each drink shown above represents one U.S. standard drink and has an equivalent amount (0.6 fluid ounces) of "pure" ethanol.

Figure 12.2 Standard Drink Amounts.

National Institutes of Alcohol Abuse and Alcoholism. Alcohol's Effect on Health: What Is A Standard Drink? Accessed July 31, 2024. https://www.niaaa.nih.gov/alcohols-effects-health/overview-alcohol-consumption/what-standard-drink

17% ethanol. Distilled spirits like gin, whisky, and vodka are about 40% ethanol. The typical drink size of each beverage type gives drinkers about 0.6 fluid ounces (or 14 grams) of pure ethanol (**Figure 12.2**).

Physiology of Brain Cells

Humans drink alcohol because it changes how their brain cells (**neurons**) function. Neurons communicate with each other by sending and receiving small organic molecules called **neurotransmitters** across tiny gaps called **synapses**. Alcohol and other **psychoactive drugs** work by increasing or decreasing the amount of neurotransmitters sent by one neuron or received by another.

There are many neurotransmitters, and they work in different areas of the brain. Most neurons communicate using **glutamate** and **gamma-aminobutyric acid (GABA)**. Glutamate mostly stimulates the receiving neurons and GABA suppresses them. Neurotransmitters with more specialized roles in specific brain regions include **dopamine** and molecules that are chemically similar to heroin and oxycodone called **endogenous opioids**.

Pathophysiology of Alcohol Use

Alcohol alters the activity of these neurotransmitters.[2] However, its effects on neurotransmitters are indirect and weak, so it takes large doses for people to feel them. While a typical dose of a directly-acting neurotransmitter drug like oxycodone is about 15 milligrams, a standard dose of ethanol (one drink) is 14 grams—nearly a thousand times as large. That much ethanol circulating in the body, repeated frequently over years, causes damage throughout the body.[3,4]

The health effects of ethanol can be put into two broad categories: those involving the brain and those involving other organ systems (**Table 12.1**).

Alcohol and the Brain

Short-Term Effects. Two key effects of alcohol are believed to be related to the neurotransmitters GABA and dopamine:

- *Sedation.* Alcohol increases the activity of GABA, which suppresses neurons. The slower brain activity gives the person who drinks a feeling of relaxation, drowsiness, and reduced anxiety, as well as a slowed reaction time, difficulty reasoning, and reduced coordination.[2,5] This effect is why drinking very large amounts of alcohol—for example, a person consuming an entire bottle of whiskey over an hour—can cause a coma or even death from alcohol overdose.

- *Euphoria.* Alcohol increases dopamine activity in the brain's **reward circuit**, which gives drinkers a feeling of pleasure known as **euphoria**. The reward circuit is a network of neurons that gives a person a pleasurable sensation for doing something that is necessary for life or reproduction, such as eating, sleeping, or sex. (The reward circuit is discussed more in Chapter 13. Use of Addictive Drugs.) This circuit uses the neurotransmitter dopamine, and the circuit can be artificially stimulated by opioids and other popular addictive drugs. It appears that alcohol causes euphoria by triggering the release of endogenous opioids.[6]

Alcohol has other important short-term effects on the brain. These effects, like sedation and

Table 12.1 Diseases and Injuries Caused by Alcohol Use

Infectious Diseases

Tuberculosis

HIV/AIDS, other sexually transmitted diseases

Lower respiratory infections

Non-communicable Diseases

Cancer: colon & rectum, breast, pancreas, liver, esophagus, mouth

Mental illness: alcohol use disorder, primary epilepsy

Chronic metabolic diseases: chronic liver disease, pancreatitis

Cardiovascular diseases: ischemic heart disease*, ischemic stroke*, hypertensive heart disease, hemorrhagic stroke

Diseases of the newborn: fetal alcohol syndrome, fetal alcohol spectrum disorder

Injuries

Motor vehicle crashes

Firearms (assault, self-harm, and unintentional harm)

Falls (unintentional, self-harm)

Poisonings

Other unintentional

*Possible J-shaped curve of effect (see text).

Data from Babor TF, Casswell S, Graham K, et al. Alcohol: No Ordinary Commodity. 3rd Edition. Oxford: Oxford University Press; 2023, and Rehm J, Gmel GE, Gmel G, et al. The relationship between different dimensions of alcohol use and the burden of disease—an update. Addiction. 2017;112(6):968-1001.

euphoria, are likely caused by changes in neurotransmitters, but their mechanisms are less well understood:

- *Disinhibition*. Everyone has desires and impulses that they have been taught to resist, like responding to anger with threats or violence. Consumption of alcohol reduces these inhibitions, a drug effect called **disinhibition**.[7,8] That is why people who have been drinking are more impulsive and more likely to take social or physical risks—for example, by saying things that are embarrassing or offensive.

- *Aggression and violence*. Studies of both animals and humans show that alcohol causes men to be more aggressive and even violent.[9,10]

Long-Term Effects. Alcohol is an addictive drug. Not everyone who drinks regularly becomes addicted to alcohol, but then not everyone who uses heroin or cocaine regularly becomes addicted to them, either. People are said to have **alcohol use disorder** (formerly called alcoholism) if they cannot stop drinking despite having adverse social, occupational, or health consequences.

When people who drink repeatedly are deprived of alcohol, their neurons experience lower-than-normal levels of activity of the neurotransmitters stimulated by alcohol. This causes some regular drinkers to have the symptoms of alcohol **withdrawal**. With dopamine levels low, people in withdrawal feel **anhedonia**, which is an inability to experience pleasure.[2,11] With GABA levels low, their brain cells become excitable, which causes them to have anxiety, tremors, and agitation.[2] At its worst, alcohol withdrawal causes a potentially-deadly condition called **delirium tremens**, which involves extremely high blood pressure, hallucinations, and seizures. Even the early symptoms of withdrawal cause regular drinkers to crave alcohol, which can lead them to behave in socially-unacceptable or self-destructive ways to get it.

Chronic alcohol consumption also causes long-term damage to the brain, including dementia. This level of brain damage does not occur with chronic consumption of most other addictive drugs.[12,13] Heavy alcohol users have difficulty with memory, learning, intellectual ability, and coordination, and scans show that their brains shrink.[14]

Drinking alcohol regularly can also lead people to have social problems like conflicts with family members and coworkers, unemployment, housing instability, and homelessness. These social problems can prompt some people to drink even more, setting up a downward spiral of dependence on alcohol and alcohol use disorder.[15]

Alcohol and the Liver

After a drink, alcohol is quickly absorbed through the lining of the stomach and small intestine into the blood, which carries it to all organs and tissues.

Alcohol travels immediately to the liver, where it is converted to a closely-related chemical called **acetaldehyde** (Figure 12.1). When the enzymes responsible for this conversion are occupied with alcohol, they are less available to metabolize other toxic chemicals. That leaves people more susceptible to the toxic effects of other drugs, including recreational drugs and cancer-causing chemicals. In addition, the metabolism of alcohol interferes with the cells' ability to metabolize fatty acids. That leads to a buildup of fats in liver cells, called **fatty liver**.[12]

Acetaldehyde is toxic to many cells.[12] Short-term damage to liver cells from acetaldehyde is called **alcoholic hepatitis**. Long-term damage to liver cells from acetaldehyde and from the excess fat leads to a condition called **cirrhosis**, in which the liver is replaced with scar tissue and stops functioning. Mortality rates from cirrhosis have been rising in the United States since 2000, in parallel with increases in consumption of **distilled spirits**.[16-18] Chronic liver disease is discussed in more detail in Chapter 7. Chronic Metabolic Diseases.

Alcohol and Injuries

Alcohol's many effects on the brain combine to increase the risk of injuries. People under the influence of alcohol are more aggressive, less perceptive of risks, more likely to take risks that they do perceive, more impulsive, slower to react to risks, and less coordinated. The biggest problem this causes is motor vehicle crashes. In the United States, 30% of car-crash deaths involve a driver who is impaired by alcohol.[19] For the same reasons, alcohol increases the risk of nearly every other type of injury, including drownings, burns, sexual assaults, intimate partner violence, and child abuse.[15,20,21] Alcohol also

plays a key role in two other major types of injury: firearm violence and suicide.[20,21] The connection to firearm violence is partly explained by alcohol's stimulation of violent behavior in men. In addition, alcohol consumption among older adults increases the risk of falls.[22,23] Firearm violence, suicide, falls, and other injuries are discussed in more depth in Chapter 6. Injuries.

Figure 12.3 shows estimates by CDC researchers of the fraction of various fatal non-traffic injuries in the United States attributable to alcohol.[21] The researchers estimate that if people did not drink alcohol, fatal non-traffic injuries as a whole would decrease by about 25%.

Alcohol and Infectious Diseases

Alcohol damages the immune system in two key ways: it weakens the gastrointestinal tract's ability to prevent bacteria from entering the bloodstream and it reduces the number and effectiveness of immune cells.[15,24] With a weakened immune system, people who drink alcohol are more susceptible to infections. The relationship between alcohol and tuberculosis is particularly strong. Experts estimate that in countries where drinking is common, about 25% of tuberculosis cases can be attributed to alcohol use.[25] Alcohol use is also associated with

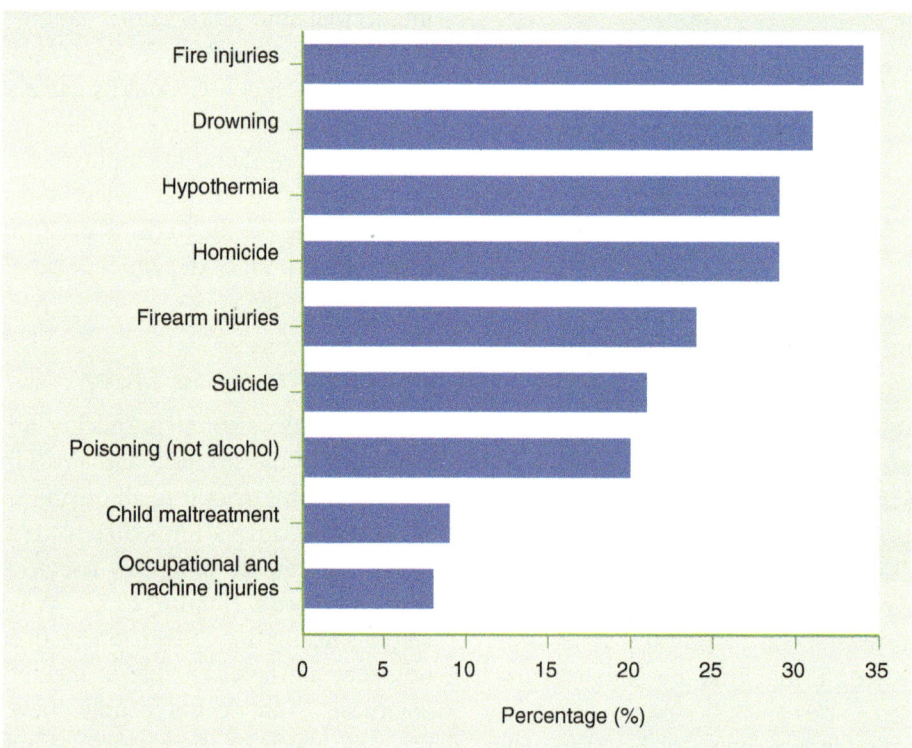

Figure 12.3 **Fractions of Different Types of Non-Traffic Fatal Injuries Attributable to Alcohol.**

Data from Alpert HR, Slater ME, Yoon Y-H et al. Alcohol consumption and 15 causes of fatal injuries: a systematic review and meta-analysis. *Am J Prev Med* 2022;63(2):286-300.

HIV/AIDS and other sexually transmitted diseases. This is in part because people who drink alcohol are more likely to take sexual risks and in part because alcohol may work together with HIV to damage the immune system.[15,26]

Alcohol and Cancer

Alcoholic beverages are classified by the U.S. Department of Health and Human Services as causing cancer, that is, they are **carcinogens**.[27] Acetaldehyde can damage DNA, and some contaminants of alcoholic beverages are also known or suspected to be carcinogens. Even people who drink no more than one drink per day have an increased risk of some cancers. An estimated 3.5% of cancer deaths in the United States (about 19,000 deaths per year) are attributable to alcohol consumption.[28,29]

The cancers most closely linked to alcohol are those involving the gastrointestinal tract, mouth and throat, liver, and breast.[28] Alcohol consumption increases the risk of colon cancer by about 50%.[12,28] The risk of breast cancer in women increases with the amount of alcohol they consume. Those drinking on average less than one drink per day have a 4% increase in risk, those averaging 1 to 3 drinks per day have about a 25% increase, and those drinking more than 3 drinks per day about a 60% increase in risk.[28]

Alcohol and Outcomes of Pregnancy

In pregnancy, alcohol crosses the placenta and damages the developing fetus. Pregnant women are more likely to have a miscarriage or a stillbirth.[30,31] If they drink heavily, they are more likely to deliver their babies preterm or with low birth weight.[32]

More important, babies who were exposed to alcohol during the pregnancy can have permanent brain damage.[33] Some of these children have a distinctive pattern of facial features called **fetal alcohol syndrome**, including a thin upper lip and a smooth ridge between the nose and upper lip (**Figure 12.4**). Many of these children also have small heads, shorter-than-average height, and lower-than-normal intelligence.[34] Studies of school-aged children have estimated that about 7 children per 1,000 in the United States have fetal alcohol syndrome.[35]

But fetal alcohol syndrome is only one of a larger group of conditions caused by alcohol exposure during pregnancy called **fetal alcohol spectrum disorders (FASD)**. Children with FASD most often do not have the physical features of fetal alcohol syndrome, but they may have other malformations. Or, more commonly, they have subtle signs of brain damage that are not noticed until they go to school. Adolescents with FASD have problems with learning, cognition, judgement, behavior, and mental illnesses.[34,36]

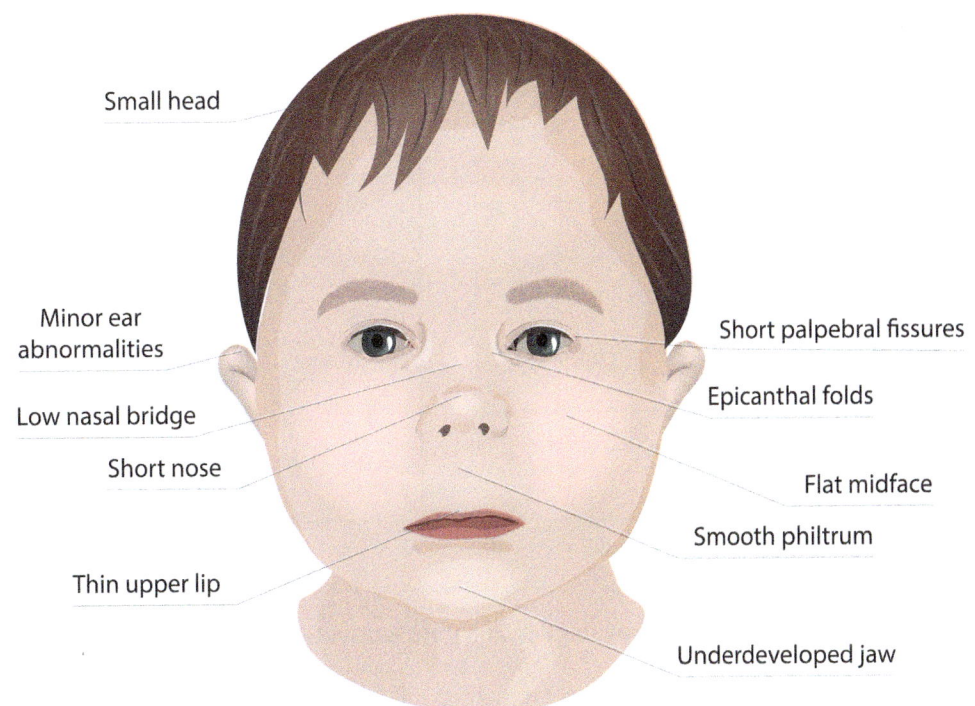

Figure 12.4 **Facial Features of Fetal Alcohol Syndrome.**
© Maniki_rus/Shutterstock

FASD is disturbingly common. Globally, about 0.8% of children have FASD, but rates are higher in Europe and the United States, where drinking is more common.[37] In the United States, conservative estimates are that between 1% and 5% of children (or approximately 30,000 to 180,000 infants born per year) have FASD.[38] The more alcohol consumed during pregnancy, the greater the risk of FASD.

Finally, young adults whose mothers drank during pregnancy are more likely to develop alcohol use disorders themselves.[39,40]

Experts recommend that women not consume any alcohol during pregnancy.[34] And because damage may occur before women even know that they are pregnant, experts recommend that women of childbearing age avoid alcohol even if they think they might become pregnant. These recommendations are not being followed: globally, about 10% of women drink alcohol during pregnancy.[41] In the United States, 14% of women report on surveys that they drank alcohol while pregnant, and 5% report binge drinking.[42]

Alcohol and the Heart

The effect of alcohol on cardiovascular disease is not fully clear, despite decades of studies. One consistent finding is that drinking alcohol increases the risk of high blood pressure and the risk of the type of stroke linked to high blood pressure known as a **hemorrhagic stroke**.[43,44] Alcohol's effect on blood pressure is reversible—that is, if people quit or reduce their drinking, their blood pressure falls.[44] But alcohol's effect on **ischemic heart disease** and ischemic stroke is complex. Many studies have found that while heavy drinkers have a higher risk of ischemic heart disease, people who drink only one to two drinks per day have a *lower* risk of ischemic heart disease and ischemic stroke than people who do not drink at all.[44-46] This is what has been called the "J-shaped" curve (**Figure 12.5**).

However, there are reasons to question whether the J-shaped curve accurately describes the risk. Most studies rely on people answering surveys to indicate how much alcohol they drink. This study design may be biased. Some heavy drinkers who are embarrassed about their drinking may claim that they do not drink. More important, people who have quit drinking because they are already experiencing symptoms of disease (so-called "sick quitters") may be classified as non-drinkers. In contrast to these survey-based studies, a study of over 500,000 persons in China, which took advantage of a biologic marker for alcohol consumption, did not find a J-shaped curve.[47] And some studies that tried to address the possible biases of traditional studies in other ways likewise did not find a J-shaped curve.[48,49] The firmest conclusion we

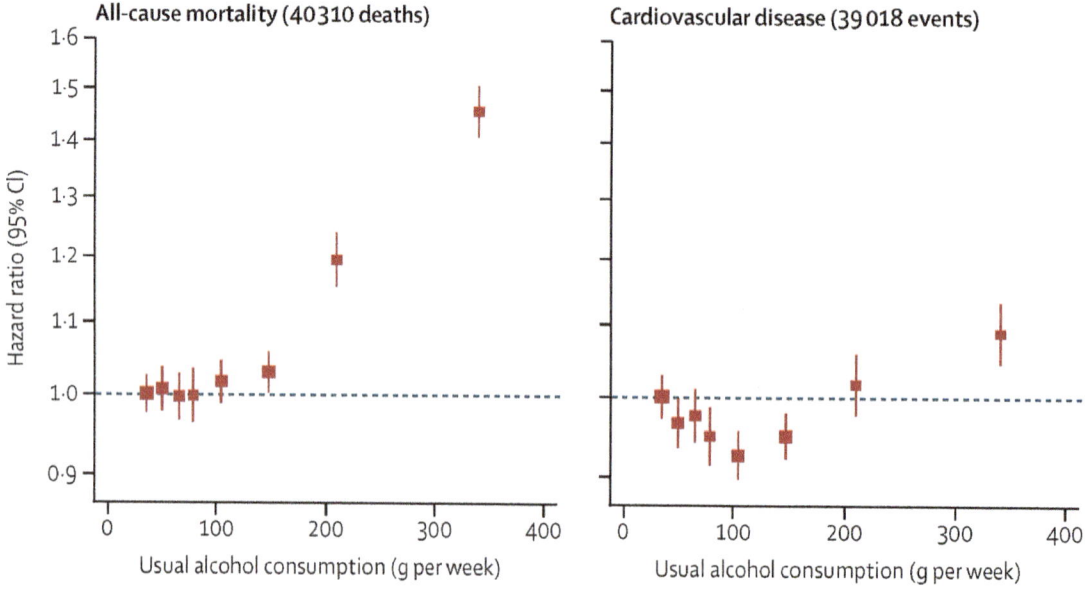

Figure 12.5 **Relationship Between Alcohol Consumption and Cardiovascular Events (Right) and All-Cause Mortality (Left).** Some studies have found that people who drink one or two alcoholic drinks per day (100–200 g per week) have a lower risk of cardiovascular disease than non-drinkers (graph on right). However, these studies do not generally show a reduced mortality in light drinkers, and they show a sharp increase in mortality in people who drink more than this (graph on left).

Wood AM, Kaptoge S, Butterworth A, et al. Risk thresholds for alcohol consumption: combined analysis of individual-participant data for 599 912 current drinkers in 83 prospective studies. The Lancet. 2018;391(10129):1513-1523.

can draw today is that drinking one to two alcoholic drinks per day *may* reduce the risk of ischemic heart disease and ischemic stroke.

Overall Health Effects of Alcohol

Studies of the effect of alcohol on mortality have some of the same complexity as studies of the effect of alcohol on ischemic heart disease. That is, some studies show a "J-shaped curve," with lower mortality risk in people who drink one drink per day.[50] However, recent studies that attempt to eliminate all possible biases do not show a lower mortality risk in light drinkers (Figure 12.5).[45,48,51]

More important, there is no question that drinking more than two drinks per day substantially increases the risk of death because of all of the other ways that alcohol damages the human body.[45,52] Even if people who drink one drink per day have a lower risk than those who abstain, enough people drink more alcohol than this that, for entire populations, the damage greatly outweighs the benefit.[50]

The CDC estimates that alcohol is responsible for 178,000 deaths per year in the United States and the World Health Organization estimates that it is responsible for 2.6 million deaths per year worldwide.[1,53] This means that alcohol consumption is responsible for more deaths worldwide than HIV/AIDS, diabetes, motor vehicle crashes, or violence.[1] In the United States, the main way that alcohol kills is through injuries, which cause of more than one-third of alcohol-attributable deaths (**Figure 12.6**).[54] Liver disease and cardiovascular disease each cause about 25% of these deaths. Globally, while injuries and liver disease are still the most common causes of alcohol-attributable deaths, infectious diseases (particularly HIV/AIDS) make up about 10%.[1]

Epidemiology: Patterns and Trends of Alcohol Use

Alcohol use is measured in populations either with data on sales of alcoholic beverages or through surveys. On surveys, a drink is considered to be 12 ounces of beer, 5 ounces of wine, or 1.5 ounces of distilled spirits (see Figure 12.2).

A little more than half of Americans over age 18 are alcohol users, defined as drinking at least one drink per month. **Binge drinking** (or **heavy episodic drinking**) is defined as drinking 5 or more drinks (for men) or 4 or more drinks (for women) on a single occasion. Binge drinking is very common: about 25% of adults in the United States report binge drinking at least once a month.[55] And about 6% of Americans report **heavy alcohol use**, which is defined as binge drinking on 5 or more days per month.[55]

Drinking is most common in young adults and falls with age after that (**Figure 12.7**). Men drink more than women (**Figure 12.8**). Whites drink more than people in other racial and ethnic groups, and—in contrast to many other risky behaviors—people with

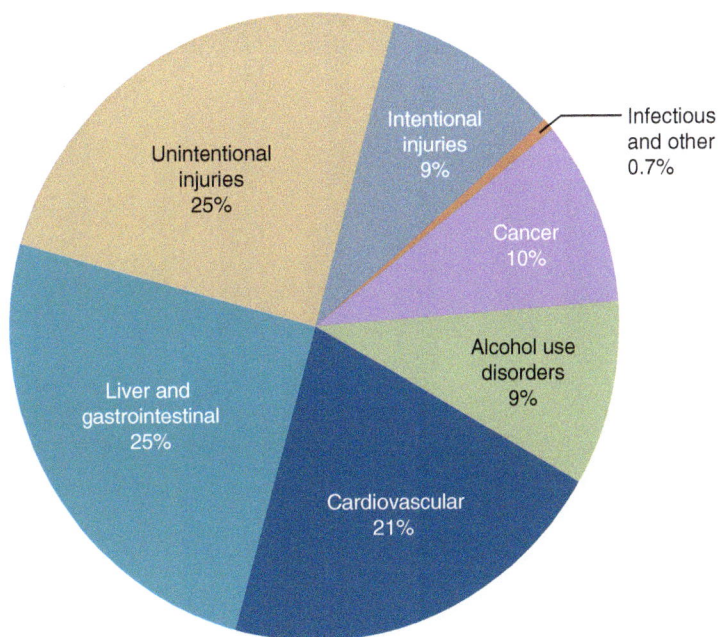

Figure 12.6 Deaths Attributable to Alcohol Use in the United States, by Disease Category, 2020–2021.

Data from Centers for Disease Control and Prevention. Alcohol-Related Disease Impact (ARDI) Application. Accessed July 8, 2024. https://nccd.cdc.gov/DPH_ARDI/Default/Default.aspx

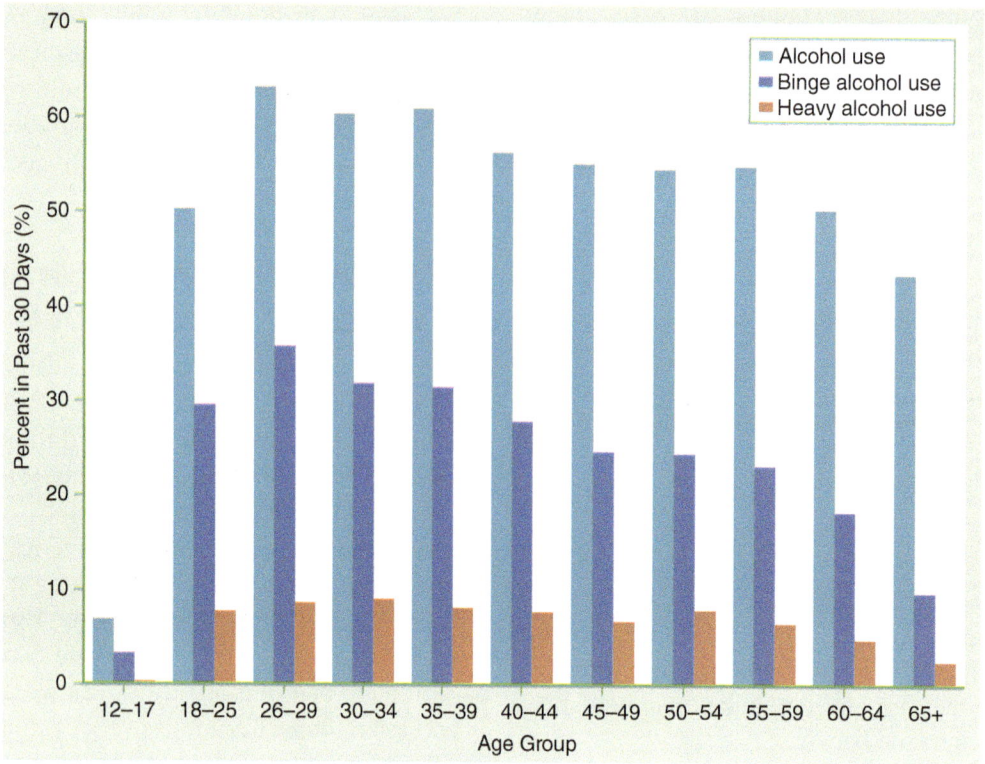

Figure 12.7 Alcohol Use in the United States by Age Group, 2022.

Data from Substance Use and Mental Health Services Administration. National Survey of Drug Use and Health: National Release for 2022. Accessed July 26, 2024. https://www.samhsa.gov/data/nsduh/national-releases

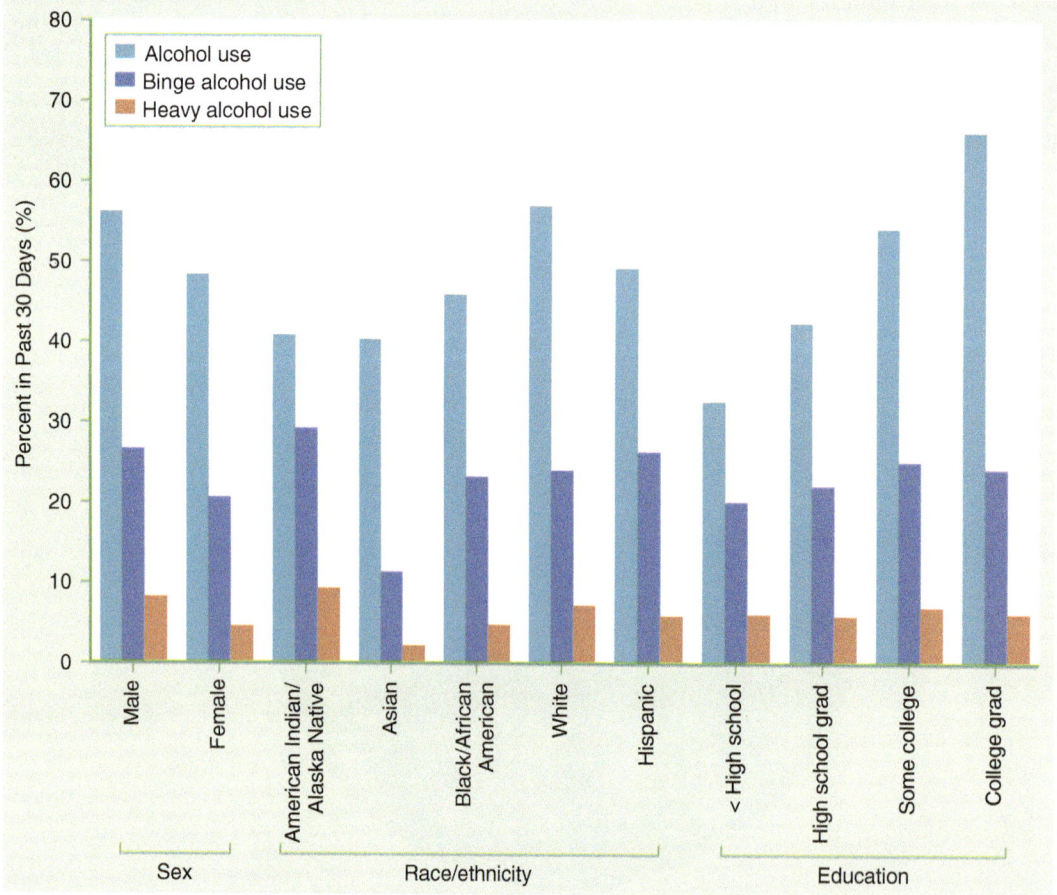

Figure 12.8 Alcohol Use Among Adults in the United States by Demographic Group, 2022.

Data from Substance Use and Mental Health Services Administration. National Survey of Drug Use and Health: National Release for 2022. Accessed July 26, 2024. https://www.samhsa.gov/data/nsduh/national-releases

higher levels of education drink more (Figure 12.8). Alcohol addiction is common: about 11% of men and 9% of women are dependent enough on alcohol that they meet the criteria for alcohol use disorder.[55]

The amount of alcohol that people drink varies greatly around the world. The places with the highest per capita alcohol consumption are Russia and Eastern European countries (about 9 liters per capita per year), with the Americas not far behind (about 7.5 liters per capita per year). The countries with the lowest consumption are in the Middle East and Eastern Mediterranean (below 1 liter per capita per year).[1] Overall, alcohol consumption is higher in higher-income countries.[1]

The distribution of alcohol consumption within a population tends to fall on a curve like those shown in **Figure 12.9**. The greatest percentage of the population drink relatively low amounts of alcohol, a smaller percent abstains, and there is a long tail on the right side of the curve of people who drink heavily.[4] The general shape of this curve is the same across populations, but the peak and the width of the curve vary markedly.

Figure 12.9 shows two hypothetical populations. Population A has a lower average alcohol consumption than population B. With the entire curve shifted,

population A also has a much smaller percent of its people who drink more than *x*—that is, heavy drinkers. This pattern is fairly consistent around the world; countries with a lower average alcohol consumption also have fewer heavy drinkers.[4,56] The goal of health policy is to shift the curve toward the left, reducing both the average consumption and the percentage of people who are heavy drinkers.

Risk Factors

Studies point to these factors as increasing alcohol use in populations (**Figure 12.10**):

- *Alcohol availability and accessibility.* Where there are more retail locations that sell alcohol (for example, bars and liquor stores), people drink more alcohol and have more alcohol-related harms like injuries, crime, and violence.[4,57] In other words, while the demand for alcohol partly determines the supply, the retail supply of alcohol also influences demand. Closely related to availability is accessibility—how easily people can obtain alcohol. The more accessible alcohol is, the more people drink. Most important to accessibility is price. Basic principles of economics hold

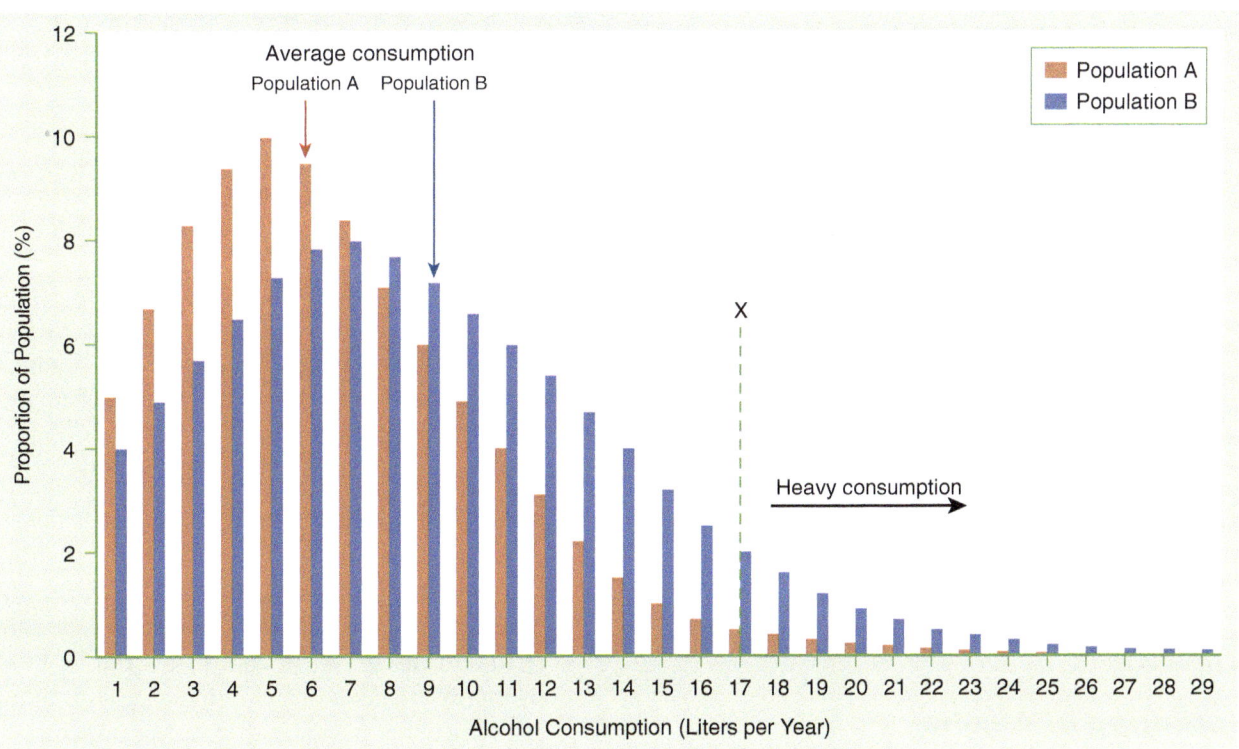

Figure 12.9 Hypothetical Distribution of Alcohol Consumption in Two Populations. Population A has a lower average alcohol consumption than population B. With the entire curve shifted, population A also has a much smaller percent of its people who drink more than *x*–that is, heavy drinkers. The goal of health policy is to shift the curve toward the left, reducing both the average consumption and the percentage of people who are heavy drinkers.

Data from Babor TF, Casswell S, Graham K, et al. Alcohol: No Ordinary Commodity. 3rd Edition. Oxford: Oxford University Press; 2023.

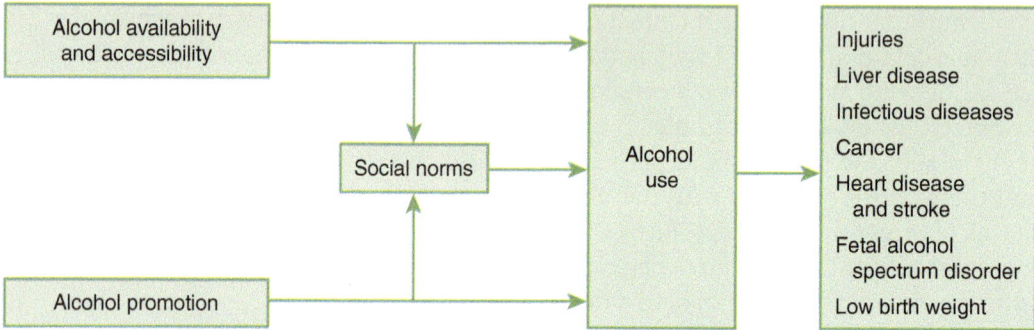

Figure 12.10 Cause-and-Effect Diagram for Alcohol Use.

with alcohol: lower prices lead to more alcohol sales, more consumption, and more alcohol-related harms.[4] For adolescents, accessibility depends on whether alcohol can legally be sold to minors and how much the law is enforced.[4]

- *Alcohol promotion.* While most countries today prohibit or limit advertising of tobacco, most still allow advertising of alcohol. Also, alcohol is promoted in many ways beyond advertising, for example, with sponsorships of sports teams and community events, product placements in movies, and social media influencer campaigns. Not surprisingly, advertising and other forms of promotion increase alcohol consumption, including hazardous drinking.[4]
- *Social norms.* Drinking alcohol is more accepted in some populations than others. Where social norms are more accepting of alcohol consumption, people drink more. For example, alcohol use is very low in Islamic countries with religious disapproval of drinking.[1] In contrast, people drink more in countries with long histories of producing wine, beer, or distilled spirits.[1] At a much smaller scale, college students in the United States drink more if they believe that alcohol use is more common and more supported by their peers.[58] The advertising and promotion of alcohol by manufacturers influences social norms by presenting drinking as popular among people that viewers admire.[59] Similarly, if there is widespread availability and accessibility of alcohol, it sends a message that alcohol use is a social norm, which encourages alcohol consumption.

Marketing of Alcohol

The availability, accessibility, and promotion of alcohol do not happen on their own. They are paid for by companies that sell alcohol. This marketing can be thought of as the most important modifiable risk factor for alcohol consumption.

The global alcohol market is increasingly controlled by a small number of multinational companies (**Table 12.2**). In the United States, more than half of sales in each category were made by the top two beer companies, the top three wine companies, and the top five spirits companies.[60] This market dominance makes advertising a good return on investment for the big companies, so they advertise heavily. For example, Anheuser-Busch InBev is the ninth largest advertiser in the world, spending more than $6 billion globally per year, not including spending for other types of promotion.[60] These big companies are now increasing their alcohol promotion in low- and middle-income countries, such as in India and Sub-Saharan Africa.[60] Both globally and locally, the alcohol companies are a large enough economic force that they influence governments to enact public policies that support alcohol sales.[4,61]

Preventive Interventions
Primary Prevention

Fortunately, much work has been done in the United States by the Community Preventive Services Task Force and globally by the World Health Organization and others to clarify the interventions that could reduce the damage caused by alcohol. Interventions that they have endorsed include (**Figure 12.11**):[4,62,63]

- *Increases in alcohol prices through taxes or minimum prices.* Raising alcohol prices leads to less drinking and less alcohol-related health damage, from motor vehicle crashes to cirrhosis to mortality from all causes[4,64,65] Alcohol prices can be raised by increasing taxes or by setting a legal minimum sales price that is higher than current prices.[4]
- *Reductions in the number of retail alcohol outlets.* Studies have generally shown that changes in the number of alcohol retail outlets (such as bars and liquor stores) have parallel effects on how much alcohol people drink and the damage caused by

Table 12.2 The Ten Largest Alcohol Companies Worldwide

Corporation	Country of Registration	Sales (billions)	Profits (billions)
Anheuser-Busch InBev	Belgium	$59.4	$5.3
Heineken	Netherlands	$32.8	$1.3
Diageo	United Kingdom	$20.4	$4.0
Asahi Group Holdings	Japan	$19.6	$1.2
Kweichow Niytau	China	$18.6	$10.9
Kirin Holdings	Japan	$15.1	$0.9
Pernod Ricard	France	$12.6	$2.2
Carlsberg	Denmark	$10.7	$5.9
Wuliangye Yibin	China	$10.3	$4.4
Constellation Brands	United States	$10.0	$1.7

Data from The Global 2000, 2024. Accessed March 21, 2025. https://www.forbes.com/lists/global2000/

alcohol. Alcohol drinking and the resulting harms of alcohol can be reduced, then, by reducing the number of retail outlets.[57,66]

- *Restrictions on the hours and days of alcohol sales.* Increasing the hours during which alcohol can be sold increases alcohol-related harms.[57,62] Likewise, increasing the days on which alcohol can be sold (generally, repealing prohibition on sales on Sundays) increases drinking and related problems, like motor vehicle crashes.[57,62] Maintaining or tightening these restrictions would help prevent those harms.

- *Dram shop liability.* In some places, the owner or server of a bar or other alcohol outlet is legally responsible for harms caused by a customer to whom they served alcohol. This is called **dram shop liability**, and it discourages bar owners and servers from selling drinks to people who are or might become intoxicated. This liability has been shown to reduce deaths from car crashes, which are often caused by drunk drivers.[67]

- *Enhanced enforcement of laws prohibiting sales to minors.* While it is illegal to sell alcohol to minors in the United States, this law is not consistently

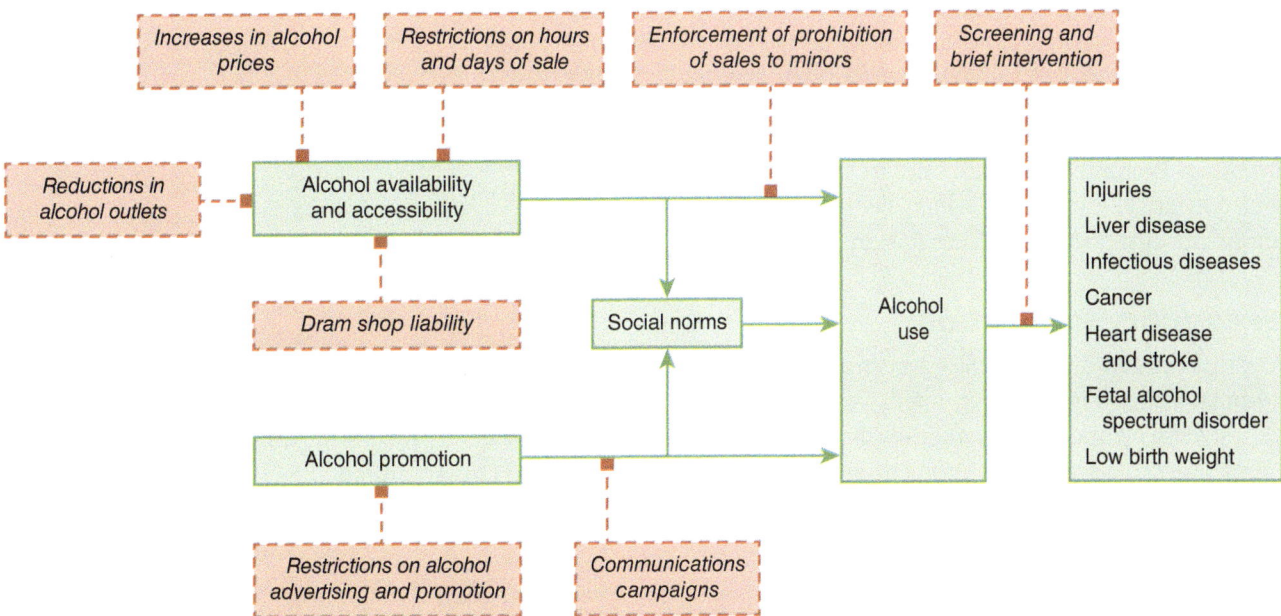

Figure 12.11 Cause-and-Effect Diagram for Alcohol Use, with Preventive Interventions.

enforced. Enforcement of these laws with compliance checks or "sting operations" at retail stores reduces alcohol sales to under age persons.[62]

In some states and countries, retail sales of some or all alcoholic beverages are or have been controlled by the government through "state stores." When alcohol sales have been turned over to private businesses, there have been large increases in alcohol sales. With this in mind, the Community Preventive Service Task Force recommends against privatization of retail alcohol sales.[62]

Alcohol use may also be reduced by countering the promotion of alcohol by manufacturers. This can be done in two ways: *prohibitions or restrictions on alcohol advertising and other promotional activities* by alcohol companies, or balancing their promotion with *communications campaigns* that educate people about the harms of alcohol use. There is not good evidence so far that advertising restrictions or communications campaigns reduce alcohol consumption, but these approaches have been very effective in reducing tobacco use.[68,69] The World Health Organization recommends that countries enact bans on alcohol advertising, sponsorship, and promotion.[63] In addition, the kind of hard-hitting counter-advertising that has been effective in reducing smoking could be tried for alcohol use.

Other interventions that have helped reduce smoking likewise could be tried to reduce alcohol use. The United States government requires alcohol companies to include warnings about health risks on their bottles. But these warnings are just words that are difficult to read and easy to ignore. Governments could instead require *graphic warning labels* containing pictures of people suffering from the harms of alcohol, like those required on cigarette packages in many countries. And *prohibitions on drinking alcohol in public places*, similar to smoke-free laws, may reduce the social acceptability of drinking. Prohibiting alcohol sales in sports stadiums and concert venues, from which people drive home afterwards, may be good places to start.

Secondary Prevention

Most of the funding by U.S. government agencies to address alcohol is used for intensive treatment for people with alcohol use disorder. While this treatment helps individuals with this problem, it cannot have a population-level benefit because only 8% of people with alcohol use disorder receive this treatment, and it does nothing for non-addicted alcohol users.[70]

For individuals who drink heavily, many studies have found that *screening and brief intervention*

programs in medical settings reduce alcohol use. This intervention involves asking individuals a few questions about their drinking habits and then offering brief tailored advice to those who admit to binge drinking.[62] The intervention can be done in person or electronically with a computer or smart phone. However, it is unclear if this intervention can reach enough heavy drinkers to affect an entire population.

Box 12.1 Summary–Prevention of Alcohol Use

- Increases in alcohol prices through taxes or minimum prices
- Reductions in the number of retail alcohol outlets
- Restrictions on the hours and days of alcohol sales
- Dram shop liability
- Enhanced enforcement of laws prohibiting sales to minors
- Prohibitions or restrictions on alcohol advertising and other promotional activities
- Communications campaigns educating about the harms of alcohol use
- Screening and brief intervention for excessive alcohol use

Box 12.2 Key Words–Alcohol Use

Acetaldehyde
Alcohol use disorder
Alcoholic hepatitis
Anhedonia
Binge drinking
Carcinogen
Cirrhosis
Delerium tremens
Dementia
Disinhibition
Distilled spirits
Dopamine
Dram shop liability
Endogenous opioids
Ethanol, ethyl alcohol
Euphoria
Fatty liver
Fermentation
Fetal alcohol spectrum disorders (FASD)
Fetal alcohol syndrome
Gamma-aminobutyric acid (GABA)
Glutamate
Heavy alcohol use
Heavy episodic drinking
Hemorrhagic stroke

Ischemic heart disease
Neuron
Neurotransmitter
Psychoactive drugs
Reward circuit
Synapse
Withdrawal

Resources–Alcohol Use

- Babor TF, Casswell S, Graham K, et al. *Alcohol: No Ordinary Commodity*. 3rd Edition. Oxford: Oxford University Press; 2023. This is a thorough review by experts on the policy approaches to reducing alcohol's harms.
- National Institute on Alcohol Abuse and Alcoholism. *Alcohol Facts and Statistics Fact Sheet*, available at https://www.niaaa.nih.gov contains useful data on alcohol use and its impacts.
- National Cancer Institute. Alcohol and cancer risk, available at https://www.cancer.gov/about-cancer/causes-prevention/risk/alcohol/alcohol-fact-sheet. This contains useful data on the cancer risks of alcohol.
- Volkow ND, Blanco C. Substance use disorders: a comprehensive update of classification, epidemiology, neurobiology, clinical aspects, treatment and prevention. *World Psychiatry*. 2023;22(2):203-229. doi:10.1002/wps.21073. This provides an excellent summary of the biology of alcohol and drug use, as well as current approaches to treatment.
- World Health Organization. *The Technical Package: A World Free from Alcohol Related Harms*, available at www.who.int. This report summarizes the WHO's strategy for addressing alcohol risks.
- World Health Organization. *WHO Global Status Report on Alcohol and Health and Treatment of Substance Abuse Disorders*, available at www.who.int. This contains an in-depth compilation of data on alcohol use and its harms globally and for each country.

References

1. World Health Organization. *WHO Global Status Report on Alcohol and Health and Treatment of Substance Abuse Disorders*. Geneva, Switzerland: World Health Organization; 2024. Accessed July 8, 2024. Available at: https://www.who.int/publications/i/item/9789240096745

2. Lovinger DM. Communication networks in the brain neurons, receptors, neurotransmitters, and alcohol. *Alcohol Res Health*. 2008;31(3):196-2014.

3. Rehm J, Gmel GE, Gmel G, et al. The relationship between different dimensions of alcohol use and the burden of disease—an update. *Addiction*. 2017;112(6):968-1001. doi:10.1111/add.13757

4. Babor TF, Casswell S, Graham K, et al. *Alcohol: No Ordinary Commodity*. 3rd ed. Oxford University Press; 2023. doi:10.1093/oso/9780192844484.001.0001

5. Volkow ND, Michaelides M, Baler R. The neuroscience of drug reward and addiction. *Physiol Rev*. 2019;99(4):2115-2140. doi:10.1152/physrev.00014.2018

6. Cruz MT, Bajo M, Schweitzer P, Roberto M, Dorris HL. Shared mechanisms of alcohol and other drugs. *Alcohol Res Health*. 2008;31(2):137-147.

7. Grant NK, MacDonald TK. Can alcohol lead to inhibition or disinhibition? Applying alcohol myopia to animal experimentation. *Alcohol Alcohol*. 2005;40(5):373-378. doi:10.1093/alcalc/agh177

8. Källmén H, Gustafson R. Alcohol and disinhibition. *Eur Addict Res*. 1998;4(4):150-162. doi:10.1159/000018948

9. Miczek KA, Debold JF, Hwa LS, Newman EL, de Almeida RMM. Alcohol and violence: Neuropeptidergic modulation of monoamine systems. *Ann N Y Acad Sci*. 2015;1349(1):96-118. doi:10.1111/nyas.12862

10. Crane CA, Godleski SA, Przybyla SM, Schlauch RC, Testa M. The proximal effects of acute alcohol consumption on male-to-female aggression: A meta-analytic review of the experimental literature. *Trauma Violence Abuse*. 2016;17(5):520-531. doi:10.1177/1524838015584374

11. Bahji A, Crockford D, El-Guebaly N. Neurobiology and symptomatology of post-acute alcohol withdrawal: A mixed-studies systematic review. *J Stud Alcohol Drugs*. 2022;83(4):461-469. doi:10.15288/jsad.2022.83.461

12. Kumar V, Abbas AK, Aster JC. Effects of alcohol. In: Kumar V, Abbas AK, Aster JC, Turner JR, eds. *Robbins & Cotran Pathologic Basis of Disease*. 10th ed. Elsevier; 2021:418-420.

13. Palm A, Vataja R, Talaslahti T, et al. Incidence and mortality of alcohol-related dementia and Wernicke-Korsakoff syndrome: A nationwide register study. *Int J Geriatr Psychiatry*. 2022;37(8). doi:10.1002/gps.5775

14. Ridley NJ, Draper B, Withall A. Alcohol-related dementia: An update of the evidence. *Alzheimers Res Ther*. 2013;5:3. doi:10.1186/alzrt157

15. Centers for Disease Control and Prevention. Alcohol use and your health. CDC. Published April 14, 2022. Accessed August 8, 2023. Available at: https://www.cdc.gov/alcohol/fact-sheets/alcohol-use.htm

16. Dang K, Hirode G, Singal AK, Sundaram V, Wong RJ. Alcoholic liver disease epidemiology in the United States: A retrospective analysis of 3 US databases. *Am J Gastroenterol*. 2020;115(1):96-104. doi:10.14309/ajg.0000000000000380

17. Slater ME, Alpert HR. Surveillance Report #120 Apparent per capita alcohol consumption: National, state, and regional trends 1977–2021. NIAAA Research Surveillance Reports. Published April 2023. Accessed March 8, 2024. Available at: https://www.niaaa.nih.gov/publications/surveillance-reports/surveillance120

18. Chen CM, Yoon YH. Surveillance Report #118. Liver cirrhosis mortality in the United States: National, state, and regional

trends, 2000–2019. NIAAA Surveillance Reports. Published February 2022. Accessed March 8, 2024. Available at https://www.niaaa.nih.gov/publications/surveillance-reports/surveillance118

19. National Highway Traffic Safety Administration. Traffic Safety Facts: A Compilation of Motor Vehicle Crash Data (Table 13). Published 2020. Accessed August 10, 2023. Available at: https://cdan.dot.gov/tsftables/tsfar.htm#

20. Branas CC, Han S, Wiebe DJ. Alcohol use and firearm violence. *Epidemiol Rev.* 2016;38(1):32-45. doi:10.1093/epirev/mxv010

21. Alpert HR, Slater ME, Yoon YH, Chen CM, Winstanley N, Esser MB. Alcohol consumption and 15 causes of fatal injuries: A aystematic review and meta-analysis. *Am J Prev Med.* 2022;63(2):286-300. doi:10.1016/j.amepre.2022.03.025

22. Xu Q, Ou X, Li J. The risk of falls among the aging population: A systematic review and meta-analysis. *Front Public Health.* 2022;10:902599. doi:10.3389/fpubh.2022.902599

23. Sun Y, Zhang B, Yao Q, et al. Association between usual alcohol consumption and risk of falls in middle-aged and older Chinese adults. *BMC Geriatr.* 2022;22(1). doi:10.1186/s12877-022-03429-1

24. Trevejo-Nunez. Alcohol as risk factor for infection. *Alcohol Res.* 2015;37(2):177-184.

25. Rehm J, Samokhvalov AV., Neuman MG, et al. The association between alcohol use, alcohol use disorders and tuberculosis (TB). A systematic review. *BMC Public Health.* 2009;9(450). doi:10.1186/1471-2458-9-450

26. Bagby G, Amedee A, Siggins R, Molina P, Nelson S, Veazey R. Alcohol and HIV effects on the immune system. *Alcohol Research.* 2015;37(2):287-297.

27. National Toxicology Program. *Report on Carcinogens, Fifteenth Edition.* 2021. Accessed August 10, 2023. Available at: https://ntp.niehs.nih.gov/whatwestudy/assessments/cancer/roc

28. National Cancer Institute. Alcohol and cancer risk. Cancer.gov. Published July 14, 2021. Accessed August 8, 2023. https://www.cancer.gov/about-cancer/causes-prevention/risk/alcohol/alcohol-fact-sheet

29. Goding Sauer A, Fedewa SA, Bandi P, et al. Proportion of cancer cases and deaths attributable to alcohol consumption by US state, 2013–2016. *Cancer Epidemiol.* 2021;71:101893. doi:10.1016/j.canep.2021.101893

30. Odendaal H, Dukes KA, Elliott AJ, et al. Association of prenatal exposure to maternal drinking and smoking with the risk of stillbirth. *JAMA Netw Open.* 2021. doi:10.1001/jamanetworkopen.2021.21726

31. Sundermann AC, Zhao S, Young CL, et al. Alcohol use in pregnancy and miscarriage: A systematic review and meta-analysis. *Alcohol Clin Exp Res.* 2019;43(8):1606-1616. doi:10.1111/acer.14124. Epub

32. Patra J, Bakker R, Irving H, Jaddoe VWV, Malini S, Rehm J. Dose-response relationship between alcohol consumption before and during pregnancy and the risks of low birthweight, preterm birth, and small for gestational age (SGA): A4 systematic review and meta-analyses. *BJOG.* 2011;118(12):1411-1421. doi:10.1111/j.1471-0528.2011.03050.x

33. Riley EP, Infante MA, Warren KR. Fetal alcohol spectrum disorders: An overview. *Neuropsychol Rev.* 2011;21(2):73-80. doi:10.1007/s11065-011-9166-x

34. Williams JF, Smith VC. Fetal alcohol spectrum disorders. *Pediatrics.* 2015;136(5):e1395-e1406. doi:10.1542/peds.2015-3113

35. May PA, Baete A, Russo J, et al. Prevalence and characteristics of fetal alcohol spectrum disorders. *Pediatrics.* 2014;134(5):855-866. doi:10.1542/peds.2013-3319

36. Astley SJ. Profile of the first 1,400 patients receiving diagnostic evaluations for fetal alcohol spectrum disorder at the Washington State Fetal Alcohol Syndrome Diagnostic & Prevention Network. *Can J Clin Pharmacol.* 2010;17(1):e132-3164.

37. Lange S, Probst C, Gmel G, Rehm J, Burd L, Popova S. Global prevalence of fetal alcohol spectrum disorder among children and youth: A systematic review and meta-analysis. *JAMA Pediatr.* 2017;171(10):948-956. doi:10.1001/jamapediatrics.2017.1919

38. May PA, Chambers CD, Kalberg WO, et al. Prevalence of fetal alcohol spectrum disorders in 4 US communities. *JAMA.* 2018;319(5):474-482. doi:10.1001/jama.2017.21896

39. Alati R, Al Mamun A, Williams GM, O'Callaghan M, Najman JM, Bor W. In utero alcohol exposure and prediction of alcohol disorders in early adulthood. *Arch Gen Psychiatry.* 2006;63(9):1009. doi:10.1001/archpsyc.63.9.1009

40. Stone AL, Becker LG, Huber AM, Catalano RF. Review of risk and protective factors of substance use and problem use in emerging adulthood. *Addict Behav.* 2012;37(7):747-775. doi:10.1016/j.addbeh.2012.02.014

41. Popova S, Lange S, Probst C, Gmel G, Rehm J. Estimation of national, regional, and global prevalence of alcohol use during pregnancy and fetal alcohol syndrome: a systematic review and meta-analysis. *Lancet Glob Health.* 2017;5(3):e290-e299. doi:10.1016/S2214-109X(17)30021-9

42. Gosdin LK, Deputy NP, Kim SY, Dang EP, Denny CH. Alcohol consumption and binge drinking during pregnancy among adults aged 18–49 Years—United States, 2018–2020. *MMWR Morb Mortal Wkly Rep.* 2022;71(1). doi:10.15585/mmwr.mm7101a2

43. Roerecke M, Tobe SW, Kaczorowski J, et al. Sex-specific associations between alcohol consumption and incidence of hypertension: A systematic review and meta-analysis of cohort studies. *J Am Heart Assoc.* 2018;7(13). doi:10.1161/JAHA.117.008202

44. Roerecke M. Alcohol's impact on the cardiovascular system. *Nutrients.* 2021;13(10). doi:10.3390/nu13103419

45. Wood AM, Kaptoge S, Butterworth A, et al. Risk thresholds for alcohol consumption: combined analysis of individual-participant data for 599,912 current drinkers in 83 prospective studies. *Lancet.* 2018;391(10129):1513-1523. doi:10.1016/S0140-6736(18)30134-X

46. Rehm J, Shield KD, Roerecke M, Gmel G. Modelling the impact of alcohol consumption on cardiovascular disease mortality for comparative risk assessments: An overview. *BMC Public Health.* 2016;16(1). doi:10.1186/s12889-016-3026-9

47. Millwood IY, Walters RG, Mei XW, et al. Conventional and genetic evidence on alcohol and vascular disease aetiology: a prospective study of 500,000 men and women in China. *Lancet.* 2019;393(10183):1831-1842. doi:10.1016/S0140-6736(18)31772-0

48. Hu C, Huang C, Li J, et al. Causal associations of alcohol consumption with cardiovascular diseases and all-cause mortality among Chinese males. *Am J Clin Nutr.* 2022;116(3). doi:10.1093/ajcn/nqac159

49. Biddinger KJ, Emdin CA, Haas ME, et al. Association of habitual alcohol intake with risk of cardiovascular disease. *JAMA Netw Open*. 2022;5(3):E223849. doi:10.1001/jamanetworkopen.2022.3849

50. Bryazka D, Reitsma MB, Griswold MG, et al. Population-level risks of alcohol consumption by amount, geography, age, sex, and year: a systematic analysis for the Global Burden of Disease Study 2020. *Lancet*. 2022;400(10347):185-235. doi:10.1016/S0140-6736(22)00847-9

51. Zhao J, Stockwell T, Naimi T, Churchill S, Clay J, Sherk A. Association between daily alcohol intake and risk of all-cause mortality: A systematic review and meta-analyses. *JAMA Netw Open*. 2023;6(3):E236185. doi:10.1001/jamanetworkopen.2023.6185

52. Griswold MG, Fullman N, Hawley C, et al. Alcohol use and burden for 195 countries and territories, 1990–2016: A systematic analysis for the Global Burden of Disease Study 2016. *Lancet*. 2018;392(10152):1015-1035. doi:10.1016/S0140-6736(18)31310-2

53. Esser MB, Sherk A, Liu Y, Naimi TS. Deaths from excessive alcohol se—United States, 2016–2021. *MMWR Morb Mortal Wkly Rep*. 2024;73(8):154-161. doi:10.15585/mmwr.mm7308a1

54. Centers for Disease Control and Prevention. Alcohol-Related Disease Impact. Centers for Disease Control and Prevention. Published 2024. Accessed July 7, 2024. Available at: https://nccd.cdc.gov/DPH_ARDI/default/Default.aspx

55. Substance Use and Mental Health Services Administration. 2022 National Survey on Drug Use and Health Detailed Tables. Published 2024. Accessed July 8, 2024. Available at: https://www.samhsa.gov/data/report/2022-nsduh-detailed-tables

56. Rossow I, Mäkelä P. Public health thinking around alcohol-related harm: Why does per capita consumption matter? *J Stud Alcohol Drugs*. 2021;82(1). doi:10.15288/jsad.2021.82.9

57. Sherk A, Stockwell T, Chikritzhs T, et al. Alcohol consumption and the physical availability of take-away alcohol: Systematic reviews and meta-analyses of the days and hours of sale and outlet density. *J Stud Alcohol Drugs*. 2018;79(1). doi:10.15288/jsad.2017.79.58

58. Krieger H, Neighbors C, Lewis MA, Labrie JW, Foster DW, Larimer ME. Injunctive norms and alcohol consumption: A revised conceptualization. *Alcohol Clin Exp Res*. 2016;40(5):1083-1092. doi:10.1111/acer.13037

59. Petticrew M, Shemilt I, Lorenc T, et al. Alcohol advertising and public health: Systems perspectives versus narrow perspectives. *J Epidemiol Community Health (1978)*. 2017;71(3):308-312. doi:10.1136/jech-2016-207644

60. Jernigan D, Ross CS. The alcohol marketing landscape: Alcohol industry size, structure, strategies, and public health responses. *J Stud Alcohol Drugs*. 2020;(Suppl 19):13-25.

61. McCambridge J, Mitchell G, Lesch M, et al. The emperor has no clothes: a synthesis of findings from the Transformative Research on the Alcohol industry, Policy and Science research programme. *Addiction*. 2023;118(3):558-566. doi:10.1111/add.16058

62. The Community Guide. Excessive Alcohol Consumption. Guide to Community Preventive Services. Published July 28, 2023. Accessed August 8, 2023. https://www.thecommunityguide.org/topics/excessive-alcohol-consumption.html

63. World Health Organization. *The SAFER Technical Package: A World Free from Alcohol Related Harms*. 2019. Accessed July 8, 2024. Available at: https://www.who.int/publications/i/item/9789241516419

64. Elder RW, Lawrence B, Ferguson A, et al. The effectiveness of tax policy interventions for reducing excessive alcohol consumption and related harms. *Am J Prev Med*. 2010;38(2):217-229. doi:10.1016/j.amepre.2009.11.005

65. Guindon GE, Zhao K, Fatima T, et al. Prices, taxes, and alcohol use: A systematic umbrella review. *Addiction*. 2022;117(12):3004-3023. doi:10.1111/add.15966

66. Campbell CA, Hahn RA, Elder R, et al. The effectiveness of limiting alcohol outlet density as a means of reducing excessive alcohol consumption and alcohol-related harms. *Am J Prev Med*. 2009;37(6):556-569. doi:10.1016/j.amepre.2009.09.028

67. Rammohan V, Hahn RA, Elder R, et al. Effects of dram shop liability and enhanced overservice law enforcement initiatives on excessive alcohol consumption and related harms: Two community guide systematic reviews. *Am J Prev Med*. 2011;41(3):334-343. doi:10.1016/j.amepre.2011.06.027

68. Siegfried N, Pienaar DC, Ataguba JE, et al. Restricting or banning alcohol advertising to reduce alcohol consumption in adults and adolescents. *Cochrane Database Systc Rev*. 2014;2017(12). doi:10.1002/14651858.CD010704.pub2

69. Young B, Lewis S, Katikireddi SV, et al. Effectiveness of mass media campaigns to reduce alcohol consumption and harm: A systematic review. *Alcohol Alcohol*. 2018;53(3):302-316. doi:10.1093/alcalc/agx094

70. National Institute on Alcohol Abuse and Alcoholism. Alcohol Facts and Statistics Fact Sheet. Published 2020. Accessed July 8, 2024. Available at: https://www.niaaa.nih.gov/sites/default/files/AlcoholFactsAndStats.pdf

CHAPTER 13

Use of Addictive Drugs

The use of addictive drugs is a public health problem that resists simple solutions.

At its core, the problem is that people like how these drugs make them feel, but when they use the drugs, they harm themselves and others. The harms can result from the drugs themselves, from the chemicals that accompany the drugs, or from the things that people do to acquire drugs. Societies have tried to limit those harms by prohibiting some drugs, only to see social harms tied to that prohibition, like violence between drug-selling gangs. The goal of a public health approach to addictive drugs should be to minimize the health damage from the combination of the drugs and the drug markets.

This chapter describes the biology and epidemiology of addictive drug use and then lays out some principles of how to minimize the damage. These principles are particularly important today, as countries are reconsidering their approach to marijuana and other addictive drugs.

Addiction and Addictive Drugs

Physiology: The Reward Circuit

The brain is a massive network of **neurons** (brain cells) connected to each other through long, wire-like structures called **axons** (**Figure 13.1**) and shorter tentacles called **dendrites**. The neurons send signals to each other, much like transistors inside a computer send signals to each other, in the form of small electrical currents that run down the axons. When the currents reach the ends of

the axons, they release packets of chemicals called **neurotransmitters** into the tiny gaps (called **synapses**) between them and dendrites of the receiving neurons. The neurotransmitters travel across the gaps and fit into **receptors** on the receiving neurons' dendrites. When a receptor receives a neurotransmitter, it either stimulates or suppresses the receiving neuron, depending on which neurotransmitter it is.

In the 1950s, researchers implanted electrodes into the brains of rats and rigged the apparatus so that rats could give their brains tiny jolts of electricity by pressing a bar. When the researchers inserted the electrodes into a brain region called the **medial forebrain bundle**, the rats pressed the bar incessantly, up to 5,000 times per hour, some until they collapsed from exhaustion.[1] The researchers had discovered the brain's **reward circuit** (or **reward pathway**), a specialized network of neurons that make the brain's owner feel pleasure. This circuit is activated when the owner does something critical to survival or procreation, like eat or mate. If rats could talk, they would probably say that when they pressed the bar, they felt a rush of pleasure, which humans call a "high" and medical experts call **euphoria**.

The researchers thought that this reward circuit might also be involved in drug addiction. Today, experts believe that all addictive drugs stimulate the reward circuit in some way.[2]

Central to the reward circuit are what can be called dopamine **reward neurons**, which live in a brain region called the **ventral tegmental area** (**Figures 13.2** and **13.3**). These reward neurons are connected through their axons to neurons in a nearby

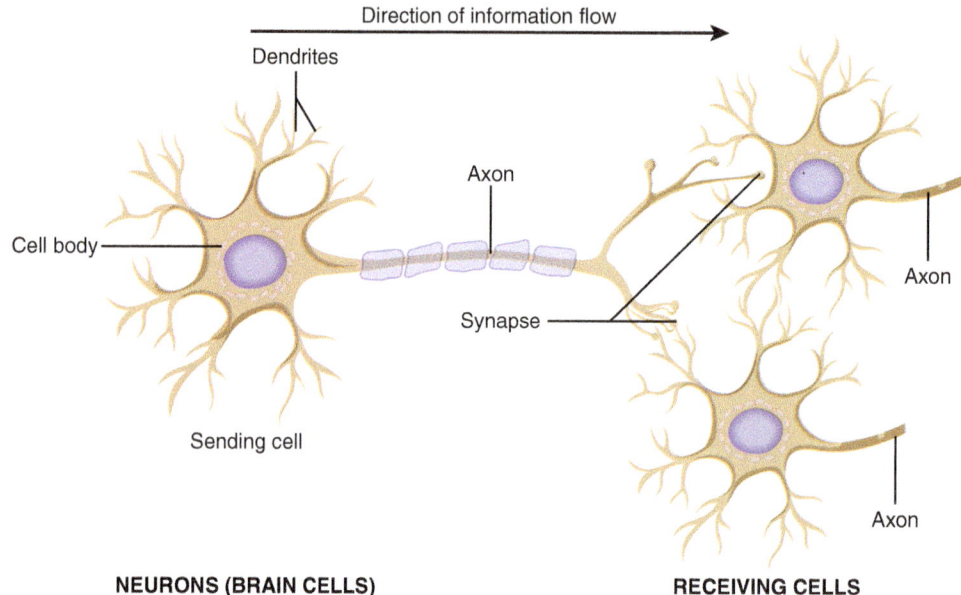

Figure 13.1 Neurons and their Connections. The brain operates by neurons sending electrical signals to each other through their axons and dendrites. The interfaces between the axon of one neuron and a dendrite of another neuron is called a synapse. The neurons communicate across the synapses by sending and receiving chemicals called neurotransmitters. These neurotransmitters play key roles in both mental illness and drug addiction.

brain region called the **nucleus accumbens**. Their axons are part of the medial forebrain bundle that was stimulated by the rat researchers. When that median forebrain bundle is stimulated with electricity, the axons behave as if the reward neurons were sending signals to the nucleus accumbens. These signals arrive as a flood of the neurotransmitter **dopamine** in the synapses between the reward neurons and the receiving neurons, which are called **medium spiny neurons** (Figure 13.3).[2]

The reward circuit has additional connections (Figure 13.2). The reward neurons in the ventral

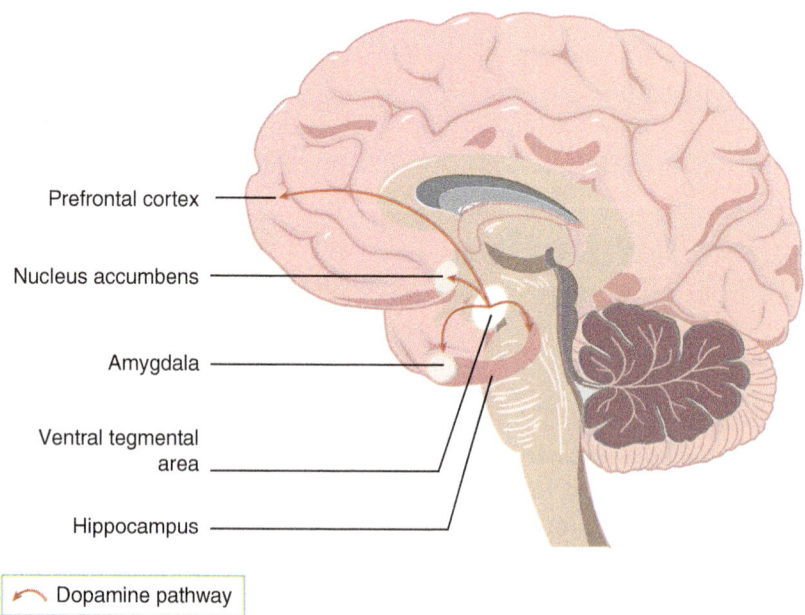

Figure 13.2 The Brain and the Reward Circuit. Central to the reward circuit are what can be called dopamine reward neurons, which live in the ventral tegmental area and are connected through their axons to neurons in the nucleus accumbens. The reward neurons in the ventral tegmental area also connect to the hippocampus and the amygdala—which are involved in memory, mood, and emotional events—and to the prefrontal cortex, which is a brain center responsible for planning and executing complex behaviors.

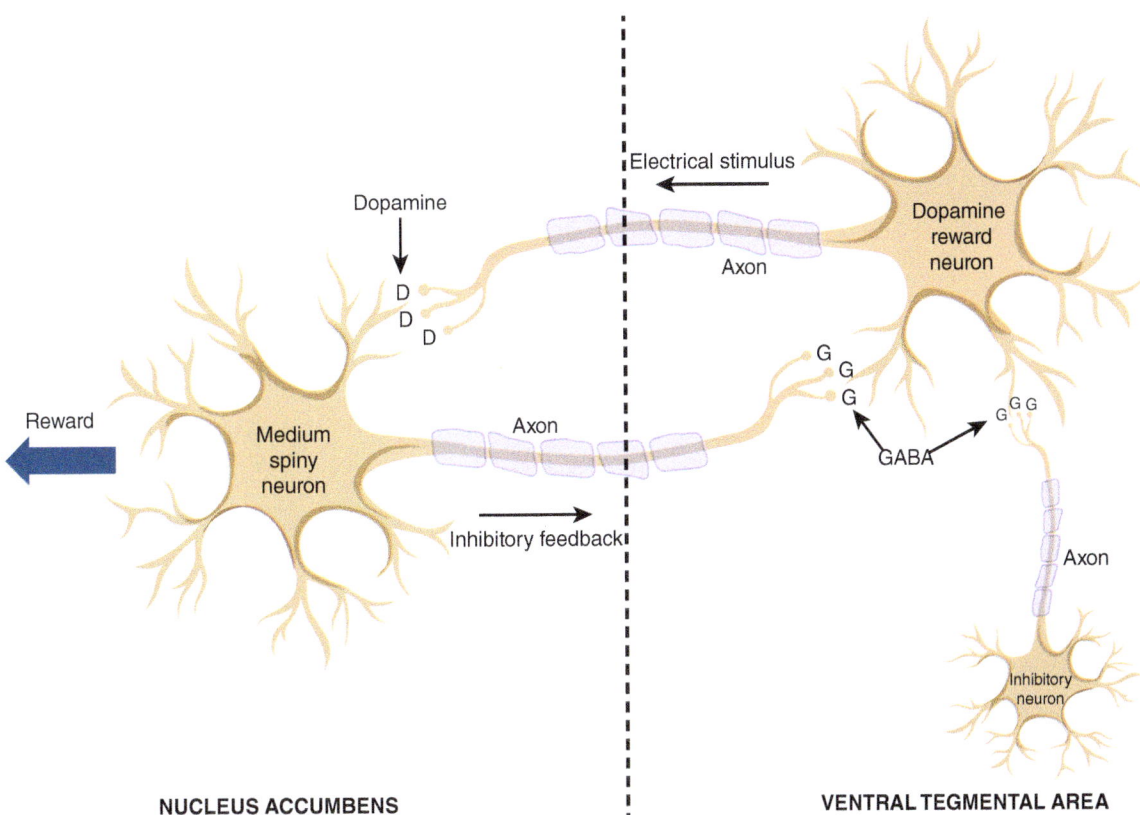

Figure 13.3 Interactions Among Neurons in the Reward Circuit. The dopamine reward neurons send electrical signals to the nucleus accumbens, where their axons release dopamine to medium spiny neurons. This causes euphoria. The medial spiny neurons in the nucleus accumbens and inhibitory neurons in the ventral tegmental area connect back to the dopamine reward neurons and dampen them by sending a neurotransmitter called GABA. This feedback prevents the positive messages from running out of control.

Data from Volkow ND, Michaelides M, Baler R. The neuroscience of drug reward and addiction. Physiol Rev. 2019;99(4):2115-2140. doi:10.1152/physrev.00014.2018

tegmental area also connect to regions of the brain called the **hippocampus** and the **amygdala**, which are involved in memory, mood, and emotional events.[2] These connections presumably enable the rat to remember what exactly the rat did to create the positive experience, for example, where he found food or a willing mate. The reward circuit also connects to the **prefrontal cortex**, which is a brain center responsible for planning and executing complex behaviors.[2] That connection presumably helps the rat find food or a mate in the future, based on what he remembers about how the rat did it before.

The reward circuit also has feedback connections. The medial spiny neurons in the nucleus accumbens and **inhibitory neurons** in the ventral tegmental area connect back to the dopamine reward neurons and dampen them by sending a neurotransmitter called **gamma-aminobutyric acid** or **GABA** (Figure 13.3).[3] This feedback inhibits the dopamine reward neuron, which prevents the positive messages from running out of control, like brakes on a car. Some addictive drugs have their stimulating effect by reducing this inhibition.

Drugs That Stimulate the Reward Circuit

People use addictive drugs for the euphoria. All addictive drugs are believed to create this feeling by stimulating this reward circuit, but they each do it in a different way.[2] **Table 13.1** lists the most popular addictive drugs and the forms in which users take the drugs. **Figure 13.4** shows where in the reward circuit these drugs work.

Here's a summary of these drugs and how they are believed to act on the reward circuit:

- *Nicotine* is in tobacco leaves and the liquids of electronic cigarettes. This drug has effects throughout the brain. Among them, nicotine stimulates the reward neurons on the ventral tegmental area, which increases their release of dopamine in the nucleus accumbens.[4]
- *Cocaine* is extracted from the leaves of the coca plant. It is sold as a powder (cocaine "salts"), which is usually absorbed through the lining of the nasal cavity ("snorted") but is sometimes dissolved and injected. Cocaine is also sold as the

Table 13.1 Summary of Popular Addictive Drugs

Drug Category	Active Ingredients Most Commonly Used	Forms Most Commonly Used	Routes of Administration
Nicotine	Nicotine	Cigarettes, cigars	Inhalation of smoke
		Leaves	Oral (chewing)
		E-cigarettes	Inhalation of vapor
Cocaine	Cocaine	Powder	Intranasal, intravenous
		Freebase (crack)	Inhalation of vapor
Stimulants	Methamphetamine, amphetamine	Powder	Ingestion, intranasal, intravenous
		Crystal	Inhalation of vapor
Opioids	Oxycodone, hydrocodone	Tablets	Ingestion, intravenous
	Heroin	Powder	Intranasal, intravenous
	Fentanyl	Powder	Intranasal, intravenous
Cannabinoids	Delta-9 tetrahydrocannabinol (THC)	Leaves	Inhalation of smoke
		E-liquids	Inhalation of vapor
		THC-infused foods & beverages	Ingestion
Benzodiazepines	Alprazolam (Xanax), Lorazepam (Ativan), Clonazepam (Klonopin), Triazolam (Halcion)	Tablet, powder	Ingestion, intravenous
Alcohol	Ethanol	Beer, wine, spirits	Ingestion

"free base" form called crack, which users heat to inhale the vapor. Cocaine directly increases the amount of dopamine in the synapses in the nucleus accumbens.[2,5] Cocaine also stimulates many other brain cells, so it causes users to be excited and hyperactive.

- **Methamphetamine** and **amphetamine** are two chemically related **stimulants**, which are often grouped together as "amphetamines" and which have effects very similar to those of cocaine.[6] Amphetamine is sold under prescription in pill form to treat attention deficit/hyperactivity disorder (ADHD), but it is also produced and sold as a powder on the illegal drug market. Methamphetamine is mostly sold in the illegal market, although there is a pharmaceutical version approved by the FDA for a few specific uses.[7,8] The powder form of these drugs can be snorted or injected, and the crystal form of methamphetamine ("crystal" or "ice") is generally smoked like crack cocaine.[7,8] There are also other stimulant drugs sold to treat ADHD that have similar

effects. In the brain, amphetamines and related stimulants act like cocaine, directly increasing the amount of dopamine in the nucleus accumbens.[2,5]

- **Tetrahydrocannabinol (THC)**, the active chemical in marijuana, is now sold in a wide variety of forms. Marijuana leaves are dried and smoked. THC that is extracted from the leaves is dissolved in fluids that are vaporized and inhaled, similar to electronic cigarettes. THC is also added to foods and beverages ("edibles") and ingested. And the drug is put in creams and salves and absorbed through the skin. THC is thought to indirectly stimulate both the reward neurons in the ventral tegmental area and the medium spiny neurons in the nucleus accumbens.[2,5]

- *Opioids* are frequently prescribed by doctors, and they are also illegally sold on the street. The opioids used the most medically are **oxycodone** and **hydrocodone** (in OxyContin and Vicodin), which people take as pills for pain. These prescription drugs are often diverted and sold illegally. The most common fully illegal opioid is heroin,

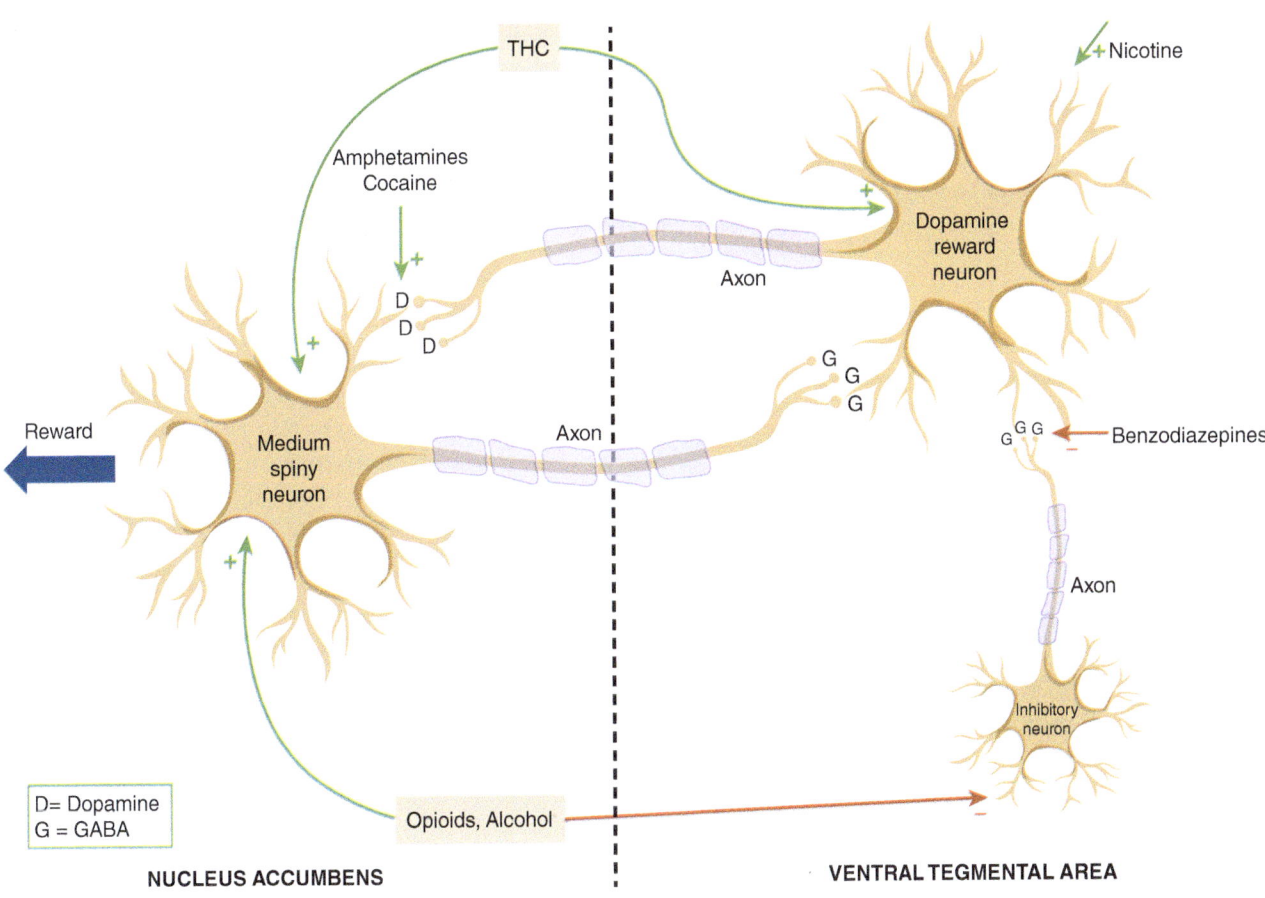

Figure 13.4 Actions of Addictive Drugs in the Reward Circuit. All addictive drugs are thought to affect the reward circuit in some way. Some stimulate the dopamine reward neurons, some stimulate the medium spiny neurons, some reduce the inhibitory feedback, and some have more than one effect. See text for more details.

Data from Volkow ND, Michaelides M, Baler R. The neuroscience of drug reward and addiction. *Physiol Rev.* 2019;99(4):2115-2140. doi:10.1152/physrev.00014.2018

which is usually sold as a powder that users snort or inject.[9] These drugs are all produced from morphine, which is extracted from the opium poppy, so they are sometimes called "semi-synthetic." In recent years, a highly potent opioid called **fentanyl**, which previously had been used only in medical care, has also been produced in illegal laboratories and sold on the street. Fentanyl is fully synthetic, that is, it is produced from chemicals instead of opium poppies. Street fentanyl is sold as a powder that is generally snorted or injected, but sometimes fentanyl is made into counterfeit tablets and ingested, and sometimes it is added to marijuana or cocaine and smoked.[10] In the brain's reward circuit, fentanyl and other opioids reduce the activity of the inhibiting neurons.[2,5] This acts like disabling the brakes on a car that is rolling downhill, speeding up the activity of the dopamine reward neurons—an effect called "disinhibition." Opioids also act directly to stimulate the neurons in the nucleus accumbens.[2,5]

- **Benzodiazepines** are a group of closely related drugs that cause relaxation and drowsiness in addition to euphoria and that are frequently used in medical care to treat anxiety. Trade names for some commonly-used benzodiazepines are Xanax, Ativan, and Klonopin.[11,12] Like prescription opioids, these drugs are often diverted to the street market. When used medically, benzodiazepines are usually taken as pills, but on the street, they may be snorted or injected.[11,12] Benzodiazepines work in the synapse between inhibitory neurons and reward neurons, and like opioids, they cause a "disinhibition" of the reward neurons.[2,5,13]

- *Alcohol* is sold and consumed in beverages, including beer, wine, spirits, and now an increasing number of mixed beverages like "wine coolers" and "hard lemonade." Unlike other addictive drugs, alcohol does not fit into specific receptors in neurons. Instead, by changing how cell membranes function, alcohol alters nearly all neurotransmitters, which profoundly affects how the brain operates. Experts believe it causes euphoria by increasing the activity of the brain's own natural opioids.[2,5]

Tolerance, Dependence and Addiction

When people first use these drugs, they simply experience the euphoria and, after the drug is fully metabolized, return to feeling normal. But after a person uses a drug many times, the neurons in the reward circuit adapt. They release less dopamine with a given dose of the drug, an effect that is called drug **tolerance**.[14] People who use drugs typically respond to tolerance by just taking larger or more frequent doses of the drug.

As the neurons adapt more, they release less dopamine than normal when the drug is *not* present. In this second stage, when users have not taken a dose, they feel depressed and/or anxious. They also have difficulty getting pleasure from everyday activities, which is known as **anhedonia**. When a person has symptoms like anxiety and anhedonia caused by stopping the use of a drug, that person is said to be experiencing **withdrawal**.[14] There are many other symptoms of withdrawal that depend on which drug the person has been using. When a person experiences withdrawal, that person is said to be **dependent** on the drug. People who are dependent on a drug can still experience euphoria by taking the drug, but it may require a large dose.

In the third stage of addiction, which may take years to occur, the reward neurons adapt further, sending normal signals only when the drug is present. In this stage, people become preoccupied with using their drug. They no longer feel euphoria after a dose; they just feel miserable when they cannot get one. Their entire lives may revolve around either using the drug, anticipating using it, or doing whatever is necessary to obtain the next dose.[2,14] They continue to use the drug regularly even when it is clear that the drug is harming them. At this point, they are fully **addicted**.

A few points about dependence and addiction are important to preventing harm from drug use in populations:

- While addiction is often discussed as all or nothing, in fact *there are varying degrees of dependence on a drug*. Some people who use drugs are fully and strongly addicted. Others may just feel unhappy when they have not taken the drug, but they can stop using it if the drug is difficult to obtain. Many people who try addictive drugs never become dependent on them, while others get fully addicted quickly. For every person who is addicted to a drug, there are many more people who use that drug but are not addicted.

- *Some drugs are more addictive than others.*[5] For example, heroin is more addictive than benzodiazepines. One index of how addictive different drugs are is the percent of those people ever using a drug who meet criteria for a **substance use disorder**. By this index, the most addictive drug is tobacco (32%), followed by heroin (23%), cocaine (17%), alcohol (15%), amphetamines (11%), marijuana (9%), and benzodiazepines (9%).[15]

- *Some routes of administration are more addictive than others.* While people can get addicted to drugs no matter how they are administered, when drugs hit the brain faster, they cause a sharper euphoria and are more addictive. Injecting heroin is more addictive than snorting it, and smoking crack is more addictive than snorting cocaine powder. Snorting, smoking, or injecting any drug is more addictive than swallowing pills.

- *People often use more than one addictive drug.* While health experts often think of addictive drugs one at a time, it is common for people to use more than one, called **polysubstance use**.[16] Common patterns are alcohol with tobacco and marijuana, or opioids with benzodiazepines.

- *People do not need to be addicted to be harmed by addictive drugs.* Even people who are just experimenting with addictive drugs can harm themselves. Cocaine can cause a fatal heart rhythm the first time someone uses it. Many people who are not addicted to alcohol get injured during a single binge drinking occasion. Many people who are not addicted to opioids die of an opioid overdose. In fact, much (perhaps most) of the damage from addictive drug use in populations involves people who are not addicted—mainly because there are so many more of them. For example, most of the population-level harms of alcohol use are experienced by people who are not the heaviest drinkers.[17]

- Some experts over-emphasize the distinction between drug *dependence* and drug *addiction* and argue that dependence is not necessarily a problem.[18] If people who are dependent on drugs show signs of withdrawal, their argument goes, these people just need another dose. By this argument, people who use drugs only have problems when they are addicted, which is defined as "the loss of control over the intense urges to take the drug, even at the expense of adverse consequences."[18] But the distinction is a fuzzy one that depends on how available the drug is. People who are dependent on opioids but can get a dose whenever they want (for example, if they have prescriptions for opioids) never "lose control" because their urges are always met. But if those same people were to be deprived of opioids, many would do risky things to get the drugs. Overemphasizing a distinction between dependence and addiction has itself caused serious damage because it endorsed the idea that people can safely take high doses of prescription opioids for chronic pain if they are "only physically dependent." That permitted pharmaceutical companies to market high doses of opioids for chronic pain, which led to many people dying unnecessarily of overdose.[19]

- *While it may not be easy, many people who use addictive drugs can quit on their own.* Medical drug treatment can be very helpful and is needed by many people addicted to drugs, but many others can stop using these drugs without it. For example, most people who quit smoking do so without medical help, despite tobacco being highly addictive.[20] For this reason, policies that make addictive drugs more difficult to obtain can reduce drug use and drug dependence in populations.

Pathophysiology of Drug Use

Addictive drugs can harm people in several different ways. Those harms can be the consequence of:

- *The drugs themselves.* Each drug has its own side effects, some of which are very dangerous. For example, alcohol damages the liver, and opioids can cause people to stop breathing.
- *Other chemicals that accompany the drugs.* For example, the chemicals in smoke from tobacco damage the lungs.
- *Behavior while intoxicated.* While users are intoxicated, they are more likely to engage in risky behavior because of poor judgement, inability to perceive risks, lack of coordination, and other drug effects like aggression. That risky behavior can have severe health consequences. For example, intoxication from alcohol or marijuana can lead to injuries from motor vehicle crashes, and intoxication from cocaine can lead to injuries from violence.
- *The route of administration.* For example, any drug that is injected will increase the risk that the user will contract HIV or other infections spread by hypodermic needles.
- *The behaviors required to obtain the drug.* For example, people who are addicted are more likely to acquire sexually transmitted diseases from prostitution or die of homicide from drug-related crime.

Table 13.2 lists the most important adverse health consequences of different drugs and the chemicals that accompany them. Summarizing:

- *Nicotine*, while addictive, is a relatively safe drug by itself. But the other chemicals that users are exposed to when they smoke or chew tobacco

Table 13.2 Most Important Adverse Health Effects of Addictive Drugs

Drug Category	Most Important Adverse Health Effects	
	Short-Term	**Long-Term**
Nicotine		Ischemic heart disease and ischemic stroke, chronic obstructive pulmonary disease, cancer
Alcohol	Injuries	Chronic liver disease, heart disease, stroke, cancer
Cocaine	Heart rhythm problems, stroke, seizures, homicide and injuries from violence	Psychosis, suicide
Stimulants	Heart rhythm problems, stroke, seizures, homicide and injuries from violence	Psychosis, suicide
Opioids	Respiratory depression (fatal overdose)	
Cannabinoids	Motor vehicle injuries	Schizophrenia and other psychoses, depression
Benzodiazepines	Injuries from sedation; Respiratory depression (fatal overdose) when combined with opioids or other drugs	

leaves are highly toxic. The most important health consequences of tobacco are **cardiovascular diseases** (heart disease and stroke), **chronic obstructive pulmonary disease**, and cancers. This is discussed in Chapter 11. Tobacco Use.

- *Alcohol* damages the body in hundreds of ways. The health consequences tied to the most deaths are unintentional and intentional injuries, chronic liver disease, heart disease, stroke, and cancer. This is discussed in Chapter 12. Alcohol Use.

- *Cocaine* can cause heart rhythm problems leading to sudden death or stroke, as well as seizures. As a stimulant, cocaine increases aggressive behavior and violence, with the injuries that often follow. And cocaine causes mental illnesses; it increases the risk of suicide and can lead to paranoia and hallucinations like those of **schizophrenia**, called **drug-induced psychosis**.[21,22]

- *Methamphetamine and amphetamine*, like cocaine, cause short-term risks of heart rhythm problems and injuries from aggressive behavior and long-term psychological risks of psychosis and suicide.[6,23]

- *Tetrahydrocannabinol (THC)*—surprisingly—has not been studied much, so its full effects are not known. However, people who use marijuana are more likely to develop schizophrenia and other forms of **psychosis**, as well as depression (discussed in Chapter 5. Mental Illnesses).[24,25] The effect of smoking marijuana on the lungs is not fully known, but the chemicals in marijuana smoke are toxic, and marijuana smokers have inflammation in the lungs.[26]

- *Opioids* have one major, severe side effect. They suppress the cells in the brain that keep people breathing, so people who take opioids may stop breathing and die from lack of oxygen. This is typically called an overdose, but many people die even with opioid prescriptions that are not considered high-dose.[27] Some opioids are more potent than others, and the more potent opioids cause more overdose deaths. The United States has had a surge in drug overdose deaths involving opioids since the 1990s (**Figure 13.5**).[28,29] The surge began with a fourfold increase in deaths involving prescription opioids like oxycodone and hydrocodone between the 1990s and 2011. That was followed by a nearly fivefold increase in deaths involving heroin between 2010 and 2016, and a more than 20-fold increase in deaths from fentanyl and related opioids from 2013 to 2022.

- *Benzodiazepines*, while addictive, are not as dangerous as opioids. However, people often use benzodiazepines in combination with opioids, both prescribed by doctors and on the street. When these two drug types are used together, they strongly suppress breathing and carry a high risk of fatal overdose.[30]

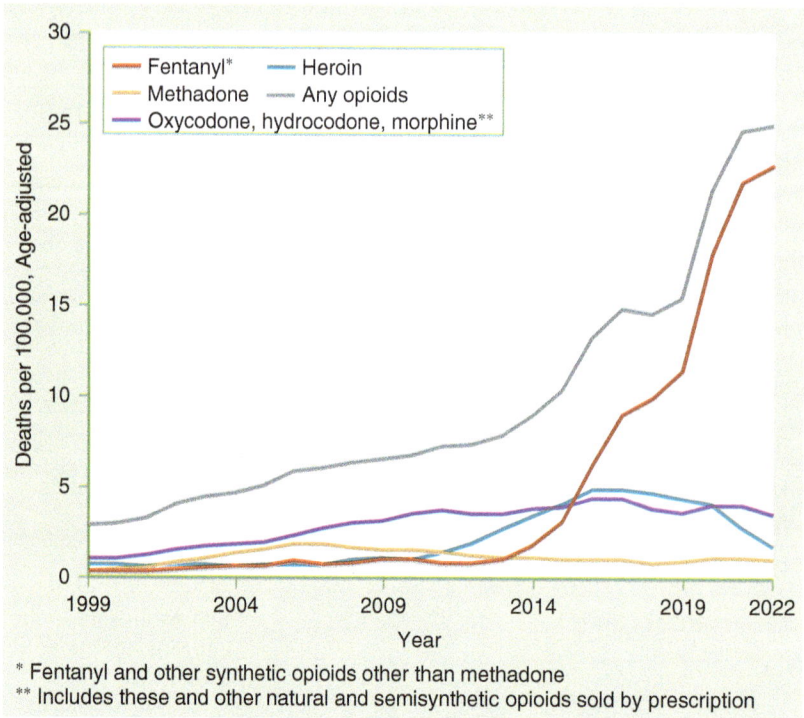

Figure 13.5 Overdose Deaths Involving Opioids in the United States, 1999–2022.

Data from Spencer MR, Garnett MF, Miniño AM. Drug Overdose Deaths in the United States, 2002-2022. NCHS Data Brief No. 491, March 2024 and NCHS Table ODMort for years 1999-2001, Accessed June 17, 2024 at https://www.cdc.gov/nchs/hus/data-finder.htm

Overall Health Effects of Addictive Drugs

Together, addictive drugs pose an enormous public health problem, with the greatest damage from drugs that are legal. Estimates vary, but the Global Burden of Disease project estimates that each year in the United States, tobacco use leads to 360,000 deaths (representing 10% of all deaths), alcohol use 110,000 deaths (3% of all deaths), and use of all other addictive drugs 110,000 deaths (3% of all deaths).[31] In other countries, illicit drugs are less used, so they are less of a public health problem—approximately 1% of deaths—but the estimate is still nearly 500,000 deaths per year worldwide.[31,32] Globally, tobacco and alcohol are responsible for similar percentages of deaths as in the United States.[31]

Social Harms of Drug Use

Drug use harms not only the people who use drugs but also others around them. The connection to injuries is particularly strong. People using alcohol or some other drugs can become aggressive, causing violent injuries to others, or clumsy, causing motor vehicle crashes that injure others, or both. Or they can injure others through crime to get money to buy drugs.[33] When parents use alcohol or drugs, they are more likely to abuse or neglect their children, which can lead to their children's own mental health problems and/or drug use problems. These social effects are difficult to quantify but are certainly large. For example, surveys show that large fractions of jail inmates committed their crimes while they were under the influence of or seeking money to buy drugs.[34]

Social Harms of Prohibition

Governments trying to limit the damage from drugs have prohibited the use and sales of some addictive drugs. Any consideration of the social harms caused by drugs should also include the harms caused by this prohibition.

Because users will pay high prices for addictive drugs, plenty of people are willing to sell drugs to them, even when legal punishments for drug sales are severe. That leads to criminal gangs, which then fight over the illegal drug markets. In 1930s America, gangs fought over the illegal market for alcohol; today they fight over illegal markets for fentanyl, heroin, cocaine, and marijuana. There is plenty to fight about because those markets are very large. Experts at the RAND Corporation estimate that the U.S. retail markets for cocaine and heroin are more than

$25 billion each and the retail market for marijuana before legalization was $40 billion.[35] Fights between drug gangs lead to homicides, including killing of innocent bystanders caught in the crossfire. And there is additional damage caused by pervasive fear in those living in neighborhoods where drug gangs shoot at each other.[33]

To make prohibition meaningful requires enforcement—that is police, courts, and jails. This enforcement creates its own social and health problems, from police-involved shootings to families broken up by the incarceration of parents.

It is difficult to quantify the social harms from prohibition and enforcement, but they are substantial. In U.S. crime statistics collected by the FBI, among homicides where circumstances were known, about 7% are estimated to be drug law-related and another 7% are gang-related, but these statistics may underestimate the problem because for many homicides the circumstances are not known or not recorded.[36] In Mexico, where an estimated 175,000 people are employed by drug gangs, these organizations are large enough to corrupt, undermine, and threaten the entire national government.[37] The drug gang wars in Mexico drove that nation's homicide rate to triple between 2007 and 2021, rising to three times that of the United States.[37]

Epidemiology: Patterns of Drug Use

Most Americans use addictive drugs at least occasionally. **Figure 13.6** shows the use of specific drugs by adults in the United States. The most commonly used drug is the one that is legal and heavily promoted—alcohol. The drugs most commonly used after alcohol are marijuana, which is now legal in much of the United States; tobacco, which is legal but has restrictions on its promotion; and medical drugs that are heavily prescribed: opioids, benzodiazepines, and stimulants. The use of drugs that are fully illegal, such as cocaine and heroin, is far lower, although people may underreport using these drugs on surveys.[38]

Each drug has its own pattern of use by age, race, and sex. For example, marijuana use is highest in young adults and is more common in men (**Figure 13.7**), but prescription opioid use is highest in older adults and is more common in women (**Figure 13.8**).[38]

Those are statistics on drug use, not drug addiction. Overall, nearly one in five adults over the age of 18 in the United States meets criteria for a

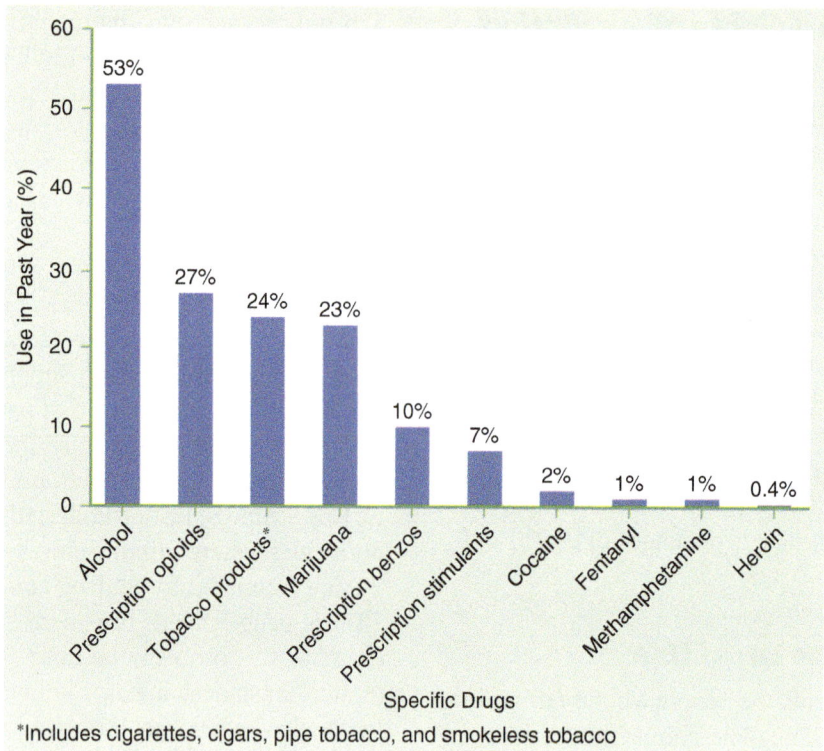

Figure 13.6 Use of Addictive Drugs by Persons Age 18+ in the United States, 2022.

Data from Substance Use and Mental Health Services Administration. National Survey of Drug Use and Health: National Release for 2022. Accessed July 26, 2024. https://www.samhsa.gov/data/nsduh/national-releases

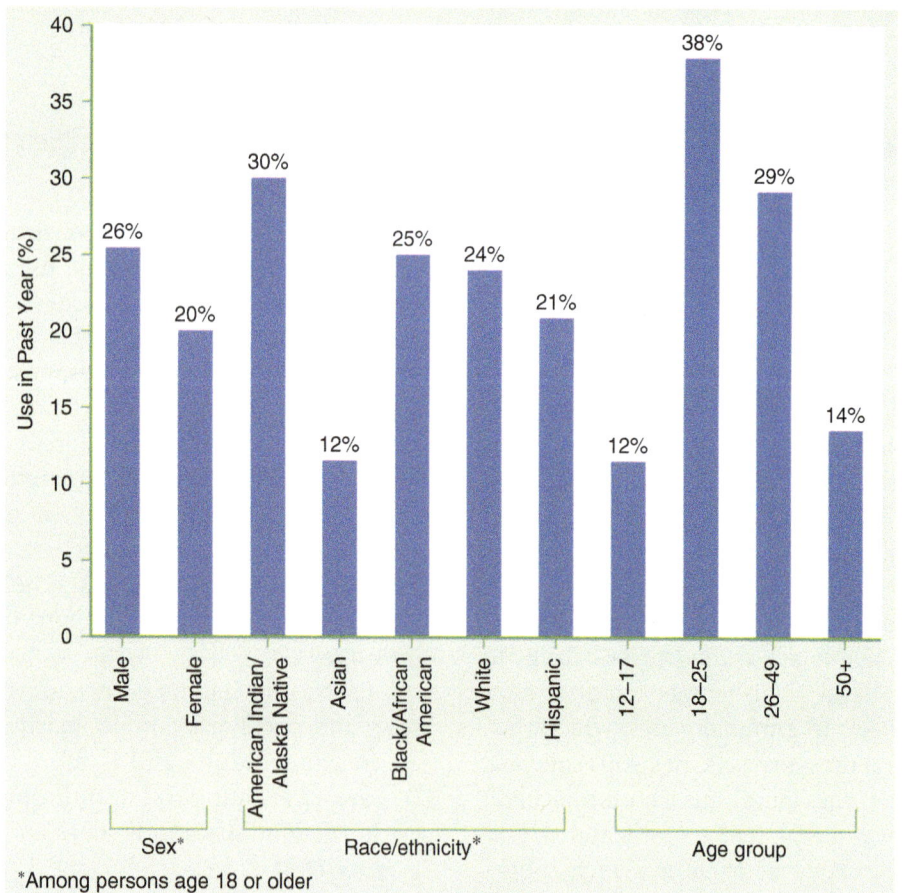

Figure 13.7 Use of Marijuana in the United States by Demographic Group, 2022.

Data from Substance Use and Mental Health Services Administration. National Survey of Drug Use and Health: National Release for 2022. Accessed July 26, 2024. https://www.samhsa.gov/data/nsduh/national-releases

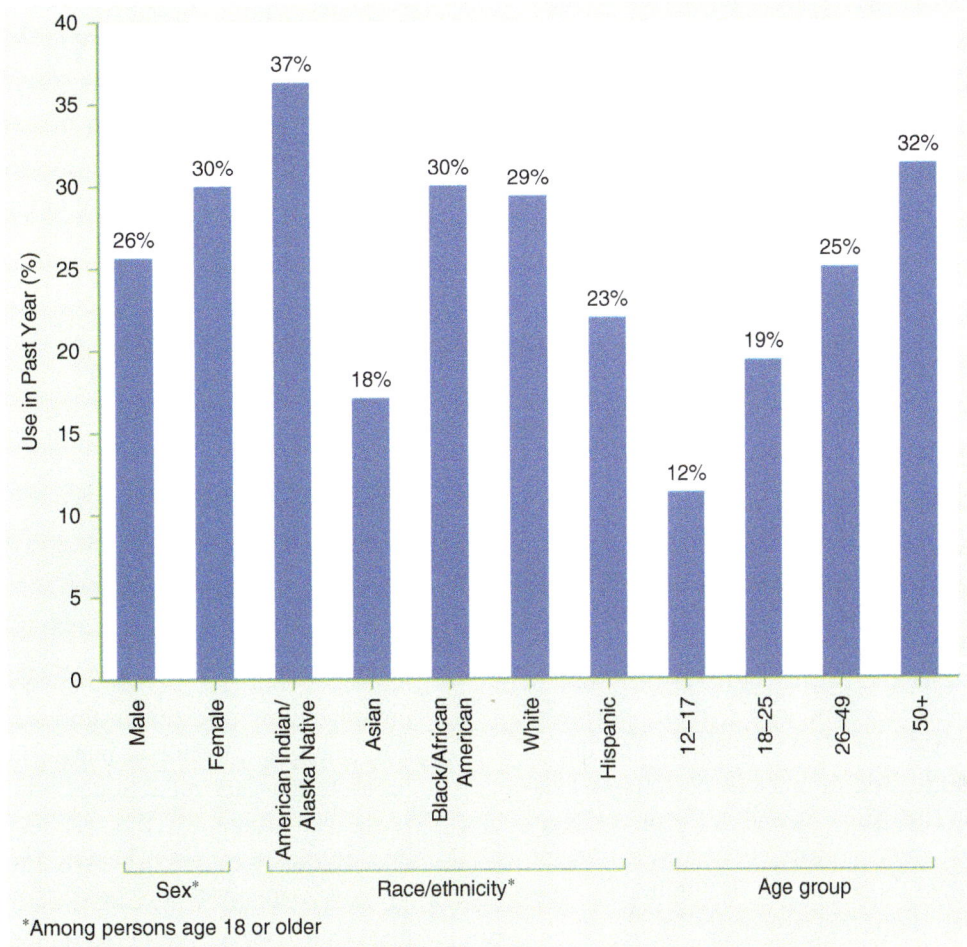

Figure 13.8 Use of Prescription Opioids in the United States by Demographic Group, 2022.

Data from Substance Use and Mental Health Services Administration. National Survey of Drug Use and Health: National Release for 2022. Accessed July 26, 2024. https://www.samhsa.gov/data/nsduh/national-releases

substance use disorder at some time over a year.[38] The most common drugs of addiction are those that are most commonly used: alcohol (11% of American adults), marijuana (7%), prescription opioids (2%), and stimulants (2%).[38]

Globally, tobacco and alcohol are the addictive drugs causing the most public health problems, followed by opioids and marijuana. Use of drugs other than alcohol and tobacco is more of a problem in the United States, Canada, Europe, Russia, and Australia than in low- and middle-income countries.[32]

Risk Factors for Drug Use

Many risk factors for drug use have been identified that, unfortunately, are not directly modifiable. For example, people are more likely to use addictive drugs if they have mental illnesses.[5] Teens are more likely to use drugs and become addicted if their peers use drugs.[39] And adults are more likely to use or become addicted to drugs if they used drugs in when they were teenagers.[2]

Risk factors that may be modifiable tend to fall into two categories: those specific to an individual's life experiences and those present in the social environment. The risk factors tied to individuals include (**Figure 13.9**):

- *Adverse childhood experiences.* Adults are more likely to use drugs if as children they were mistreated or raised by parents who were violent or used drugs.[5,39,40]
- *Lack of family/social support during childhood.* Adults raised with low levels of support or guidance from their parents are also more likely to use addictive drugs.[2,5,40]

Factors in the environment that increase the risk of drug use include:

- *Drug product design.* Drugs that are easier to administer, more potent, or absorbed more rapidly are more addictive. Examples of more addictive drug products introduced in recent years are high-dose OxyContin pills, high-potency marijuana, THC vapes, and illicit fentanyl.

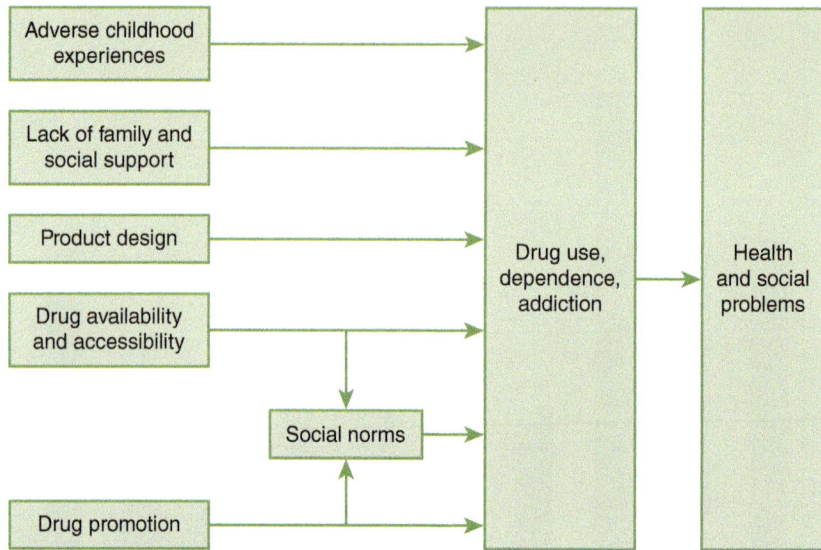

Figure 13.9 Cause-and-Effect Diagram for Addictive Drug Use.

- *Availability and accessibility of drugs.* The use of drugs is related to how easy it is for people to obtain and use them.[2,5,40] Availability and accessibility includes the number of persons or locations selling the drugs, as well as the price. Drugs that are legal are usually much more available and accessible than those that are prohibited.

- *Social norms.* Populations can be more or less supportive of the use of specific drugs. These norms strongly influence how many individuals will try or become addicted to these drugs.[2,5,39,40] Social norms change over time. For example, in the United States today, social norms are turning against cigarette smoking; a smoker who is in a crowd of people, even outdoors, is unlikely to light up. But alcohol use tends to be broadly supported; a person surrounded by others who are drinking feels embarrassed *not* to drink alcohol. Social norms around drug use are in turn influenced by drugs' legal status, availability, and promotion. As marijuana use is increasingly legalized and promoted, social norms around its use are more supportive, and use is increasing. The use of illicit drugs like heroin and cocaine, for which social norms are less supportive, is relatively low. Social norms around different drugs are not tracked consistently, but they are tied to how risky people consider different drugs to be. As **Figure 13.10** shows, Americans generally believe heroin and cocaine use is very risky, tobacco and alcohol use are somewhat less risky, and regular marijuana use is not risky. These perceptions do not match the actual risks.

- *Promotion.* Some drugs are actively promoted by manufacturers, and this promotion increases use. For example, alcohol is heavily advertised and promoted in the United States, which causes people to drink more.[41] In the past 30 years, prescription opioids have been heavily promoted to and by physicians, and this promotion led to sharp increases in use of these drugs. Marijuana use is increasingly advertised and promoted by marijuana producers and retailers.

Preventive Interventions

The effect of these drugs on the brain's reward circuit is so powerful that there will always be people who use addictive drugs. But addressing the modifiable risk factors may reduce or limit the use of these drugs, as well as their health and social consequences (**Figure 13.11**).

Primary Prevention

These interventions directed toward children may limit or reduce drug use in adults over the long term. However, these are intensive interventions that may be hard to bring to scale for entire populations:

- *Prevention of child abuse and child maltreatment.* There are many reasons to prevent maltreatment of children, but a large one is that it should reduce the number of people who develop alcohol or drug use problems as adults. While there are governmental and nongovernmental organizations already working on child abuse prevention, they may need more support.

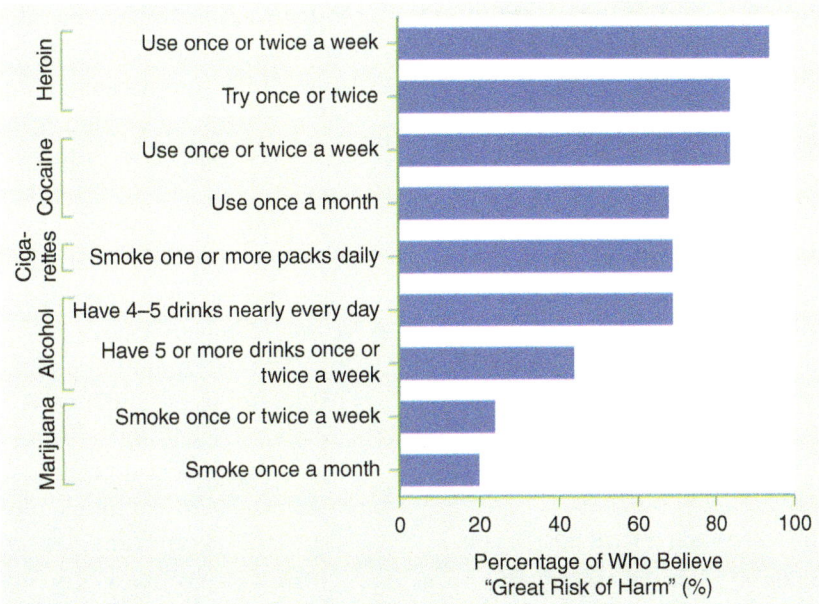

Figure 13.10 **Perceived Risk of Different Drugs in the United States, 2022.**

Data from Substance Use and Mental Health Services Administration. National Survey of Drug Use and Health: National Release for 2022. Accessed July 26, 2024. https://www.samhsa.gov/data/nsduh/national-releases

- *Family support.* Future drug addiction may be reduced by providing more support for families that have parents dealing with their own alcohol or drug abuse problems, mental illnesses, domestic violence, or other problems.
- *Family-based prevention education.* Programs in which parents are given training to help their

adolescent children avoid substance use have been effective.[42]

These policy interventions may change the environment to limit or reduce use:

- *Restrictions on drug use:* Restricting the use of drugs in certain places (such as prohibiting

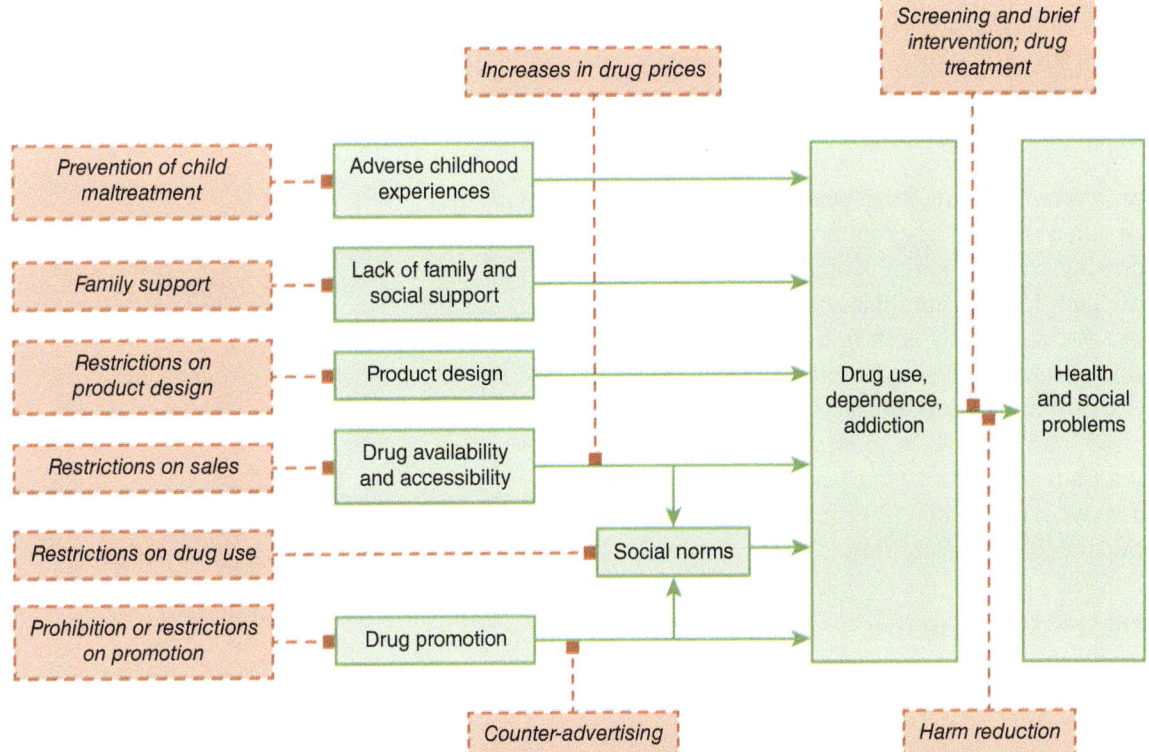

Figure 13.11 **Cause-and-Effect Diagram for Addictive Drug Use, With Preventive Interventions.**

smoking in restaurants or drinking in public places) can limit use and influence social norms to be less supportive.

- *Restrictions on drug sales.* Prohibiting sales of currently legal addictive drugs would likely reduce consumption but create a harmful illegal market, like that for alcohol in the 1930s and for cocaine and heroin today. However, restricting but not prohibiting sales may limit the size of the illegal market while also keeping consumption low. Examples of how sales can be restricted are by a prescription system, by selling drugs only through a small number of government-operated outlets, or by limiting the number, location, and hours of sales of private retail outlets.

- *Increases in drug prices.* When drugs cost more, people use them less, even when the drugs are addictive. That economic principle holds true not just for cigarettes and alcohol but also for illicit drugs like heroin and cocaine.[43-45] The retail price of tobacco, alcohol, and other legal drugs can be raised through taxes or legally enforced minimum prices. The retail price of illicit drugs rises with more enforcement of drug prohibitions.[46]

- *Restrictions on drug product design.* There is no practical way to limit the design of illegal drugs, but public policies can regulate legal drugs. The design of alcohol, tobacco, and prescription drug products is already regulated by the federal government. These regulations can be modified to limit the addictiveness of these drugs, for example, by reducing the dose or potency of nicotine, THC, or opioids.

- *Prohibition or restrictions on promotion.* The restriction on advertising of cigarettes probably has been a key reason that smoking rates have fallen so much since the 1970s. Prohibiting or restricting advertising and promotion of other legal addictive drugs like alcohol, marijuana, and prescription drugs should similarly limit or reduce their use.

- *Counter-advertising.* Just as advertising is effective, so is **counter-advertising**—for example, the ads produced by the CDC to discourage smoking. Counter-advertising may likewise be able to help reduce use of other addictive drugs that now have supportive social norms.

Secondary Prevention

These secondary prevention interventions may also help limit drug use or the harms of drugs:

- **Screening, brief intervention, and referral to treatment (SBIRT).** Public health and drug treatment agencies developed this intervention in the 1990s. People who go to medical clinics are screened for use of alcohol or other drugs, counseled briefly if they admit to risky use, and if appropriate, referred for more in-depth alcohol or drug treatment. This process persuades heavy drinkers to reduce their alcohol consumption on average by 10–15%.[47,48] It may help people using other drugs, too.[49]

- *Drug treatment.* There are various approaches to medical treatment to help people with addiction to alcohol or other drugs. All forms of treatment involve individual or group counseling. For those dependent on opioids, *medication-assisted treatment* also includes medications that prevent the symptoms of withdrawal without causing euphoria. The value of drug treatment is limited, though, by how many people it can reach.

- *Harm reduction.* Many people who are addicted to drugs will not or cannot undergo drug treatment. With this in mind, interventions called **harm reduction** have been developed to help people using drugs avoid the worst consequences. Most commonly, they include *provision of sterile hypodermic needles* so that the drug users do not become infected with HIV. Many organizations take on *distribution of naloxone*, an antidote to opioids. If a person stops breathing because of opioids and a bystander administers the drug naloxone, the opioid effects are reversed immediately and the person starts breathing again. Some organizations also operate *safe injection facilities*, in which addicted drug users

---

Box 13.1 Summary–Prevention of Use of Addictive Drugs

- Primary Prevention
  - Prevention of child abuse and child maltreatment
  - Family support
  - Restrictions on drug use
  - Restrictions on drug sales
  - Increases in drug prices
  - Restrictions on drug product design
  - Prohibition or restrictions on promotion
  - Counter-advertising
- Secondary Prevention
  - Screening, brief intervention, and referral to treatment
  - Drug treatment
  - Harm reduction

Box 13.2 Key Words

Addicted, addiction
Amphetamine
Amygdala
Anhedonia
Axon
Benzodiazepines
Cardiovascular disease
Chronic obstructive pulmonary disease
Counter advertising
Dendrite
Dependence, dependent
Dopamine
Drug-induced psychosis
Euphoria
Fentanyl
Gamma-aminobutyric acid (GABA)
Harm reduction
Hippocampus
Hydrocodone
Inhibitory neurons
Medial forebrain bundle
Medium spiny neurons
Methamphetamine
Neuron
Neurotransmitter
Nucleus accumbens
Oxycodone
Polysubstance use
Prefrontal cortex
Psychosis
Receptor
Reward circuit, reward pathway
Reward neuron
Schizophrenia
Screening, brief intervention, and referral to
 treatment (SBIRT)
Stimulants
Substance use disorder
Synapse
Tetrahydrocannabinol (THC)
Tolerance
Ventral tegmental area
Withdrawal

administer their drugs under medical supervision so that if they overdose, there are people standing by who can resuscitate them with naloxone. Like drug treatment, these harm reduction programs, while valuable, can help only a fraction of people using drugs.

Resources

- The Substance Use and Mental Health Services Administration conducts the annual National Survey on Drug Use and Health, which provide the best population-level statistics on drugs in the United States. Annual summary reports and detailed tables are available at https://www.samhsa.gov/data/data-we-collect/nsduh-national-survey-drug-use-and-health
- Volkow ND, Blanco C. Substance use disorders: a comprehensive update of classification, epidemiology, neurobiology, clinical aspects, treatment and prevention. *World Psychiatry*. 2023;22(2):203-229. doi:10.1002/wps.21073. This is a very technical, detailed, comprehensive summary of current thinking on substance use disorders.
- The National Institute on Drug Abuse produces detailed summaries of biomedical research on specific drugs at https://nida.nih.gov/research-topics/publications/research-reports
- The Drug Enforcement Administration maintains a series of fact sheets on illicit drugs sold in the United States at https://www.dea.gov/factsheets
- Degenhardt L, Charlson F, Ferrari A, et al. The global burden of disease attributable to alcohol and drug use in 195 countries and territories, 1990–2016: a systematic analysis for the Global Burden of Disease Study 2016. *Lancet Psychiatry*. 2018;5(12): 987-1012. doi:10.1016/S2215-0366(18)30337-7. This is an epidemiologic overview of health problems from alcohol and drug abuse around the world.

References

1. Olds J. Satiation effects in self-stimulation of the brain. *J Comp Physiol Psychol*. 1958;51(6):675-678.
2. Volkow ND, Michaelides M, Baler R. The neuroscience of drug reward and addiction. *Physiol Rev*. 2019;99(4): 2115-2140. doi:10.1152/physrev.00014.2018
3. Volkow ND, Morales M. The brain on drugs: From reward to addiction. *Cell*. 2015;162(4):712-725. doi:10.1016/j.cell.2015.07.046
4. Office of the Surgeon General. *How Tobacco Smoke Causes Disease: The Biology and Behavioral Basis for Smoking-Attributable Disease: A Report of the Surgeon General.*

Department of Health and Human Services; 2010. Accessed December 11, 2024. Available at: https://www.ncbi.nlm.nih.gov/books/NBK53017/
5. Volkow ND, Blanco C. Substance use disorders: a comprehensive update of classification, epidemiology, neurobiology, clinical aspects, treatment and prevention. *World Psychiatry*. 2023;22(2):203-229. doi:10.1002/wps.21073
6. National Institute on Drug Abuse. Methamphetamine Research Report. Published 2022. Accessed November 15, 2023. Available at: https://nida.nih.gov/publications/research-reports/methamphetamine/overview

7. Drug Enforcement Administration. *Drug Fact Sheet: Methamphetamine.* Published 2020. Accessed July 10, 2024. Available at: https://www.dea.gov/factsheets

8. Drug Enforcement Administration. *Drug Fact Sheet: Amphetamines.* Published 2020. Accessed July 10, 2024. Available at: https://www.dea.gov/factsheets

9. Drug Enforcement Administration. *Drug Fact Sheet: Heroin.* Published 2020. Accessed July 10, 2024. Available at: https://www.dea.gov/factsheets

10. Drug Enforcement Administration. *Drug Fact Sheet: Fentanyl.* Published 2022. Accessed July 10, 2024. Available at: https://www.dea.gov/factsheets

11. Drug Enforcement Administration. *Drug Report: Benzodiazepines.* Published 2023. Accessed July 10, 2024. Available at: https://www.dea.gov/factsheets

12. Drug Enforcement Administration. *Drug Fact Sheet: Benzodiazepines.* Published 2020. Accessed July 10, 2024. Available at: https://www.dea.gov/factsheets

13. Tan KR, Brown M, Labouébe G, et al. Neural bases for addictive properties of benzodiazepines. *Nature.* 2010;463 (7282):769-774. doi:10.1038/nature08758

14. Koob GF. Neuroanatomy of Addiction. In: Brownell KD, Gold MS, eds. *Food and Addiction: A Comprehensive Handbook.* Oxford University Press; 2012:20-29.

15. Anthony JC, Warner LA, Kessler RC. Comparative epidemiology of dependence on tobacco, alcohol, controlled substances, and inhalants: Basic findings from the National Comorbidity Survey. *Exp Clin Psychopharmacol.* 1994;2(3):244-268. doi:10.1037/1064-1297.2.3.244

16. Connor JP, Leung J, Chan GCK, Stjepanović D. Seeking order in patterns of polysubstance use. *Curr Opin Psychiatry.* 2023;36(4):263-268. doi:10.1097/YCO.0000000000000881

17. Sherk A, Churchill S, Cukier S, Grant SC, Shield K, Stockwell T. Distributions of alcohol use and alcohol-caused death and disability in Canada: Defining alcohol harm density functions and new perspectives on the prevention paradox. *Addiction.* 2024;119(4):696-705. doi:10.1111/add.16414

18. Szalavitz M, Rigg KK, Wakeman SE. Drug dependence is not addiction—and it matters. *Ann Med.* 2021;53(1):1989-1992. doi:10.1080/07853890.2021.1995623

19. Bohnert ASB, Valenstein M, Bair MJ, et al. Association between opioid prescribing patterns and opioid overdose-related deaths. *JAMA.* 2011;305(13):1315-1321.

20. Caraballo RS, Shafer PR, Patel D, Davis KC, McAfee TA. Quit methods used by US adult cigarette smokers, 2014–2016. *Prev Chronic Dis.* 2017;14(4). doi:10.5888/pcd14.160600

21. National Institute on Drug Abuse. Cocaine Research Report. Published 2020. Accessed November 15, 2023. Available at: https://nida.nih.gov/publications/research-reports/cocaine/what-cocaine

22. Peacock A, Tran LT, Larney S, et al. All-cause and cause-specific mortality among people with regular or problematic cocaine use: A systematic review and meta-analysis. *Addiction.* 2021;116(4):725-742. doi:10.1111/add.15239

23. Stockings E, Tran LT, Santo T, et al. Mortality among people with regular or problematic use of amphetamines: A systematic review and meta-analysis. *Addiction.* 2019;114(10):1738-1750. doi:10.1111/add.14706

24. Gobbi G, Atkin T, Zytynski T, et al. Association of cannabis use in adolescence and risk of depression, anxiety, and suicidality in young adulthood: A systematic review and meta-analysis. *JAMA Psychiatry.* Published online 2019. doi:10.1001/jamapsychiatry.2018.4500

25. Marconi A, Di Forti M, Lewis CM, Murray RM, Vassos E. Meta-analysis of the association between the level of cannabis use and risk of psychosis. *Schizophr Bull.* 2016;42(5):1262-1269. doi:10.1093/schbul/sbw003

26. Committee on the Health Effects of Marijuana. *The Health Effects of Cannabis and Cannabinoids: An Evidence Review and Research Agenda.* Vol 15. National Academies of Sciences, Engineering, and Medicine; 2017. doi:10.17226/24625

27. Coyle DT, Pratt CY, Ocran-Appiah J, Secora A, Kornegay C, Staffa J. Opioid analgesic dose and the risk of misuse, overdose, and death: A narrative review. *Pharmacoepidemiol Drug Saf.* 2018;27(5):464-472. doi:10.1002/pds.4366

28. Spencer MR, Garnett MF, Miniño AM. Drug overdose deaths in the United States, 2002–2022. *NCHS Data Brief.* 2024;(491):1-8.

29. National Center for Health Statistics. Overdose mortality statistics: ODMort Table. Centers for Disease Control. Published 2024. Accessed July 10, 2024. Available at: https://www.cdc.gov/nchs/hus/data-finder.htm

30. National Institute on Drug Abuse. Benzodiazepines and Opioids. Published 2022. Accessed November 15, 2023. Available at: https://nida.nih.gov/research-topics/opioids/benzodiazepines-opioids

31. Global Burden of Disease Collaboration. Global Burden of Disease tool—GBD Results. Published 2024. Accessed April 18, 2025. Available at: https://vizhub.healthdata.org/gbd-results

32. Degenhardt L, Charlson F, Ferrari A, et al. The global burden of disease attributable to alcohol and drug use in 195 countries and territories, 1990–2016: A systematic analysis for the Global Burden of Disease Study 2016. *Lancet Psychiatry.* 2018;5(12):987-1012. doi:10.1016/S2215-0366(18)30337-7

33. Caulkins JP, Kleiman MAR. *How Much Crime Is Drug-Related? History, Limitations, and Potential Improvements of Estimation Methods.* Published 2014. Accessed July 10, 2024. Available at: https://www.ojp.gov/pdffiles1/nij/grants/246404.pdf

34. Dorsey T. *Drugs and Crime Facts.* Published 2006. Accessed July 10, 2024. Available at: https://bjs.ojp.gov/content/pub/pdf/dcf.pdf

35. Kilmer B, Everingham SS, Caulkins JP, et al. *How Big Is the U.S. Market for Illegal Drugs?* Published 2014. Accessed July 10, 2024. Available at: https://www.rand.org/pubs/research_briefs/RB9770.html

36. Federal Bureau of Investigation. Crime in the United States—2019. FBI Uniform Crime Reports. Published 2019. Accessed July 9, 2024. Available at: https://ucr.fbi.gov/crime-in-the-u.s/2019/crime-in-the-u.s.-2019/tables/expanded-homicide-data-table-12.xls

37. Prieto-Curiel R, Maria Campedelli G, Hope A. Reducing cartel recruitment is the only way to lower violence in Mexico. *Science (1979).* 2023;381:1312-1316.

38. Substance Use and Mental Health Services Administration. 2022 National Survey on Drug Use and Health Detailed Tables. Published 2022. Accessed July 8, 2024. Available at: https://www.samhsa.gov/data/report/2022-nsduh-detailed-tables

39. Degenhardt L, Grebely J, Stone J, et al. Global patterns of opioid use and dependence: Harms to populations, interventions, and future action. *Lancet.* 2019;394(10208):1560-1579. doi:10.1016/S0140-6736(19)32229-9

40. Stone AL, Becker LG, Huber AM, Catalano RF. Review of risk and protective factors of substance use and problem use

in emerging adulthood. *Addict Behav.* 2012;37(7):747-775. doi:10.1016/j.addbeh.2012.02.014

41. Babor TF, Casswell S, Graham K, et al. *Alcohol: No Ordinary Commodity.* 3rd ed. Oxford University Press; 2023. doi:10.1093 /oso/9780192844484.001.0001

42. Allen ML, Garcia-Huidobro D, Porta C, et al. Effective parenting interventions to reduce youth substance use: A systematic review. *Pediatrics.* 2016;138(2). doi:10.1542/peds.2015 -4425

43. Gallet CA. Can price get the monkey off our back? A meta-analysis of illicit drug demand. *Health Econ.* 2014;23(1):55-68. doi:10.1002/hec.2902

44. Chaloupka FJ, Wechsler H. Price, tobacco control policies and smoking among young adults. *J Health Econ.* 1997;16: 359-373.

45. Wagenaar AC, Salois MJ, Komro KA. Effects of beverage alcohol price and tax levels on drinking: A meta-analysis of 1003 estimates from 112 studies. *Addiction.* 2009;104(2): 179-190. doi:10.1111/j.1360-0443.2008.02438.x

46. Caulkins JP. *Effects of Prohibition, Enforcement and Interdiction on Drug Use.* Published 2014. Accessed April 4, 2025. Available at: http://www.globalcommissionondrugs.org/Report

47. Kaner EFS, Beyer FR, Muirhead C, et al. Effectiveness of brief alcohol interventions in primary care populations. *Cochrane Database Syst Rev.* 2018;2018(2). doi:10.1002/14651858 .CD004148.pub4

48. Bertholet N, Daeppen JB, Wietlisbach V, Fleming M, Burnand B. Reduction of alcohol consumption by brief alcohol intervention in primary care systematic review and meta-analysis. *Arch Intern Med.* 2005;165:986-995.

49. Substance Use and Mental Health Services Administration. *Evidence Supporting the Effectiveness of SBIRT.* Published 2011. Accessed July 10, 2024. Available at: https://www .samhsa.gov/sbirt

CHAPTER 14

Nutrition

This chapter covers the most important nutritional problems today, grouping them in two categories: 1) **undernutrition** and 2) consumption of foods linked to chronic diseases, which this chapter will refer to as **dietary risks**. Both of these problems qualify as **malnutrition**.[1]

Undernutrition—not consuming enough nutrients—mainly occurs today in pregnant women and children in low- and middle-income countries. Dietary risks involve people eating foods that the human body is not well designed to handle. People become ill with diseases like diabetes and heart disease from eating these less healthful foods over many years.

It is tempting to view these two problems as opposites: under- and "over-nutrition." But the two problems can occur together in populations, households, and even individuals.[2] This is called the **double burden of malnutrition**, and it is found most in historically low-income countries in which highly processed food has become widely available.

Few people grow their own food today. Most people buy most of their food from retail stores, and that food is produced by manufacturers. Therefore, human health is heavily influenced by how foods are manufactured, where and how they can be purchased, the cost of these foods, and how these foods are marketed. The food industry is increasingly producing food that is highly processed and built from refined carbohydrates, sugar, and fats.[3] There are advantages to this type of food: it is inexpensive and reliable to produce, is dense in calories, has a long shelf life, and is relatively safe from contamination. These features are valuable when millions of children worldwide are dying from undernutrition. But, as discussed later in this chapter, highly processed food based on refined carbohydrates, and saturated fats also causes obesity,

heart disease, and cancer. A central challenge to improving global health is to improve the food system so that it delivers food that everyone can afford but that does not carry these health risks.

Before discussing nutritional health problems, some background on nutrition is needed.

Nutrients

Foods contain **macronutrients** and **micronutrients**. Macronutrients are very large molecules that supply the body with energy and the biochemical building blocks of tissues. Micronutrients are small chemical compounds that the body needs and that its cells cannot synthesize, so they must be obtained from food; these include minerals and organic chemicals called **vitamins**.

There are three types of macronutrients: **long-chain carbohydrates**, **proteins**, and **fats**.

- **Carbohydrates** are molecules with the chemical formula $Cm(H_2O)n$ where m is the number of carbon atoms and n is the number of water molecules incorporated in the molecule. Carbohydrates include **monosaccharides** (most of which have six carbon atoms), **disaccharides** (which are two monosaccharides joined together) and **polysaccharides** (which are chains of more than two monosaccharides). Long-chain carbohydrates are very long polysaccharides built from thousands of monosaccharide subunits. Most of these monosaccharide subunits are **glucose**, which is the monosaccharide that circulates in the blood and supplies energy to cells. The main long-chain carbohydrate in food that humans eat is **starch** (**Figure 14.1**), which is the storage form of glucose used most by plants, such as wheat, corn, rice, and potatoes.

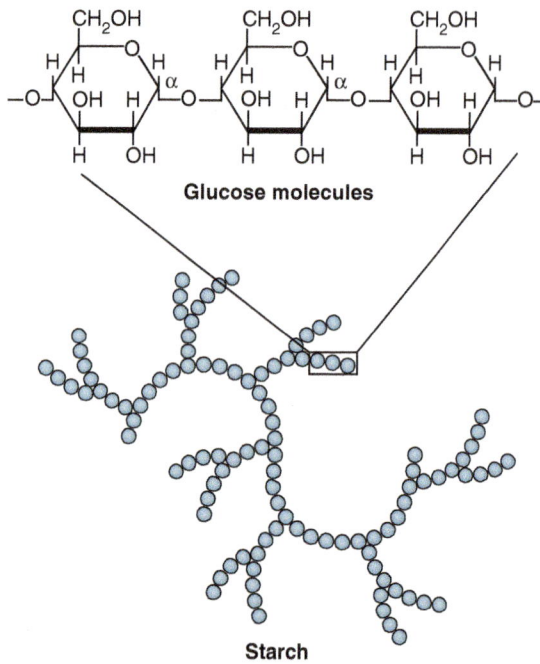

Glucose molecules

Starch

Figure 14.1 The Structure of Starch. The main carbohydrate that humans eat is called starch. It is composed of extensive webs and chains of linked molecules of glucose.

- Proteins are long chains of **amino acid** subunits, which are then twisted and "folded" in complex ways to do specific jobs in cells (**Figure 14.2**). Proteins are the key building blocks of many of the structures in the body, particularly muscle. **Enzymes**, which catalyze the key biochemical reactions in the body, are also proteins. Meat and seafood are good sources of proteins, as are beans.

- Fats are **triglycerides**, which are molecules composed of three **fatty acids** (medium-sized or long chains of carbon atoms) linked to a compound called glycerol (**Figure 14.3**). Both animal fats and plant oils are triglycerides.

Humans need about 30 different micronutrients. The ones that are most important to population health today are vitamin A, **folate** (also called vitamin B_9), vitamin D, iron, iodine, zinc, and calcium.[4] If people do not consume enough of these micronutrients, they can develop various illnesses, from anemia to blindness.

Box 14.1 Key Words—Nutrition

Amino acid
Carbohydrates
Dietary risks
Disaccharides
Double burden of malnutrition
Enzyme
Fats
Fatty acids
Folate
Glucose
Long-chain carbohydrates
Macronutrients
Malnutrition
Micronutrients
Monosaccharides
Polysaccharides
Proteins
Starch
Triglycerides
Undernutrition
Vitamin

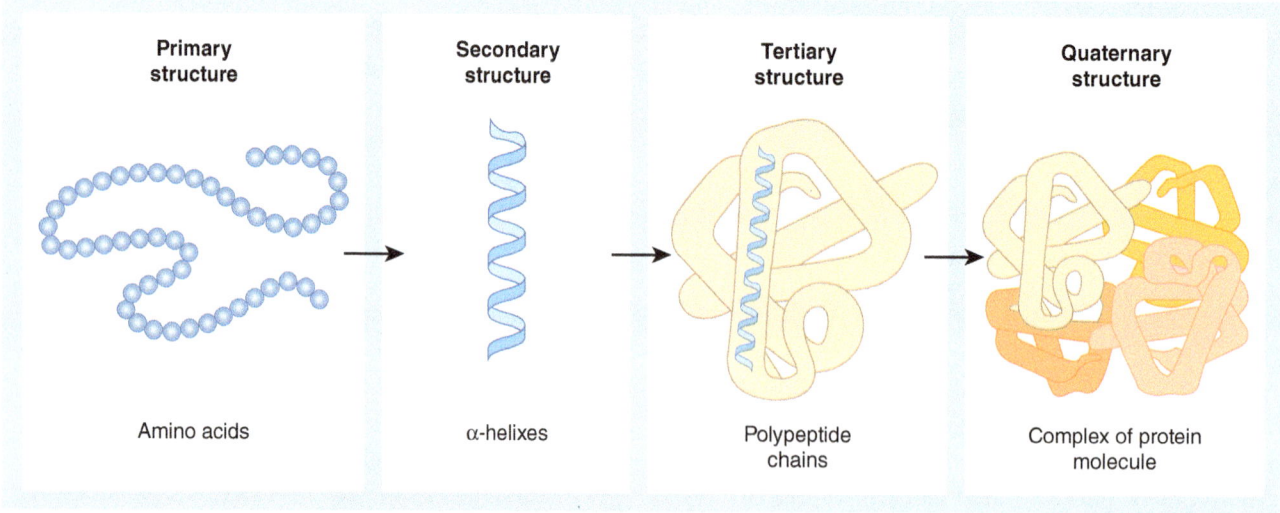

Primary structure	Secondary structure	Tertiary structure	Quaternary structure
Amino acids	α-helixes	Polypeptide chains	Complex of protein molecule

Figure 14.2 The Structure of Proteins. Proteins are long chains of amino acid subunits, which are then twisted and "folded" in complex ways to do specific jobs in cells.

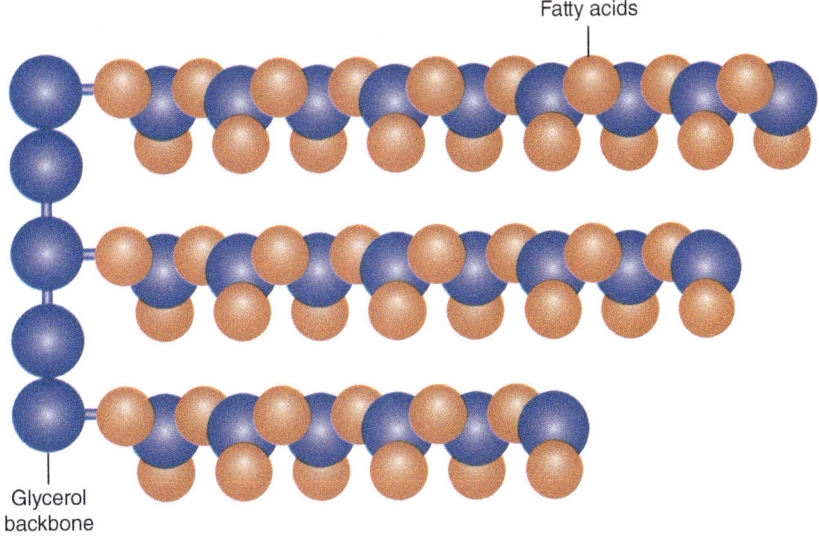

Figure 14.3 The Structure of Triglycerides. Triglycerides, also known as fats, are molecules composed of three fatty acids connected to a molecule called glycerol.

Maternal and Child Undernutrition

Introduction

While rates are falling, undernutrition of mothers and children remains a major cause of death in low- and middle-income countries. It is ranked first among risk factors for disability-adjusted life years lost worldwide (see Figure 1.9 in Chapter 1. Disease Prevention and Populations). This problem should continue to gradually shrink as economies develop further, but many interventions can reduce the problem now.

Pathophysiology of Undernutrition of Mothers and Young Children

The 1,000 days from when a human embryo is conceived until the child reaches their second birthday is a time of extremely rapid growth and development. During this time, the mother and the infant or young child need a large and steady supply of macronutrients and micronutrients to build tissues. For example, during pregnancy, a woman's need for protein may increase by 30% and for folate may increase by 50%.[5] If there are not enough stores of macronutrients and micronutrients at the beginning of pregnancy or the mother does not take in enough during pregnancy, the fetus may not develop fully or in a healthy way.

Pregnancy tends to deplete women of nutrients. Because of that, women who become pregnant again soon after a delivery are more likely to be undernourished in the subsequent pregnancy, which can lead to undernutrition in the next fetus and child.[6,7]

The nutrition of infants and young children is closely tied to the nutritional status of their mothers.[8] Infants are healthiest if they consume the mother's breast milk. Infants grow rapidly, typically doubling their birth weight in the first six months of life and tripling it by a year. A child is called **stunted** if the child's length or height falls to more than two standard deviations below the median for age.[9] A child is called **wasted** if the child's weight falls to more than two standard deviations below the median for length or height. **Growth faltering** means either stunting or wasting.[9]

Underlying all maternal and child undernutrition in low-income countries is poverty—not the relative poverty seen in high-income countries but absolute poverty, in which people do not have enough food or enough money to buy food. Poverty tends to cause diets that are insufficient in quantity, leading to shortages of macronutrients, or that are insufficient in variety, leading to shortages of micronutrients. Poverty is an important nutritional risk not just during pregnancy but also before pregnancy because much growth and development of the fetus happens in the first few weeks of gestation.

The Consequences of Maternal and Child Undernutrition

Undernutrition has severe consequences for both mothers and children.

Undernutrition during pregnancy increases the risk of **fetal growth restriction** (inadequate growth of the fetus during pregnancy), **preterm birth** (before 37 weeks gestation), and **low birth weight** (less than 2,500 grams).[10-13] And pregnant women who have narrow diets are more likely to have a child with **congenital malformations**.[14-17] These health problems are discussed more in Chapter 10. Diseases of the Newborn.

Children with stunting or wasting before age two are about two or three times as likely to die in early childhood, respectively.[8,18,19] Undernutrition weakens the immune system, and the final event that kills these children is usually an infection, particularly diarrheal disease, lower respiratory tract infection, or measles.[9,18,19] Children with stunting who live to become adults have less cognitive development, get less schooling, and have a lower income.[8,20-22]

While inadequate growth during pregnancy and early childhood is mainly caused by shortages of macronutrients, there are also specific health problems caused by shortages of micronutrients. The most important micronutrient deficiencies in mothers and children globally today are summarized in **Table 14.1**:[19,23]

- *Vitamin A* is essential for the eyes and the body's immune system. Children who do not take in enough vitamin A can lose their sight and develop

Table 14.1 Key Biologic Functions and Health Risks of Deficiencies of Micronutrients Most Important in Maternal and Child Undernutrition

Vitamin or Mineral	Key Biologic Function	Health Risks of Deficiency
Vitamin A	Vision	Vision loss
	Immune function	Infections
	Growth and development	Mortality in children
Folate (folic acid)	Brain development	Neural tube defects
	Red blood cell formation	Anemia
	Cell growth	
Vitamin D	Bone growth and strength	Weak and deformed bones
	Calcium absorption	Calcium deficiency
	Immune function	
	Muscle function	
	Nervous system function	
Calcium	Bone and teeth formation	Weak bones
	Constriction and relaxation of blood vessels	High blood pressure
		Pre-eclampsia in pregnant women
Iodine	Thyroid hormone production	Reduced growth
		Intellectual disability
		Goiter (swelling of the thyroid gland)
Iron	Hemoglobin (carrying oxygen in blood)	Anemia
	Brain development	
Zinc	Immune function	Infections
	Growth and development	Reduced growth
	Cell growth	Preterm birth
		Mortality in children

infections, particularly measles and diarrheal diseases.[24] About one-fourth of children in low- and middle-income countries are thought to have levels of vitamin A that are too low.[9] Giving vitamin A supplements to children with undernutrition significantly improves their chances of survival. Vitamin A is discussed more in Chapter 9. Infectious Diseases.

- *Folate* is a vitamin that is needed to make new cells, and it appears particularly important to the early development of the brain.[4] Women who have low levels of folate when they become pregnant are more likely to have infants with **neural tube defects**.[17] The connection of folate deficiency to neural tube defects is discussed more in Chapter 10. Diseases of the Newborn.

- *Vitamin D* helps the body build strong bones by increasing the absorption of the mineral calcium. This vitamin is also important for the immune system, muscles, and nerves. Humans make vitamin D in the skin when it is exposed to sunlight, but the amount made varies by how direct the sunlight is, skin tone, and other factors.[4] Vitamin D deficiency is believed to be very common in low- and middle-income countries in Asia, the Middle East, and Africa, as well as in immigrants from those areas living elsewhere.[25]

- *Calcium* deficiency in pregnant women increases their risk of high blood pressure and a disease called **pre-eclampsia**.[12,20] Pre-eclampsia is discussed in Chapter 10. Diseases of the Newborn.

- *Iodine* is needed by the **thyroid gland**. The thyroid gland regulates the speed of metabolism, and it is essential for infants' growth and brain development.[4] In the past, in some regions of the world, severe iodine deficiency was a very common cause of intellectual disability.[9] In most of the world today, salt is fortified with iodine, so severe iodine deficiency is rare.[9] However, a lesser degree of iodine deficiency is very common and may cause less noticeable problems with children's brain growth and behavior.[9]

- *Iron* is a mineral that is needed by cells to make **hemoglobin**, the protein that carries oxygen in red blood cells. People with low levels of iron have **anemia**, that is, not enough hemoglobin and red blood cells. Iron is also needed for brain development.[19] Iron deficiency is extremely common across the globe: about 40% of children and pregnant women in low- and middle-income countries have anemia, and the cause is iron deficiency in about one-third of the children and one-half of the pregnant women.[9]

- *Zinc* is a mineral that is needed for healthy pregnancies and that helps the immune system work.[4] Pregnant women with zinc deficiency are more likely to deliver babies preterm, and infants who have zinc deficiency have more infectious diseases, less growth, and higher mortality.[4,9] More than half of children in sub-Saharan Africa have low levels of zinc.[9] When children have a bout of diarrhea, they lose more zinc than normal and have a reduced ability to absorb it. Zinc deficiency can be avoided by giving pregnant women and children in low-income countries zinc supplements, and giving children additional zinc after diarrheal illnesses.[4,26]

Shortages of macronutrients and micronutrients have devastating effects on children in low- and middle-income countries. An estimated 45% of child deaths globally are caused by stunting, wasting, poor growth of the fetus, deficiencies of vitamin A or zinc, and inadequate breastfeeding.[19]

Epidemiology: Patterns and Trends

Undernutrition in children is gradually improving, but this condition is still distressingly common. The hardest-hit countries are those with the lowest incomes, such as India, Bangladesh and those in sub-Saharan Africa. These countries are making progress, though. With economic development, the percentage of young children who are stunted in these areas fell roughly in half from 1990 to 2020 (**Figure 14.4**).[27]

In low- and middle-income countries, growth faltering is a population-level problem, reflected by a shift in the entire distribution curve for height or weight compared to well-nourished populations (**Figure 14.5**).[28]

Risk Factors

Risk factors for undernutrition in mothers and children include (**Figure 14.6**):

- *Poverty*. The most important risk factor is living in poverty.[8,29] This is mostly because these families simply do not have enough food. However, there may also be risks from other factors closely tied to poverty, such as not having electricity at home, not having access to clean drinking water or sanitation, and using smoke-producing fuels for heating and cooking at home.[8,29] Also, *low maternal education* is associated with child undernutrition;[8,29] it is not clear if this is just a marker of poverty or if education of women independently helps protect children from undernutrition.

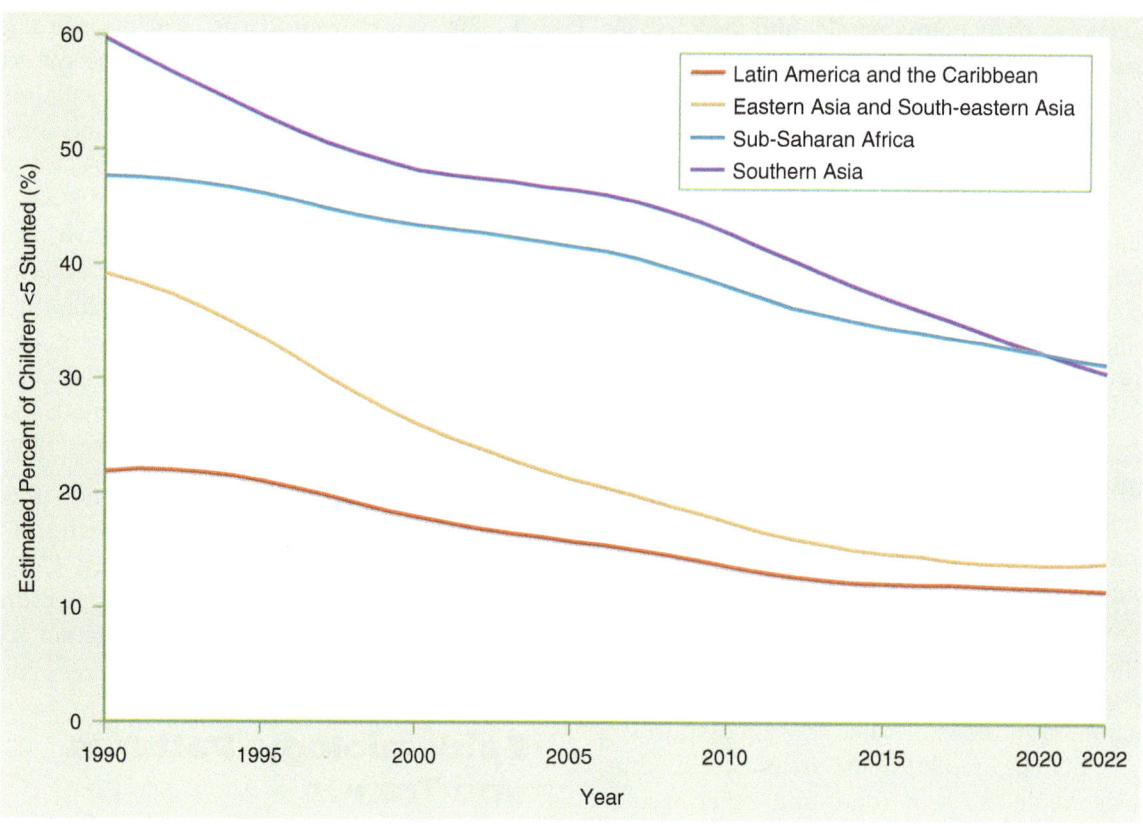

Figure 14.4 **Trends in the Estimated Prevalence of Stunting in Children Under 5 in Low-Income U.N. Regions.**

Data from World Health Organization. The Global Health Observatory. World Health Organization. Published 2023. Accessed August 1, 2024. https://www.who.int/data/gho/data/indicators/indicator-details/GHO/gho-jme-stunting-prevalence

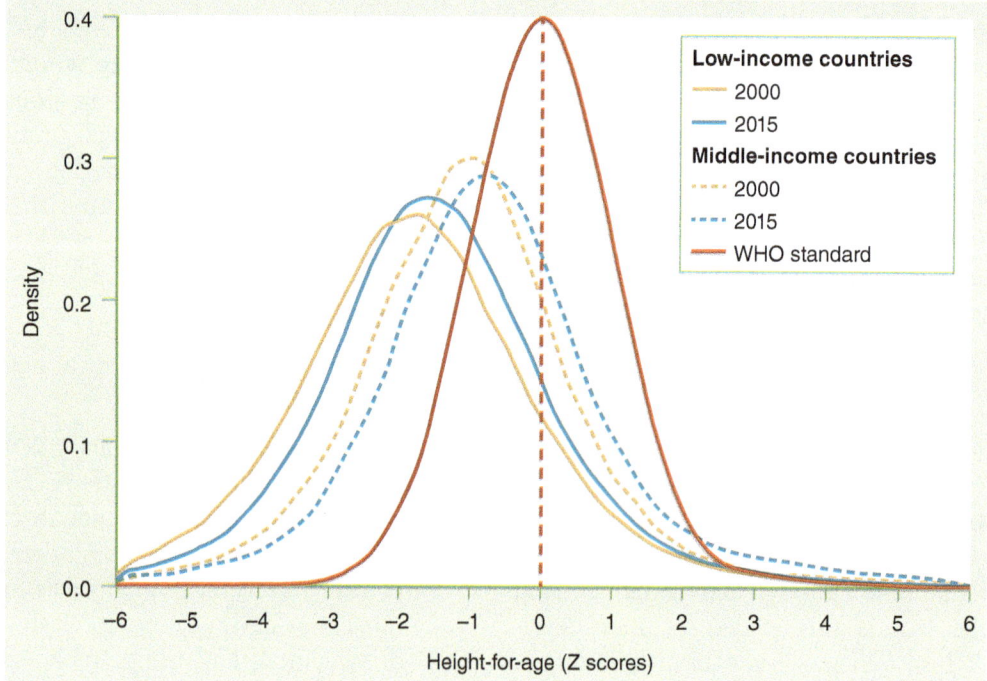

Figure 14.5 **Height for Age in Low- and Middle-income Countries for Children Under Age 5, 2000 and 2015.**

In low- and middle-income countries, growth faltering is a population-level problem. It is reflected by a shift in the entire growth distribution curve compared to well-nourished populations.

Reproduced from Victora CG, Christian P, Vidaletti LP, Gatica-Domínguez G, Menon P, Black RE. Revisiting maternal and child undernutrition in low-income and middle-income countries: variable progress towards an unfinished agenda. *Lancet.* 2021;397(10282):1388-1399. doi:10.1016/S0140-6736(21)00394-9

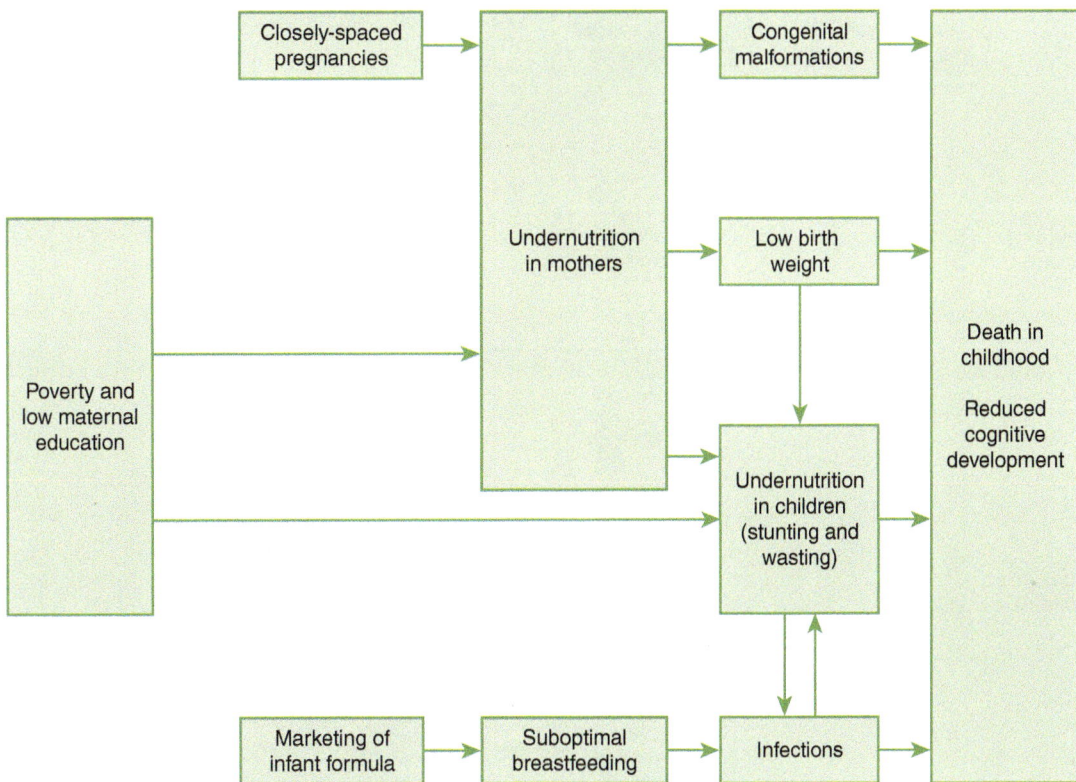

Figure 14.6 Cause-and-Effect Diagram for Maternal and Child Undernutrition. Undernutrition in mothers and children is primarily caused to poverty. Undernutrition in mothers often leads to undernutrition in infants and young children. However, other risk factors contribute to the problem, including closely-spaced pregnancies, the marketing of infant formula, and infections in children.

- *Closely-spaced pregnancies.* A mother needs time to restore nutrients before another pregnancy. Closely spaced pregnancies increase the risk of preterm birth, low birth weight, stunting, and wasting.[6,30] For example, in a study in Ghana, infants born less than 24 months after a previous child were twice as likely to be stunted or wasted as those born 48 more months afterward.[6]

- *Infections.* Malnutrition in young children is closely tied to infections, especially those causing diarrheal diseases. Children who are malnourished are more likely to develop diarrheal diseases, and children suffering from diarrheal diseases are more likely to become malnourished.[31-33] Diarrheal diseases and their connection to undernutrition are discussed more in Chapter 9. Infectious Diseases.

- *Suboptimal breastfeeding.* The World Health Organization recommends that all babies take in only breastmilk for the first six months and continue to breastfeed until their second birthday.[34] Breastfeeding helps protect infants from gastrointestinal and respiratory infections.[35] In low-income countries, infants who are not breastfed in the first 6 months are several times more likely to die, and children age 6–23 months who are not breastfed are about twice as likely to die.[35] In low- and middle-income countries today, less than half of infants under 6 months of age are exclusively breastfed.[34,35]

- *Marketing of infant formula.* Companies that make infant formulas promote artificial feeding in many ways, such as giving free formula to parents through hospitals, advertising to parents, and sponsoring organizations of pediatricians.[36] This marketing is effective—that is, it reduces breastfeeding.

Preventive Interventions

Because the cause of undernutrition is so clear, in theory the solution is also clear: give adult women and children additional nutrients. The difficulty lies in doing this sustainably for hundreds of millions of people.

Specific interventions that address the known risk factors for undernutrition are (**Figure 14.7**):

- *Economic development.* With poverty the fundamental cause of undernutrition, the best long-term solution is to end poverty. The global reduction in stunting shows that economic development alone can succeed, but it can take many years to occur.

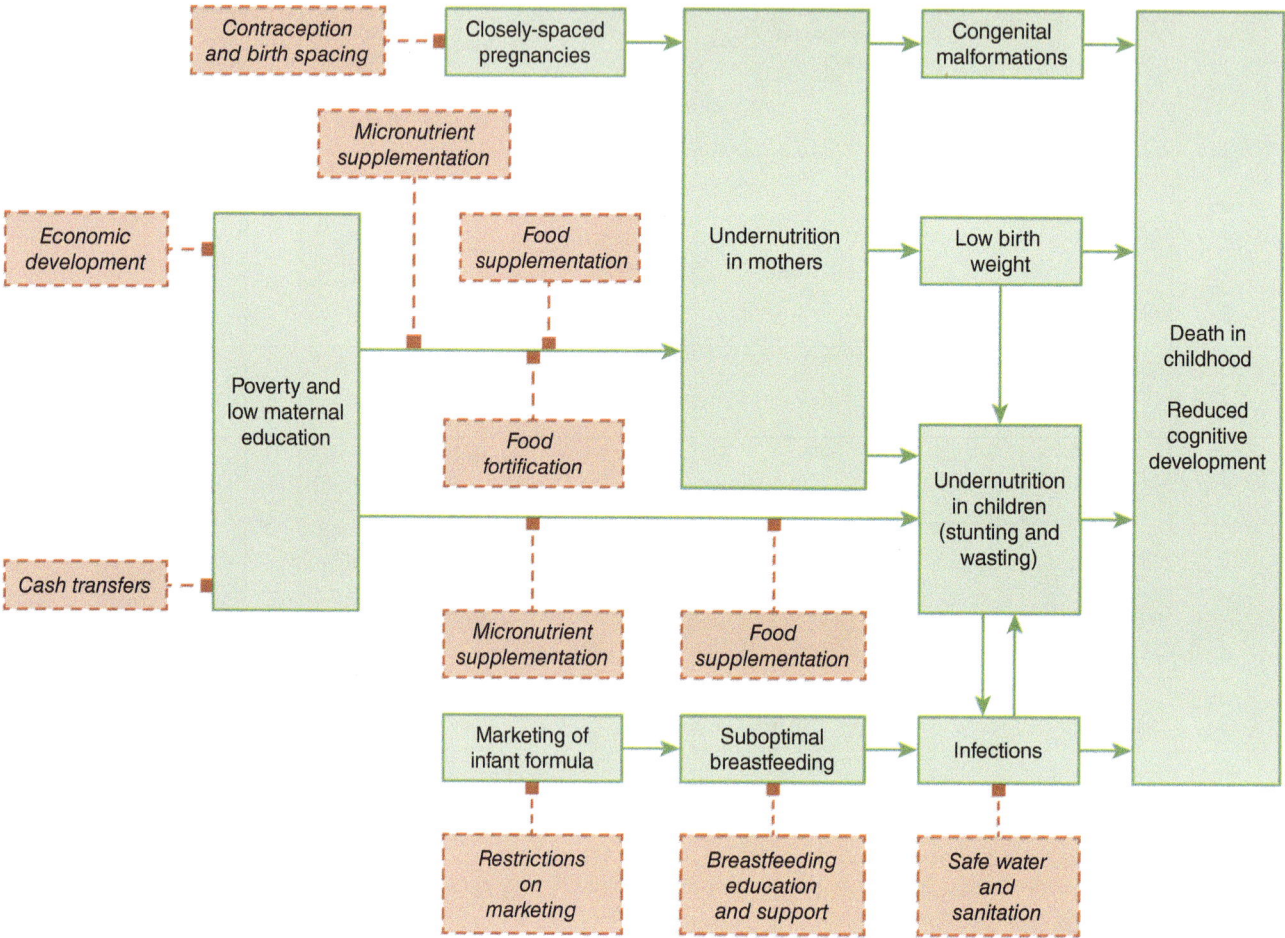

Figure 14.7 Cause-and-Effect Diagram for Maternal and Child Undernutrition, with Preventive Interventions.

- *Cash transfer.* A quicker solution to families living in poverty is simply to give them money. These are called **cash transfer** programs, and many countries in Latin America, Africa, and Asia operate them. Some programs provide money unconditionally and some are conditional—that is, they require families to take steps, such as having their children vaccinated to continue receiving payments.[37] These programs work extremely well. Even small amounts of money, such as $10–$30 per person per month, increase children's food intake and improve their health, including reducing child mortality.[37,38]

- *Food supplementation in pregnancy.* Programs in low-income countries that have given pregnant women supplementary food that is specifically tailored to pregnancy have reduced low birth weight; they have also reduced **stillbirth** (death of a fetus between the 20th week of pregnancy and delivery).[12] More general food supplementation programs for pregnant women have likewise helped, reducing low birth weight as well as wasting and stunting in their children.[12] In the United States, pregnant women who have

low incomes or nutritional risk factors qualify for food supplements through a federal program called the Special Supplemental Nutrition Program for Women, Infants, and Children (informally called WIC).

- *Micronutrient supplementation for pregnant women and other women of reproductive age.* Pregnant women can also be given supplements, not of food, but instead of key micronutrients. Supplementing women with multivitamins that include iron and folic acid has significantly reduced stillbirths, neural tube defects, and low birth weight.[12] The World Health Organization recommends that all pregnant women take iron and folic acid. The WHO also recommends that pregnant women living in areas where diets are likely to be deficient in vitamin A and calcium take supplements with these nutrients.[12,20] Ideally, supplements should also be taken by those who might become pregnant, including teenage girls. Taking folic acid supplements starting *before* pregnancy has been shown to reduce neural tube defects.[12]

- *Food fortification.* It is not realistic to expect that those who might become pregnant will take vitamin supplements consistently. To ensure that everyone is protected, some countries "fortify" common foods (like grains) with key micronutrients, particularly folic acid, iron, iodine, and vitamin A. This fortification has reduced health problems like anemia and neural tube defects.[39]

- *Contraception and birth spacing* enables women to restore their body's nutrients after pregnancy so that they have healthier subsequent pregnancies. Programs that make contraceptives available and encourage women to have more time between births have led to reductions in stunting in children.[12]

- *Breastfeeding education and support.* Programs that educate people about the benefits of breastfeeding have significantly boosted the number who breastfeed their babies.[12]

- *Restrictions on marketing of infant formula.* To restrict the marketing of formula, the World Health Organization has adopted an International Code of Marketing of Breast-milk Substitutes.[40] In addition, the WHO and UNICEF have developed criteria for delivery hospitals to be publicly designated as "baby-friendly" by not participating in the marketing of infant formula to their patients.[41] Babies born at hospitals that follow these "baby-friendly" rules are more likely to be exclusively breastfed.[42]

- *Food supplementation for infants and children.* In many low- and middle-income countries there are programs that give supplementary food to infants and young children who are no longer exclusively breastfed. While not all of these programs have had an impact on undernutrition, one review found that programs that were targeted to the poorest families reduced stunting and wasting.[12] In the United States, children in low-income families can receive government-funded foods through the WIC program.

- *Micronutrient supplementation for infants and young children.* Programs that give children in low-income countries supplements of key micronutrients have been very successful. Vitamin A supplementation by itself has reduced mortality in children, and zinc supplementation has reduced infectious diseases.[12] Programs that supplement infants and young children with multiple micronutrients have been associated with reductions in anemia, stunting, and mortality.[12]

- *Safe water and sanitation.* The close connection between diarrheal diseases and undernutrition suggests that just giving families access to clean water and sanitation may reduce undernutrition.

So far, though, low-cost programs to improve water quality and sanitation that have been evaluated have not had an impact on children's growth.[9]

Box 14.2 Summary–Prevention of Maternal and Child Undernutrition

- Economic development
- Cash transfers
- Food supplementation in pregnancy
- Micronutrient supplementation for pregnant women and women of reproductive age
- Food fortification
- Contraception and birth spacing
- Breastfeeding education and support
- Restrictions on marketing of infant formula
- Food supplementation for infants and children
- Micronutrient supplementation for infants and young children.
- Safe water and sanitation

Box 14.3 Key Words–Maternal and Child Undernutrition

Anemia
Cash transfer
Congenital malformations
Fetal growth restriction
Growth faltering
Hemoglobin
Low birth weight
Neural tube defect
Pre-eclampsia
Preterm birth
Stillbirth
Stunted, stunting
Thyroid gland
Wasted, wasting

Resources–Maternal and Child Undernutrition

- Victora CG, Christian P, Vidaletti LP, Gatica-Domínguez G, Menon P, Black RE. Revisiting maternal and child undernutrition in low-income and middle-income countries: variable progress towards an unfinished agenda. *The Lancet.* 2021;397(10282):1388-1399. doi:10.1016/S0140-6736(21)00394-9
- Keats EC, Das JK, Salam RA, et al. Effective interventions to address maternal and child malnutrition: an update of the evidence. *Lancet Child Adolesc Health.* 2021;5(5):367-384. doi:10.1016/S2352-4642(20)30274-1

Dietary Risks

Pathophysiology of Dietary Risks

Dietary risks are more complicated than undernutrition because they involve eating the wrong types of foods—not enough of certain foods and too much of others.

The foods that are most strongly linked to preventable illnesses in the United States are listed in **Table 14.2**. The table also shows rough estimates of the number of deaths that can be attributed to consumption of these foods.[43,44] This table illustrates a few key points:

- There is much overlap among the foods that increase the risk of cardiovascular disease,

Table 14.2 **Estimates of Attributable Risks of Deaths and Strength of Evidence for Most Important Dietary Risk Factors, United States**

This table summarizes how many deaths in the United States can be attributed to different dietary risk factors. For those that have not been estimated, the table summarizes the strength of the scientific evidence that these risk factors cause these health problems.

Dietary risk factor		Cardiovascular disease	Obesity and type 2 diabetes	Colon cancer	Breast cancer	All deaths
Too much	Red meat	**	*	**	*	***
	Processed meat	***	**	*	+	***
	Refined grains	++	+		+	++
	Sugar-sweetened beverages and foods	*	*	+	+	*
	Saturated fatty acids	+	+	+		
	Cholesterol	++	+			
	Sodium	***	+			***
Not enough	Seafood	***	+	+		***
	Whole grains	***	*	**	+	****
	Fruits	***	*	+	+	***
	Vegetables	***	+	+	+	***
	Legumes	***	+	+		***
	Nuts	*	*			*
	Milk (low fat)	++	+	*		*
	Polyunsaturated fatty acids	*	+			*
	Potassium	++				
All dietary factors		****	***	***	*	*****

Attributable deaths in GBD analysis
*0–10,000
**10,000–25,000
***25,000–75,000
****75,000–300,000
*****>300,000

Evidence, for those not included in GBD analysis
+Moderate evidence
++Strong evidence

Data from Global Burden of Disease Collaboration, Institute for Health Metrics and Evaluation. GBD Results Tool. Published July 12, 2023. Accessed July 14, 2024. https://vizhub.healthdata.org/gbd-results/ and U.S. Department of Agriculture. USDA Nutrition Evidence Systematic Review. USDA. Published 2023. Accessed July 14, 2024. https://nesr.usda.gov/

diabetes, colon cancer, and breast cancer. For example, over-consumption of red meat and under-consumption of whole grains are risks for all of these diseases.

- The foods that are over-consumed and under-consumed often fall naturally into pairs, such as too many refined grains and not enough whole grains. These pairs give insight into the mismatch between what Americans eat and what humans' bodies are designed to handle. For example, humans are better equipped to digest whole grains than refined grains, need more potassium and less sodium, and would be healthier eating less meat and more seafood.
- The foods that are over-consumed tend to be highly processed, and the foods that are under-consumed tend to be unprocessed. Refined grains, processed meats, sugar-sweetened beverages, and sodium are the products of factories, but fruits, vegetables (and the potassium in them), and whole grains grow on farms.
- The overall effect on health from these dietary risks is very large. The Global Burden of Disease project estimates that 350,000 deaths per year in the United States are attributable to all dietary risks combined, which places dietary risks alongside tobacco as the top killers in America. About 240,000 diet-related deaths result from cardiovascular disease alone.

Other chapters discuss the biologic connections between these foods and specific illnesses, but a few key relationships are summarized here:

Sugar-sweetened Beverages

Sugar-sweetened beverages contain many calories, which by itself can lead to obesity. But dissolved sugar is not (as is often claimed) just "empty calories." These beverages cause chronic diseases.[45] The monosaccharides and disaccharides are digested and absorbed by the intestines very quickly, causing a very rapid rise in blood glucose.[45] The body responds to this rapid rise in blood glucose by releasing large amounts of the hormone **insulin** (see Chapter 7. Chronic Metabolic Diseases). The primary role of insulin is to regulate blood glucose levels, but high insulin levels also cause the body to store fat. By promoting fat storage, regular consumption of sugar-sweetened beverages can cause cells to become resistant to insulin, which can lead to type 2 diabetes.[45,46]

Sugar-sweetened beverages are thought to increase the risk of heart disease and stroke because the repeated high levels of insulin can raise the levels of cholesterol and triglycerides in the blood.[46-48] That promotes **atherosclerosis**, the clogging of the arteries with cholesterol that underlies cardiovascular disease.

Beverages are the largest source of sugar in the American diet, but added sugars in foods may pose some similar risks.[44,49,50]

Refined Grains and Whole Grains

Refined grains act like sugar-sweetened beverages. Because the refining process strips grains of **fiber** (food components than cannot be digested), the carbohydrates in grains are rapidly digested into glucose, causing a rapid rise in blood glucose and a large insulin response.[46] Whole grains, in which the carbohydrates are still encased in fiber, are thought to have the opposite effect, slowing the rise in blood glucose and reducing insulin levels.

Whole grains also reduce the risk of colon cancer. Experts believe this is because the dietary fiber in whole grains is metabolized in the colon into compounds that reduce cell proliferation.[51]

Fruits, Vegetables, and Legumes

Fruits, vegetables, and legumes help prevent obesity and diabetes. This may be simply because they have a low **energy density** (calories per gram) or because they do not cause a rapid rise in blood glucose or a spike in insulin levels.[46] The lower insulin levels also reduce the risk of cardiovascular disease.[46,52,53]

These foods may prevent heart disease and stroke in other ways, too. Fruits, vegetables, and legumes tend to be rich in potassium and magnesium, which lower blood pressure. They also contain chemicals that are **antioxidants**, which prevent **oxidation** of fats.[53] (When fats in the body undergo oxidation, it may cause inflammation in the blood, which increases the risk of atherosclerosis.)[54]

It is unclear how fruits, vegetables, and legumes reduce the risk of cancer, but the fiber, minerals, and other organic compounds in them may protect against the transformation of normal cells into cancer cells.

Fatty Acids

Saturated fatty acids increase the risk of heart disease and stroke because, compared to polyunsaturated fatty acids, they tend to raise blood cholesterol levels, increasing the risk of atherosclerosis.[55]

Red Meat and Processed Meat

Red meat (including beef, pork, and lamb) and processed meat (such as bacon, hot dogs, sausage, and lunch meats) are thought to increase the risk of cardiovascular disease in several ways:

- They contain high levels of saturated fats.
- They contain **heme**, a compound in red blood cells. When heme is in food, it is thought to cause the oxidation of fats.[54]
- Processed meat is high in sodium, so it raises blood pressure.

Red meat and processed meat are thought to increase the risk of cancer through heme. Heme stimulates the formation in the colon of "N-nitroso compounds," which are **carcinogenic** (cause cancer), and processed meat contains nitrates and nitrites that have the same effect. In addition, cooking meats at high temperatures produces chemicals that are carcinogenic.[54]

It is not clear why red meat and processed meat are associated in epidemiologic studies with an increased risk of obesity and diabetes.[54,56]

Nuts and Seeds

Nuts and seeds are thought to reduce the risk of cardiovascular disease in ways similar to fruits, vegetables, and legumes. They contain fiber that prevents a spike in blood glucose, and they contain antioxidants. In addition, nuts and seeds tend to contain more polyunsaturated fatty acids and less saturated fatty acids.[57]

Sodium and Potassium

Sodium tends to increase blood pressure and potassium tends to reduce it.[58] For more on this, see Chapter 2. Heart Disease and Stroke.

Epidemiology: Patterns and Trends in Dietary Risks

There are large differences between the foods that are known to be healthy and what Americans eat. The American Heart Association (AHA) has developed a score for the healthfulness of a person's diet, based on how close that person is to consuming the recommended amounts of eight key foods and food components. Four healthy food components are scored on a scale of 0 to 10, and four unhealthy food components are scored 10 to 0 (with less consumption given a higher score). The component scores are then added, giving a final score between 0 to 80, with 80 a perfectly healthy diet.[59] In 2017–2020, the average AHA diet score for Americans was a very low 36.7.[60]

Figure 14.8 shows the average scores for each of the food components from 1999 to 2020.[60] Americans' diets were furthest from recommendations in whole grains and in fish and shellfish, with average scores between 2 and 3. They were only slightly better in fruits, vegetables, nuts, seeds, legumes, sodium, and saturated fat. Scores for sugar-sweetened beverages were the highest in 2017–20, as Americans increasingly avoided sugary drinks. Overall, diets became only slightly healthier during these years.

Figure 14.9 shows average total AHA diet scores by demographic group in 2017–2020. The average score was higher for Asians than for other racial and ethnic groups, higher for people with more income, and higher for older adults. However, these differences were very small compared to the gap between every group's diet and what is recommended.[60]

Risk Factors for Unhealthy Diets

People choose to eat what they like from the available options, but their eating choices are influenced by many factors, including (Figure 14.10):

- *Availability and accessibility.* The more available and accessible a food item is, the more people will eat it. Obviously, if a food item is not available at all, no one will eat it, and if it is available, people have the option to eat it. But even small differences in how available and accessible a food item is can make big differences in how much people buy and eat it.[61,62] Nearly all grocery stores devote much more shelf space to unhealthy items than to healthy items.[63] And unhealthy snack foods are placed not just in grocery stores but also alongside the cash registers of most other types of retail stores, such as pharmacies, gasoline stations, and hardware stores.[64]

  The price of foods also matters. Not surprisingly, when prices of food items are higher, people buy and eat less of them, and vice versa.[65,66] On average, a 10% change in the price of foods is accompanied by a 6%–12% change in sales in the opposite direction.[65]

- *Food product design.* While the healthiest foods grow from the ground and need little processing, the foods that people eat are increasingly highly processed products that are designed in laboratories and produced in factories. The design of these products has a big impact on consumption.[61] Specifically, the diets and health of consumers are influenced by:

  - *Ingredients,* such as sodium, potassium, sugar, refined grains, and added fats.

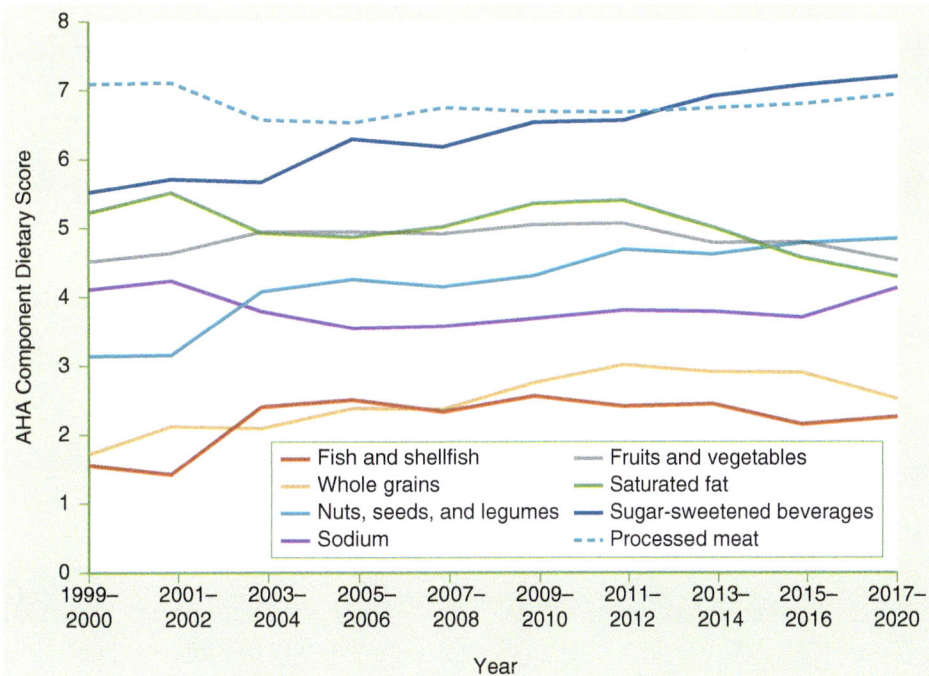

Figure 14.8 **Trends in Dietary Component Quality Scores Among Adults in the United States, 1999–2020.** Trends in scores showing consumption of four healthy diet components and four unhealthy diet components. Scores are on a scale of 0 to 10; for healthy components higher scores reflect more consumption, and for unhealthy components higher scores reflect less consumption. Americans' diets were furthest from recommendations in whole grains and in fish and shellfish. Scores for sugar-sweetened beverages increased during this time as Americans increasingly avoided sugary drinks.

Data from Liu J, Mozaffarian D. Trends in Diet Quality Among U.S. Adults From 1999 to 2020 by Race, Ethnicity, and Socioeconomic Disadvantage. Ann Intern Med. June 2024. doi:10.7326/M24-0190

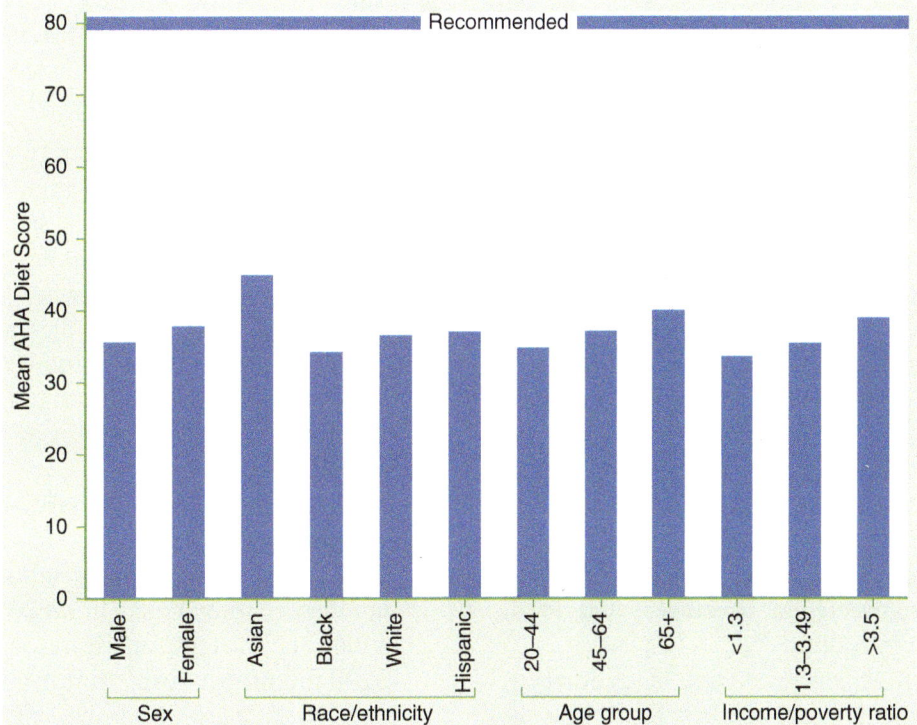

Figure 14.9 **AHA Diet Quality Score for American Adults by Demographic Group, 2017–20.** Trends in scores of total diet quality by sex, race/ethnicity, income, and age group. Total scores are the sum of eight dietary component scores and fall on a scale of 0 (least healthy) to 80 (most healthy).

Data from Liu J, Mozaffarian D. Trends in Diet Quality Among U.S. Adults From 1999 to 2020 by Race, Ethnicity, and Socioeconomic Disadvantage. Ann Intern Med. June 2024. doi:10.7326/M24-0190

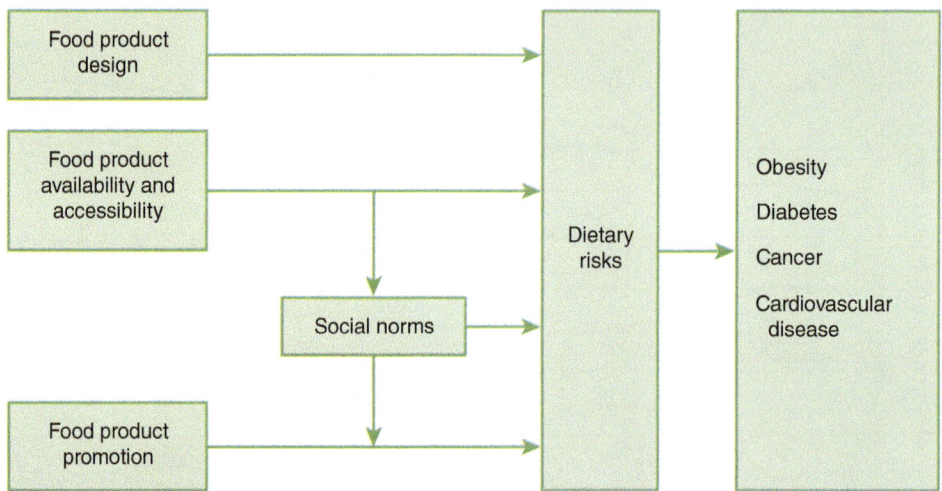

Figure 14.10 Cause-and-Effect Diagram for Dietary Risks.

- *Processing,* such as whether grains are whole or refined.
- *Portion sizes.* People tend to consume the full amount of a product sold as a single portion, regardless of how large that portion is.[67] During the sharp increase in obesity from 1980 through 2010, portion sizes of packaged foods and items sold at fast food restaurants grew two- to five-fold.[68,69]
- *Packaging and labeling.* Packaging and labeling are central to how all products are marketed, and they greatly influence people's choices.[61] For example, foods with names and packaging that hint at healthfulness (such as fruit-flavored sugary drinks, or crackers labeled as "low fat") can attract consumers by persuading them that the foods are healthier.
- *Food product promotion.* The food industry spends more than $10 billion a year advertising packaged foods and restaurants.[70] Coca-Cola and PepsiCo alone spend more than $1.3 billion.[70] Companies advertise and promote their food products not just in the general media but also inside food stores to encourage people to buy them on impulse.[71] Nearly all food advertising promotes foods that Americans consume too much of: red meat, processed meat, refined grains, sugar-sweetened beverages, and foods that are high in sodium.[70]
- *Social norms.* As with smoking and drinking, social norms influence people's eating. People often eat food with others, and they tend to eat the type and amount of foods that others around them are eating or consider to be normal.[72]

These social norms are in turn influenced by the availability of different types of food and by promotion of food items.

Preventive Interventions

Unfortunately, there are few success stories of interventions that have reduced dietary risks in entire populations. But, by understanding the risk factors for unhealthy eating, we can list interventions that may work.

Many of these interventions involve changes in government policy and programs. The U.S. government is already heavily involved in shaping America's food system, often in ways that encourage unhealthy eating. The most important government food programs are:

- The farm commodity program, which provides about $6 billion per year in subsidies and price guarantees to agribusinesses to grow "commodity" crops—mostly corn, wheat, soybeans, and sugar. Because these subsidies are tied to how much these businesses produce, this program encourages the overproduction of these commodity crops, which reduces prices and encourages over-consumption.[73-75]
- The **Supplemental Nutrition Assistance Program (SNAP**, formerly called Food Stamps), which provides financial benefits to low-income families to buy food. In 2024, SNAP served about one in eight Americans, at a cost of about $100 billion per year.[76] Unfortunately, the foods purchased with SNAP benefits are not very healthy. Nearly 20% of the benefits are used to buy sugar-sweetened beverages, desserts, salty snacks, candy, and sugar.[77]

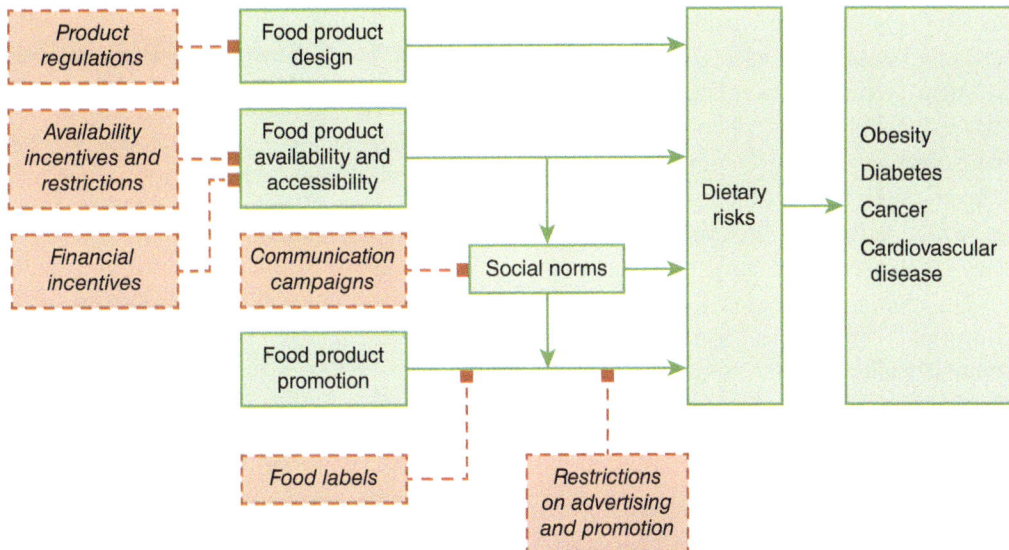

Figure 14.11 Cause-and-Effect Diagram for Dietary Risks, with Preventive Interventions.

- The National School Lunch Program and School Breakfast Program, through which the U.S. government pays for most school meals for children in America. In 2010, Congress passed improved nutrition standards for school foods by setting minimum amounts for fruits, vegetables, and whole grains (and for meat), and maximum amounts for sodium and saturated fat.[78]

- Regulation of food safety by the Food and Drug Administration (FDA). These regulations are mostly designed to prevent bacterial contamination of food, which is not a large public health problem today. However, the FDA has prohibited some disease-causing food additives like trans fat, and it has the authority to regulate other food additives to reduce disease risks.

With this current government involvement in mind, interventions that may improve diet at the population level include (**Figure 14.11**):

- *Food labels.* The FDA requires manufacturers to label the back of food packages with information about ingredients and calories, but these labels are extremely hard for most people to interpret. The FDA could instead require manufacturers to put simpler labels on the front of food packages. In the early 2020s, many other countries tried simple front-of-pack labels. Some labels inform people about several food components, with each component color-coded (called "multiple traffic light" labels) and some give more explicit warnings, such as the system used in Chile (**Figure 14.12**).[79-81] In addition to helping consumers make healthier choices, the systems may encourage manufacturers to produce healthier foods to avoid negative labels.

- *Financial incentives:* Financial incentives could be used to encourage healthier food production or promotion. These incentives could be applied at various levels of the food system: farmers, manufacturers, retailers, or consumers. For example, the subsidies to grow wheat, corn, and sugar could be changed to subsidies to grow fruits and

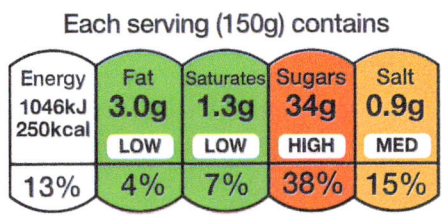

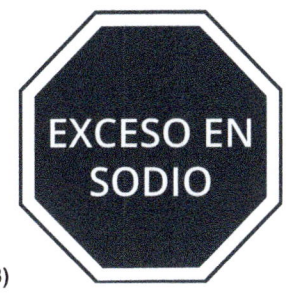

Figure 14.12 Front-of-pack Nutrition Labels Used in the **(A)** the United Kingdom (left) and **(B)** Chile (right).

(A) Department of Health and Social Care, 'Guide to creating a front of pack (FoP) nutrition label for pre-packed products sold through retail outlets', GOV.UK, 2016; **(B)** © EveVectors/Shutterstock

vegetables. Or the SNAP program could restrict the use of financial benefits for extremely unhealthy items like sugar-sweetened beverages and/or give extra dollar value of benefits when they are used to buy fruits and vegetables. Or unhealthy items could be taxed, such as a tax on sugar-sweetened beverages, which is in place in several U.S. cities. Where they have been tried, financial incentives have worked, changing people's food purchases or consumption.[65,82-86] Sugary-drink taxes have been particularly effective: in U.S. cities they have been followed not only by reductions in soda consumption but also by reductions in children's body mass index (BMI) compared to cities without these taxes.[87-89]

- *Availability incentives and restrictions.* Policies could provide incentives or restrictions to increase the availability of healthy foods and reduce the over-abundance of the unhealthiest foods. These have been proven successful in schools. School policies to increase the availability of fruits, vegetables, and water and to restrict snack foods and sugary drinks have improved children's diets and reduced childhood obesity.[90] Similar approaches could be tried in stores. For example, grocery stores could be given incentives to increase their shelf space of fruits and vegetables and to limit the shelf space for the unhealthiest foods. Sales of unhealthy foods could be prohibited in non-food retailers like gasoline stations and hardware stores. Food availability changes have been tried for sugar-sweetened beverages—for example, prohibiting them on children's menus at restaurants, and they have worked, prompting people to choose healthier beverages instead.[84]

- *Product regulations.* Government regulations on foods could be updated to prevent the leading causes of death today: heart disease, cancer, and diabetes. For example, regulations could prohibit companies from selling the unhealthiest items (such as foods with dangerously high levels of sodium) or require that certain items use whole rather than refined grains.

- *Restrictions on advertising and promotion.* Advertising and promotion of cigarettes is restricted in the United States, and this advertising restriction has helped reduce smoking. Similarly restricting the advertising of particularly unhealthy foods may help reduce how much people consume them.

- *Communications campaigns.* Public health organizations can run communications campaigns in the mass media to discourage unhealthy foods and encourage healthy foods.[91]

Box 14.4 **Summary–Prevention of Dietary Risks**

- Food labels
- Financial incentives
- Availability incentives and restriction
- Product regulations
- Restrictions on advertising and promotion
- Communications campaigns

Box 14.5 **Key Words–Dietary Risks**

Antioxidant
Atherosclerosis
Carcinogen, carcinogenic
Energy density
Fiber
Heme
Insulin
Oxidation
Supplemental Nutrition Assistance Program
(SNAP)

Resources–Dietary Risks

- *The Scientific Report of the 2020 Dietary Guidelines Advisory Committee: Advisory Report to the Secretary of Agriculture and Secretary of Health and Human Services.* This report provides the detailed scientific evidence behind the Dietary Guidelines for Americans.
- Mozaffarian D. Dietary and Policy Priorities for Cardiovascular Disease, Diabetes, and Obesity. *Circulation.* 2016;133(2):187-225. doi:10.1161 /CIRCULATIONAHA.115.018585. This is a highly detailed review of the nutritional risks for obesity, diabetes, and cardiovascular disease.
- Congressional Research Service. *Farm Bill Primer: What Is the Farm Bill?* https://crsreports.congress .gov
- Healthy Eating Research (at https://healthyeat ingresearch.org) is a program that conducts research and produces reports on policy, systems, and environmental strategies to promote healthy eating among children.
- Hollands GJ, Carter P, Anwer S, et al. Altering the availability or proximity of food, alcohol, and tobacco products to change their selection and consumption. *Cochrane Database of Systematic Reviews.* 2019 Aug 27;8(8):CD012573. doi: 10.1002/14651858.CD012573.pub2

References

1. World Health Organization. Malnutrition. World Health Organization. Published March 1, 2024. Accessed October 24, 2024. Available at: https://www.who.int/news-room/fact-sheets/detail/malnutrition/

2. Popkin BM, Corvalan C, Grummer-Strawn LM. Dynamics of the double burden of malnutrition and the changing nutrition reality. *Lancet.* 2020;395(10217):6574. doi:10.1016/S0140-6736(19)32497-3

3. Pan American Health Organization, World Health Organization. *Ultra-Processed Food and Drink Products in Latin America: Trends, Impact on Obesity, Policy Implications.* PAHO/WHO; 2015.

4. Centers for Disease Control and Prevention (CDC). Micronutrient facts. Published February 1, 2022. Accessed November 30, 2023. Available at: https://www.cdc.gov/nutrition/micronutrient-malnutrition/micronutrients/index.html

5. United States Department of Agriculture. DRI calculator for healthcare professionals. National Agricultural Library. Published 2024. Accessed July 11, 2024. Available at: https://www.nal.usda.gov/human-nutrition-and-food-safety/dri-calculator

6. Essilfie G, Kofinti RE, Asmah EE. Reducing stunting and underweight through mother's birth spacing: Evidence from Ghana. *BMC Pregnancy Childbirth.* 2024;24(1):624. doi:10.1186/s12884-024-06824-1

7. Dewey KG, Cohen RJ. Does birth spacing affect maternal or child nutritional status? A systematic literature review. *Matern Child Nutr.* 2007;3(3):151-173. doi:10.1111/j.1740-8709.2007.00092.x

8. Mertens A, Benjamin-Chung J, Colford JM, et al. Causes and consequences of child growth faltering in low-resource settings. *Nature.* 2023;621(7979):568-576. doi:10.1038/s41586-023-06501-x

9. Victora CG, Christian P, Vidaletti LP, Gatica-Domínguez G, Menon P, Black RE. Revisiting maternal and child undernutrition in low-income and middle-income countries: variable progress towards an unfinished agenda. *Lancet.* 2021;397(10282):1388-1399. doi:10.1016/S0140-6736(21)00394-9

10. Ramakrishnan U, Grant F, Goldenberg T, Zongrone A, Martorell R. Effect of women's nutrition before and during early pregnancy on maternal and infant outcomes: A systematic review. *Paediatr Perinat Epidemiol.* 2012;26(Suppl 1):285-301. doi:10.1111/j.1365-3016.2012.01281.x

11. Bryce E, Gurung S, Tong H, et al. Population attributable fractions for risk factors for spontaneous preterm births in 81 low- and middle-income countries: A systematic analysis. *J Glob Health.* 2022;12:04013. doi:10.7189/jogh.12.04013

12. Keats EC, Das JK, Salam RA, et al. Effective interventions to address maternal and child malnutrition: an update of the evidence. *Lancet Child Adolesc Health.* 2021;5(5):367-384. doi:10.1016/S2352-4642(20)30274-1

13. Goldenberg RL, Culhane JF, Iams JD, Romero R. Epidemiology and causes of preterm birth. *Lancet.* 2008;371(9606):75-84. doi:10.1016/S0140-6736(08)60074-4

14. Botto LD, Krikov S, Carmichae SL, Munger RG, Shaw GM, Feldkamp ML. Lower rate of selected congenital heart defects with better maternal diet quality: A population-based study. *Arch Dis Child Fetal Neonatal Ed.* 2016;101(1):F43-F49. doi:10.1136/archdischild-2014-308013

15. Carmichael SL, Yang W, Feldkamp ML, et al. Reduced risks of neural tube defects and orofacial clefts with higher diet quality. *Arch Pediatr Adolesc Med.* 2012;166(2):121-126. doi:10.1001/archpediatrics.2011.185

16. Carmichael SL, Yang W, Gilboa S, et al. Elevated body mass index and decreased diet quality among women and risk of birth defects in their offspring. *Birth Defects Res A Clin Mol Teratol.* 2016;106(3):164-171. doi:10.1002/bdra.23471

17. Crider KS, Qi YP, Yeung LF, et al. Folic acid and the prevention of birth defects: 30 years of opportunity and controversies. *Annu Rev Nutr.* 2022;42:423-452. doi:10.1146/annurev-nutr-043020

18. Olofin I, McDonald CM, Ezzati M, et al. Associations of suboptimal growth with all-cause and cause-specific mortality in children under five years: A pooled analysis of ten prospective studies. *PLoS One.* 2013;8(5). doi:10.1371/journal.pone.0064636

19. Black RE, Victora CG, Walker SP, et al. Maternal and child undernutrition and overweight in low-income and middle-income countries. *Lancet.* 2013;382(9890):427-451. doi:10.1016/S0140-6736(13)60937-X

20. Christian P, Mullany LC, Hurley KM, Katz J, Black RE. Nutrition and maternal, neonatal, and child health. *Semin Perinatol.* 2015;39(5):361-372. doi:10.1053/j.semperi.2015.06.009

21. Victora CG, Adair L, Fall C, et al. Maternal and child undernutrition 2 maternal and child undernutrition: consequences for adult health and human capital. *Lancet.* 2008;371:340-357. doi:10.1016/S0140

22. Adair LS, Fall CHD, Osmond C, et al. Associations of linear growth and relative weight gain during early life with adult health and human capital in countries of low and middle income: Findings from five birth cohort studies. *Lancet.* 2013;382(9891):525-534. doi:10.1016/S0140-6736(13)60103-8

23. National Institutes of Health, Office of Dietary Supplements. Dietary supplement fact sheets. National Institutes of Health. Published November 8, 2022. Accessed October 29, 2024. Available at: https://ods.od.nih.gov/factsheets/list-all/

24. World Health Organization. Vitamin A deficiency. World Health Organization. Published 2020. Accessed April 14, 2024. Available at: https://www.who.int/data/nutrition/nlis/info/vitamin-a-deficiency

25. Roth DE, Abrams SA, Aloia J, et al. Global prevalence and disease burden of vitamin D deficiency: A roadmap for action in low-and middle-income countries. *Ann N Y Acad Sci.* 2018;1430(1):44-79. doi:10.1111/nyas.13968

26. Dhingra U, Kisenge R, Sudfeld CR, et al. Lower-dose zinc for childhood diarrhea—a randomized, multicenter trial. *N Engl J Med.* 2020;383(13):1231-1241. doi:10.1056/nejmoa1915905

27. World Health Organization. The Global Health Observatory. Published 2023. Accessed August 1, 2024. Available at: https://www.who.int/data/gho/data/indicators/indicator-details/GHO/gho-jme-stunting-prevalence

28. Roth DE, Krishna A, Leung M, Shi J, Bassani DG, Barros AJD. Early childhood linear growth faltering in low-income and middle-income countries as a whole-population condition: analysis of 179 Demographic and Health Surveys from 64 countries (1993–2015). *Lancet Glob Health.* 2017;5:e1249-e1257.

29. Amadu I, Seidu AA, Duku E, et al. Risk factors associated with the coexistence of stunting, underweight, and wasting in children under 5 from 31 sub-Saharan African countries. *BMJ Open.* 2021;11(12). doi:10.1136/bmjopen-2021-052267

30. Hassen TA, Harris ML, Shifti DM, et al. Effects of short inter-pregnancy/birth interval on adverse perinatal outcomes in Asia-Pacific region: A systematic review and meta-analysis. *PLoS One.* 2024;19(7 July). doi:10.1371/journal.pone.0307942

31. Brown KH. Diarrhea and Malnutrition. *J Nutr.* 2003;133(1):328S-332S. doi:10.1093/jn/133.1.328S

32. Acosta AM, De Burga RR, Chavez CB, et al. Relationship between growth and illness, enteropathogens and dietary intakes in the first 2 years of life: Findings from the MAL-ED birth cohort study. *BMJ Glob Health.* 2017;2(4). doi:10.1136/bmjgh-2017-000370

33. Checkley W, Buckley G, Gilman RH, et al. Multi-country analysis of the effects of diarrhea on childhood stunting. *Int J Epidemiol.* 2008;37(4):816-830. doi:10.1093/ije/dyn099

34. World Health Organization. Infant and Young Child Feeding. Published December 20, 2023. Accessed October 24, 2024. Available at: https://www.who.int/news-room/fact-sheets/detail/infant-and-young-child-feeding

35. Victora CG, Bahl R, Barros AJD, et al. Breastfeeding in the 21st century: epidemiology, mechanisms, and lifelong effect. *Lancet.* 2016;387:475-490. Available at: http://mics

36. Piwoz EG, Huffman SL. Impact of marketing of breast-milk substitutes on WHO-recommended breastfeeding practices. *Food Nutr Bull.* 2015;36(4):373-386. doi:10.1177/0379572115602174

37. Huda TM, Alam A, Tahsina T, et al. Shonjibon cash and counselling: a community-based cluster randomised controlled trial to measure the effectiveness of unconditional cash transfers and mobile behaviour change communications to reduce child undernutrition in rural Bangladesh. *BMC Public Health.* 2020;20(1). doi:10.1186/s12889-020-09780-5

38. Richterman A, Millien C, Bair EF, et al. The effects of cash transfers on adult and child mortality in low- and middle-income countries. *Nature.* 2023;618(7965):575-582. doi:10.1038/s41586-023-06116-2

39. Keats EC, Neufeld LM, Garrett GS, Mbuya MNN, Bhutta ZA. Improved micronutrient status and health outcomes in low-and middle-income countries following large-scale fortification: Evidence from a systematic review and meta-Analysis. *Am J Clinl Nutr.* 2019;109(6):1696-1708. doi:10.1093/ajcn/nqz023

40. World Health Organization. International code for marketing of breast-milk substitutes. Published 1981. Accessed October 28, 2024. Available at: https://www.who.int/publications/i/item/9241541601

41. World Health Organization. Promoting Baby-friendly Hospitals. Published 2024. Accessed October 28, 2024. Available at: https://www.who.int/activities/promoting-baby-friendly-hospitals

42. Venancio SI, Saldiva SRDM, Escuder MML, Giugliani ERJ. The Baby-Friendly Hospital Initiative shows positive effects on breastfeeding indicators in Brazil. *J Epidemiol Community Health (1978).* 2012;66(10):914-918. doi:10.1136/jech-2011-200332

43. Global Burden of Disease Collaboration, Institute for Health Metrics and Evaluation. GBD Results. Published May 16, 2024. Accessed April 19, 2025. Available at: https://vizhub.healthdata.org/gbd-results/

44. U.S. Department of Agriculture. USDA Nutrition Evidence Systematic Review. USDA. Published 2024. Accessed July 14, 2024. Available at: https://nesr.usda.gov/

45. Malik VS, Hu FB. Sugar-sweetened beverages and cardiometabolic health: An update of the evidence. *Nutrients.* 2019;11(8). doi:10.3390/nu11081840

46. Mozaffarian D. Dietary and policy priorities for cardiovascular disease, diabetes, and obesity. *Circulation.* 2016;133(2):187-225. doi:10.1161/CIRCULATIONAHA.115.018585

47. Ludwig DS, Ebbeling CB. The carbohydrate-insulin model of obesity: Beyond "calories in, calories out." *JAMA Intern Med.* 2018;178(8):1098-1103. doi:10.1001/jamainternmed.2018.2933

48. Swaminathan S, Dehghan M, Raj JM, et al. Associations of cereal grains intake with cardiovascular disease and mortality across 21 countries in prospective urban and rural epidemiology study: Prospective cohort study. *The BMJ.* 2021;372. doi:10.1136/bmj.m4948

49. Te Morenga LA, Howatson AJ, Jones RM, Mann J. Dietary sugars and cardiometabolic risk: Systematic review and meta-analyses of randomized controlled trials of the effects on blood pressure and lipids. *Am J Clinl Nutr.* 2014;100(1):65-79. doi:10.3945/ajcn.113.081521

50. Debras C, Chazelas E, Srour B, et al. Total and added sugar intakes, sugar types, and cancer risk: Results from the prospective NutriNet-Santé cohort. *Am J Clin Nutr.* 2020;112(5):1267-1279. doi:10.1093/ajcn/nqaa246

51. American Institute of Cancer Research, World Cancer Research Fund. Diet, nutrition, physical activity and colorectal cancer. Published 2018. Accessed July 2, 2023. Available at: https://dietandcancerreport.org

52. Fardet A. New hypotheses for the health-protective mechanisms of whole-grain cereals: What is beyond fibre? *Nutr Res Rev.* 2010;23(1):65-134. doi:10.1017/S0954422410000041

53. Miller V, Mente A, Dehghan M, et al. Fruit, vegetable, and legume intake, and cardiovascular disease and deaths in 18 countries (PURE): A prospective cohort study. *Lancet.* 2017;390(10107):2037-2049. doi:10.1016/S0140-6736(17)32253-5

54. Rohrmann S, Linseisen J. Processed meat: The real villain? *Proc Nutr Soc.* 2016;75(3):233-241. doi:10.1017/S0029665115004255

55. Sacks FM, Lichtenstein AH, Wu JHY, et al. Dietary fats and cardiovascular disease: A presidential advisory from the American Heart Association. *Circulation.* 2017;136(3):e1-e23. doi:10.1161/CIR.0000000000000510

56. Kim Y, Keogh J, Clifton P. A review of potential metabolic etiologies of the observed association between red meat consumption and development of type 2 diabetes mellitus. *Metabolism.* 2015;64(7):768-779. doi:10.1016/j.metabol.2015.03.008

57. Kim Y, Keogh JB, Clifton PM. Benefits of nut consumption on insulin resistance and cardiovascular risk factors: Multiple potential mechanisms of actions. *Nutrients.* 2017;9(11). doi:10.3390/nu9111271

58. Whelton PK, Carey RM, Aronow WS, et al. 2017 guideline for the prevention, detection, evaluation, and management

of high blood pressure in adults. *J Am Coll Cardiol.* 2018;71(19). doi:10.1016/j.jacc.2017.11.006

59. Rehm CD, Peñalvo JL, Afshin A, Mozaffarian D. Dietary intake among US Adults, 1999–2012. *JAMA.* 2016;315(23):2542-2553. doi:10.1001/jama.2016.7491

60. Liu J, Mozaffarian D. Trends in diet quality among U.S. adults from 1999 to 2020 by race, ethnicity, and socioeconomic disadvantage. *Ann Intern Med.* June 2024. doi:10.7326/M24-0190

61. Cohen DA, Babey SH. Contextual influences on eating behaviours: Heuristic processing and dietary choices. *Obes Rev.* 2012;13(9):766-779. doi:10.1111/j.1467-789X.2012.01001.x

62. Hollands GJ, Carter P, Anwer S, et al. Altering the availability or proximity of food, alcohol, and tobacco products to change their selection and consumption. *Cochrane Database of Syst Rev.* 2019;8(8):CD12573. doi:10.1002/14651858.cd012573.pub2

63. Farley TA, Rice J, Bodor JN, Cohen DA, Bluthenthal RN, Rose D. Measuring the food environment: Shelf space of fruits, vegetables, and snack foods in stores. *J Urban Health.* 2009;86(5):672-682. doi:10.1007/s11524-009-9390-3

64. Farley TA, Baker ET, Futrell L, Rice JC. The ubiquity of energy-dense snack foods: A national multicity study. *Am J Public Health.* 2010;100(2):306-311. doi:10.2105/AJPH.2009.178681

65. Afshin A, Peñalvo JL, Gobbo L Del, et al. The prospective impact of food pricing on improving dietary consumption: A systematic review and meta-analysis. *PLoS One.* 2017;12(3). doi:10.1371/journal.pone.0172277

66. Andreyeva T, Long MW, Brownell KD. The impact of food prices on consumption: A systematic review of research on the price elasticity of demand for food. *Am J Public Health.* 2010;100(2):216-222. doi:10.2105/AJPH.2008.151415

67. Hollands GJ, Shemilt I, Marteau TM, et al. Portion, package or tableware size for changing selection and consumption of food, alcohol, and tobacco. *Cochrane Database of Syst Rev.* 2015;2017(3). doi:10.1002/14651858.CD011045.pub2

68. Young LR, Nestle M. Expanding portion sizes in the US marketplace: Implications for nutrition counseling. *J Am Diet Assoc.* 2003;103(2):231-240. doi:10.1053/jada.2003.50027

69. Young LR, Nestle M. Portion sizes of ultra-processed foods in the United States, 2002 to 2021. *Am J Public Health.* 2021;111(12):2223-2226. doi:10.2105/AJPH.2021.306513

70. Harris JL, Frazier WI, Kumanyika S, Ramirez AG. Increasing disparities in unhealthy food advertising targeted to Hispanic and Black youth. Published 2019. Accessed December 11, 2024. Available at: https://uconnruddcenter.org/wp-content/uploads/sites/2909/2020/09/TargetedMarketingReport2019.pdf

71. Cohen DA, Collins R, Hunter G, Ghosh-Dastidar B, Dubowitz T. Store impulse marketing strategies and body mass index. *Am J Public Health.* 2015;105:1446-1452. doi:10.2105/AJPH.2014.302220

72. Robinson E, Thomas J, Aveyard P, Higgs S. What everyone else is eating: A systematic review and meta-analysis of the effect of informational eating norms on eating behavior. *J Acad Nutr Diet.* 2014;114(3):414-429. doi:10.1016/j.jand.2013.11.009

73. Congressional Research Service. *Farm Bill Primer: What Is the Farm Bill?* Published 2023. Accessed December 7, 2025. Available at: https://crsreports.congress.gov

74. Congressional Research Service. *Farm Bill Primer: Farm Safety Net Programs.* Published 2022. Accessed April 7, 2025. Available at: https://crsreports.congress.gov

75. Congressional Research Service. *Farm Commodity Provisions in the 2018 Farm Bill (P.L. 115–334).* Published 2019. Accessed April 7, 2025. Available at: https://crsreports.congress.gov

76. Food and Nutrition Service, U.S. Department of Agriculture. SNAP Data Tables. Accessed June 6, 2025. Available at https://www.fns.usda.gov/pd/supplemental-nutrition-assistance-program-snap

77. Franckle RL, Moran A, Hou T, et al. Transactions at a northeastern supermarket chain: Differences by Supplemental Nutrition Assistance Program use. *Am J Prev Med.* 2017;53(4):e131-e138. doi:10.1016/j.amepre.2017.06.019

78. Congressional Research Service. *School Meals and Other Child Nutrition Programs: Background and Funding.* Published 2022. Accessed April 7, 2025. Available at: https://crsreports.congress.gov

79. Talati Z, Egnell M, Hercberg S, Julia C, Pettigrew S. Consumers' perceptions of five front-of-package nutrition labels: An experimental study across 12 countries. *Nutrients.* 2019;11(8). doi:10.3390/nu11081934

80. Talati Z, Egnell M, Hercberg S, Julia C, Pettigrew S. Food choice under five front-of-package nutrition label conditions: An experimental study across 12 countries. *Am J Public Health.* 2019;109(12):1770-1775. doi:10.2105/AJPH.2019.305319

81. Taillie LS, Bercholz M, Popkin B, Rebolledo N, Reyes M, Corvalán C. Decreases in purchases of energy, sodium, sugar, and saturated fat 3 years after implementation of the Chilean food labeling and marketing law: An interrupted time series analysis. *PLoS Med.* 2024;21(9):e1004463. doi:10.1371/journal.pmed.1004463

82. Harnack L, Oakes JM, Elbel B, Beatty T, Rydell S, French S. Effects of subsidies and prohibitions on nutrition in a food benefit program: A randomized clinical trial. *JAMA Intern Med.* 2016;176(11):1610-1618. doi:10.1001/jamainternmed.2016.5633

83. French SA, Rydell SA, Mitchell NR, Michael Oakes J, Elbel B, Harnack L. Financial incentives and purchase restrictions in a food benefit program affect the types of foods and beverages purchased: Results from a randomized trial. *Int J Behav Nutr Phys Act.* 2017;14(1). doi:10.1186/s12966-017-0585-9

84. von Philipsborn P, Stratil JM, Burns J, et al. Environmental interventions to reduce the consumption of sugar-sweetened beverages and their effects on health. *Cochrane Database Syst Rev.* 2019;2019(6). doi:10.1002/14651858.CD012292.pub2

85. Bleich SN, Dunn CG, Soto MJ, et al. Association of a sweetened beverage tax with purchases of beverages and high-sugar foods at independent stores in Philadelphia. *JAMA Netw Open.* 2021. doi:10.1001/jamanetworkopen.2021.13527

86. Teng AM, Jones AC, Mizdrak A, Signal L, Genç M, Wilson N. Impact of sugar-sweetened beverage taxes on purchases and dietary intake: Systematic review and meta-analysis. *Obes Rev.* 2019;20(9):1187-1204. doi:10.1111/obr.12868

87. Young DR, Hedderson MM, Sidell MA, et al. City-level sugar-sweetened beverage taxes and youth body mass index percentile. *JAMA Netw Open*. 2024;7(7):e2424822. doi:10.1001/jamanetworkopen.2024.24822

88. Flynn J. Do sugar-sweetened beverage taxes improve public health for high school aged adolescents? *Health Econ*. 2023;32(1):47-64. doi:10.1002/hec.4609

89. Flynn J. Soda taxes, consumption, and health outcomes for high school students. *Econ Lett*. 2024;234. doi:10.1016/j.econlet.2023.111507

90. Wethington HR, Finnie RKC, Buchanan LR, et al. Healthier food and beverage interventions in schools: four Community Guide systematic reviews. *Am J Prev Med*. 2020;59(1):e15-e26. doi:10.1016/j.amepre.2020.01.011

91. Farley TA, Halper HS, Carlin AM, Emmerson KM, Foster KN, Fertig AR. Mass media campaign to reduce consumption of sugar-sweetened beverages in a rural area of the United States. *Am J Public Health*. 2017;107(6):989-995. doi:10.2105/AJPH.2017.303750

CHAPTER 15

Physical Inactivity

From our species' days as hunter-gatherers into the industrial revolution, humans have had to exert themselves to catch, collect, grow, or earn money for food. But coming out of the industrial revolution and into the information age, humans have gradually engineered physical activity out of their daily lives. In high-income countries and increasingly around the world, agriculture is now mostly the work of tractors, manufacturing the work of robots, construction the work of heavy machinery, and transportation the work of automobiles. Much of the physical labor in the past ranged from unpleasant to back-breaking, so this mechanization represents progress. But a consequence is that humans are now getting sick and dying early because they are not as physically active as evolution has designed them to be. For modern humans to live to their full potential, physical activity must again become part of their daily lives.

Physical Activity and Inactivity

Skeletal Muscles

Skeletal muscles are the tissues that animals use to move their bodies. They typically span across **joints**, and when given small electrical signals from nerves, they suddenly shorten (contract), moving one bone relative to others. Physical activity is the repeated contraction of skeletal muscles.

Skeletal muscles are composed of packets of two different types of fibers (**Figure 15.1**). **Type 1 fibers** (sometimes called slow-twitch) do not have much power, but they can contract repeatedly without tiring, for example, when a person walks. **Type 2 fibers** (sometimes called fast-twitch) provide more power than Type 1 fibers, but they tire within about

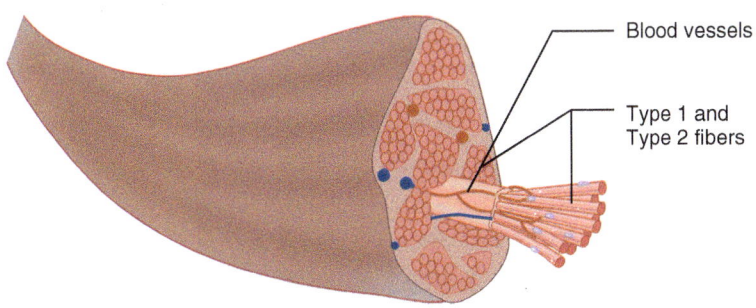

Blood vessels

Type 1 and Type 2 fibers

Figure 15.1 Muscle Fibers. Skeletal muscles are composed of packets of two different types of fibers. Type 1 fibers (sometimes called slow-twitch) do not have much power, but they can contract repeatedly without tiring, for example, when a person walks. Type 2 fibers (sometimes called fast-twitch) provide more power than Type 1 fibers, but they tire within about a minute.

a minute. Type 2 fibers are activated when muscles contract against resistance, such as when a person lifts weights or sprints.

Types of Physical Activity

Most physical activity falls into two types: **aerobic activity**, in which muscles contract repeatedly for more than a few minutes against low resistance, and **strengthening activity**, in which muscles contract a small number of times against higher resistance.[1] These types can be thought of as focusing on Type 1 and Type 2 muscle fibers, respectively. Of these types, aerobic activity has a longer list of proven health benefits.[1] Other types of physical activity include balance training, flexibility training, bone-strengthening activity, and brief high-intensity **anaerobic physical activity**.[1]

Domains of Physical Activity

Researchers studying physical activity in populations often group it into four **physical activity domains** based on the circumstances in which it occurs:[1]

- *Occupational* physical activity is part of people's work, such as stocking shelves, serving food, lifting items in a factory, or working in agricultural fields.
- *Household* physical activity takes place in and around the home, such as cooking, cleaning, or raking leaves.
- *Transportation* physical activity involves traveling to work, school, or on errands, usually by walking, but sometimes by bicycling.
- *Leisure-time* physical activity is any activity that people choose to do for health or pleasure when not at work, such as sports, going for a walk or working out at a gym.

Measuring Aerobic Physical Activity

Physical activity ranges in **intensity**, or how much energy is expended to do it. The intensity is expressed in units called the **metabolic equivalent of task, or MET**, where 1.0 MET is 1 kilocalorie per kilogram of body weight per hour, which is about the amount of energy that a person expends while sitting entirely still. Researchers have measured and compiled the intensity required for hundreds of different types of physical activity;[2] examples are shown in **Table 15.1**. For example, standing in line requires 1.3 METs, sweeping the floor expends 3.3 METs, bicycling at a

Table 15.1 Intensity of Different Types of Activity in METs

Major Heading	Activity	METs
Inactivity	Sitting still, watching television	1.0
	Standing in line	1.3
	Sitting, fidgeting feet	1.8
Music activities	Playing piano, sitting	2.3
	Playing trumpet, standing	2.5
Sexual activity	Having sex	3.0
Home activities	Cooking, light effort	2.0
	Cleaning, sweeping	3.3
Occupation	Sitting, computer work	1.3
	Nursing patient care	3.3
	Yardwork	4.0
	Carpentry, moderate effort	4.3
	Farming, moderate effort	4.8
	Shoveling, digging ditches	7.3
Lawn & garden	Mowing lawn, walking, moderate effort	5.5
Walking	Walking slowing (2.5 mph)	3.0
	Walking moderately (2.8-3.4 mph)	3.8
	Walking briskly (3.5 to 3.9 mph)	4.8
	Walking very briskly (4.0 to 4.4 mph)	5.5
Dancing	Ballet, modern, or jazz class	5.0
Conditioning exercise	Yoga	2.3
	Circuit training, moderate effort	5.0
	Aerobics, general	7.3
Bicycling	Bicycling, easy pace	4.3
	Bicycling, moderate pace	7.0
	Bicycling, vigorous effort	10.0
Running	Running 12 min/mile	8.5
	Running 10 min/mile	9.3
	Running 7.5 min/mile	11.8

Data from Ainsworth B. Compendium of Physical Activities. Published 2024. Accessed July 15, 2024. https://pacompendium.com/

moderate pace 7.0 METs, and running at 10 minutes per mile 9.3 METs.[2,3]

Light physical activity requires between 1.6 and 2.9 METs, **moderate physical activity** (such as walking) requires 3.0 to 5.9 METs, and **vigorous physical activity** (such as jogging) requires 6.0 or more METs.[4] One simple way to estimate the intensity of an activity is this: When people do moderate physical activity, they can usually talk but not sing. When people do vigorous activity, they cannot say more than a few words without stopping to catch their breath. **Sedentary behavior** is the opposite of physical activity. It is defined as behavior that requires less than 1.5 METs. It involves sitting, typically while watching television, reading, working at a computer, or driving.

To summarize physical activity over a week, researchers often calculate total "minutes" of **moderate-to-vigorous activity** in which each minute of vigorous activity is counted as two minutes of moderate activity. Another common summary measure is a **MET-Hour**, calculated by multiplying the METs of different activities by the hours spent doing them and then summing across activity types. For example, an adult who spends ½ hour riding a bicycle (at 7.0 METs) in the morning and ½ hour walking (at 3.8 METs) in the evening expends 5.4 MET-Hours that day (½ × 7.0 + ½ × 3.8 = 5.4).

For many years, measuring physical activity levels in populations could only be done with surveys in which people reported the time they spent in various activities.[5] But in the mid-2000s, researchers began using body-worn **accelerometers** to measure physical activity in large numbers of people. When they did, they found that people reported far more physical activity on surveys than the accelerometers measured. For example, on a national survey, American adults reported an average of 325 minutes per week of moderate activity, but the accelerometers that they wore registered only 45 minutes.[6] That means that interpreting any report about a population's physical activity requires first understanding how the activity was measured. Today's physical activity guidelines are still based on data from surveys, but in the future, they are likely to be based on accelerometer measurements.

Biologic Effects of Physical Activity

Physical activity reduces the risk of many different diseases, but the biologic mechanisms behind these health benefits are complex and not well understood.

When skeletal muscles contract repeatedly, their metabolism generates small and large compounds that indirectly stimulate the muscles to build more proteins and other cell structures, as well as to improve how the muscle fibers function.[7] This is the training effect, and it produces skeletal muscles that are bigger and stronger. The heart is also a muscle, and it responds similarly: A heart that is exercised becomes stronger and can pump a larger volume of blood.[8]

This makes evolutionary sense. When muscles are underused, they shrink, probably so that the body can avoid wasting energy and nutrients on them. Activating those tissues through exercise is a signal that these muscles are needed, so the body diverts resources to strengthen them.

But the biologic benefits of physical activity go far beyond stronger skeletal muscles and heart muscle. For example, exercise improves the health and functioning of cells lining the arteries, which may partly explain why physical activity reduces the risk of heart disease and stroke.[9] Exercise promotes the growth of and improves the function of brain cells.[10] And exercise slows down many of the normal aging processes of the body's cells.[9]

One specific effect of physical activity helps the entire body. Exercise increases cells' sensitivity to the hormone **insulin**.[11] That makes it easier for the blood sugar **glucose** to move from the blood into metabolically-active cells, especially those in muscle and the liver. The opposite of insulin sensitivity is **insulin resistance**, which happens in people who are physically inactive. When cells become resistant to insulin, the body responds by just releasing more insulin, so insulin levels in the blood rise. Insulin resistance and high levels of insulin in the blood are central to the development of obesity, diabetes, and their consequences, as discussed in Chapter 7. Chronic Metabolic Diseases.

Health Risks of Physical Inactivity

Physical activity is often described as an added benefit to health, as if being inactive were natural. But instead, it is natural for all animals, including humans, to be active, so it is probably better to think of physical *inactivity* as a health *risk*. People who are physically inactive are more likely to develop:

- *Obesity and type 2 diabetes.* Inactive people are more likely to gain body fat.[1] And because it causes insulin resistance, physical inactivity also increases the risk of diabetes, separate from its effect on obesity.[11,12]

- *Hypertension, heart disease, and stroke.*[1] Compared to the most physically active people, those who are inactive are more likely to develop high blood pressure or damage to the heart or brain caused by narrowed arteries called **ischemic heart disease** or **ischemic stroke**.[1] Inactive people are about 40% more likely to die of heart disease or stroke than people who walk just 40 minutes or more per day.[1] This effect of inactivity may result from insulin resistance (which leads to higher levels of fats in the blood), from damage to the lining of arteries, or from a reduction in the network of very small arteries that supply oxygen to tissues.[8,13]

- *Cancer* of the colon, breast, bladder, endometrium, esophagus, stomach, and kidney, and perhaps other cancers as well.[1] There are four possible explanations for the connection to cancer. First, the high levels of insulin present in inactive people stimulate active cells to proliferate, which increases cancer risk. Second, people who are physically inactive have constant low-level **inflammation**; that is, activation of their immune system, which has been linked to cancer. Third, despite the inflammation, inactivity may inhibit the immune cells responsible for killing cancer cells. And fourth, the increased body fat resulting from inactivity produces the female hormone **estrogen**, which increases the risk of breast cancer.[14]

- *Dementia.* Older adults who are inactive do less well on tests of cognition and are more likely to develop **dementia**.[1,15] Inactivity harms the brain in both direct and indirect ways. The brain seems to behave like a muscle, growing in strength when stimulated during physical activity and weakening if left inactive.[1,15-17] And inactivity increases **atherosclerosis** (narrowing of the arteries) in the arteries that supply blood to the brain, which increases the risk of dementia.[15]

- *Depression.*[1] People who are inactive are about 20% more likely to experience depression, and when people who are sedentary become more active, their symptoms of depression improve.[18-20] The biologic mechanisms behind this benefit are not clear, but exercise has effects on stress hormones, the growth of brain cells, and the immune system, all of which play a role in depression.[10]

- *Musculoskeletal problems.* The weaker muscles in people who are inactive can result in various **musculoskeletal problems**. For example, people with weaker leg muscles are more likely to develop **osteoarthritis** of the knee.[21,22] Inactivity may also increase the risk of chronic low back pain.[23,24]

- *Falls and fractures in older adults.* Older adults with weaker muscles are more likely to have major falls and to break their bones if they do fall.[1,25]

Overall, people who are physically inactive do not live as long. The relationship between activity and mortality is a curve that is steepest at the lowest levels of activity (**Figure 15.2**); that is, the people who see the biggest health benefit are those who change from being completely inactive to being only minimally active. For example, compared to those who are inactive, people taking up a weekly habit of walking slowly for only one hour a week, getting 3.0 MET-Hours of physical activity, have a 20% reduction in mortality.[1] Those who follow the minimum recommendations by walking slowly 2.5 hours per week reduce their mortality rate by more than 30%. Beyond that, the improvement gets smaller, but the graph suggests that there is some additional benefit up to at least 22.5 MET-Hours per week, and maybe well beyond that.[1] Separately, a study in which people wore accelerometers on their wrists found that the mortality-reduction benefits of walking continued up to about 10,000 steps per day, which translates to about 40–45 MET-Hours per week, depending on their stride length and pace.[26]

Sedentary behavior carries its own serious health risks, separate and apart from just not engaging in moderate or vigorous activity. People who sit for more than eight hours per day, unless they are unusually active the rest of the day, have about a 50% increased risk of dying from heart disease or stroke, and about a 25% increase in mortality overall.[1,27]

The Limits of Physical Activity's Health Benefits

There are limits to the health benefits of physical activity, and even some risks.

First, some studies have found that occupational physical activity, unlike leisure-time physical activity, does not decrease and may actually increase the risks of heart disease and mortality.[28] This has been called the **physical activity paradox**, and the reasons for it are not known. Maybe this surprising relationship is because physical activity on the job is repetitive, stressful, or uninterrupted by rest breaks.

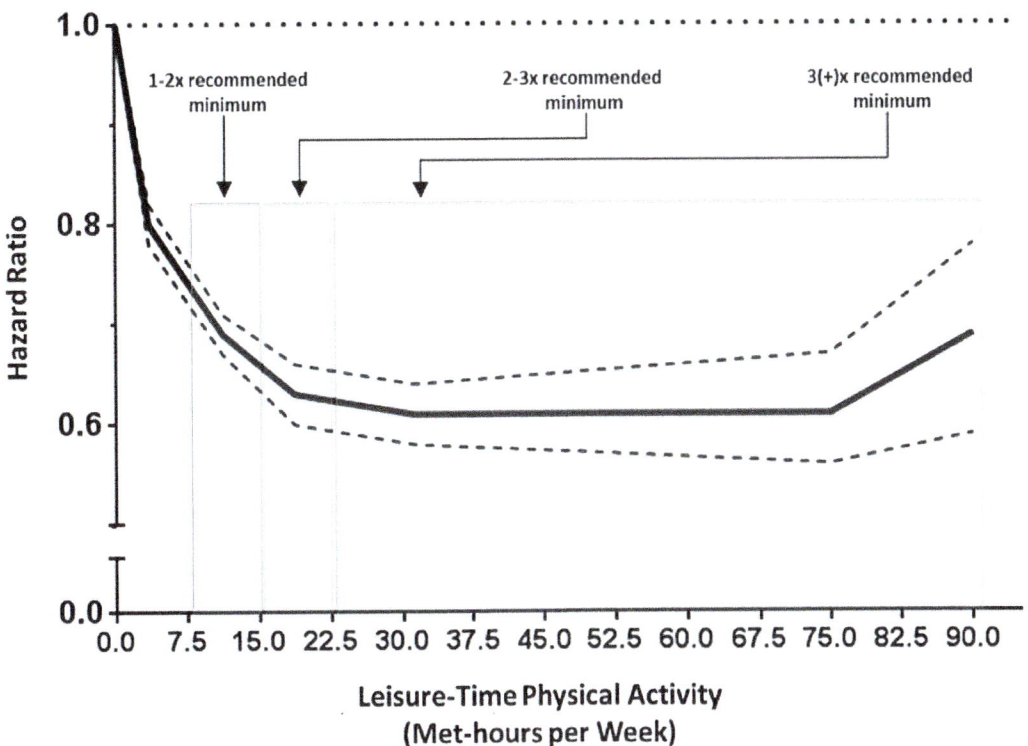

Figure 15.2 **Relationship Between Physical Activity and Mortality from All Causes.** The people who see the biggest health benefit from physical activity are those who change from being completely inactive to being only minimally active. Those who follow the minimum recommendations by walking slowly 2½ hours per week reduce their mortality rate by more than 30%. Beyond that, the benefit is smaller, but is an additional reduction in mortality up to at least 22.5 MET-Hours per week.

Physical Activity Guidelines Advisory Committee. 2018 Physical Activity Guidelines Advisory Committee Scientific Report. Washington, DC; 2018. Accessed July 17, 2024. https://health.gov/healthypeople/tools-action/browse-evidence-based-resources/2018-physical-activity-guidelines-advisory-committee-scientific-report

Second, physical activity is not an antidote to other health risks. Even among people who are physically active, those who smoke still are more likely to get cancer, those who have diets high in saturated fats still develop atherosclerosis, and those who consume too much sodium still develop high blood pressure.

Third, exercise reduces but does not eliminate the health risks of sedentary behavior.

Fourth, there appear to be health risks to extremely high levels of exercise. For example, endurance athletes who exercise for more than 75 MET-Hours per week can develop heart rhythm problems and may have an increase in mortality compared to those who meet the minimum recommendations (Figure 15.2).[1,29,30] That is a lot of exercise, though. It translates to running about 7–8 hours per week, or about 50–60 miles per week, depending on the pace.

Recommended Physical Activity Levels

The U.S. Department of Health and Human Services (HHS) and the World Health Organization (WHO) recommend that adults each week get 150–300 minutes of moderate-intensity or 75–150 minutes of vigorous-intensity aerobic activity or an equivalent combination.[4,31] That translates to a minimum of about 8 MET-Hours per week, and more typically, 10–20 MET-Hours of activity per week, depending on the intensity of the activities people choose.

It does not require vigorous exercise to get either the minimum or maximum activity. Walking is a very health-promoting form of activity, expending between 3.0 and 5.5 METs, depending on the pace. And walking is probably the type of physical activity that humans have historically done the most. Hunter-gatherer groups that maintain their traditional habits get very healthy levels of physical activity—about 55–70 MET-Hours of activity per week—mostly by just walking.[32]

HHS recommends that children get at least 60 minutes per day of moderate or vigorous physical activity. HHS and the WHO also recommend that adults do muscle-strengthening activities two to three days per week, and that children incorporate muscle-strengthening and bone-strengthening activity into their 60 minutes at least three days per week.[31]

Epidemiology: Patterns and Trends in Physical Activity

While many people think of physical activity only as deliberate exercise, around the world most people get most of their activity on the job or through household chores (**Figure 15.3**).[5] Transportation activity (mostly walking) is the next most common domain, and leisure-time physical activity is the least used. As country incomes rise, people and employers buy more labor-saving devices, so people are less physically active at work, in the home, or when traveling. People living in higher-income countries get more leisure-time physical activity than people in lower- and middle-income countries, but the increase is not nearly enough to compensate for the loss of occupational and household activity.[5]

Globally, about three-fourths of adults get the recommended minimum amount of aerobic physical activity. Inactivity is twice as common in high-income countries as it is in low-income countries and is increasing over time.[33,34]

In the United States, occupational and household physical activity have been decreasing at least since the 1960s, but 50% of activity is still occupational, 28% household, and 15% is leisure-time.[35] In this car-dependent country, only 2% of activity is through transportation.[36]

As activity in these other domains falls, leisure-time activity is gradually increasing in the United States. From 1998 to 2018, the percentage of adults who said on surveys they met the minimum guidelines increased, and the percent who engaged in no leisure-time aerobic physical activity fell (**Figure 15.4**).[37,38] The percentage who said they were inactive was higher among Blacks, Hispanics, people with less education, and older adults (**Figure 15.5**).[37,38]

But children are not doing as well; only 27% of U.S. teenagers report getting 60 minutes of physical activity per day.[39]

And even as people are exercising more in their leisure time, they are also spending more time in sedentary behavior—that is, sitting.[40] American adults on average sit for 6.4 hours per day and teens sit for 8.2 hours per day.[41] While many people are essentially forced to sit as part of their jobs, much sitting is optional. During nonwork and non-school hours, more than half of American adults and teens use computers for more than 1 hour a day, and nearly two-thirds watch television or videos for more than 2 hours a day.[41]

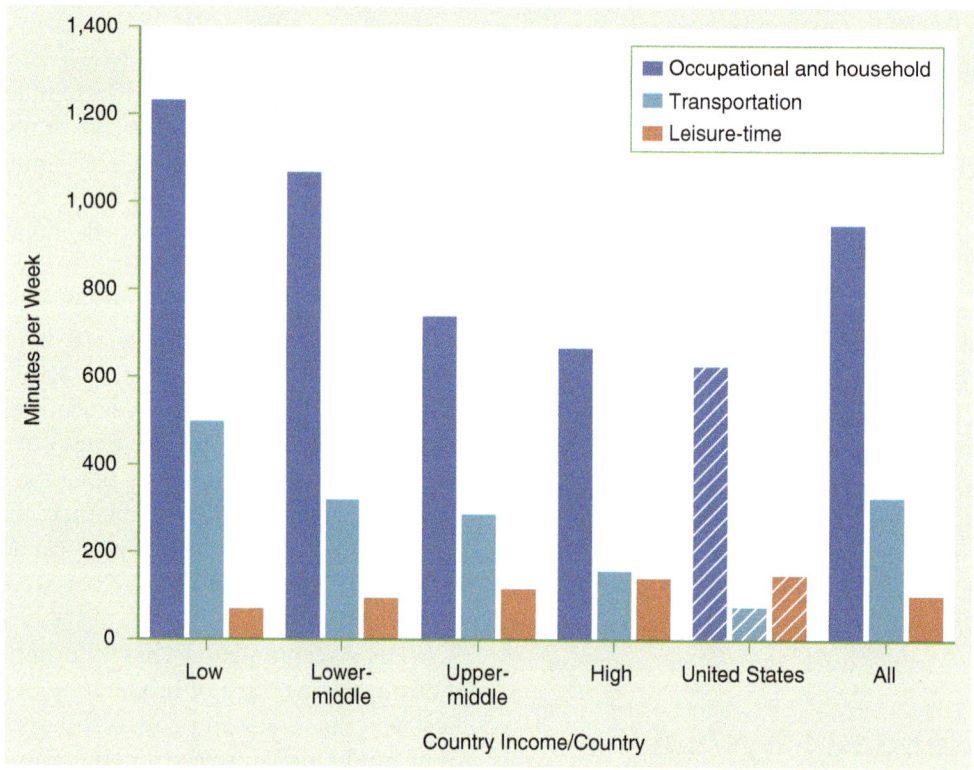

Figure 15.3 Self-Reported Physical Activity by Domain and Country Income. In higher-income countries, people engage in less physical activity at work, at home, and during transportation. They are more physically active in their leisure time, but not nearly enough to compensate.

Data from Strain T, Wijndaele K, Garcia L, et al. Levels of domain-specific physical activity at work, in the household, for travel and for leisure among 327 789 adults from 104 countries. *Br J Sports Med.* 2020;54(24):1488-1497. doi:10.1136/bjsports-2020-102601

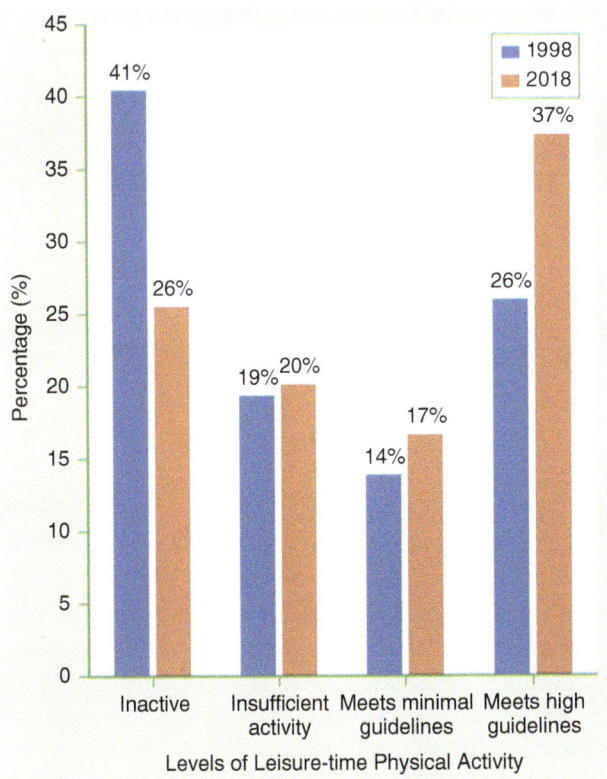

Figure 15.4 **Percent of U.S. Adults Engaging in Different Levels of Leisure-time Physical Activity, 1998 vs. 2018.**

Data from Whitfield GP, Hyde ET, Carlson SA. Participation in leisure-time aerobic physical activity among adults, national health interview survey, 1998-2018. *J Phys Act Health.* 2021;18(1):S25-S36. doi:10.1123/JPAH.2021-0014

Risk Factors for Physical Inactivity

People are physically inactive because of historic changes in the designs of communities and the availability of machines and devices, or what has been called the **built environment**. Features of the built environment that have been linked to physical inactivity can be grouped into a few categories (**Figure 15.6**):

- *Automobiles* and the infrastructure for them. Cars inhibit the physical activity of both drivers and the people around them.[42-44] Driving is a sedentary behavior that American car owners do about one hour a day, and people who own cars are much less physically active than those who do not.[44,45] In addition, streets that could be used for walking or socializing are filled with cars, often moving dangerously fast.[46] To avoid getting hit, people tend to avoid those streets, and the alternative is often a sedentary behavior. Studies show that where there is more car traffic, both adults and children are less physically active.[42,43]

- *Lack of infrastructure for walking and bicycling.* Even with car traffic, people can safely walk outdoors if there are sidewalks and other infrastructure for pedestrians. When this infrastructure is lacking, people are less likely to walk and less physically active.[43] Similarly, where there is a lack of infrastructure for bicycling, people are less likely to ride bikes.[43]

- *Lack of destinations near residences.* While plenty of people walk just for exercise or pleasure, it is more convenient if they can also walk to do errands. People are more likely to walk if there are destinations for errands like grocery stores, restaurants, and churches within walking distance of their homes.[43] Children are more likely to walk or bike to school where there are shorter distances

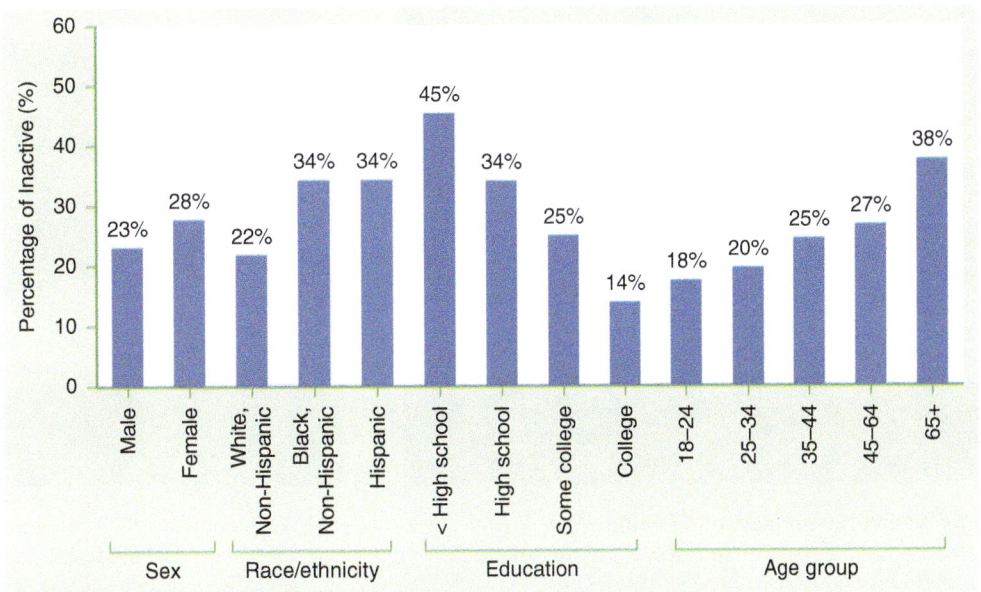

Figure 15.5 **Self-reported Physical Inactivity in the United States by Demographic Group, 2018.**

Data from Whitfield GP, Hyde ET, Carlson SA. Participation in leisure-time aerobic physical activity among adults, national health interview survey, 1998-2018. *J Phys Act Health.* 2021;18(1):S25-S36. doi:10.1123/JPAH.2021-0014

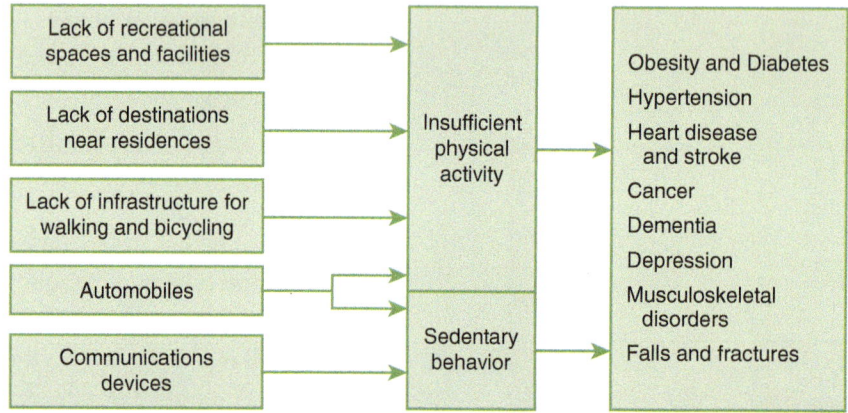

Figure 15.6 Cause-and-Effect Diagram for Physical Inactivity.

between home and schools.[42,43,47] In urban and suburban areas, the distances between homes and destinations are shaped by laws and regulations on **land use**. Land use rules (called **zoning** rules) specify the type of buildings and activities allowed in each zone of a community. For example, land can be "zoned" for only one use, like single-family homes, multi-family buildings, commercial businesses, or factories. This is called **single-use zoning**. Alternatively, land can be zoned for multiple uses, which is called **mixed land use** or **mixed-use zoning**. With single-use zoning, store and workplaces are prohibited in residential neighborhoods (**Figure 15.7A**), so most people live beyond walking distance from destinations.

- *Lack of recreational spaces and facilities.* People are less likely walk or be physically active in other ways if there are no nearby places to exercise, play, or socialize like parks, greenspaces, playgrounds, and recreational facilities.[43] Children are less active if schoolyards are locked or unavailable for recreation after school.[42]

- *Communications devices,* such as televisions, computers, and smart phones. While no one is required to watch videos, play computer games, or scroll through social media posts, these devices are designed to grab and hold people's attention, and nearly everyone is captured by them. When people use these communications devices, they are almost always sedentary.[48,49]

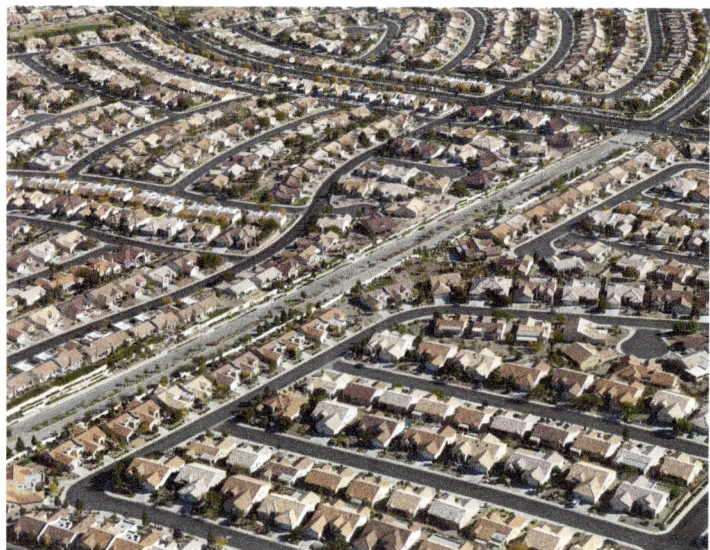
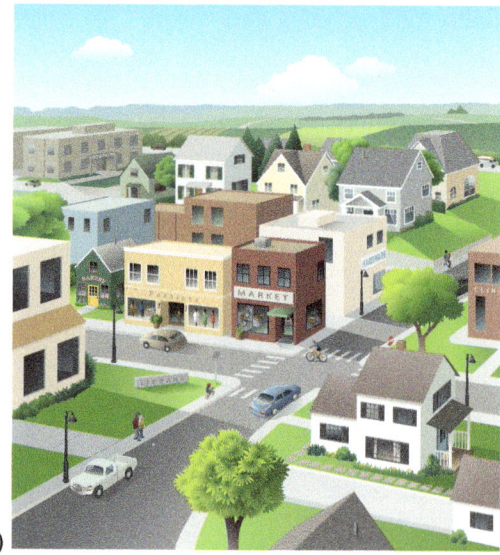

(A) (B)

Figure 15.7 Single-use versus mixed-use Zoning. With single-use zoning **(A)** stores and workplaces are prohibited in residential neighborhoods, so people cannot walk to destinations. With mixed-use zoning **(B)** destinations are within walking distance of residences.

(A) © iofoto/Shutterstock; (B) © skeeg/DigitalVision Vectors/Getty Images.

Preventive Interventions

Promotion of physical activity in populations is much harder than it is in individuals or small groups.

For individuals and small groups, many approaches succeed. Exercise classes reliably increase people's physical activity.[1] Feedback devices like pedometers or accelerometers help motivate people, as do programs that deliver encouragement by computer or smart phones.[1] Social supports like organized walking groups and buddy systems are likewise helpful.[50] But these programs are difficult to bring to scale for entire populations and to sustain over time.

Attempts to increase physical activity in populations include:

- *Community-wide mobilization campaigns.* Some organizations have successfully mobilized entire communities to be more active through campaigns that combine messages in the media, workplaces, neighborhoods, and medical clinics. However, these campaigns are difficult to carry out and sustain, and they have generally worked only if they have reached a majority of community members over time.[1,51,52] Some organizations have tried standalone media campaigns encouraging people to be physically active. While some of these campaigns have had small successes, most have failed to increase physical activity, maybe because most people already know that they should exercise.[53,54]
- *Point-of-decision prompts.* An extraordinarily simple change increases people's use of stairs: signs at the spot where they must choose between stairs and escalators.[43] Unfortunately, the effect of these prompts on population-wide physical activity is extremely small.[55]

Attempts to promote physical activity specifically in children include:

- *School-based physical activity programs* through expanded or revised physical education classes or recess. These programs are reliably effective.[1] Many communities have requirements for a minimum number of minutes of physical education that are not followed by schools. Where there are limits in space or time in the school day, classroom-based physical activity sessions have been a successful substitute.[1]
- *Safe routes to school programs* that combine walking and bicycling infrastructure improvements with promotion and traffic enforcement. These programs have increased the number of children who walk or bike to school.[56]

Because it is difficult for physical activity programs to reach entire populations, public health experts have gravitated to changing the built environment to make it easier for people to walk, bicycle, or exercise. While these changes typically have a small impact on each individual, they can touch many people. And the additional activity needed by most people is not much: A person can meet the minimum guidelines for 150 minutes of aerobic activity by taking only two 15-minute walking trips each weekday.

Changes to the built environment that have been shown to increase physical activity or that have that potential include (**Figure 15.8**):

- *Infrastructure for walking and bicycling.* Streets can be changed to accommodate walkers and bicyclists. Both adults and children walk more if there are sidewalks and walking trails and are more likely to bicycle if there are bike lanes, bike trails, bikeshare systems, and bike storage facilities.[42,43] Parents are more likely to allow children to walk or bike for transportation if there are safety features like traffic lights, crosswalks, and traffic calming devices.[42] Similarly, people are more likely to take public transit (which always involves walking) if public transit systems are more extensive and more convenient.[43] Street lighting also seems to promote walking by giving people a sense of safety at dawn and dusk.[43]
- *Closure of streets to automobiles.* Some communities organize "play streets" or "summer streets" in which street blocks or entire corridors are closed to car traffic for a day or more. These can increase physical activity, but their overall benefit is small because they are so temporary.[42] Some European cities are experimenting with "superblocks" that permanently prohibit automobile traffic in small, dense neighborhoods; their impact on physical activity is not yet known.
- *Mixed land use.* Zoning rules can be changed to allow mixed land use, so that destinations are built within walking distance of homes (**Figure 15.7B**).
- *Recreational facilities.* Parks and playgrounds can be built within residential neighborhoods, and schoolyards can be unlocked so that they become playgrounds during non-school hours.[43]

Finally, it is difficult to influence sedentary behavior when so much of work takes place at computer workstations and attention-grabbing devices are always in our pockets. We need new ideas on how to reverse the trend of increasing sedentary behavior caused by these communications devices.

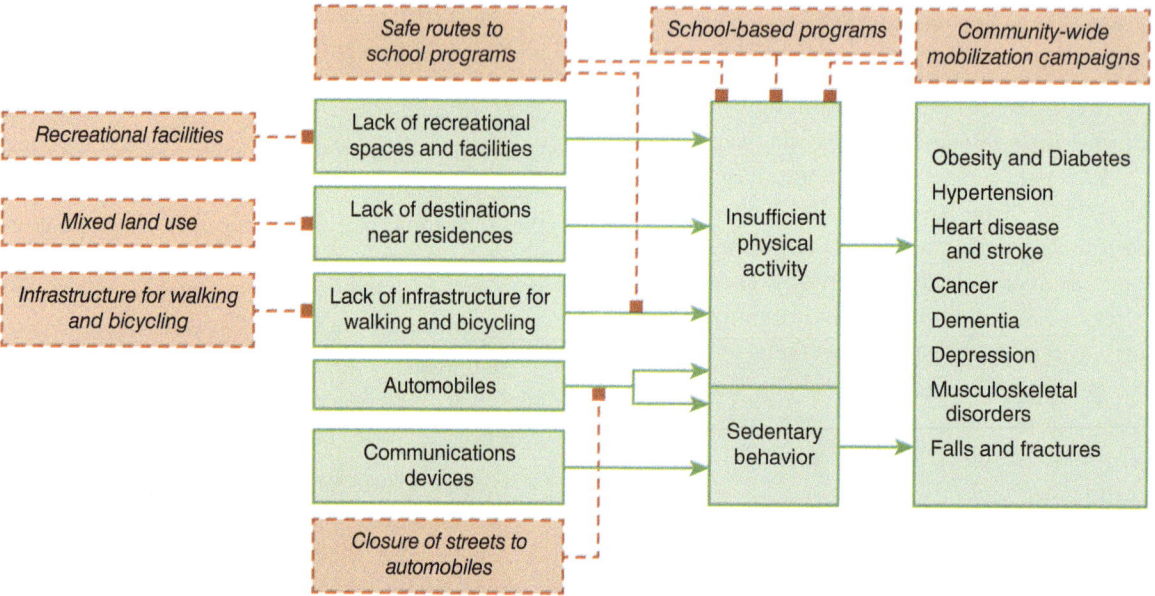

Figure 15.8 **Cause-and-Effect Diagram for Physical Inactivity, with Preventive Interventions.**

Box 15.1 Summary–Prevention of Physical Inactivity

- Community-wide mobilization campaigns
- School-based physical activity programs
- Safe routes to school programs
- Infrastructure for walking and bicycling
- Closure of streets to automobiles
- Mixed land use
- Recreational facilities

Box 15.2 Key Words

Accelerometer
Aerobic activity
Anaerobic physical activity
Atherosclerosis
Built environment
Dementia
Estrogen
Glucose
Inflammation
Insulin
Intensity (of physical activity)
Ischemic heart disease
Ischemic stroke
Joints
Land use
Light physical activity
Metabolic Equivalent of Task (MET)
MET-Hour
Mixed land use or mixed-use zoning
Moderate physical activity

Moderate-to-vigorous activity
Musculoskeletal
Osteoarthritis
Physical activity domains
Physical activity paradox
Sedentary behavior
Single-use zoning
Skeletal muscles
Strengthening activity
Type 1 muscle fibers
Type 2 muscle fibers
Vigorous physical activity
Zoning

Resources

- The *Physical Activity Guidelines for Americans*, produced by the Office of Disease Prevention and Health Promotion in the U.S. Department of Health and Human Services, available at https://health.gov/our-work/nutrition-physical-activity/physical-activity-guidelines, provides easily-understandable background on the health benefits of physical activity, the recommended amounts and types of physical activity, and ways to promote physical activity at the individual and community level.
- Physical Activity Guidelines Advisory Committee. *2018 Physical Activity Guidelines Advisory Committee Scientific Report*, available at https://health.gov/our-work/nutrition-physical-activity/physical-activity-guidelines/current-guidelines/scientific-report. This is an extensive, detailed summary of the scientific research underpinning the Physical

Activity Guidelines for Americans. It contains information on both the health effects and the community determinants of physical activity.

- Ainsworth B, Haskell W, Herrmann S. *Compendium of Physical Activities.* https://pacompendium.com. This contains MET values of different types of physical activity.

- Prince SA, Lancione S, Lang JJ, et al. Examining the state, quality, and strength of the evidence in the research on built environments and physical activity among adults: An overview of reviews from high income countries. *Health Place.* 2022;77. doi:10.1016/j.healthplace.2022.102874, and Prince SA, Lancione S, Lang JJ, et al. Examining the state, quality, and strength of the evidence in the research on built environments and physical activity among children and youth: An overview of reviews from high income countries. *Health Place.* 2022;76. doi:10.1016/j.healthplace.2022.102828. These are up-to-date summaries of the research on the impact of the built environment on physical activity.

References

1. Physical Activity Guidelines Advisory Committee. 2018 Physical Activity Guidelines Advisory Committee Scientific Report. Published 2018. Accessed July 17, 2024. Available at: https://health.gov/healthypeople/tools-action/browse-evidence-based-resources/2018-physical-activity-guidelines-advisory-committee-scientific-report

2. Ainsworth B. Compendium of Physical Activities. Published 2024. Accessed July 15, 2024. Available at: https://pacompendium.com/

3. Herrmann SD, Willis EA, Ainsworth BE, et al. 2024 Adult Compendium of Physical Activities: A third update of the energy costs of human activities. *J Sport Health Sci.* 2024;13(1):6-12. doi:10.1016/j.jshs.2023.10.010

4. Department of Health and Human Services. Physical Activity Guidelines for Americans 2nd ed. Published 2018. Accessed July 17, 2024. Available at: https://health.gov/healthypeople/tools-action/browse-evidence-based-resources/physical-activity-guidelines-americans-2nd-edition

5. Strain T, Wijndaele K, Garcia L, et al. Levels of domain-specific physical activity at work, in the household, for travel, and for leisure among 327 789 adults from 104 countries. *Br J Sports Med.* 2020;54(24):1488-1497. doi:10.1136/bjsports-2020-102601

6. Tucker JM, Welk GJ, Beyler NK. Physical activity in U.S. adults: Compliance with the physical activity guidelines for Americans. *Am J Prev Med.* 2011;40(4):454-461. doi:10.1016/j.amepre.2010.12.016

7. Viña J, Sanchis-Gomar F, Martinez-Bello V, Gomez-Cabrera MC. Exercise acts as a drug; The pharmacological benefits of exercise. *Br J Pharmacol.* 2012;167(1):1-12. doi:10.1111/j.1476-5381.2012.01970.x

8. Tucker WJ, Fegers-Wustrow I, Halle M, Haykowsky MJ, Chung EH, Kovacic JC. Exercise for primary and secondary prevention of cardiovascular disease: JACC focus seminar 1/4. *J Am Coll Cardiol.* 2022;80(11). doi:10.1016/j.jacc.2022.07.004

9. Carapeto PV, Aguayo-Mazzucato C. Effects of exercise on cellular and tissue aging. *Aging.* 2021;13(10). doi:10.18632/aging.203051

10. Kandola A, Ashdown-Franks G, Hendrikse J, Sabiston CM, Stubbs B. Physical activity and depression: Towards understanding the antidepressant mechanisms of physical activity. *Neurosci Biobehav Rev.* 2019;107. doi:10.1016/j.neubiorev.2019.09.040

11. Grøtved A, Rimm EB, Willett WC, Andersen LB, Hu FB. A prospective study of weight training and risk of type 2 diabetes mellitus in men. *Arch Intern Med.* 2012;172(17):1306-1312. doi:10.1001/archinternmed.2012.3138

12. Stocks B, Zierath JR. Post-translational modifications: The signals at the intersection of exercise, glucose uptake, and insulin sensitivity. *Endocr Rev.* 2022;43(4):654-677. doi:10.1210/endrev/bnab038

13. Pierce GL, Donato AJ, Larocca TJ, Eskurza I, Silver AE, Seals DR. Habitually exercising older men do not demonstrate age-associated vascular endothelial oxidative stress. *Aging Cell.* 2011;10(6):1032-1037. doi:10.1111/j.1474-9726.2011.00748.x

14. Larson EA, Dalamaga M, Magkos F. The role of exercise in obesity-related cancers: Current evidence and biological mechanisms. *Semin Cancer Biol.* 2023;91:16-26. doi:10.1016/j.semcancer.2023.02.008

15. Dintica CS, Yaffe K. Epidemiology and risk factors for dementia. *Psychiatr Clin North Am.* 2022;45(4):677-689. doi:10.1016/j.psc.2022.07.011

16. Livingston G, Huntley J, Sommerlad A, et al. Dementia prevention, intervention, and care: 2020 report of the Lancet Commission. *Lancet.* 2020;396(10248):413-446. doi:10.1016/S0140-6736(20)30367-6

17. Chen C, Nakagawa S. Physical activity for cognitive health promotion: An overview of the underlying neurobiological mechanisms. *Ageing Res Rev.* 2023;86. doi:10.1016/j.arr.2023.101868

18. Schuch FB, Vancampfort D, Firth J, et al. Physical activity and incident depression: A meta-analysis of prospective cohort studies. *Am J Psychiatry.* 2018;175(7):631-648. doi:10.1176/appi.ajp.2018.17111194

19. Choi KW, Stein MB, Nishimi KM, et al. An exposure-wide and mendelian randomization approach to identifying modifiable factors for the prevention of depression. *Am J Psychiatry.* 2020;177(10):944-954. doi:10.1176/appi.ajp.2020.19111158

20. Kandola AA, del Pozo Cruz B, Osborn DPJ, Stubbs B, Choi KW, Hayes JF. Impact of replacing sedentary behaviour with other movement behaviours on depression and anxiety symptoms: A prospective cohort study in the UK Biobank. *BMC Med.* 2021;19(1). doi:10.1186/s12916-021-02007-3

21. Hunter DJ, Bierma-Zeinstra S. Osteoarthritis. *Lancet.* 2019;393(10182). doi:10.1016/S0140-6736(19)30417-9

22. Whittaker JL, Runhaar J, Bierma-Zeinstra S, Roos EM. A lifespan approach to osteoarthritis prevention. *Osteoarthritis Cartilage.* 2021;29(12):1638-1653. doi:10.1016/j.joca.2021.06.015

23. Shiri R, Falah-Hassani K. Does leisure time physical activity protect against low back pain? Systematic review and meta-analysis of 36 prospective cohort studies. *Br J Sports Med.* 2017;51(19):1410-1418. doi:10.1136/bjsports-2016-097352

24. Knezevic NN, Candido KD, Vlaeyen JWS, Van Zundert J, Cohen SP. Low back pain. *Lancet.* 2021;398(10294):78-92. doi:10.1016/S0140-6736(21)00733-9

25. Rubenstein LZ. Falls in older people: epidemiology, risk factors, and strategies for prevention. *Age Ageing.* 2006;35-S2: ii37-ii41.

26. Del Pozo Cruz B, Ahmadi MN, Lee IM, Stamatakis E. Prospective associations of daily step counts and intensity with cancer and cardiovascular disease incidence and mortality and all-cause mortality. *JAMA Intern Med.* 2022;182(11):1139-1148. doi:10.1001/jamainternmed.2022.4000

27. Ekelund U, Steene-Johannessen J, Brown WJ, et al. Does physical activity attenuate, or even eliminate, the detrimental association of sitting time with mortality? A harmonised meta-analysis of data from more than 1 million men and women. *Lancet.* 2016;388(10051). doi:10.1016/S0140-6736(16) 30370-1

28. Holtermann A, Schnohr P, Nordestgaard BG, Marott JL. The physical activity paradox in cardiovascular disease and all-cause mortality: The contemporary Copenhagen General Population Study with 104 046 adults. *Eur Heart J.* 2021;42(15). doi:10.1093/eurheartj/ehab087

29. O'Keefe JH, Patil HR, Lavie CJ, Magalski A, Vogel RA, McCullough PA. Potential adverse cardiovascular effects from excessive endurance exercise. In: *Mayo Clin Proc.* Vol 87. Elsevier Ltd; 2012:587-595. doi:10.1016/j.mayocp .2012.04.005

30. Arem H, Moore SC, Patel A, et al. Leisure time physical activity and mortality: A detailed pooled analysis of the dose-response relationship. *JAMA Intern Med.* 2015;175(6):959-967. doi:10.1001/jamainternmed.2015.0533

31. World Health Organization. WHO guidelines on physical activity and sedentary behavior. Published 2020. Accessed December 11, 2024. Available at: https://www.who.int /publications/i/item/9789240015128

32. Pontzer H, Wood BM, Raichlen DA. Hunter-gatherers as models in public health. *Obes Rev.* 2018;19:24-35. doi:10 .1111/obr.12785

33. Guthold R, Stevens GA, Riley LM, Bull FC. Worldwide trends in insufficient physical activity from 2001 to 2016: A pooled analysis of 358 population-based surveys with 1·9 million participants. *Lancet Glob Health.* 2018;6(10):e1077-e1086. doi:10.1016/S2214-109X(18)30357-7

34. World Health Organization. Physical activity fact sheet. Published 2021. Accessed July 17, 2024. Available at: https:// www.who.int/publications/i/item/WHO-HEP-HPR-RUN-2021.2

35. Ng SW, Popkin BM. Time use and physical activity: A shift away from movement across the globe. *Obes Rev.* 2012;13(8):659-680. doi:10.1111/j.1467-789X.2011.00982.x

36. Saint-Maurice PF, Berrigan D, Whitfield GP, et al. Amount, type, and timing of domain-specific moderate to vigorous physical activity among US adults. *J Phys Act Health.* 2021;18(S1):S114-S122. doi:10.1123/JPAH.2021-0174

37. Watson KB, Whitfield G, Chen TJ, Hyde ET, Omura JD. Trends in aerobic and muscle-strengthening physical activity by race/ethnicity across income levels among US adults, 1998-2018. *J Phys Act Health.* 2021;18(1):S45-S52. doi:10.1123/JPAH.2021-0260

38. Whitfield GP, Hyde ET, Carlson SA. Participation in leisure-time aerobic physical activity among adults, national health interview survey, 1998-2018. *J Phys Act Health.* 2021; 18(1):S25-S36. doi:10.1123/JPAH.2021-0014

39. Katzmarzyk PT, Lee IM, Martin CK, Blair SN. Epidemiology of physical activity and exercise training in the United States. *Prog Cardiovasc Dis.* 2017;60(1). doi:10.1016/j.pcad.2017 .01.004

40. Ussery EN, Whitfield GP, Fulton JE, et al. Trends in self-reported sitting time by physical activity levels among US adults, NHANES 2007/2008-2017/2018. *J Phys Act Health.* 2021;18(1):S74-S83. doi:10.1123/JPAH.2021-0221

41. Yang L, Cao C, Kantor ED, et al. Trends in sedentary behavior among the US population, 2001-2016. *JAMA.* 2019;321(16):1587-1597. doi:10.1001/jama.2019.3636

42. Prince SA, Lancione S, Lang JJ, et al. Examining the state, quality and strength of the evidence in the research on built environments and physical activity among children and youth: An overview of reviews from high income countries. *Health Place.* 2022;76. doi:10.1016/j.healthplace.2022.102828

43. Prince SA, Lancione S, Lang JJ, et al. Examining the state, quality and strength of the evidence in the research on built environments and physical activity among adults: An overview of reviews from high income countries. *Health Place.* 2022;77. doi:10.1016/j.healthplace.2022 .102874

44. Anderson ML, Lu F, Yang J. Physical activity and weight following car ownership in Beijing, China: Quasi-experimental cross-sectional study. *BMJ.* 2019;367. doi:10.1136/bmj.l6491

45. Shoham DA, Dugas LR, Bovet P, et al. Association of car ownership and physical activity across the spectrum of human development: Modeling the Epidemiologic Transition Study (METS). *BMC Public Health.* 2015;15(1). doi:10.1186/s12889-015-1435-9

46. Rosén E, Stigson H, Sander U. Literature review of pedestrian fatality risk as a function of car impact speed. *Accid Anal Prev.* 2011;43(1):25-33. doi:10.1016/j.aap.2010.04.003

47. Carlin A, Perchoux C, Puggina A, et al. A life course examination of the physical environmental determinants of physical activity behaviour: A "Determinants of Diet and Physical Activity" (DEDIPAC) umbrella systematic literature review. *PLoS One.* 2017;12(8). doi:10.1371/journal.pone .0182083

48. O'Donoghue G, Perchoux C, Mensah K, et al. A systematic review of correlates of sedentary behaviour in adults aged 18-65 years: A socio-ecological approach. *BMC Public Health.* 2016;16(1). doi:10.1186/s12889-016-2841-3

49. Fennell C, Barkley JE, Lepp A. The relationship between cell phone use, physical activity, and sedentary behavior in adults aged 18-80. *Comput Human Behav.* 2019;90:53-59. doi:10.1016/j.chb.2018.08.044

50. Kassavou A, Turner A, French DP. Do interventions to promote walking in groups increase physical activity? A meta-analysis. *Int J Behav Nutr Phys Act.* 2013;10. doi:10.1186/1479-5868-10-18

51. Mummery WK, Brown WJ. Whole of community physical activity interventions: Easier said than done. *Br J Sports Med.* 2009;43(1). doi:10.1136/bjsm.2008.053629

52. Baker PR, Francis DP, Soares J, Weightman AL, Foster C. Community wide interventions for increasing physical activity. *Cochrane Database Syst Rev.* 2015;2017(6). doi:10 .1002/14651858.CD008366.pub3

53. Brown DR, Soares J, Epping JM, et al. Stand-alone mass media campaigns to increase physical activity. *Am J Prev Med*. 2012;43(5). doi:10.1016/j.amepre.2012.07.035

54. Lankford T, Wallace J, Brown D, Soares J, Epping JN, Fridinger F. Analysis of physical activity mass media campaign design. *J Phys Act Health*. 2014;11(6). doi:10.1123/jpah.2012-0303

55. Wu S, Cohen D, Shi Y, Pearson M, Sturm R. Economic analysis of physical activity interventions. *Am J Prev Med*. 2011;40(2):149-158. doi:10.1016/j.amepre.2010.10.029

56. Community Preventive Services Task Force. Physical activity: interventions to increase active travel to school. Published April 30, 2019. Accessed September 10, 2023. Available at: https://www.thecommunityguide.org/pages/tffrs-physical-activity-interventions-increase-active-travel-school.html

CHAPTER 16

Social Disadvantage

This chapter discusses the health risks of poverty, social inequality, and racial discrimination. These social factors have profound and far-reaching impacts on disease and mortality. However, their impacts are often indirect, involving more than just a lack of money or other resources. The mechanisms involved are still not fully understood, but enough is known to outline general approaches to prevention.

The Health Risks of Social Disadvantage

History and Terms

In the 1970s, epidemiologists in England published studies showing that government workers in lower ranks had higher mortality rates than those ranking above them in the workplace hierarchy (**Figure 16.1**).[1,2] The researchers could not explain the mortality gaps by poverty because all the workers had decent incomes and job security. They could not explain the mortality gaps by differences in access to health care, either, because, like all British citizens, everyone in their study could get health care through the National Health Service.[2] The researchers labeled these mortality differences **health inequalities**. Their surprising findings set off what has become an international movement to address these inequalities.

A similar movement occurred in the United States, only it focused more on differences in health among racial groups. Using the term **health disparities**, public health officials highlighted the higher rates of disease and mortality in Black Americans compared to Whites.[3] As part of their response, health officials in the 1990s established the National Center for Minority Health and Health Disparities at the National Institutes of Health and Offices of Minority Health in each of the other large federal health agencies.[4,5]

Also in the 1990s, researchers published studies showing that health was also linked to social factors beyond income and race, like education, unemployment, workplace conditions, and neighborhood characteristics. They called their research area **social epidemiology** and the factors they studied the **social determinants of health**.[6] The list of social determinants has grown over time to explicitly name **racial discrimination** and racism, as well as to include other social factors like housing stability

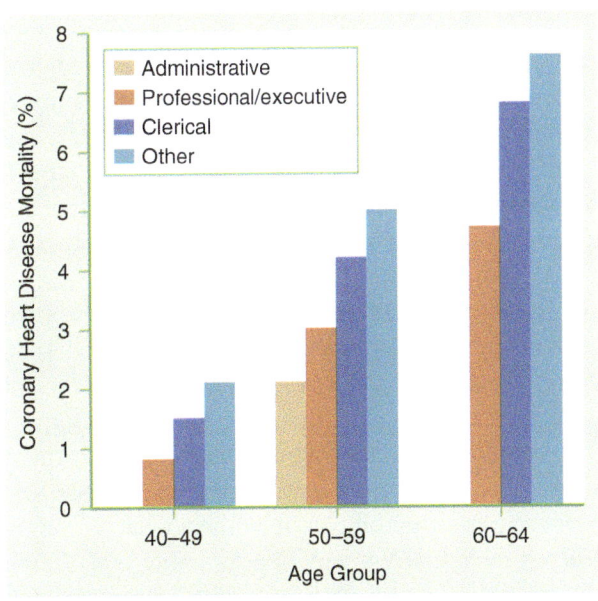

Figure 16.1 Differences in Mortality from Coronary Heart Disease in British Civil Servants by Occupation Class.

Data from Marmot MD, Rose G, Shipley M, Hamilton PJS. Employment grade and coronary heart disease in British civil servants. *J Epi Comm Health* 1978;32:244-249. doi:10.1136/jech.32.4.244

and (by some definitions) access to medical care.[7] The United States Department of Health and Human Services now defines the social determinants of health very broadly as the "conditions in the environment where people are born, live, learn, work, play, worship, and age."[8]

In the 2000s, researchers and advocates on both sides of the Atlantic began to speak more of **health equity**.[3,9,10] At first, they defined health equity as the elimination of avoidable health inequalities and health disparities. Now, the CDC defines it more broadly as "the state in which everyone has a fair and just opportunity to attain their highest level of health."[7] This shift in terms was tied to the idea that eliminating health disparities would require more than just giving everyone equal opportunities. It would require giving extra help for groups dealing with the consequences of historical discrimination, such as African Americans and American Indians/Alaska Natives. More recently, the list of groups deserving extra help under the concept of health equity has been expanded beyond racial minority groups and those with less money to include those with disabilities, people with limited English proficiency, and others.[7]

Defining Social Disadvantage

It is not possible for one chapter to cover all the social determinants of health or every social group under CDC's health equity umbrella. Instead, this chapter will limit itself to one core observation of social epidemiology: the link between disease and social disadvantage. This chapter defines **social disadvantage** as being in a social group that has less resources, autonomy, and power than other social groups.

In most societies, resources, autonomy, and power are not equally distributed. Some people and some groups have more resources, particularly income and wealth, than others. Some have more autonomy—that is, they have more ability to choose for themselves how to live their lives. And some people have more power—the ability to tell others what to do. The studies by social epidemiologists show consistently that people in groups with less wealth, autonomy, and power are sicker and die younger.[6,11]

In most countries, resources, autonomy, and power are measured by factors such as income, education, and employment; people with less income or education and people who are unemployed have social disadvantage and adverse health consequences as a result. In the United States, resources, autonomy, and power can also often be measured by race. One example: African Americans have less wealth, autonomy, and power than White Americans, not just because they have a lower average income but also because of historical and current racial discrimination. Racial discrimination is the imposition of barriers to education, employment, and other aspects of society based on a person's race. American Indians and Alaska Natives have similarly endured racial discrimination and live with its health consequences.

There is no known biological reason that Americans of African descent or American Indians should be less healthy than Americans in other racial groups. They are less healthy, ultimately, because of social disadvantage.

Mechanisms: The State of the Science

Very few experts would question the fact that social disadvantage causes disease and death, but experts do not understand exactly *how* it has that effect. It is difficult to study the impacts of large social factors that have indirect effects and that exert those effects over lifetimes. The next sections will cover this complex issue by first summarizing the data linking social disadvantage to poor health, then discussing the puzzling findings from research on the topic, and then proposing mechanisms that might explain those findings.

Patterns and Trends: The Relationship of Social Disadvantage to Health

Income, Education, and Employment

Figure 16.2 shows life expectancy for 18-year-olds in the United States by family income and by their highest achieved educational level. The differences are very large: people with the lowest incomes have an expected age of death about 11 years less than those with the highest.[12,13] And adults who did not complete high school have an expected age of death that is nearly 15 years less than those with Master's degrees or more education.[12] There are similar relationships of income and education to other general measures of health of a population, such as infant mortality, self-rated health, and the percent of people with chronic diseases.[11]

Employment also has a big effect on health. Adults who are unemployed have nearly twice the mortality rate of those who are employed, even after taking

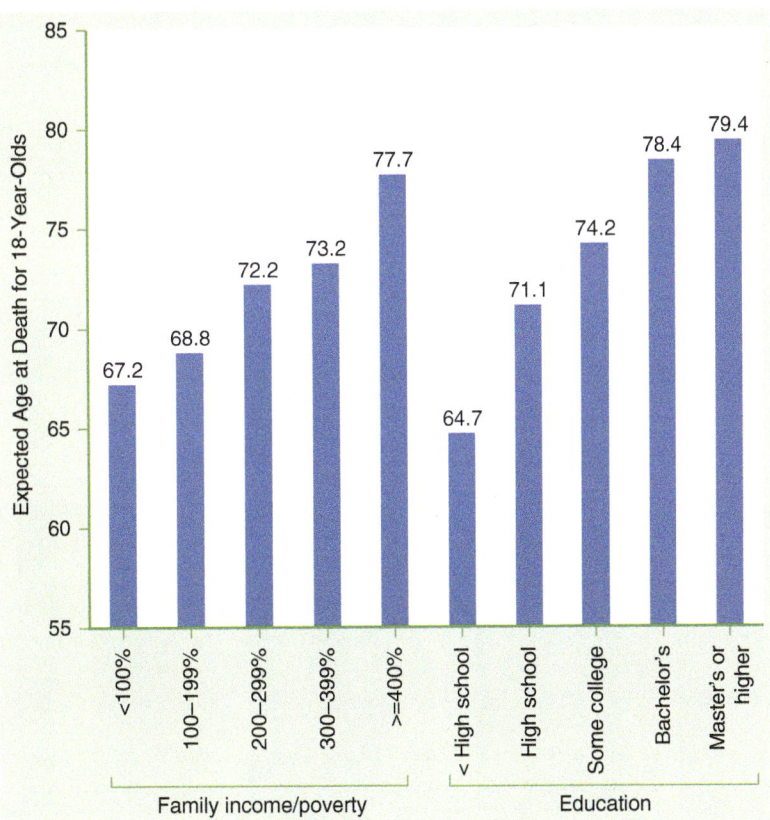

Figure 16.2 Life Expectancy by Family Income and by Education in the United States, 1997–2014. Life expectancy is higher in groups with more education or more income.

Data from Singh G, Lee H. Marked Disparities in Life Expectancy by Education, Poverty Level, Occupation, and Housing Tenure in the United States, 1997–2014. International Journal of Maternal and Child Health and AIDS (IJMA). 2020;10(1):7-18. doi:10.21106/ijma.402

into account pre-existing illnesses. The health risks of unemployment are greater in men than in women and greater in younger than older adults.[14,15]

The connection of social disadvantage to disease is not unique to the United States. People with lower levels of income and education and people who are unemployed have higher mortality rates throughout Europe and Scandinavia, even in countries in which everyone has access to medical care and which have generous social programs.[14,16]

Race

Figure 16.3 shows life expectancy at birth by race and Hispanic ethnicity in the United States. (The numbers here are not directly comparable to those in Figure 16.2 because the metric and time periods are different.)[17] Non-Hispanic Black Americans have a life expectancy nearly five years less than that of Non-Hispanic Whites. This is not the largest racial health disparity, though. The racial group with the lowest life expectancy is American Indians/Alaska Natives, and the group with the highest life expectancy is Asians. The gap between these two groups is strikingly high at more than 16 years.[17]

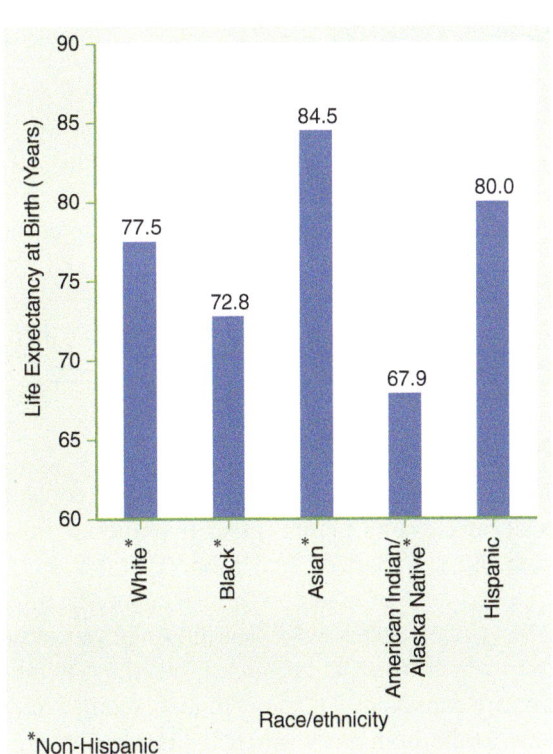

Figure 16.3 Life Expectancy at Birth in the United States by Race/Ethnicity, 2022.

Data from Arias E, Kochanek KD, Xu J, Tejada-Vera B. Provisional Life Expectancy Estimates for 2022. *NVSS Vital Statistics Rapid Release.* 2023;31:1-16.

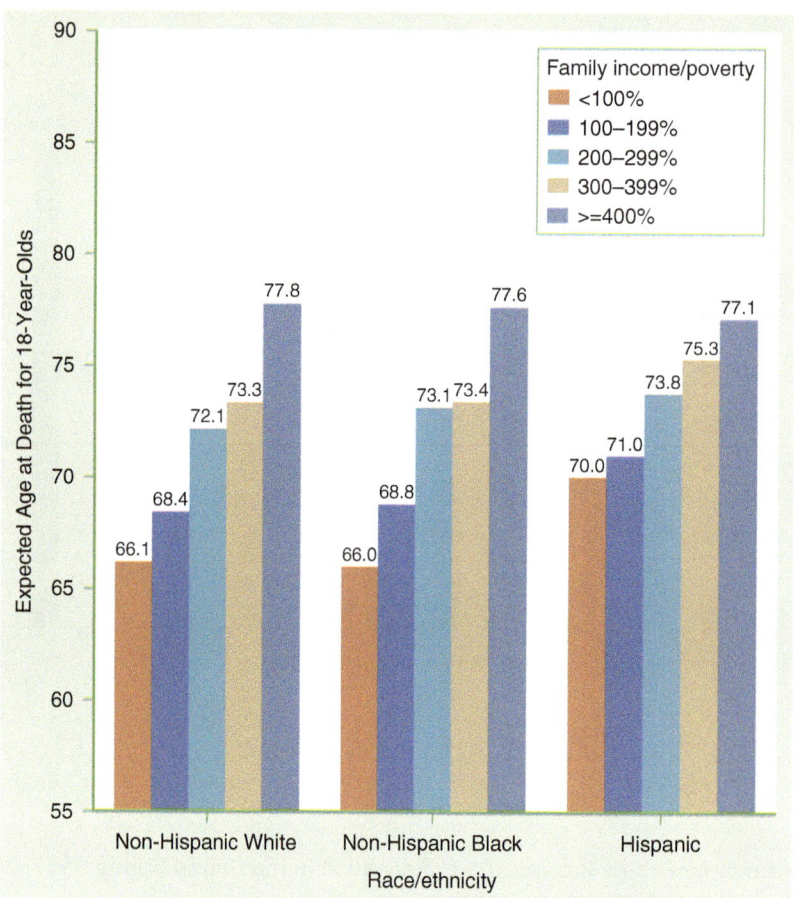

Figure 16.4 **Life Expectancy in the United States by Family Income and Race/Ethnicity, 1997–2014.** Life expectancy is higher in groups with more education or more income, even within racial groups.

Data from Singh G, Lee H. Marked Disparities in Life Expectancy by Education, Poverty Level, Occupation, and Housing Tenure in the United States, 1997–2014. International Journal of Maternal and Child Health and AIDS (IJMA). 2020;10(1):7-18. doi:10.21106/ijma.402

In addition, *within* individual racial groups, there are differences in life expectancy by income, education, and employment. For example, Black people with lower incomes have a much lower life expectancy than Black people with higher incomes, and White people with lower incomes have a much lower life expectancy than White people with higher incomes (**Figure 16.4**).[11]

Disparities in Diseases

What diseases shorten the life spans in people with social disadvantage? Surprisingly, most diseases. **Table 16.1** summarizes data from several sources on racial and income-based disparities in specific diseases in the United States.[11,18-25] The findings vary according to which data source is used, but the general patterns are consistent. People with less income are more likely to die from cardiovascular disease, cancer, diabetes, chronic lung disease, and respiratory infections; are more likely to live with musculoskeletal disorders; and are more likely to rate themselves on surveys as

unhealthy. In fact, there are only a few diseases and injuries that are *not* more common in people with lower incomes. The relationship of minority race and ethnicity to these diseases is less consistent, but similar.

People with lower education and people who are unemployed likewise have increased mortality rates from a long list of diseases, although unemployment is especially strongly linked to mortality related to alcohol and drug use.[15,26-28]

Trends in Social Disadvantage and Its Health Effects

Social inequalities in the United States are increasing. While the U.S. economy is growing and average incomes are rising, almost all of the rise in the past 50 years has benefited those who were already well off, and incomes of the people with the lowest incomes remain stagnant (**Figure 16.5**).[29] In 1967, the top 5% of earners, made on average, 17.6 times as much money as people in the lowest quintile; in 2022 that ratio had increased to 31.

Table 16.1 Summary of Association of Diseases and Conditions with Income and Race

People with less income and people in specific racial minority groups (African-Americans and American Indians/Alaska Natives) are at higher risk for diseases and conditions caused by very different biologic mechanisms.

	Increased Risk		
	Low vs. High Income	**Black vs. White**	**AI/AN vs. White**
Cardiovascular disease	✓	✓	
Cancer	✓*	✓	
Diabetes	✓	✓	✓
Injuries			
Unintentional ("accidents")	✓	✓	✓
Self-harm (suicide)	✓		
Violence (homicide)	✓	✓	✓
Chronic lung disease	✓		
Respiratory infections	✓	✓	
Low birth weight and infant mortality	✓	✓	✓
Musculoskeletal disorders			
Osteoarthritis	✓		✓
Low back pain	✓	✓	✓
Self-rated fair or poor health	✓	✓	✓

AI/AN = American Indian/Alaska Native
*Except Breast

And while life expectancy has been increasing, the gap in life expectancy between those with high incomes and those with low incomes has been widening. Between 2001 and 2014, the difference in life expectancy for men between the top 25% and bottom 25% rose from 8.7 to 9.7 years (**Figure 16.6**).[13]

Income for all racial groups in the United States has been rising over the past 50 years, but income gaps between races continue. In fact, from 1972 to 2022, the difference in median household income between White and Black people widened slightly, from $25,800 to $27,560.[29]

The White-Black gap in life expectancy at birth since 1900 is shown in (**Figure 16.7**). This gap has narrow substantially over these 120 years, but it persisted through the overdose death crisis that started in about 2000 and widened during the COVID-19 pandemic in the early 2020s.[17,30]

Around the world, the distribution of income varies markedly by country. The income gap between those on the higher end of the distribution and those on the lower end is generally higher in countries with worse health statistics. **Figure 16.8** shows income inequality by country, measured as the estimated percent of total national income received by the top 10% of earners.[31] In the most equal countries, which are in northern Europe, Scandinavia, and Oceania, the top 10% receive about 30% of national income. In the most unequal countries, such as India and those in Southern Africa, Latin America, and the Middle East, the top 10% receive between 55% and 60% of national income. The United States is among the most unequal of high-income countries, with the top 10% receiving 48% of national income.

The income gap has been growing in most high-income countries since 1980 (**Figure 16.9**).[31] More important, this graph shows that income inequality is not a constant feature of any society; it changes over time.

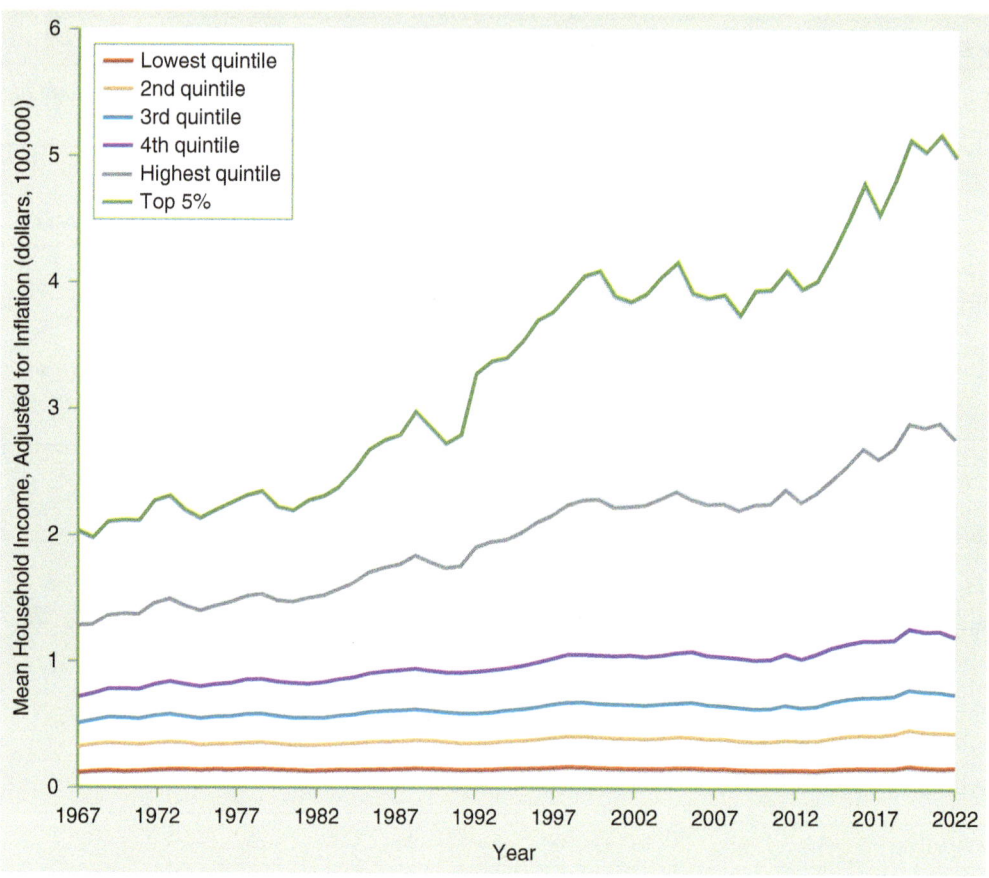

Figure 16.5 Trends in Income Inequality in the United States.

Data from Guzman G, Kollar M, US Census Bureau. Income in the United States: 2022. Current Population Reports. 2023;[P60-279]. Table A-4b.

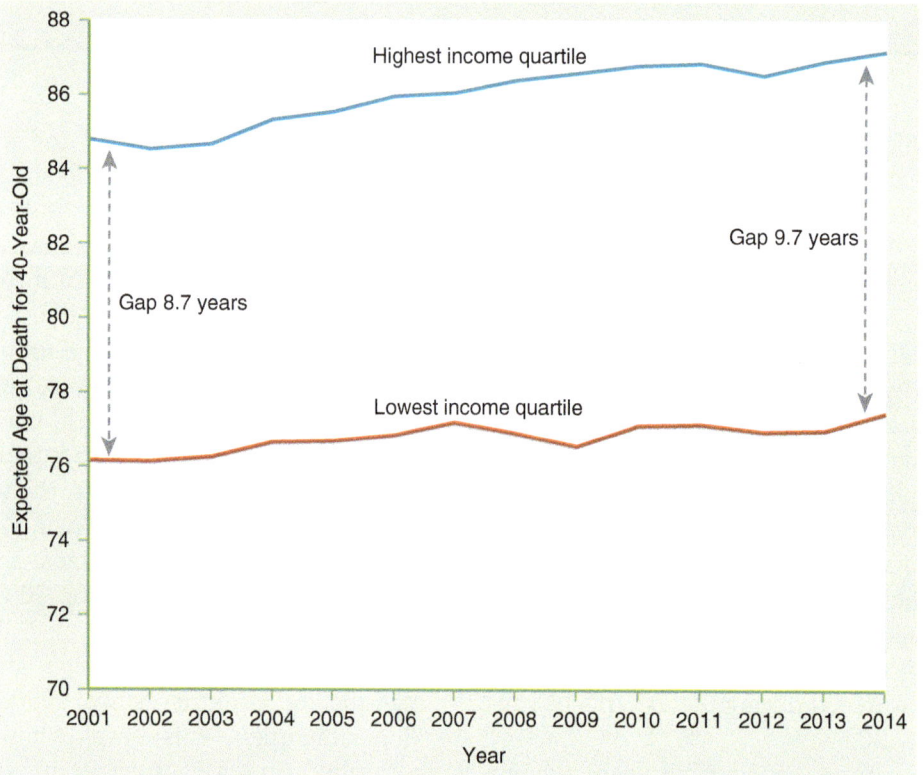

Figure 16.6 Trends in Life Expectancy for Men by Income Quartile, United States, 2001–2014.

Data from Chetty R, Stepner M, Abraham S, et al. The association between income and life expectancy in the United States, 2001–2014. JAMA - Journal of the American Medical Association. 2016;315(16):1750-1766. Data obtained from shttps://healthinequality.org/data/

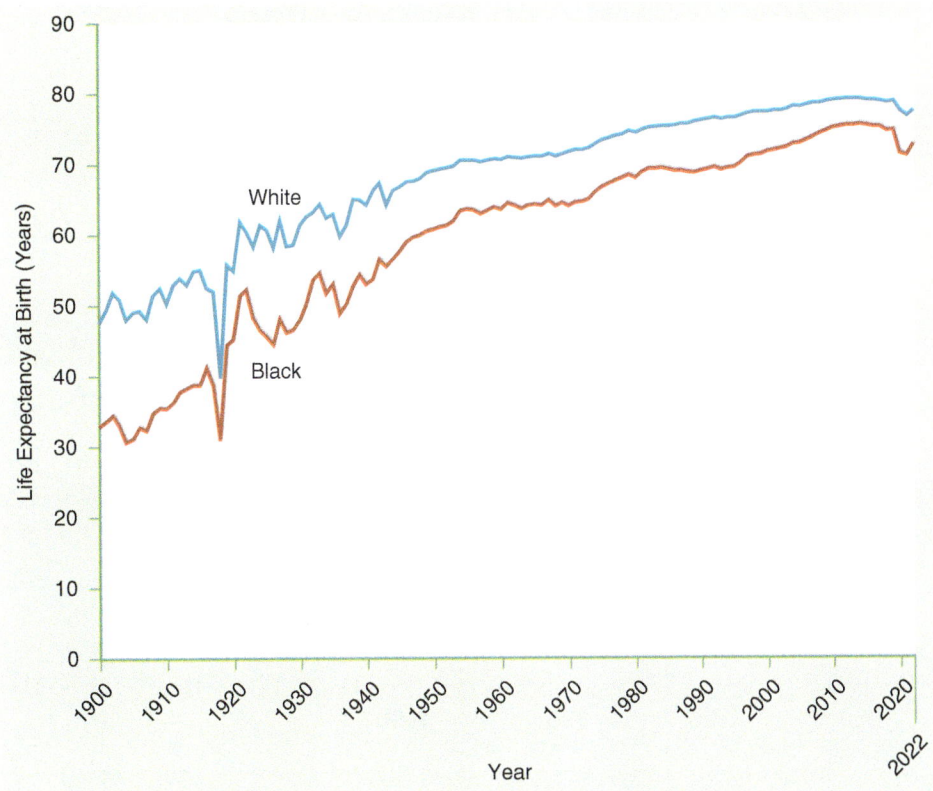

Figure 16.7 Trends in Life Expectancy at Birth in White and Black people, United States 1900–2022.

Data from Arias E, Xu J, Kochanek K. United States Life Tables, 2021. National Vital Statistics Reports. 2023;72(12):1-64 and Arias E, Kochanek KD, Xu J, Tejada-Vera B. Provisional Life Expectancy Estimates for 2022. *NVSS Vital Statistics Rapid Release*. 2023;31:1-16.

Pathophysiology: How Social Disadvantage Causes Disease

Puzzling Patterns of Social Disadvantage

Any explanation for how social disadvantage ultimately causes disease and death must account for several puzzling patterns:

- *Non-specificity of effect:* The health damage caused by social disadvantage is biologically nonspecific. That is, health disparities are found for diseases with very different biologic mechanisms. The biologic mechanisms of heart disease, respiratory infections, low back pain, and homicides are completely different. How could a person's income, education, or race have such diverse biologic effects?

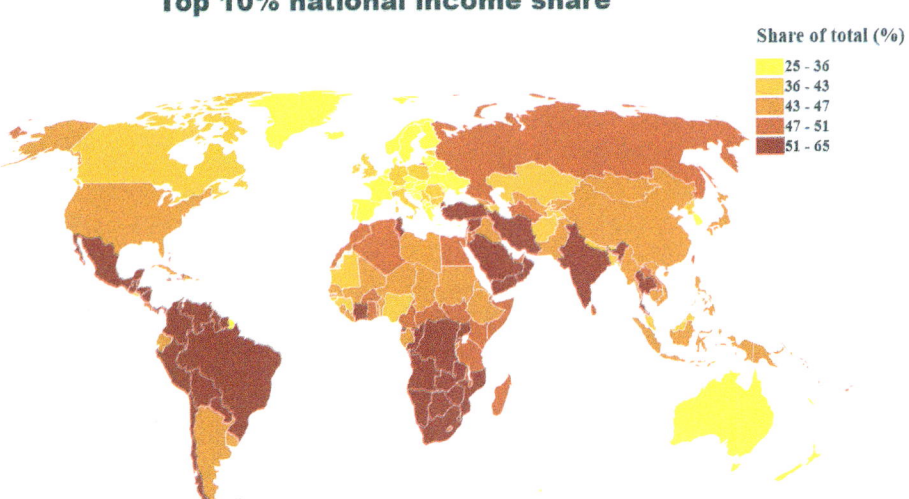

Figure 16.8 Income Inequality by Country, 2022.

Top 10% national income share

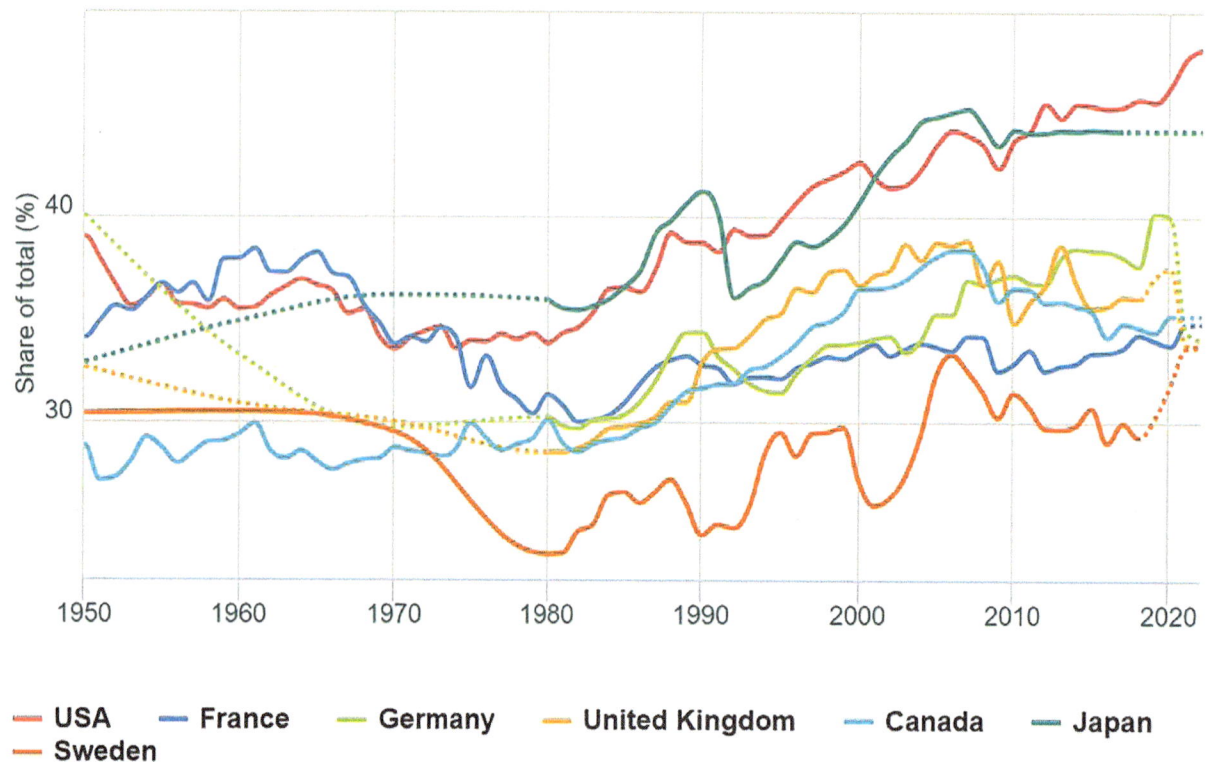

USA — **France** — **Germany** — **United Kingdom** — **Canada** — **Japan** — **Sweden**

Figure 16.9 **Trends in Income Inequality in Selected High-Income Countries Since 1950.** Income inequality is rising within most high-income countries since 1980.

- *Relative effect and the gradient:* The higher rates of disease and death and not just linked to poverty. Instead, there is a gradient of health across the entire range of social advantage in which, at every level, those with more advantage are healthier. This is shown in Figure 16.1 and also **Figure 16.10**, which is from a study that linked U.S. income tax records to mortality data.[13] Even people at the 90th percentile for income, who by global or historical standards are rich, have a shorter life expectancy than people who have even higher incomes.[11,13] In addition, some studies show that, among developed countries, higher mortality is associated less with *median* income than with the *inequality* of income.[32,33] These studies suggest that the determinants of an individual's health include not just *absolute* income but also *relative* income, that is, how many people earn more than that individual. Why should the income of others have an impact on the health of an individual?

- *Neighborhood effect:* Adverse health effects are linked not just to *individual* social disadvantage

but also to *neighborhood* disadvantage.[11,13] That is, people who live in lower-income neighborhoods are less healthy than people with similar incomes who live in higher-income neighborhoods.[34]

- *Life-course effect:* The effect of social disadvantage plays out over a lifetime. Adults who grew up in families with lower incomes are more likely to be ill and more likely to die young, even after taking into account their income as adults.[35,36]

- *Inter-generational effect:* The negative impact of social disadvantage even seems to be partially passed down from one generation to another. Children of parents who were socially disadvantaged before they were born are more likely to develop disease than those of more advantaged parents, even after taking into account their own income.[37,38]

- *Effect on health-related behavior:* People with social disadvantage tend to have unhealthier habits.[39-43] For example, in data from the CDC's Behavioral Risk Factor Surveillance System (**Figure 16.11**), people with lower incomes are

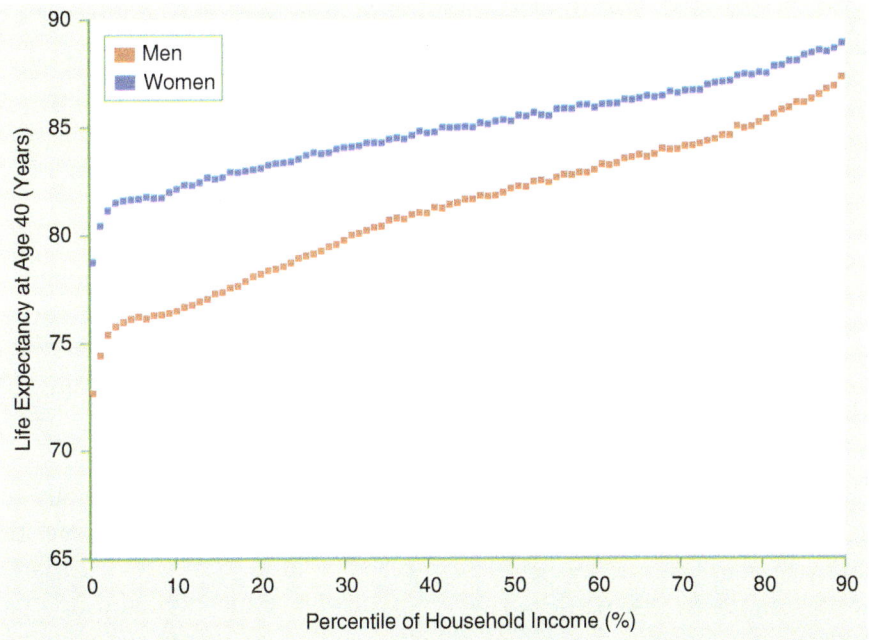

Figure 16.10 **Life Expectancy at Age 40 by Income in the United States.** Across the entire range of income, those with higher incomes have higher life expectancies.

Data from Chetty R, Stepner M, Abraham S, et al. The association between income and life expectancy in the United States, 2001–2014. JAMA - Journal of the American Medical Association. 2016;315(16):1750-1766. Data obtained from shttps://healthinequality.org/data/

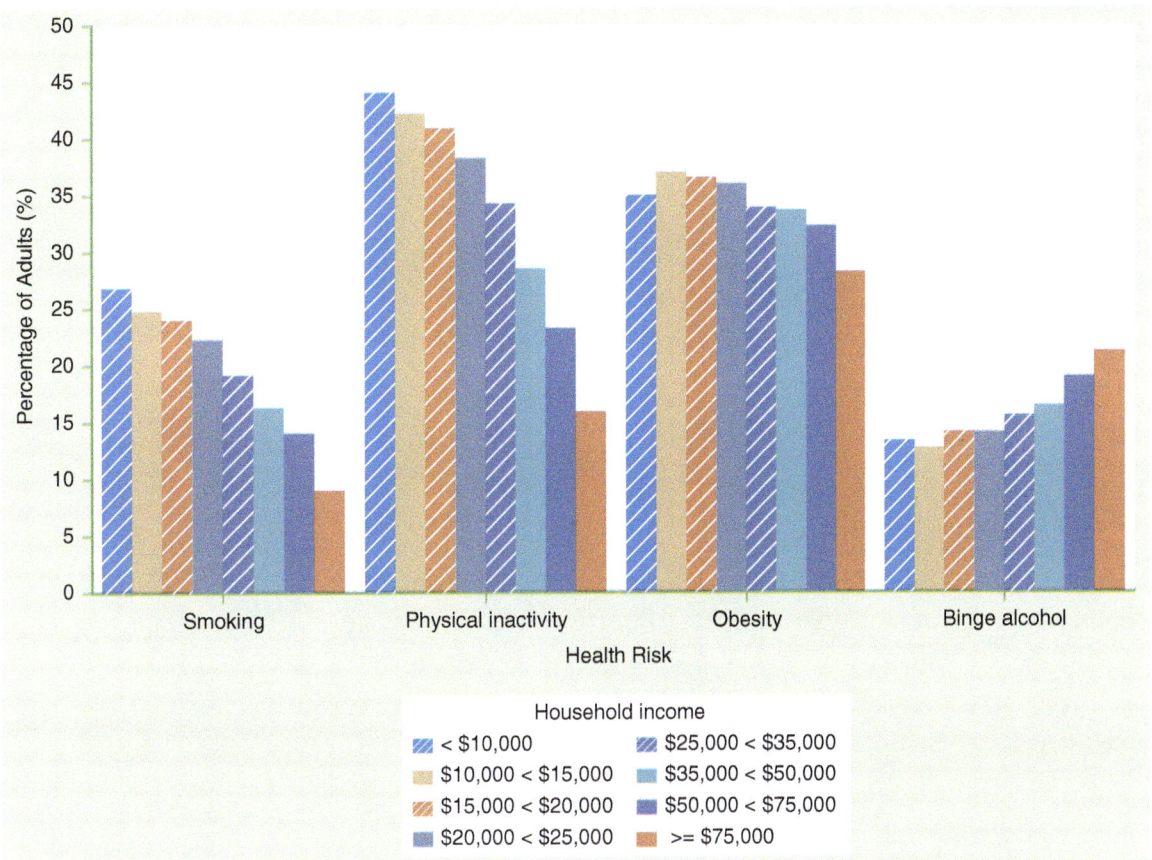

Figure 16.11 **Behavioral Health Risks Among Adults in the United States by Household Income, 2019.** People who have lower incomes are more likely to practice behavior that is unhealthy for several (but not all) key health-related behaviors.

Data from Centers for Disease Control and Prevention. Behavioral Risk Factor Surveillance System. Accessed January 6, 2024. https://www.cdc.gov/brfss/index.html. Data analysis using Web Enabled Analysis Tool (WEAT).

much more likely to smoke, be physically inactive, and be obese (a marker for an unhealthy diet). Similarly, African Americans and American Indians/Alaska Natives are more likely than Whites or Asians to smoke, be physically inactive, and be obese (**Figure 16.12**).[40,43-47] The pattern is not completely consistent, though. People with higher incomes are more likely to binge drink alcohol. The differences by income for smoking and physical inactivity are particularly large. Interpersonal violence is another behavior that is unhealthy (for the victim, bystanders, and the perpetrator), and lower-income neighborhoods also have higher levels of gun violence.[48,49] There are two puzzling aspects of these findings. First, it is not clear why having less income should make someone adopt unhealthy habits, especially when some of the habits (particularly smoking) are expensive to maintain. Second, studies show that these behaviors, while very important to health, do not fully explain the socioeconomic differences in mortality.[39,50]

The Impact of Medical Care

Before proposing mechanisms by which social disadvantage causes health inequalities, it is worth discussing one key factor that—perhaps surprisingly—does *not* seem to be an important mechanism: access to medical care.

Four facts demonstrate that differences in access to medical care do not explain why people with social disadvantage are less healthy and die younger. First, most deaths cannot be prevented by medical care.[51,52] Best estimates are that optimal medical care has the potential to prevent only 27% of deaths.[52] Second, geographic areas that have more medical resources like hospitals and doctors do not have lower mortality rates from these treatable diseases.[53] Third, there are big differences in mortality by income, education, and occupational rank, even in populations where everyone has equal access to medical care—such as those British government workers.[2,16] And fourth, differences in access to medical care cannot explain several of the puzzling

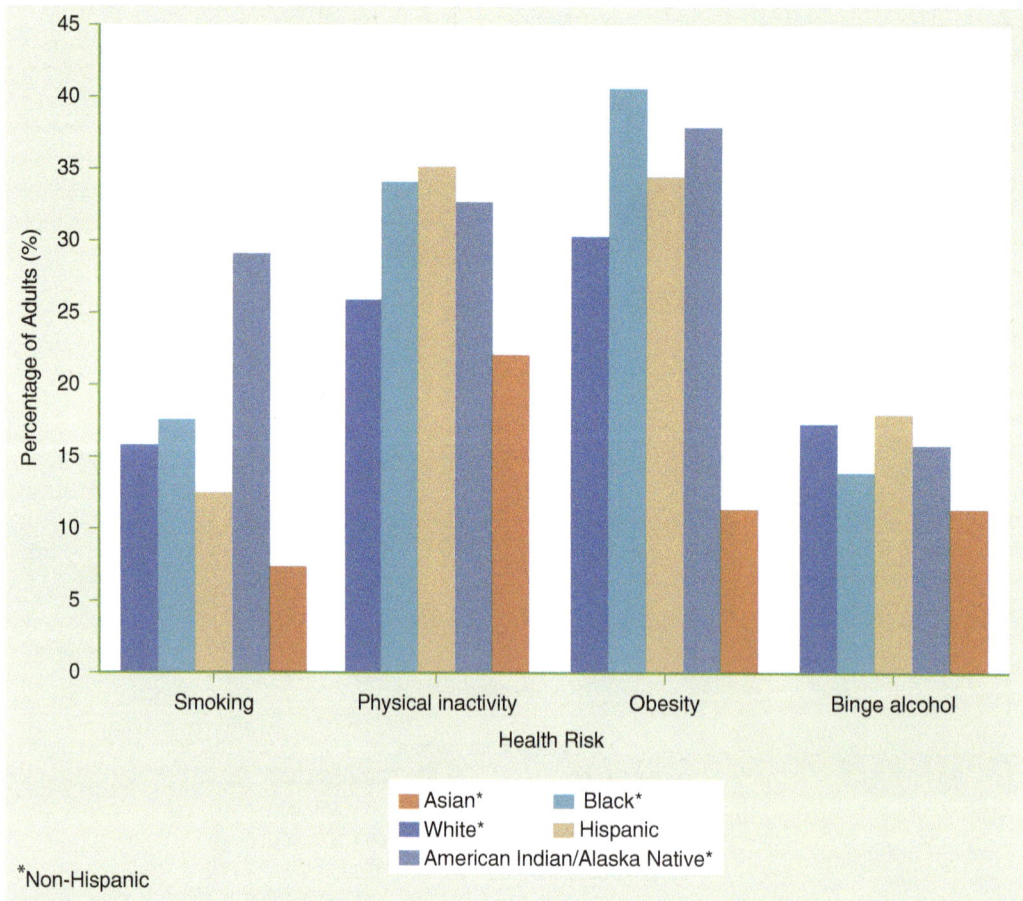

Figure 16.12 **Behavioral Health Risks Among Adults in the United States by Race/Ethnicity, 2019.** The patterns for health-related behavior are less consistent by race and ethnicity than they are by income, but people with social disadvantage still tend to have unhealthier habits.

Data from Centers for Disease Control and Prevention. Behavioral Risk Factor Surveillance System. Accessed January 6, 2024. https://www.cdc.gov/brfss/index.html. Data analysis using Web Enabled Analysis Tool (WEAT).

patterns listed above, such as the neighborhood effect, the life course effect, or the inter-generational effect. For these reasons, most experts do not view lack of access to medical care as an important cause of health inequalities, and most plans to reduce health inequalities in higher-income countries do not emphasize medical care.[32,54-57]

Certainly, in the United States, people with less income or people in racial minority groups often have difficulty accessing primary medical care. And people in racial minority groups often do not receive equal or optimal medical treatment for their illnesses.[58] These problems should be fixed. But fixing those problems is very unlikely to meaningfully reduce health disparities by race or income.

Possible Mechanisms for Health Effects of Social Disadvantage

Experts have proposed several possible mechanisms to explain the connection between social disadvantage and disease. These are theories, and all are unproven. While each one would not explain all patterns of health disparities, together they may come close.

- *Access to resources and opportunities:* Those with social disadvantage have less access to many resources and opportunities—not just money but also knowledge, power, and helpful social networks.[59] People who have more of these resources and opportunities use them to maximize their success and happiness, which usually also means minimizing health risks. Money and power can buy safer neighborhoods, quieter streets, better housing, cleaner air, cleaner water, and jobs that are less physically demanding. While this theory is easy to understand, it may not explain the full gradient in health risk; it is difficult to argue that people with high incomes in the richest nation on earth are less healthy than those with even higher incomes because they lack resources.
- *Stress.* **Stress** is a response by the body to a threat that the person feels cannot be overcome or handled. By this theory, people with less money, education, or rank in the workplace are forced to follow the demands of others, causing constant, low-level, psychological stress. Some experts use the term **allostatic load** for the chronic, daily stress of living with social disadvantage.[60] Psychological stress is known to activate brain cells and hormones in ways that can be harmful over the long term, increasing susceptibility to many different diseases, from infections to cancer.[61] Also, people may cope

with stress by using drugs like nicotine, alcohol, or opioids to lift their mood, which may explain some of the link between poverty and unhealthy behaviors.[62] Some pediatricians argue that stress experienced in childhood (which they label "toxic stress") is especially damaging because it interferes with children's brain development and increases the likelihood that when these children are adults, they will have unhealthy behaviors, physical illness, and mental illnesses.[63] Studies have shown that children growing up in households in which parents are neglectful, abusive, violent, or using drugs are more likely as adults to have depression and anxiety and to use drugs themselves.[64-66] This stress theory is appealing because it might help explain the gradient in health across income levels: in a country with a large gap between those with high and low incomes, nearly everyone deals with those who are richer than they are, and that interaction can be stressful. Those in the bottom ranks feel the stress the most. The damage from toxic stress in childhood might also explain the life-course effect of social disadvantage and its far-ranging biologic effects. So far, though, researchers have had difficulty confirming this theory by measuring stress hormones in people with different levels of social disadvantage.[67]
- *Social cohesion:* Humans are social animals who help each other. The degree to which people trust each other, help each other, and work together to solve common problems has been called **social cohesion**. At one extreme, neighborhoods with low social cohesion are violent. At the other extreme, in neighborhoods with high social cohesion, people look out for each other, helping friends and neighbors avoid health risks. According to this theory, the greater the gap between those with high and low incomes, the less social cohesion. And when there is less social cohesion, people are more likely to be exposed to things that are harmful and to receive less help from others.[68] While this theory makes intuitive sense, it is a little hard to believe that a lack of trust within a community could lead to such profound and wide-ranging damage to the individuals within it.
- *Environments and working conditions:* People with lower incomes or education have less freedom to choose where they live or work. They may have no choice but to live in less-desirable homes and neighborhoods and work in less-desirable jobs. That leaves them more exposed to health risks

in the home (for example, lead paint, pests), at work (physical demands, toxic chemicals), in their neighborhoods (traffic noise, liquor stores, street violence), and in their communities (air pollution). This theory is easy to understand, but it needs more studies to confirm it, and it does not fully explain the life-course effect or inter-generational effect.

These four theories overlap, and the factors that they highlight relate to each other. For example, people with less resources and opportunities are more likely to be exposed to unhealthy environments and working conditions. People in unhealthy environments may experience more stress. And people who are stressed by their living and working conditions may be less likely to trust or help their neighbors.

The "Piling On" of Diseases, Injuries, and Health Risks

The damaging effects of social disadvantage may "pile on" to each other. That is, people with social disadvantage may experience the cumulative effect of many different psychological and physical "injuries," each of which increases the likelihood of other injuries and each of which interferes with the recovery from others.[69] This "piling on" can happen in several ways:

- *Biologically*, the consequences of one illness or injury increase the risk of or interfere with the recovery from other illnesses or injuries. For example, people with diabetes are more likely to die from cancer.[70]
- *Behaviorally*, the adverse effects of unhealthy behaviors promote the adoption of other unhealthy behaviors. For example, people who

smoke consume more alcohol than nonsmokers do, and people using alcohol or drugs are more likely to be violent.[71,72]

- *Socially*, lower-income neighborhoods contain unhealthy conditions and influences that adversely reinforce each other. For example, the people in poverty are more likely to live in neighborhoods where they experience the stress of witnessing community violence *and* in social networks with others under psychological stress.[73,74] And people living in neighborhoods with concentrated poverty are more likely to have biologic markers of stress.[75]
- *Across the life course*, adverse exposures starting at birth accumulate and make subsequent adverse exposures more likely and more harmful. Children exposed to stressful situations are more likely as adults to adopt unhealthy behaviors and develop chronic disease.[76-78]
- *Inter-generationally*, the struggles of parents dealing with stress or illness increase the risk that their children will develop similar problems. For example, women who are stressed, unhealthy, or use tobacco or other drugs during pregnancy are more likely to deliver babies with low birth weight. In turn, low birth weight increases the child's risk of developing many chronic diseases as an adult.[37,79]

Risk Factors: A Model Summarizing Possible Mechanisms

Figure 16.13 is a cause-and-effect model for social disadvantage that incorporates these theories. The model shows what some experts have called

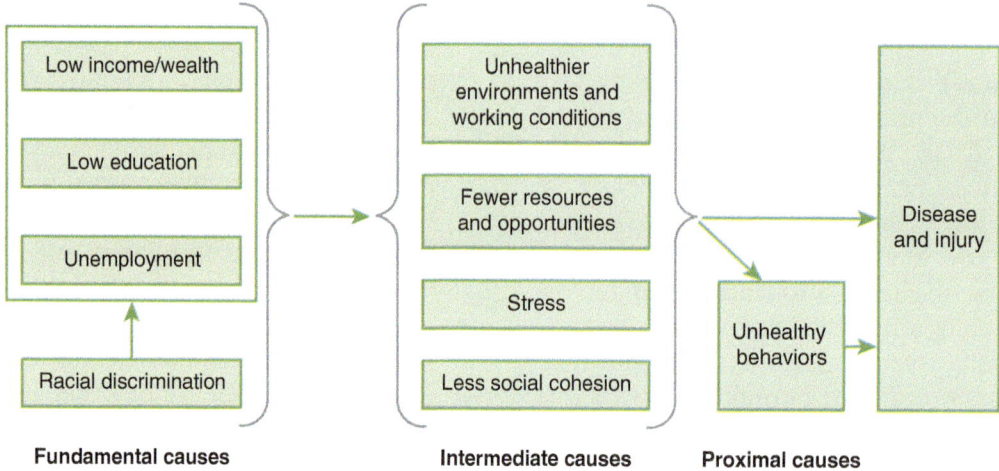

Fundamental causes   **Intermediate causes**   **Proximal causes**

Figure 16.13 **Cause-and-Effect Diagram for the Health Impact of Social Disadvantage.**

the "fundamental causes" of lower income/wealth, lower education, unemployment, and past and current racial discrimination.[59] Obviously, these fundamental causes are closely related. For example, people who are unemployed have less income and people with lower levels of education are more likely to lose their jobs. People in racial groups that face discrimination have barriers to education, employment, and income.

These fundamental causes combine to produce four overlapping intermediate causes: *unhealthier environments and working conditions, fewer opportunities and resources, psychological stress*, and, at a group level, *less social cohesion*.

The four intermediate causes in turn combine to promote *unhealthy behaviors*, particularly smoking, drug use, physical inactivity, unhealthy eating habits, and interpersonal violence. For example, people with lower incomes are more likely to have unhealthy diets if they are dealing with the stress of unpaid bills and difficult working conditions *and* if they are living in neighborhoods in which the grocery stores stock mostly unhealthy foods. These four intermediate causes also have direct effects on health, for example, from dangerous or toxic exposures in homes, neighborhoods, and workplaces, and from chronic stress causing disease-promoting hormonal responses.

These fundamental, intermediate, and proximal causes exert their effects over years and over the course of individual lives. Health risks during pregnancy and in early childhood have lifelong impacts. That means it is especially important to prevent these risks for women who are pregnant (or may become pregnant) and for children.

Preventive Interventions

The model offers two types of approaches to improve the health in people with social disadvantages: 1) address the fundamental causes, that is, reduce gaps in income, education, and employment, and eliminate racial discrimination, and 2) address the intermediate and proximal causes, that is, improve the conditions of daily living of those with social disadvantage and work to reduce unhealthy behaviors (**Figure 16.14**).

The first of these two approaches could include:

- *Reduction of gaps in income and wealth.* Today, many economists are even more concerned than public health experts are about rising income inequality, and they have proposed several policy solutions.[80] For example, income gaps can be narrowed by increases in the minimum wage, support for union bargaining power, and more-progressive income taxes. Wealth gaps can be narrowed by financially supporting home ownership among persons with low incomes and by placing taxes on high-level wealth.

- *Expansion of access to education.* Education helps individuals earn a decent living and overcome many other barriers to health. Education also benefits society as a whole, enough that it is justified to provide education at public expense. Because the benefits play out over a lifetime, education is particularly important in early childhood. For example, public health experts have promoted universal or expanded early childhood education.[81] Educational gaps for teenagers and adults can be narrowed by providing free vocational and adult education and by reducing (or eliminating) tuition at public colleges and universities.

- *Reduction in unemployment:* Employment helps people in ways beyond the money that they make in wages. It can offer structure, a sense of purpose, social connection, and more diverse social networks. Various government policies, from lower interest rates to infrastructure projects, can affect the number of people who are employed.[82] The people who need jobs the most are those who are the most socially disadvantaged.

- *Affirmative action* in education and employment: Racial groups that have long faced discrimination—particularly African Americans and American Indians/Alaska Natives—deserve opportunities in education and employment that have been denied to them and their parents in the past.

The second approach of improving the conditions of daily living for the socially disadvantaged includes:

- *Healthier environments and working conditions.* The model suggests that people with social disadvantage are more vulnerable to unhealthy conditions at home or at work. These conditions can be addressed through policies on healthier housing, transportation, the built environment, air pollution, employment, and workplaces. Some of these policies are covered in other chapters of this book, and others are covered in textbooks on environmental and occupational health.

- *Support for racial and economic integration.* People with low incomes or affected by racial discrimination often are concentrated within low-income neighborhoods. This segregation tends to exacerbate

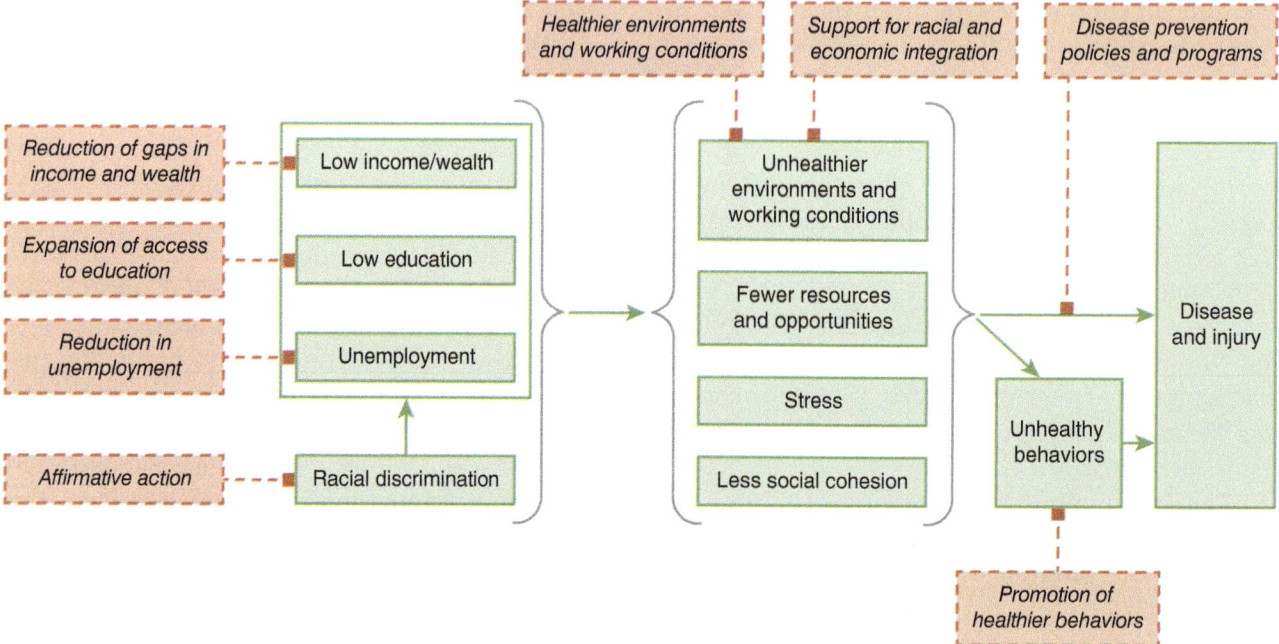

Figure 16.14 Cause-and-Effect Diagram for the Health Impact of Social Disadvantage, with Preventive Interventions.

the social "piling on" of the harms of social disadvantage. One way to lessen this problem is to make it easier for people to live in any neighborhood, for example by eliminating zoning rules that prohibit multi-family housing.

- *Promotion of healthier behaviors:* Policies and programs to promote healthier behaviors are often not thought of as addressing the social determinants of health. However, because people with social disadvantage are more likely to adopt unhealthy behaviors, these initiatives disproportionately benefit them. The behaviors that matter most to health are smoking, dietary risks, alcohol consumption, use of other drugs, and physical inactivity. Other chapters in this book cover strategies to promote healthier behaviors. They include not just educational messages but also policies to increase the availability of healthy products and to limit the marketing of unhealthy products.

- *Other disease prevention policies and programs.* Disadvantaged groups are at higher risk for nearly every disease, injury, and unhealthy condition. For that reason, all the preventive interventions identified in other chapters of this book, if they are well directed, have the potential to help people with social disadvantage and to reduce health disparities. To realize that potential, though, the interventions must be implemented in ways that ensure they especially reach and help people in disadvantaged groups.

Many of these interventions are difficult to put in place, practically and politically. But health disparities by income are growing. Reducing the social disadvantage that drives those health disparities—or even preventing it from getting worse—is worth the effort.

Box 16.1 Summary–Prevention of Health Effects of Social Disadvantage

- Reduction of gaps in income and wealth
- Expansion of access to education
- Reduction in unemployment
- Affirmative action in education and employment
- Healthier environments and working conditions
- Support for racial and economic integration
- Promotion of healthier behaviors
- Other disease prevention policies and programs

Box 16.2 Key Words–Social Disadvantage

Allostatic load
Health disparities
Health equity
Health inequalities
Racial discrimination
Social cohesion
Social determinants of health
Social disadvantage
Social epidemiology
Stress

Resources–Social Disadvantage

- Braveman P, Egerter S, Williams DR. The social determinants of health: Coming of age. *Annu Rev Public Health*. 2011;32:381-398. doi:10.1146/annurev-publhealth-031210-101218
- Berkman L, Kawachi I, Glymour M, eds. *Social Epidemiology*. 2nd ed. Oxford University Press; 2014. This book contains 15 chapters summarizing concepts and research findings on health disparities and the social determinants of health.
- Braveman P. Defining Health Equity. *J Natl Med Assoc*. 2022;114(6):593-600. doi:10.1016/j.jnma.2022.08.004
- Shonkoff JP, Garner AS, Siegel BS, et al. The lifelong effects of early childhood adversity and toxic stress. *Pediatrics*. 2012;129(1). doi:10.1542/peds.2011-2663
- Evans GW, Kim P. Multiple risk exposure as a potential explanatory mechanism for the socioeconomic status-health gradient. *Ann N Y Acad Sci*. 2010;1186:174-189. doi:10.1111/j.1749-6632.2009.05336.x. This paper explains and tests the idea that social disadvantage exerts its effects through multiple, cumulative adverse exposures ("piling on").
- The *World Inequality Database* provides estimates on inequalities in income and wealth at https://wid.world.
- Opportunity Insights is a group of economists that summarize their research on inequalities of income and opportunity in the United States at https://opportunityinsights.org.
- Marmot M, Friel S, Bell R, Houweling TA, Taylor S. Closing the gap in a generation: health equity through action on the social determinants of health. *Lancet*. 2008;372(9650):1661-1669. doi:10.1016/S0140-6736(08)61690-6. This paper summarizes the World Health Organization's plans to address the social determinants of health at a global level.
- Marmot M. *Fair Society, Healthy Lives (2010)* and *Health Equity in England: The Marmot Review 10 Years On (2020)* describe a detailed, evidence-based plan for reducing social disadvantage and its health effects in England. Many of the principles and ideas are applicable to the United States and other high-income countries. These reports are available at https://www.instituteofhealthequity.org.
- Bhatt A, Kolb M, Ward O. How to Fix Economic Inequality? An Overview of Policies for the United States and Other High-Income Countries. Peterson Institute for International Economics. https://www.piie.com/microsites/how-fix-economic-inequality. This is an in-depth report and set of recommendations on income inequality from a nonpartisan group of economists.

References

1. Davey Smith G, Egger M. Socioeconomic differentials in wealth and health. *BMJ*. 1993;307(6912):1085-1086. doi:10.1136/bmj.307.6912.1085
2. Marmot MG, Rose G, Shipley M, Hamilton PJ. Employment grade and coronary heart disease in British civil servants. *J Epidemiol Community Health (1978)*. 1978;32(4):244-249. doi:10.1136/jech.32.4.244
3. Braveman P. Defining health equity. *J Natl Med Assoc*. 2022;114(6):593-600. doi:10.1016/j.jnma.2022.08.004
4. Office of Minority Health. Institute and Offices of Minority Health/Health Equity at HHS. Department of Health and Human Services. Published 2024. Accessed July 18, 2024. Available at: https://minorityhealth.hhs.gov/offices-minority-health-hhs
5. National Institute on Minority Health and Health Disparities. History - NIMHD Celebrates 10 Year Anniversary in 2020. National Institutes of Health. Published 2024. Accessed July 18, 2024. Available at: https://www.nimhd.nih.gov/about/overview/history/
6. Berkman LF, Kawachi I, Glymour MM. Social Epidemiology. 2nd ed. Oxford University Press; 2014.
7. Centers for Disease Control and Prevention. What is health equity? Centers for Disease Control and Prevention. Published June 11, 2024. Accessed July 18, 2024. Available at: https://www.cdc.gov/health-equity/what-is/index.html
8. Office of Assistant Secretary for Health. Social determinants of health. healthy people 2030. Published 2023. Accessed October 3, 2024. Available at: https://health.gov/healthypeople/priority-areas/social-determinants-health
9. Liu Y. Understanding and setting up the process for health equity. *Bull World Health Organ*. 2000;78(1):82-83.
10. Braveman P. Health disparities and health equity: Concepts and measurement. *Annu Rev Public Health*. 2006;27:167-194. doi:10.1146/annurev.publhealth.27.021405.102103
11. Braveman PA, Cubbin C, Egerter S, Williams DR, Pamuk E. Socioeconomic disparities in health in the United States: What the patterns tell us. *Am J Public Health*. 2010;100(Suppl 1). doi:10.2105/AJPH.2009.166082
12. Singh G, Lee H. Marked disparities in life expectancy by education, poverty level, occupation, and housing tenure in the United States, 1997–2014. *Int J Matern Child Health AIDS*. 2020;10(1):7-18. doi:10.21106/ijma.402
13. Chetty R, Stepner M, Abraham S, et al. The association between income and life expectancy in the United States, 2001–2014. *JAMA*. 2016;315(16):1750-1766. doi:10.1001/jama.2016.4226

14. Roelfs DJ, Shor E, Davidson KW, Schwartz JE. Losing life and livelihood: A systematic review and meta-analysis of unemployment and all-cause mortality. *Soc Sci Med.* 2011;72(6):840-854. doi:10.1016/j.socscimed.2011.01.005

15. Nie J, Wang J, Aune D, et al. Association between employment status and risk of all-cause and cause-specific mortality: A population-based prospective cohort study. *J Epidemiol Community Health.* 2020;74(5):428-436. doi:10.1136/jech-2019-213179

16. Mackenbach JP, Stirbu I, Roskam AJR, et al. Socioeconomic inequalities in health in 22 European countries. *N Engl J Med.* 2008;358(23):2468-2481. doi:10.1056/nejmsa 0707519

17. Arias E, Kochanek KD, Xu J, Tejada-Vera B. Provisional life expectancy estimates for 2022. *NVSS Vital Statistics Rapid Release.* 2023;31:1-16.

18. Chandrasekhar R, Sloan C, Mitchel E, et al. Social determinants of influenza hospitalization in the United States. *Influenza Other Respir Viruses.* 2017;11(6):479-488. doi:10.1111/irv.12483

19. Howard G, Anderson RT, Russell G, Howard VJ, Burke GL. Race, Socioeconomic status, and cause-specific mortality. *Ann Epidemiol.* 2000;10:214-223.

20. Steenland K, Hu S, Walker J. All-cause and cause-specific mortality by socioeconomic status among employed persons in 27 US states, 1984–1997. *Am J Public Health.* 2004;94(6):1037-1042. doi:10.2105/AJPH.94.6.1037

21. Steenland K, Halperin W, Hu S, Walker JT. Deaths due to injuries among employed adults: The effects of socioeconomic class. *Epidemiology.* 2003;14(1):74-79. doi:10.1097/00001648-200301000-00017

22. Dwyer-Lindgren L, Kendrick P, Kelly YO, et al. Cause-specific mortality by county, race, and ethnicity in the USA, 2000–19: a systematic analysis of health disparities. *Lancet.* 2023;402(10407):1065-1082. doi:10.1016/S0140 -6736(23)01088-7

23. Hasin DS, Sarvet AL, Meyers JL, et al. Epidemiology of adult DSM-5 major depressive disorder and its specifiers in the United States. *JAMA Psychiatry.* 2018;75(4):336-346. doi:10.1001/jamapsychiatry.2017.4602

24. Chiarotto A, Koes BW. Nonspecific Low Back Pain. *N Engl J Med.* 2022;386(18):1732-1740. doi:10.1056/nejmcp 2032396

25. Waterman BR, Belmont PJ, Schoenfeld AJ. Low back pain in the United States: Incidence and risk factors for presentation in the emergency setting. *Spine Jl.* 2012;12(1):63-70. doi:10.1016/j.spinee.2011.09.002

26. Gutin I, Hummer RA. Occupation, employment status, and "despair"-associated mortality risk among working-aged U.S. adults, 1997–2015. *Prev Med.* 2020;137:106129. doi:10 .1016/j.ypmed.2020.106129

27. Saul C, Lange S, Probst C. Employment status and alcohol-attributable mortality risk: A systematic review and meta-analysis. *Int J Environ Res Public Health.* 2022;19(12):7354. doi:10.3390/ijerph19127354

28. Mackenbach JP, Kulhánová I, Bopp M, et al. Variations in the relation between education and cause-specific mortality in 19 European populations: A test of the "fundamental causes" theory of social inequalities in health. *Soc Sci Med.* 2015;127:51-62. doi:10.1016/j.socscimed.2014.05.021

29. Guzman G, Kollar M, US Census Bureau. Income in the United States: 2022. *Current Population Reports.* 2023; (P60-279).

30. Arias E, Xu J, Kochanek K. United States Life Tables, 2021. *National Vital Statistics Reports.* 2023;72(12):1-64. Accessed April 8, 2024. Available at: https://www.cdc.gov /nchs/products/index.htm

31. World Inequality Database. World Inequality Database. Published 2024. Accessed January 25, 2024. Available at: https://wid.world

32. Pickett KE, Wilkinson RG. Income inequality and health: A causal review. *Soc Sci Med.* 2015;128:316-326. doi:10 .1016/j.socscimed.2014.12.031

33. Wilkinson RG, Pickett KE. Income inequality and socioeconomic gradients in mortality. *Am J Public Health.* 2008;98(4):699-704. doi:10.2105/AJPH.2007.109637

34. Winkleby MA, Cubbin C. Influence of individual and neighbourhood socioeconomic status on mortality among Black, Mexican-American, and White women and men in the United States. *J Epidemiol Community Health (1978).* 2003;57(6):444-452. doi:10.1136/jech.57.6.444

35. Galobardes B, Lynch JW, Davey Smith G. Is the association between childhood socioeconomic circumstances and cause-specific mortality established? Update of a systematic review. *J Epidemiol Community Health (1978).* 2008;62(5): 387-390. doi:10.1136/jech.2007.065508

36. Galobardes B, Lynch JW, Smith GD. Childhood socioeconomic circumstances and cause-specific mortality in adulthood: Systematic review and interpretation. *Epidemiol Rev.* 2004;26:7-21. doi:10.1093/epirev/mxh008

37. Calkins K, Devaskar SU. Fetal origins of adult disease. *Curr Probl Pediatr Adolesc Health Care.* 2011;41(6):158-176. doi:10.1016/j.cppeds.2011.01.001

38. Halliday TJ, Mazumder B, Wong A. The intergenerational transmission of health in the United States: A latent variables analysis. *Health Econ.* 2020;29(3):367-381. doi:10 .1002/hec.3988

39. Nandi A, Glymour MM, Subramanian SV. Association among socioeconomic status, health behaviors, and all-cause mortality in the United States. *Epidemiology.* 2014;25(2): 170-177. doi:10.1097/EDE.0000000000000038

40. Cornelius ME, Loretan CG, Jamal A, et al. Tobacco product use among adults—United States, 2021. *MMWR Morb Mortal Wkly Rep.* 2023;72(18):475-483.

41. Collins SE. Associations between socioeconomic factors and alcohol outcomes. *Alcohol Res.* 2016;38(1):83-94.

42. Ogden CL, Lamb MM, Carroll MD, Flegal KM. Obesity and socioeconomic status in adults: United States, 2005–2008. *NCHS Data Brief.* 2010;50:1-8.

43. Watson KB, Whitfield G, Chen TJ, Hyde ET, Omura JD. Trends in aerobic and muscle-strengthening physical activity by race/ethnicity across income levels among US adults, 1998–2018. *J Phys Act Health.* 2021;18(1): S45-S52. doi:10.1123/JPAH.2021-0260

44. Whitfield GP, Hyde ET, Carlson SA. Participation in leisure-time aerobic physical activity among adults, national health interview survey, 1998–2018. *J Phys Act Health.* 2021;18(1):S25-S36. doi:10.1123/JPAH.2021-0014

45. Ogden CL, Fryar CD, Martin CB, et al. Trends in obesity prevalence by race and Hispanic origin - 1999–2000 to 2017–2018. *JAMA.* 2020;324(12):1208-1210. doi:10.1001 /jama.2020.14590

46. Bohm MK, Liu Y, Esser MB, et al. Binge drinking among adults, by select characteristics and state—United States, 2018. *MMWR Morb Mortal Wkly Rep.* 2021;70(41): 1441-1446.

47. Blackwell DL, Villarroel MA. Age-adjusted percentages of adults aged ≥18 years who are current regular drinkers of alcohol, by sex, race, and hispanic origin—National Health Interview Survey, 2016. *MMWR Morb Mortal Wkly Rep*. 2018;67(10):315.

48. Barrett JT, Lee LK, Monteaux MC, Farrell CA, Hoffmann JA, Fleegler EW. Association of county-level poverty and inequities with firearm-related mortality in US youth. *JAMA Pediatr*. 2022;176(2):E214822. doi:10.1001/jama pediatrics.2021.4822

49. Kim D. Social determinants of health in relation to firearm-related homicides in the United States: A nationwide multilevel cross-sectional study. *PLoS Med*. 2019;16(12):e1002978. doi:10.1371/journal.pmed.1002978

50. Lantz PM, House JS, Lepkowski JM, Williams DR, Mero RP, Chen J. Socioeconomic factors, health behaviors, and mortality: Results from a nationally representative prospective study of US adults. *JAMA*. 1998;279(21):1703-1708. doi: 10.1001/jama.279.21.1703

51. Plug I, Hoffmann R, Artnik B, et al. Socioeconomic inequalities in mortality from conditions amenable to medical interventions: Do they reflect inequalities in access or quality of health care? *BMC Public Health*. 2012;12:346. doi:10.1186/1471-2458-12-346

52. Schoenbaum SC, Schoen C, Nicholson JL, Cantor JC. Mortality amenable to health care in the United States: The roles of demographics and health systems performance. *J Public Health Policy*. 2011;32(4):407-429. doi:10.1057/jphp .2011.42

53. Mackenbach JP, Bouvier-Colle MH, Jougla E. "Avoidable" mortality and health services: a review of aggregate data studies. *J Epidemiol Community Health*. 1990;44(2):106-111. doi:10.1136/jech.44.2.106

54. Adler N. Socioeconomic disparities in health: Pathways and policies. *Health Aff*. 2002;21(2):60-76.

55. Braveman P, Egerter S, Williams DR. The social determinants of health: Coming of age. *Annu Rev Public Health*. 2011;32:381-398. doi:10.1146/annurev-publhealth-031210 -101218

56. Marmot M, Friel S, Bell R, Houweling TA, Taylor S. Closing the gap in a generation: health equity through action on the social determinants of health. *Lancet*. 2008;372(9650):1661-1669. doi:10.1016/S0140-6736(08) 61690-6

57. Marmot M. Fair Society, Healthy Lives: The Marmot Review. Institute of Health Equity. Published 2010. Accessed July 20, 2024. Available at: https://www.instituteofhealth equity.org/resources-reports/fair-society-healthy-lives-the -marmot-review

58. Institute of Medicine. *Unequal Treatment*. Smedly BD, Stith AY, Nelson AR, eds. National Academies Press; 2003. doi:10.17226/12875

59. Phelan JC, Link BG, Tehranifar P. Social conditions as fundamental causes of health inequalities: Theory, evidence, and policy implications. *J Health Soc Behav*. 2010; 51(1_suppl):S28-S40. doi:10.1177/0022146510383498

60. Ribeiro AI, Amaro J, Lisi C, Fraga S. Neighborhood socioeconomic deprivation and allostatic load: A scoping review. *Int J Environ Res Public Health*. 2018;15(6):1092. doi:10.3390/ijerph15061092

61. Wilkinson R. *Unhealthy Societies: The Afflictions of Inequality*. Routledge; 1996.

62. Koob GF. Neuroanatomy of addiction. In: Brownell KD, Gold MS, eds. *Food and Addiction: A Comprehensive Handbook*. Oxford University Press; 2012:20-29.

63. Shonkoff JP, Garner AS, Siegel BS, et al. The lifelong effects of early childhood adversity and toxic stress. *Pediatrics*. 2012;129:e232-e246. doi:10.1542/peds.2011-2663

64. Kessler RC, McLaughlin KA, Green JG, et al. Childhood adversities and adult psychopathology in the WHO world mental health surveys. *Br J Psychiatry*. 2010;197(5):378-385. doi:10.1192/bjp.bp.110.080499

65. Gardner MJ, Thomas HJ, Erskine HE. The association between five forms of child maltreatment and depressive and anxiety disorders: A systematic review and meta-analysis. *Child Abuse Negl*. 2019;96:104082. doi:10.1016/j .chiabu.2019.104082

66. Volkow ND, Blanco C. Substance use disorders: a comprehensive update of classification, epidemiology, neurobiology, clinical aspects, treatment and prevention. *World Psychiatry*. 2023;22(2):203-229. doi:10.1002/wps .21073

67. Dowd JB, Simanek AM, Aiello AE. Socio-economic status, cortisol, and allostatic load: A review of the literature. *Int J Epidemiol*. 2009;38(5):1297-1309. doi:10.1093/ije /dyp277

68. Kawachi I, Kennedy BP, Lochner K, Prothrow-Stith D. Social capital, income inequality, and mortality. *Am J Public Health*. 1997;87(9):1491-1498.

69. Evans GW, Kim P. Multiple risk exposure as a potential explanatory mechanism for the socioeconomic status-health gradient. *Ann N Y Acad Sci*. 2010;1186:174-189. doi:10.1111/j.1749-6632.2009.05336.x

70. Zhao XB, Ren GS. Diabetes mellitus and prognosis in women with breast cancer: A systematic review and meta-analysis. *Medicine (United States)*. 2016;95(49):e5602. doi:10.1097/MD.0000000000005602

71. Zimmerman RS, Warheit GJ, Ulbrich PM, Auth JB. The relationship between alcohol use and attempts and success at smoking cessation. *Addict Behav*. 1990;15(3):197-207. doi:10.1016/0306-4603(90)90063-4

72. Zacny JP. Behavioral aspects of alcohol-tobacco interactions. *Recent dev Alcohol*. 1990;8:205-219.

73. Gibson CL, Morris SZ, Beaver KM. Secondary exposure to violence during childhood and adolescence: Does neighborhood context matter? *Justice Quarterly*. 2009;26(1): 30-57. doi:10.1080/07418820802119968

74. Casciano R, Massey DS. Neighborhood disorder and anxiety symptoms: New evidence from a quasi-experimental study. *Health Place*. 2012;18(2):180-190. doi:10.1016/j.health place.2011.09.002

75. Iyer HS, Hart JE, James P, et al. Impact of neighborhood socioeconomic status, income segregation, and greenness on blood biomarkers of inflammation. *Environ Int*. 2022;162:107164. doi:10.1016/j.envint.2022.107164

76. Dube SR, Anda RF, Felitti VJ, Edwards VJ, Croft JB. Adverse childhood experiences and personal alcohol abuse as an adult. *Addict Behav*. 2002;27:713-725.

77. Campbell JA, Walker RJ, Egede LE. Associations between adverse childhood experiences, high-risk behaviors, and morbidity in adulthood. *Am J Prev Med*. 2016;50(3): 344-352. doi:10.1016/j.amepre.2015.07.022

78. Anda RF, Croft JB, Felitti VJ, et al. Adverse childhood experiences and smoking during adolescence and adulthood.

JAMA. 1999;282(17):1652-1658. doi:10.1001/jama.282.17.1652

79. Valero De Bernabé J, Soriano T, Albaladejo R, et al. Risk factors for low birth weight: A review. *Eur J Obstet Gynecol Reprod Biol.* 2004;116(1):3-15. doi:10.1016/j.ejogrb.2004.03.007

80. Bhatt A, Kolb M, Ward O. How to Fix Economic Inequality? An overview of policies for the United States and other high-income countries. Peterson Institute for International Economics. Published December 17, 2020. Accessed January 25, 2024. Available at: https://www.piie.com/microsites/how-fix-economic-inequality

81. Hahn RA, Barnett WS, Knopf JA, et al. Early childhood education to promote health equity: A community guide systematic review. *J Public Health Manag Pract.* 2016;22(5):E1-E8. doi:10.1097/PHH.0000000000000378

82. Bivens J. Recommendations for creating jobs and economic security in the U.S. Making sense of debates about full employment, public investment, and public job creation. Economic Policy Institute. Published March 27, 2018. Accessed July 20, 2024. Available at: https://www.epi.org/publication/creating-jobs-and-economic-security/

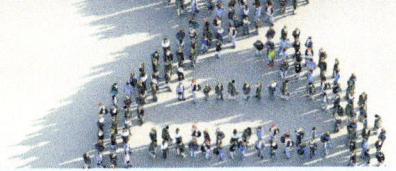

Glossary

A

Accelerometer A device that can be worn on the body to objectively measure physical activity

ACE inhibitor A type of antihypertensive that blocks certain hormones secreted by the kidneys

Acetaldehyde Chemical (with the formula C_2H_4O) that is the most common product of the metabolism of ethanol

Acute HIV infection Illness characterized by fever and other symptoms that can occur in the first few weeks of an infection with HIV

Acid-fast, acid-fast bacilli Retaining a stain even after being washed with acid. Acid-fast bacilli are rod-shaped bacteria that have this property, like *Mycobacterium tuberculosis*.

Acinus, acini (of the pancreas) Tiny bulbs in the pancreas that produce enzymes for digestion

Acquired immunity Adaptive immunity

Acquired immunodeficiency syndrome (AIDS) A disease caused by the human immunodeficiency virus characterized by a greatly weakened immune system and opportunistic infections

Active tuberculosis Disease caused by an infection with *Mycobacterium tuberculosis* that is characterized by fever, night sweats, cough, and weight loss

Acute bloody diarrhea An episode of diarrhea in which blood is present in the feces, also called dysentery

Acute glomerulonephritis A condition with sudden onset that involves inflammation of the glomeruli and reduced kidney function

Acute infection An infection that ends after the immune system responds to it

Acute low back pain Low back pain that begins suddenly and that resolves in less than six weeks

Acute Respiratory Distress Syndrome (ARDS) A life-threatening condition of the lungs characterized by protein-containing fluid in the alveoli and low blood oxygen levels

Acute watery diarrhea An episode of diarrhea that lasts several hours or days in which blood is not seen in the feces

Adaptive immunity The capability of the immune system to remember, recognize, and combat specific infectious agents in a tailored way

Addicted, addiction Addiction is a disorder characterized by a persistent and intense urge to continue to use a drug despite negative consequences of that use. A person with addiction is said to be addicted.

Adenocarcinoma A malignant tumor of gland cells, that is, cells that normally secrete a fluid or compound

Adenoma A benign tumor of gland cells, that is, cells that normally secrete a fluid or compound

Adenovirus type 40 or 41 A virus that is a common cause of diarrheal disease

Adipocyte A cell in adipose tissue that stores fats

Aerobic activity Physical activity in which muscles contract repeatedly for more than a few minutes against low resistance

Aerosol A suspension of small liquid or solid particles in air

Afferent arterioles The arterioles between the large arteries supplying the kidney and the glomerular capillaries

Agoraphobia A mental disorder characterized by anxiety about being in crowded public settings or out of the home

Air exchanges (or air changes) per hour The calculated average number of times that the total air volume in a defined space is replaced each hour

Air pollution The presence of gases, liquids, or particles in air that are not commonly present in air and that have adverse effects on humans or the natural environment

Airways The channels through which air enters and leaves the body

Albumin A protein present in high levels in the blood

Albumin-creatinine ratio (ACR) An index of kidney health that measures the amount of protein that is excreted into the urine relative to the amount of creatinine excreted

Alcohol use disorder A medical condition characterized by an impaired ability to stop using alcohol despite adverse social, occupational, or health consequences of drinking

Alcoholic hepatitis Inflammation of the liver caused by the toxic effect of alcohol

Alcoholic liver disease Fatty liver or hepatitis caused by consumption of alcohol

Allergen A biologic substance that triggers an inflammatory (allergic) response in a person with allergy

Allergic Of, characterized by, or caused by an allergy

Allergy A condition in which the immune system responds to exposure to even small amounts of specific biologic substances with a disproportionate and unhealthy inflammatory reaction

Allostatic load The "wear and tear" on the body caused by chronic stress

Alveolus (of the breast) *plural* **alveoli** The terminus of a breast duct

Alveolus (of the lung), plural alveoli The tiny air sac(s) at the end of airways in the lung, through which oxygen and carbon dioxide diffuse

Alzheimer's disease A disease that gradually causes dementia, usually in persons over age 65 but sometimes in younger adults

Ambient air pollution Air pollution that is present outdoors

Amino acid A small organic compound that contains an amino group (NH_2) and a carboxylic acid group (COOH) and that serves as the building block for proteins

Amnion The inner membrane surrounding the fetus

Amniotic fluid The fluid inside the amnion that surrounds the fetus

Amphetamine An addictive stimulant drug that increases dopamine activity in the nucleus accumbens

Amygdala A region of the brain thought to be central to the brain's storage of memories of threatening and emotion-producing events

Amyloid beta fragments Small waste products of a protein used in the brain

Amyloid plaques Large clumps of amyloid beta fragments that damage neurons and are characteristic of Alzheimer's disease

Anaerobic Capable of living without oxygen

Anaerobic physical activity High-intensity physical activity that exceeds the capacity of the cardiovascular system to provide enough oxygen to sustain. Anaerobic physical activity can be maintained for only about 2 to 3 minutes.

Anemia A condition involving insufficient levels of red blood cells or hemoglobin

Anencephaly A neural tube defect in which the brain does not develop

Anhedonia An inability to experience pleasure

Annulus fibrosus The tough, fibrous tissue that forms the outer ring of an intervertebral disc

Anopheles The genus of mosquitos that carries the malaria parasite

Anopheles funestus A species of *Anopheles* mosquito that is responsible for spreading malaria in Africa

Anopheles gambiae A species of *Anopheles* mosquito that is responsible for spreading malaria in Africa

Anopheles stephensi A species of *Anopheles* mosquito that can transmit malaria and that prefers urban environments

Anthropogenic Produced by the activity of humans

Antibiotic A chemical produced by an organism (such as a mold) that kills bacteria

Antibody, antibodies Specialized proteins secreted by immune cells that combat invading organisms

Antidepressants Medications used to treat depression

Antigen A substance that stimulates a response by the immune system

Antigenic drift Small changes in the genetic makeup of viruses that may reduce the effectiveness of an immune response

Antigenic shift Large changes in the genetic makeup of viruses that may render an immune response ineffective

Antihypertensive Drug that reduces blood pressure in people with high blood pressure

Antimalarial drug A drug that can cure malaria

Antioxidant A compound that can prevent the oxidation of other compounds, typically by giving up its own electrons

Antipsychotic medications Drugs used to treat the symptoms of psychosis that reduce dopamine activity in the brain

Antiviral medication Medication used to treat a viral infection that works by interfering with the functioning of a virus

Anxiety Fear of or uneasiness about an event or situation that might happen in the near future

Anxiety disorder A mental disorder characterized by anxiety that is out of proportion to the threat, severe or persistent, or disruptive of a person's ability to function

ApoE4 A gene that greatly increases the risk of Alzheimer's disease

Apoptosis Programmed death of a cell

ARB antihypertensive A type of antihypertensive that blocks certain hormones secreted by the kidneys

Artemisinin An antimalarial drug extracted from a plant that grows in China

Artemisinin-based combination therapy (ACT) Recommended treatment for malaria that involves a combination of antimalarial drugs, at least one of which is chemically related to artemisinin

Arterial roads Major streets or highways that connect cities or towns in rural areas or that connect different geographic sections within urban areas

Arterioles The smallest branches of arteries that connect them to capillaries

Artery Blood vessel that transports blood from the heart to organs and tissues

Arthritis A condition involving inflammation of the joints.

Articular cartilage The cartilage that covers the ends of bones in a synovial joint

Assault Intentional injury directed at another person

Asthma A disease of the lung in which the airways become inflamed and narrowed, causing cough and difficulty breathing, and that is characterized by periodic asthma attacks

Asthma action plan A written plan used by physicians, families, and others, such as school staff, to help persons with asthma take the right medicines at the right time

Asthma attack A sudden worsening of symptoms of asthma

Atherosclerosis A condition characterized by numerous cholesterol-containing plaques in different arteries

Atherosclerotic cardiovascular disease Disease of any organ system caused by atherosclerosis, including ischemic heart disease, ischemic stroke, and peripheral artery disease; Also called ischemic cardiovascular disease

Atherosclerotic cardiovascular risk (ASCVD risk) The probability that an individual will experience a heart attack, stroke, or other serious adverse consequence of atherosclerosis in the next 10 years

Atherosclerotic heart disease Ischemic heart disease

Attributable risk An estimate of the number of deaths, YLL, or DALYs that can be attributed to a risk factor

Autoimmune diseases Diseases caused by the immune system inappropriately attacking the host's own cells

Automatic emergency braking A system in automobiles that senses impending front crashes and sounds an alarm and/or applies the brakes

Axon An extremely long extension of a neuron that interfaces with other neurons or muscles and that sends signals to them

B

B lymphocytes Immune cells that produce antibodies

Bacillus, *plural* bacilli Bacteria shaped like rods

Background check A process by which a firearm retailer checks with government databases to ensure that a potential purchaser is not legally prohibited from purchasing a firearm

Bacterial vaginosis A condition in which the vagina is mainly colonized by *Gardnerella vaginalis* and other anaerobic bacteria instead of *Lactobaccillus.*

Bacterium, *plural* bacteria A single-celled organism in the kingdom Bacteria

Barrel (of a firearm) The tube in a gun through which a bullet travels when fired

BCG Commonly-used abbreviation for Bacillus Calmette-Guerin, a vaccine used to prevent tuberculosis

Behavioral norm A behavior of individuals expected or accepted as normal by a group of people

Behavioral risk factor A risk factor for disease that is a behavior that individual people engage in, such as smoking, eating unhealthy food, or being sedentary

Benign (neoplasm) A neoplasm that does not invade surrounding tissue or distant sites

Benzodiazepines A class of sedative-hypnotic drugs that cause sedation (drowsiness), induce sleep, and reduce anxiety. Examples include Xanax, Ativan, Tranxene, and Klonopin.

Beta cells Specialized cells in the pancreas that produce insulin

Bile A liquid produced by the liver and stored in the gall bladder that is directed to the interior of the intestines to help with the absorption of fats

Bile acids The acids in bile that help the intestines absorb fats

Binge drinking Consuming five or more drinks (for men) or four or more drinks (for women) within a two-hour period

Biomass Organic substance such as wood, dung, or plant materials that is burned as fuel for cooking or heat

Biosphere The layer on the earth's surface supporting life and all of the living organisms within it

Bipolar disorder A disorder characterized by periods of depression and other periods of mania

Birth defects Structural abnormalities present at birth that affect how the body appears or functions

Bisphosphonates A group of drugs that treats osteoporosis by slowing the resorption of bone

Blood meal The small amount of blood extracted from an animal or human by an insect bite

Blood pressure Force of blood pressing against the walls of the arteries

Body mass index (BMI) A measure of weight for height, calculated as weight in kilograms divided by height in meters squared

Bone cysts Small, fluid-filled spaces near the ends of bones that are found in advanced osteoarthritis

Bone spurs Small outgrowths of bone that develop in joints with arthritis; Also called osteophytes

Bowman's capsule A cup-like structure that surrounds the glomerulus and receives filtrate from the capillaries in it

Brain stem The part of the brain that connects the spinal cord to the higher structures, and that regulates involuntary actions like heartbeat and breathing

BRCA1, BRCA2 Genes that repair damaged DNA and that, when defective, put a woman at extremely high risk of developing breast cancer

Bronchi The larger airways in the lung, connecting the trachea to the bronchioles

Bronchial tree The entire branched network of airways, including the trachea, bronchi, and bronchioles

Bronchioles The smallest branches of the respiratory tract, which connect bronchi to alveoli

Bronchodilators Medications that cause smooth muscle cells in the walls of bronchioles to relax, increasing the diameter of airways and air flow

Bronchus, *plural* bronchi The larger airways in the respiratory tract, connecting the trachea to the bronchioles

Built environment The features of the physical environment built by people and influencing the behavior of people, such as the layout of streets, the designs of buildings, the infrastructure for different modes of transportation, land use, and the types of recreational facilities present

Buprenorphine An opioid (drug chemically related to heroin) that can be taken by mouth and that is used for medication-assisted treatment of opioid addiction

C

Caliber The diameter of a gun barrel or bullet, measured in inches or millimeters

Cancer Malignant neoplasm

Capillaries The tiniest blood vessels, which bridge between the smallest branches of arteries (arterioles) and the smallest branches of veins (venules)

Capsid The protein coating of DNA or RNA in a virus

Carbohydrates Molecules with the chemical formula $(CH_2O)n$ where n is the number of carbon atoms in the molecule. Carbohydrates include monosaccharides (which have 3 to 6 carbon atoms), disaccharides (which are two monosaccharides joined together), and polysaccharides (which are chains of more than two monosaccharides)

Carcinogen Substance or radiation that promotes the development of cancer

Carcinogenic Having the ability to initiate or promote the development of cancer

Carcinoma Cancer that arises from epithelial cells

Cardiac output The volume of blood pumped by the heart per minute

Cardiovascular Relating to the heart or blood vessels

Cardiovascular disease Disease involving the heart and/or blood vessels

Cartilage A spongy type of tissue that provides structural support in some organs (for example, the large airways in the lungs) and that covers the ends of bones in synovial joints

Cartridge A unit of ammunition that includes a bullet, powdered propellant, and a primer, stored in a metal casing

Cash transfer Programs to alleviate poverty involving regular cash payments

Casing The metal container of an ammunition cartridge

CD4 surface protein A protein found on the surface of helper T lymphocytes and regulatory T lymphocytes

Cell The smallest structural unit of an organism that is capable of independent functioning, consisting of cytoplasm, usually one nucleus, and other organelles, surrounded by a cell membrane.

Cell-mediated immunity Immunity involving cytotoxic T lymphocytes

Central nervous system The brain and the spinal cord

Central vein (of the liver) The vein at the center of a liver lobule that receives blood filtered by the lobule and directs the blood toward the heart

Cerebellum A part of the brain that lies behind the brain stem and below the cerebral cortex, and that is responsible for coordinating voluntary movements

Cerebral cortex The highest, outermost layer of the brain, responsible for planning and directing complex movements, interpreting the images sent by the eyes and ears, speaking and interpreting the speech of others, learning, and "thought"

Cerebral malaria Damage to the brain caused by malaria that can rapidly lead to coma and death

Cervical Part of or relating to the neck

Cervix The narrow neck-like opening of the uterus

Chamber (of a firearm) The space in the back end of a firearm's barrel in which the ammunition is fired

Chemoprevention (for breast cancer) The use of drugs that reduce the production or effects of estrogen to prevent breast cancer

Chemoprevention (for malaria) The use of antimalarial drugs to prevent malaria infection in a person or a population

Chicanes Curves deliberately added to roads to slow traffic

Chloroquine A synthetic antimalarial drug that is chemically related to quinine

Cholesterol An organic compound that occurs in all animal tissues and that is needed to form cell membranes as well as many other functions; Abnormally high levels of cholesterol in the blood cause atherosclerosis

Chondrocytes Cells that live in and support the health of cartilage

Chorion The outer membrane surrounding the fetus

Chromosomal defects Birth defects caused by an abnormal number of chromosomes

Chronic bronchitis Disease of the lung characterized by inflammation and narrowing of small airways, excess mucus production in airways, and obstruction to air flow

Chronic infection An infection that persists for months or years despite attempts by the immune system to cure it

Chronic kidney disease A disease of the kidneys characterized by either an abnormally low estimated glomerular filtration rate (GFR) or an abnormally high urine albumin-creatinine ratio (ACR)

Chronic liver disease A condition of the liver characterized by progressive deterioration of liver function for more than six months

Chronic low back pain Low back pain that persists for six weeks or more or that recurs episodically

Chronic obstructive pulmonary disease A chronic disease of the lung characterized by production of sputum, inflammation of lung tissue, and destruction of lung tissue

Chronic pancreatitis A condition characterized by chronic inflammation of the pancreas, usually resulting from long-term heavy alcohol use

Chronic traumatic encephalopathy (CTE) A rare disorder of the brain caused by repeated, mild head injuries and that involves cognitive impairment

Cirrhosis A condition in which the liver has been replaced by scar tissue that separates small clusters of regrown hepatocytes

Cleft lip A congenital malformation characterized by a split or gap in the upper lip

Cleft palate A congenital malformation characterized by a split or gap in the palate (roof of the oral cavity)

Clubfoot A congenital malformation in which one or both feet are rotated inward

Coccus, *plural* cocci A sphere-shaped bacterium

Coccyx A small triangular bone below the sacrum that is the low end of the spine

Cofactor (for HIV transmission) A factor that increases the risk of transmission of HIV when a person is exposed to the virus

Cognition Mental processes involved in gaining knowledge and understanding, including attention, perception, learning, memory, and language

Cognitive Involving mental processes needed to gain knowledge and understand, including attention, perception, learning, memory, and language

Cognitive behavioral therapy A form of psychotherapy designed to change a person's problematic thought processes and behaviors through a combination of cognitive and behavioral techniques

Cognitive impairment Reduced ability to think, reason, remember, or learn

Cognitive reserve Spare capacity of the brain that enables a person to maintain cognitive abilities even if some neurons are lost

Collagen A protein that maintains the structure of connective tissues

Collector roads Streets that provide intracounty travel in rural areas or that connect neighborhoods to arterial roads in urban areas

Colon The part of the large intestine that extends from the final portion of the small intestine to the rectum

Colonoscope, colonoscopy A flexible instrument that can be inserted through the anus to the entire length of the colon to view the interior and to remove tissue (colonoscope); the procedure involving use of the colonoscope to view the interior of the colon and remove polyps (colonoscopy)

Colorectal Relating to either the colon or the rectum

Combination antiretroviral therapy (cART) Treatment of HIV infection with a combination of antiviral drugs that interfere with the enzymes used by retroviruses

Component cause A factor that works in combination with other factors to create a sufficient cause for a disease

Concussion A temporary disruption of brain function resulting from a blow to the head

Conditioned fear response A fear response that is triggered by a stimulus that has become associated with a threatening event through repeated experiences

Congenital abnormalities Structural abnormalities present at birth that affect how the body appears or functions

Congenital anomalies Structural abnormalities present at birth that affect how the body appears or functions

Congenital disorders Structural or functional abnormalities present at birth that affect how the body appears or functions

Congenital heart defects Defects in the structure of the heart present at birth

Congenital malformations Structural abnormalities present at birth that affect how the body appears or functions

Congestive heart failure Failure of the heart to pump sufficient blood to the body's organs and tissues due to weakening of heart muscle

Constrict Become narrower

Contact tracing The process of interviewing a person who has a contagious disease to identify those persons who may have been exposed to the infection though contact with that person ("contacts") and then finding those contacts to provide medical treatment or take preventive actions

Coronary arteries Arteries supplying blood to the heart muscle

Corticosteroids Medications chemically similar to the hormone cortisol that reduce inflammation, among many other biologic effects

Cortisol A steroid hormone secreted in response to stress

Counter-advertising Media messages designed to deter people from using a specific product

Creatinine A chemical waste product of the metabolism of muscle cells, which is excreted in urine and which is used to measure kidney function

Criteria air pollutants Six air pollutants regulated by the EPA to protect human health

Crypts Tiny recesses in the tissue that lines the intestines

CT colonography A radiographic test that detects abnormal growths in the intestines

Cytotoxic T lymphocytes Immune cells that kill host cells that have been altered by specific foreign invaders

DDT Abbreviation for the chemical dichlorodiphenyltrichloroethane, which kills insects and was used widely in the attempt to eradicate malaria in the 1950s and 1960s

Deforming rounds Bullets designed to expand or break into fragments when they hit a target

Degenerative joint disease Osteoarthritis

Dehydration A condition in which the body does not have enough fluids to maintain healthy organ systems

Delerium tremens Condition caused by alcohol withdrawal, which involves spikes in blood pressure, hallucinations, and seizures, and which can be fatal

Delusions Fixed false beliefs

Dementia A condition of the brain characterized by loss of cognitive abilities to the extent that it interferes with a person's routine activities

Dendrite A short, branched extension of a neuron that interfaces with other neurons and receives signals from them

Dependence, dependent A condition in which a person must continue to take a certain drug to avoid withdrawal

Depression A condition characterized by a persistently negative mood, often accompanied by physical symptoms

Determinant (of a disease) Risk factor for a disease

Diabetes A disease characterized by abnormal insulin levels and high blood glucose levels

Diagnostic and Statistical Manual of Mental Disorders (DSM) A manual used by psychiatrists to consistently diagnose, name, and classify mental illnesses

Dialysis A procedure through which water, electrolytes, and small chemical compounds are artificially filtered to maintain healthy amounts and concentrations of body fluids

Diarrhea The passage of three or more loose or watery stools per day

Diarrheal (or diarrhoeal) diseases Diseases caused by infectious agents characterized by frequent liquid stools

Diastolic blood pressure Minimum blood pressure in the pulse cycle

Dietary risks Consumption of foods that promote illness

Dilate Expansion of the internal diameter

Directly-observed therapy (DOT) A system for assuring that a person follows a prescribed course of medical treatment by having that person swallow medications under the observation of another person

Disability-adjusted life years (DALYs) A metric of the disease burden of a population that combines years of life lost (YLL) with years lived with disability

Disaccharides Carbohydrates in which two monosaccharides are joined

Disinhibition A loss or reduction in normal inhibitions

Dislocated hip A condition in which the end of the femur (thigh bone) does not fully sit within the hip joint; Some babies are born with this problem, which is then called a congenital dislocated hip or congenital hip dysplasia

Distant cancer stage Stage of cancer in which cancer cells are spread to tissues distant from the organ of cancer origin

Distilled spirits Alcoholic beverage made by distillation to increase the alcohol content

Dopamine A neurotransmitter involved in the nucleus accumbens (part of the brain's reward system)

Double burden of malnutrition The combination of undernutrition and overweight or other conditions caused by consumption of unhealthy foods

Down Syndrome Trisomy 21

Dram shop liability A policy in which the owner or server of a bar or other alcohol outlet is legally responsible for harms caused by a customer to whom they served alcohol

Driveway access points Places where vehicles can enter a roadway between intersections

Droplet nuclei Small particles that remain in the air after water evaporates from airborne droplets

Drug-induced psychosis Psychosis that is induced by drug use and that resolves with discontinuation of drug use

Dry snuff A powder made from tobacco leaves that delivers nicotine through the lining of the nose

Duct (of the breast) Tiny channel through which milk flows from a breast lobule to the nipple

Ductal carcinoma in situ (DCIS) Breast cancer in which the cancer cells are confined to the milk duct

Duodenum The initial section of the small intestine, connecting the stomach to the jejunum

Dysentery Diarrhea in which blood is present in the feces, also called acute bloody diarrhea

Dysthymia A disorder characterized by persistently negative mood most of the time for at least two years (now called persistent depressive disorder)

E

E-cigarette An electronic device containing nicotine in a liquid that, when a user draws on it, delivers vaporized nicotine to the user's lungs

Eclampsia A disease characterized by a combination of pre-eclampsia and either seizures or coma

Ecosystem A system of living organisms, their physical environment, and their interactions in a specific location

Ectopic pregnancy A dangerous condition of pregnancy in which the fertilized egg implants in the fallopian tubes instead of the uterus

Efferent arterioles The arterioles that receive blood that has been filtered from the glomerular capillaries

Electronic nicotine delivery system (ENDS) An electronic device containing nicotine in a liquid that, when a user draws on it, delivers vaporized nicotine to the user's lungs. Commonly known as an e-cigarette.

Electronic stability control systems Systems designed to prevent vehicles traveling at high speeds from steering too little or too much

Elevated blood pressure A blood pressure with systolic value between 120 and 129 mm Hg and diastolic value below 80 mm Hg

Elimination of malaria The complete interruption of local spread of malaria in a defined geographic area

Emphysema Disease of the lung characterized by a decrease in the number and increase in the size of alveoli

Encephalocele A neural tube defect in which the brain protrudes through an opening in the skull

Endocrine pancreas The parts of the pancreas that produce and secrete insulin and other hormones that regulate blood glucose levels

Endocrine-disrupting chemicals Environmental chemicals that disrupt the release or action of hormones

Endogenous opioids Naturally occurring neurotransmitters in the brain that have similar effects to opioid drugs

Endothelium, endothelial cells Tissue that lines blood vessels and the cells that make up that tissue

Endotoxins Compounds contained within bacteria that are released when the bacteria are killed and that when released are damaging toxic to human cells

End-stage kidney disease or end-stage renal disease (ESRD) A disease of the kidney in which the estimated glomerular filtration rate (GFR) is less than 15 ml/min, adjusted for body size

Energy density The number of available calories in a food divided by the weight

Enteroaggregative E. coli A strain of *Escherichia coli* that damages the intestinal epithelium

Enteroinvasive E. coli A strain of *Escherichia coli* that invades the intestinal epithelium

Enteropathogenic E. coli A strain of *Escherichia coli* that damages the intestinal epithelium

Enterotoxigenic E. coli A strain of *Escherichia coli* that produces a toxin which stimulates fluid secretion into the intestines, a common cause of "traveler's diarrhea"

Envelope (of a virus) The outermost layer of a virus

Environmental risk factor A characteristic of an environment that increases a person's risk of disease

Enzyme A protein that acts as a catalyst for specific biochemical reactions in living organisms

Epithelium, epithelial cells The cellular tissue lining an organ and the cells that comprise that tissue

Eradication of malaria Permanent reduction to zero of the worldwide incidences of infection caused by human malaria parasites

Erythrocytes Red blood cells

Erythrocytic cycle The cycle of reproduction of *Plasmodium* that takes place in erythrocytes (red blood cells)

Esophagus The tube connecting the mouth to the stomach

Estrogen A group of hormones present in women more than men that promote the development of female sexual characteristics and that regulate cells in the breast and female reproductive system, among many other effects

Estrogen receptor (ER) A receptor on breast epithelial cells or cancer cells that fits estrogen

Ethanol, ethyl alcohol Chemical (with the formula CH_3-CH_2-OH) that is the active ingredient of alcoholic beverages

Euphoria A sensation of pleasure created by the reward circuit in the brain in response to certain positive behaviors or drugs

Executive function Mental processes that enable a person to plan and to achieve goals, such as organizing tasks, keeping track of details, managing time, and solving problems

Exocrine pancreas The parts of the pancreas that produce, secrete, and transport enzymes for digestion

Exo-erythrocytic cycle The cycle of reproduction of *Plasmodium* that takes place in liver cells

Expiration The expelling of air from the lungs

Extinction (of a conditioned responses) The process by which a stimulus that has become associated with an event is no longer paired with it

F

Facet joint Joint between facets of two adjacent vertebrae

Facets Spikes extending from vertebrae that form joints with spikes from adjacent vertebrae

Fall risk-increasing drugs (FRIDs) Drugs shown to increase the risk of falls, including benzodiazepines, other sedative-hypnotics, opioids, and antidepressants; Some experts also include other drugs, such as those used to treat high blood pressure, heart problems, and diabetes

Fasting The metabolic condition in place when a person has not consumed food in the previous 12 or more hours

Fat cells Specialized cells that take up and store triglycerides

Fats Organic compounds composed of glycerol bound to three fatty acids; Also called triglycerides

Fatty acids Organic compounds made of long chains of carbon atoms, which bond with glycerol to form triglycerides

Fatty liver An abnormal condition in which hepatocytes (liver cells) store excess amounts of fats

Fear response A response to a real or perceived threat characterized by fear, attentiveness, and physical changes, such as a rapid heart rate

Fecal immunochemical test (FIT) A test for blood in feces based on antibodies that recognize human hemoglobin

Fecal-oral route A route of transmission of infectious agents in which fecal particles from one person are ingested into the mouth of another person

Fentanyl A highly potent opioid drug

Fermentation Metabolism of sugars by micro-organisms under low-oxygen conditions

Fetal Alcohol Spectrum Disorders (FASD) A group of birth defects and brain problems caused by a fetus' exposure to alcohol during the pregnancy

Fetal alcohol syndrome A birth defect caused by exposure of a fetus to alcohol during the pregnancy, which includes thin upper lip, flat ridge between the nose and upper lip, and other abnormal facial features, often accompanied by shorter-than-normal height, small head size, and lowered intelligence

Fetal growth restriction A condition in which a fetus grows more slowly than expected; Different organizations use different specific definitions for this term, but many define it as an estimated weight of the fetus (based on an ultrasound) that is below the 10th percentile for gestational age

Fiber (in food) Components of food that cannot be digested or absorbed

Filtrate (in the kidney) The fluid received by Bowman's capsule and the renal tubule as a result of filtration by the glomerulus

Filtration (in the kidney) The first step of cleansing body fluids carried out by the kidney, in which fluid flows from the glomerular capillaries into Bowman's capsule

Fine particle air pollution Air pollution involving fine particles of 2.5 microns or less suspended in the air

Firearm identification Technology built into firearms that allow bullets or casings to be traced to specific firearms

Firearm trafficking The illegal purchase or sale of firearms

Firing pin A pin in a firearm that when struck passes impact to a cartridge in the chamber, causing the gun to fire

Folate, folic acid A vitamin (also called Vitamin B9) found in green leafy vegetables that is necessary for DNA synthesis and cell growth

Fomite An object people touch that can become contaminated with pathogens by one person and that can then pass those pathogens to another person

Forced expiratory volume 1 (FEV₁) The maximum volume of air that can be expired in one second after a maximal inspiration

Forced vital capacity (FVC) The maximum volume of air that can be expired after a maximal inspiration

Formaldehyde A chemical with the formula CH_2O that is considered a carcinogen

Framework Convention on Tobacco Control A multinational treaty specifying steps that countries will take to reduce smoking and use of other tobacco products

Free base form of nicotine The form of nicotine that does not include an additional hydrogen ion, more readily absorbed into biologic tissues than the ionic form

Fungus, *plural* fungi Organism(s) in the kingdom Fungi, including yeast, mold, and mushrooms

G

GAD-2 and GAD-7 Two versions of brief questionnaires used to screen for anxiety disorders

Gametocyte The life stage of *Plasmodium* that is transmitted from humans to mosquitoes by a mosquito bite and that reproduces sexually in mosquitoes

Gamma-aminobutyric acid (GABA) A neurotransmitter that tends to suppress the receiving neuron

Gas exchange The diffusion of oxygen from the lung's alveoli into the blood and carbon dioxide from the blood into the lung's alveoli

Gastroenteritis Inflammation of the stomach and/or small intestines, usually causing vomiting and/or diarrhea

Gastrointestinal tract The pathway by which food enters the body, nutrients are extracted from food, and wastes are expelled, including the mouth, esophagus, stomach, small intestine, and large intestine (colon and rectum)

Gastroschisis A congenital malformation in which the intestines protrude through an opening in the abdominal wall

Generalized anxiety disorder A mental disorder characterized by anxiety about routine activities, such as performance at work or school

Genital infections Infections involving a man's penis or a woman's vagina or cervix

Genital ulcer An open sore in the genital area

Gestation The period of development of an embryo and fetus until birth

Ghrelin A hormone secreted by the stomach that stimulates appetite

Gland A specialized cell or group of cells that secretes a fluid or compound

Glomerular filtration rate (GFR) The rate at which fluid is filtered by the kidneys, expressed as milliliters per minute, adjusted for body size

Glomerulonephritis An abnormal condition of the kidney characterized by inflammation of the glomeruli

Glomerulus, *plural* glomeruli A small tuft of specialized capillaries in the nephron

GLP-1 agonist Drug that mimics the effect of the hormone glucagon-like peptide 1 (GLP-1) on the brain

Glucagon-like peptide 1 (GLP-1) A hormone secreted by the small intestine that reduces appetite

Glucose A monosaccharide that circulates in the blood and in cells and that is central to energy storage and metabolism

Glutamate A neurotransmitter that tends to stimulate the receiving neuron

Glycemic index A measure of how quickly blood glucose levels rise after eating a specific food

Glycerol A small organic compound that, when bonded to three fatty acids, forms a triglyceride

Glycogen A storage form of glucose present in liver cells and in muscle

Glycoproteins Proteins linked to oligosaccharides (complex sugars) that are often found on the surface of cells or viruses

Glycosylated hemoglobin A measure of the percentage of hemoglobin in the blood coated by glucose molecules. Also called hemoglobin A1c or glycated hemoglobin.

Granuloma A small lump of chronically inflamed tissue usually association with an infection

Grip safety (on a firearm) A safety feature that prevents a gun from firing if a lever on the grip is not squeezed

Growth faltering Either stunting or wasting

Guaiac fecal occult blood test (gFOBT) A chemical test that can detect blood in feces in amounts lower than can be recognized visually

Gut microbiome The bacteria and other microorganisms that inhabit the interior of the intestines

H

Hallucinations Perceptions—that is, things that people see, hear, smell, taste, or feel—that do not have an objective source

Handgun A firearm designed to be held and fired with one hand

Harm reduction Policies and practices designed to reduce the harm of people's continued use of drugs

Health disparities Differences in rates of disease incidence, prevalence, or mortality by level of income, education, or employment, or by race/ethnicity; This term is used more in the United States and there it most often refers to differences by race/ethnicity

Health equity The state in which everyone has a fair and just opportunity to attain their highest level of health

Health inequalities Differences in rates of disease incidence, prevalence, or mortality by level of income, education, or employment, or by race/ethnicity; This term is used more in Europe than in the United States, and there it most often refers to differences by income or education

Heavy alcohol use Binge drinking at least once per month

Heavy episodic drinking Consuming five or more drinks (for men) or four or more drinks (for women) within a two-hour period (binge drinking)

Helper T lymphocytes Immune cells that stimulate and assist other immune cells to attack invaders

Heme An organic chemical compound contained in blood that carries iron

Hemodialysis Dialysis in which blood flows out of an artery into a machine that exchanges the fluid in it, thereby removing wastes and toxins

Hemoglobin A protein present in red blood cells that contains heme and carries oxygen

Hemoglobin A1c (HbA1c) A measure of the percent of hemoglobin in the blood coated by glucose molecules; Also called glycosylated hemoglobin or glycated hemoglobin

Hemorrhage Discharge of blood from blood vessels into tissues or out of the body

Hemorrhagic stroke Stroke caused by rupture (bursting) of an artery supplying the brain

Hepatic fibrosis The presence of scar tissue in the liver

Hepatitis Inflammation of the liver from any cause

Hepatitis viruses Viruses that have an affinity for the liver

Hepatocellular cancer Cancer that originates in hepatocytes

Hepatocyte The cell that conducts the main functions of the liver, also called a liver cell

HER2 cancer Type of breast cancer that expresses the HER2 receptor

Herniate (v), herniation (n) Protrude abnormally through an opening or weakness in a surrounding tissue

Hib vaccine A vaccine against the bacterium *Haemophilus influenzae* Type B

High-density lipoproteins (HDL) Lipoproteins that are associated with a reduced risk of atherosclerosis, often called "good cholesterol"

Hippocampus A brain center within the limbic system that is involved in long-term memory and learning

Homicide Injury intentionally directed by one person toward another that causes death

Hormone A chemical compound produced by a group of cells that circulates in the blood and alters the functioning of other cells or organs

Hormone-replacement therapy Treatment of women who have symptoms after menopause with medications that contain estrogen and progesterone

Household air pollution Air pollution that is generated indoors and is present indoors in households

Human epidermal growth factor receptor (HER2) A receptor on breast epithelial cells or cancer cells that fits human epidermal growth factor

Human immunodeficiency virus (HIV) A retrovirus that causes immune deficiency and AIDS

Humoral immunity Immunity involving B lymphocytes and antibodies

Hydrocodone An opioid drug frequently sold by prescription

Hygiene hypothesis The theory that children who are not exposed to diverse microbes in infancy are more likely to develop allergy

Hypertension Condition in which the blood pressure is high enough to create a substantial risk of heart disease, stroke, or kidney damage

Hypertensive cardiovascular disease Damage to or weakening of the heart and blood vessels caused by long-standing high blood pressure

Hypertensive heart disease Damage to or weakening of the heart caused by longstanding high blood pressure

Hypnozoites The life stage of *Plasmodium* that remains dormant inside liver cells

Hypochlorite A negative ion with the chemical formula ClO. It is the active ingredient in household bleach

Hypothalamus A brain center within the limbic system that controls the release of many of the body's hormones, which regulate other organs—among many other functions, the hypothalamus is activated in a stressful event, and it prompts a release of stress hormones; It also regulates appetite and energy expenditure

Iatrogenic preterm birth A preterm birth induced by or conducted by a medical provider to protect the health of the mother or fetus

IgE A type of antibody that is present in high levels in persons with allergy

Ignition interlock devices Devices that prevent a vehicle from being started if the potential driver has a high breath alcohol level

Ileum The third section of the small intestine, connecting the jejunum to the large intestine

Immune system A group of cells that the body maintains to recognize and combat invading pathogens like bacteria or viruses

Immunoglobulins Antibodies

Incidence, incidence rate Incidence—the number of new cases of disease in a population per unit time. Incidence rate—incidence divided by the size of the population at risk

Indoor residual spraying Spraying of long-acting insecticides on interior surfaces of houses to prevent malaria

Infection The invasion of body tissue by a pathogen that causes injury to the tissue

Infectious agents A life form or virus that causes an infectious disease

Inflammation A response by the body's immune system involving migration of immune cells and molecules to the site of an infection or cell damage

Influenza virus A virus that infects the lungs and respiratory tract

Inhibitory neurons Neurons that inhibit or suppress the activity of other neurons

Innate immunity The capability of the immune system to combat infectious agents immediately and in a nonspecific way

Inspiration The drawing of air into the lungs

Insulin A hormone produced by the pancreas that helps regulate glucose levels in blood by promoting the cellular uptake and storage of glucose

Insulin receptors Compounds in the membranes of liver, muscle, and fat cells that fit insulin as a lock fits a key and that alter the cells' handling of glucose and fatty acids

Insulin resistance A condition in which cells do not alter their metabolism of glucose and fats normally in response to insulin

Insulin sensitivity The degree to which insulin changes cells' metabolism of glucose and fats

Insulin-like growth factor (ILGF) A hormone similar to insulin that promotes the growth of various cell types

Integrase An enzyme used by retroviruses to integrate their DNA into the DNA of host cells

Integrated pest management A science-based approach to reducing pests in a building or other site through combined actions to avoid attracting them, prevent them from entering, and kill those that enter

Intelligent speed assistance A system in a vehicle that warns drivers or reduces power to the engine if the vehicle travels faster than the speed limit

Intensity (of physical activity) The energy expenditure to perform a physical activity per unit time, often measured in Metabolic Equivalents of Task (METs)

Intent (of an injury) The intent of the person who produced the injury, also known as the manner; The intent of an injury can be intentional directed at self, intentional directed at another person, unintentional, or legal intervention

Intentional injury Injury that was caused intentionally by a person directed at him/herself or another person

Interferon-gamma release assay (IGRA) A blood test that measures immunity to *Mycobacterium tuberculosis*

Intermittent preventive treatment of malaria in infants Treatment of infants and children in the first two years of life with antimalarial drugs to prevent malaria or its adverse consequences (now called perennial malaria chemoprophylaxis)

Intermittent preventive treatment of malaria in pregnancy Treatment of pregnant women with antimalarial drugs, regardless of whether they are infected with *Plasmodium*, to prevent malaria or its adverse consequences in them and their infants

Intermittent preventive treatment of malaria in school-aged-children Treatment of children aged 5 to 15 years with antimalarial drugs to prevent malaria or its adverse consequences

Intervention An action taken to reduce the likelihood of a disease's occurrence by reducing the presence of a risk factor or limiting its ability to cause disease

Intervertebral disc Cartilage that lies between two vertebral bodies

Intrauterine growth restriction A condition in which a fetus grows more slowly than expected, as measured by weight for gestational age below the 10th percentile

Intrauterine infection Infection of the amnion and/or chorion

Invasive carcinoma (of the breast) Breast cancer in which the cancer cells have invaded tissue beyond the tissue of cancer origin

Ionic form of nicotine The form of nicotine that has an additional hydrogen ion, not as readily absorbed into biologic tissues as the free base form

Irritant A substance that irritates or causes inflammation in a tissue (for example, the lung's airways)

Ischemia Condition in which tissues do not receive sufficient oxygen and nutrients because of a restriction in blood flow to them

Ischemic cardiovascular disease Disease of any organ system caused by atherosclerosis, including ischemic heart disease, ischemic stroke, and peripheral artery disease; Also called atherosclerotic cardiovascular disease

Ischemic heart disease Condition involving damage to the heart from a restriction of blood flow to heart tissue

Ischemic stroke Sudden damage to an area of the brain from an obstruction of blood flow to it

Isoniazid (INH) An antimicrobial drug commonly used in combination with other drugs to treat latent tuberculosis infection or active tuberculosis

J

Jejunum The second section of the small intestine, connecting the duodenum to the ileum

Joint The interface between two or more bones

Joint capsule The tough, fibrous tissue that encases a synovial joint

Joint space The gap between the articular cartilage of adjacent bones in synovial joints, which is normally filled by synovial fluid

K

Kaposi sarcoma A type of cancer seen in people with AIDS

L

Land use The types of buildings or activities allowed on parcels of land, usually determined by the zone in which they are located

Large intestine The section of the gastrointestinal tract between the small intestine and the anus

Larva, *plural* larvae The life stage of an insect that hatches from an egg, that actively feeds, and that does not have wings

Larvicides Chemical or biologic agents that kill the larval form of insects

Latent TB infection A condition in which a person harbors living *Mycobacterium tuberculosis* organisms but has no signs of active tuberculosis disease

Legal intervention Injury resulting from a law enforcement officer acting in the line of duty

Leptin A hormone secreted by adipocytes that are laden with fat which suppresses appetite

Ligament A dense band of tissue that connects bones to other bones

Light physical activity Physical activity requiring between 1.6 and 3.0 METs

Limbic system An interconnected group of structures at the base of the brain that are involved in memory and emotion

Lipoproteins A clump of cholesterol, certain proteins, and other compounds that circulates in the blood

Liver lobule The functional unit of the liver, containing a central vein, rows of hepatocytes that radiate from the central vein, and sinusoids between them

Lobe (of the breast) One of about 15-20 sections of the breast, which produces milk in a woman who is lactating

Lobule (of the breast) Tiny section of a breast lobe

Localized cancer stage Stage of cancer in which all cancer cells are confined to the organ in which the cancer originated

Long gun A rifle or a shotgun

Long-chain carbohydrates Carbohydrates made of hundreds or thousands of monosaccharide subunits

Low birth weight Birth weight below 2,500 grams

Low-density lipoproteins (LDL) Lipoproteins that carry the most cholesterol in the blood and that are associated with atherosclerosis, often called "bad cholesterol"

Low-dose computed tomography (LDCT) A type of digital x-ray technique that can detect tumors

Lower respiratory infections (LRI) Infections involving the bronchi, bronchioles, and alveoli of the lung

Lumbar Part of or relating to the spine between the thorax and sacrum

Lumen The interior channel of the gastrointestinal tract

Luminal cancer Type of breast cancer that expresses ER and not HER2

Lupus Common term for the disease systemic lupus erythematosus, a disease in which the immune system attacks the body's own tissues, including those in the kidney

Lymph node A round mass of tissue composed mainly of lymphocytes (a type of immune cell); part of the immune system

Lymphocyte A type of cell that is a key part of the immune system

Lymphoma A cancer that originates in lymphocytes

M

Macromolecules Very large molecules; in biology, typically refers to molecules that carry genetic information (DNA and RNA), proteins, long-chain carbohydrates, or lipids

Macronutrients Nutrients that supply energy and structural components to the body: carbohydrates, fats, and proteins

Macrophage A large cell that is part of the immune system and that is responsible for phagocytosis of infectious agents or foreign substances

Macrovascular complications of diabetes Damage to the large and medium-sized arteries (also called atherosclerosis) caused by diabetes, and can cause heart disease or stroke

Magazine (relating to a firearm) A device in a gun used to store ammunition

Magazine disconnect safety A safety feature that prevents a gun from firing if the magazine has been removed

Major congenital malformations Congenital malformations that have significant medical, social, or cosmetic consequences

Major depression, major depressive disorder A disorder defined as having a persistently negative mood nearly every day for at least two weeks, in combination with other psychological and/or physical symptoms severe enough to interfere with the ability to carry out routine activities of living

Malignant (neoplasm) A neoplasm that has invaded or is capable of invading other tissues

Malnutrition Altered growth or less-than-optimal health caused either by insufficient intake of food or by excess consumption of foods that promote illness; includes undernutrition, micronutrient deficiencies, overweight, and diet-related chronic diseases

Mania A condition characterized by an abnormally positive mood, including features such as talkativeness, impulsiveness, and unrealistic optimism

Manner (of an injury) The intent of the person who produced the injury. The manner of an injury can be intentional—directed at self, intentional—directed at another person, unintentional, or legal intervention.

Mass drug administration (for malaria prevention) Treatment of every child and adult in a defined geographic area with antimalarial drugs over a short period of time to interrupt transmission of *Plasmodium*

Mechanism (of an injury) The physical action or sequence of actions that induces an injury, for example, a motor vehicle crash, stabbing, or poisoning

Medial forebrain bundle A pathway containing axons that connect different areas of the brain, including the ventral tegmental area and the nucleus accumbens

Median barriers Physical barriers between lanes of traffic flowing in opposing directions

Medically-indicated preterm birth A preterm birth induced by or conducted by a medical provider to protect the health of the mother or fetus

Medication-assisted treatment Treatment of drug addiction that involves the use of medications, such as methadone and buprenorphine

Medium spiny neurons Neurons located in the nucleus accumbens that are involved in the reward circuit

Memory (in the immune system) The ability of the immune system to quickly recognize a specific antigen that the body has previously encountered and respond to it in a specific way

Menthol A chemical found in mint leaves that causes a "cool" or "numbing" sensation in the mouth and throat

Mercury A metal that, in organic form, can accumulate in fish and cause disease for those who eat the fish

Merozoite The life stage of *Plasmodium* that is released into the blood when schizonts rupture

Metabolic Equivalent of Task (MET) A unit of energy expenditure by the body per unit time related to the type of physical activity taking place, where 1.0 MET is the energy expended while sitting entirely still

Metabolic risk factor A feature of a human's biologic functioning that indicates that he or she is at increased risk for developing a disease

Metabolic Syndrome A syndrome characterized by central obesity, high blood sugar, high blood triglycerides, low HDL cholesterol, and high blood pressure

Metastasize, metastasis, metastatic Metastasize (v.) to spread (cancer) to a distant body site; Metastasis (n.) a colony of cancer cells that has spread to a distant body site; Metastatic (adj.) having metastasized

Metformin A drug that lowers blood glucose levels and that is commonly used to treat diabetes

Methadone An opioid (drug chemically related to heroin) that can be taken by mouth and that is used for medication-assisted treatment of opioid addiction

Methamphetamine An addictive stimulant drug that increases dopamine activity in the nucleus accumbens

MET-Hour A measure of total energy expenditure for physical activity that is the sum of the products of the METs required for different activities and the hours spent engaging in each of them

Microbes Microorganisms, including bacteria, fungi, protozoa, and algae

Microbiome The community of bacteria and other microorganisms that inhabit a specific location, such as the intestines, respiratory tract, or vagina

Microbiome, gut The bacteria and other microorganisms that inhabit the interior of the intestines

Microcephaly Abnormally small head size

Micronutrients The approximately 30 vitamins and minerals needed in small amounts for health and that must be obtained from food

Microorganisms Organisms too small to be seen with the naked eye

Microstamping A proprietary firearm identification technology required for new guns sold in California

Microvascular complications of diabetes Damage to the tiny arteries caused by diabetes, which causes kidney disease, vision loss, and damage to nerves

Microvillus, *plural* **microvilli** Microscopic hair-like structures on the lumen side of epithelial cells lining the intestines

Middle East Respiratory Syndrome (MERS) A respiratory illness caused by the MERS-CoV coronavirus, which caused an outbreak in Saudi Arabia in 2012

Mild cognitive impairment Difficulties with learning, memory, or language that are not severe enough to interfere with a person's routine activities

Minerals In the context of nutrition, minerals needed in small amounts by human cells for metabolism and growth that must be obtained from food

Minor congenital malformations Congenital malformations that have no or limited medical, social, or cosmetic consequences

Mitosis The process by which a cell duplicates its genes and splits into two genetically identical daughter cells

Mixed land use or mixed-use zoning Rules that allow a mix of land uses within zones, for example, allowing single-family residential, multi-family residential, and commercial buildings

Mode(s) of transportation The means by which people are transported from place to place, such as private motor vehicles, buses, trains, bicycles or by walking

Moderate physical activity Physical activity requiring between 3.0 and 6.0 METs

Moderate-to-vigorous activity Physical activity requiring 3.0 or more METs, usually measured in "minutes", which are calculated as the actual minutes engaging in vigorous activity multiplied by two plus the actual minutes engaging in moderate physical activity

Monoamines A group of chemically-related neurotransmitters, including serotonin, norepinephrine, and dopamine

Monosaccharides Carbohydrates that have 3 to 6 carbon atoms

Monounsaturated fatty acids Fatty acids in which one pair of carbon atoms are double-bonded to each other so that less than the maximum number of hydrogen atoms are present

Mood A prevailing positive or negative emotion and interpretation of events and conditions

Mood disorder An illness characterized by periods of time with abnormally and persistently positive or negative mood

Morbidity Occurrence of a disease that may or may not be fatal, or the rate of the disease occurrence in a specified population

Mortality, mortality rate The number of deaths in a population (mortality), or the number of deaths divided by the number of people in the population (mortality rate); These may refer to deaths from specific diseases or death from all causes

Mosquirix The commercial name for the RTS,S/AS01 malaria vaccine

Mucous membranes Moist membranes lining body parts exposed to outside air, including those in the mouth, nose, eyes, respiratory tract, and urogenital tract

Multi-modal transport and land use planning Planning of communities, neighborhoods, and transportation systems to give people options for travel modes beyond other than private motor vehicles

Muscle-strengthening exercise or physical activity Physical activity in which muscles contract a small number of times against resistance

Musculoskeletal disorders Diseases and abnormal conditions involving the bones, joints, muscles, ligaments, and tendons

Mutation Change in the genetic material of an organism

Muzzle The open end of a gun barrel from which bullets are fired

Myocardial infarction Sudden damage to heart muscle caused by blockage of a coronary artery, commonly known as a "heart attack"

N

Natural killer (NK) lymphocyte A cell that is part of the immune system and that kills host cells that appear stressed or abnormal

Negative symptoms of schizophrenia Symptoms that involve lack of motivation, lack of interest, and withdrawal from others

Neoplasm An abnormal growth of tissue arising from a single cell that has acquired damage to its genes, also called a tumor

Nephron The central functional unit of the kidney, which includes a glomerulus, the Bowman's capsule, and a renal tubule

Nerve root The initial segment of a nerve leaving the brain or spinal cord

Nerves Extensions of neurons (nerve cells) that send electrical signals to control muscle action or to communicate sensation to the brain

Nervous system The organ system that includes the brain, spinal cord, and peripheral nerves

Neural tube Structure in an embryo created by a disc of cells folding over onto itself that develops into the brain and spinal cord

Neural tube defects Malformations of the brain or spinal cord caused by failure of the neural tube to close

Neurofibrillary tangles Large clumps of tau proteins that develop in persons with Alzheimer's disease

Neuron A cell in the brain or spinal cord that sends and receives signals from other neurons

Neurotransmitter A chemical released by one neuron and taken up by another neuron across a synapse that sends a signal to the receiving neuron

Nicotine An alkaloid chemical produced by *Nicotiana tabacum* (the tobacco plant) that when taken as a drug is both pleasurable and addictive

Nicotine-replacement therapy FDA-approved medications that safely deliver nicotine to tobacco users who are trying to quit

Night blindness A condition characterized by difficulty seeing in dim light

Nitrites Chemicals added as preservatives to meat that may increase the risk of cancer

N-nitrosamines Chemicals that contain a nitroso group and an amine group, many of which are known to cause cancer

NNK An N-nitrosamine in tobacco smoke that is carcinogenic in the pancreas

Non-alcoholic fatty liver disease (NAFLD) Liver steatosis, hepatitis, or steatohepatitis that is not caused by a virus or by alcohol consumption

Non-alcoholic steato-hepatitis (NASH) Steato-hepatitis that is not caused by alcohol consumption

Non-communicable diseases Chronic diseases that are not caused by infectious agents, such as ischemic heart disease, diabetes, chronic obstructive pulmonary disease, and chronic kidney disease

Non-point sources (of air pollution) Sources of air pollution other than large industrial operations, such as homes, farms, and small commercial operations like dry cleaners

Nonspecific low back pain Low back pain in the absence of abnormalities visible on x-ray, MRI, or other imaging

Norepinephrine A neurotransmitter involved in regulating appetite, sex drive, concentration, and mood

Normal blood pressure A blood pressure with systolic value below 120 mm Hg and diastolic value below 80 mm Hg

Norovirus A virus that is a common cause of diarrheal disease

Nucleus accumbens A region of the brain that produces a sense of pleasure, as part of the brain's reward system

Nucleus pulposus The soft, gel-like center of an intervertebral disc

Obesity A condition characterized by excess body fat, defined at the population level as a body mass index above 30.0 kg/m²

Obsessive-compulsive disorder A mental disorder characterized by unwanted thoughts and fears (obsessions) that lead people to do repetitive behaviors (compulsions), such as compulsive washing of hands because of fears of germs

Occupational asthma Asthma that is triggered by substance(s) encountered during an occupation

One gun a month laws Laws prohibiting the purchasing by an individual of more than one gun in a month

Opioid replacement Treatment of opioid addiction with opioids that can be given by mouth, such as methadone or buprenorphine

Opioids A class of drugs either derived from the opium poppy or synthesized to have a similar effect of stimulating opioid receptors in the brain, causing euphoria, drowsiness, pain relief, slowed breathing, and addiction

Opportunistic infections Infections occurring in a person with immune deficiency caused by organisms that a healthy immune system can ordinarily contain

Oral Glucose Tolerance Test (OGTT) A test for diabetes in which glucose levels in blood are measured two hours after a person consumes a standard amount of glucose

Oral rehydration solution A solution containing water, sodium, and glucose in specified ratios that is ingested by persons with diarrhea to replace lost fluids

Organ A group of different tissues working together to perform a complex biologic function

Organ system A group of organs working together to serve a complex biologic function (for example, the small intestine is an organ, and the gastrointestinal system is an organ system)

Organism An individual unit of life, (such as a bacterium, plant, or animal) composed of a single cell or a group of differentiated cells in which organs work together to carry out the various processes of life

Orofacial cleft Cleft lip and/or cleft palate

Osmosis Diffusion of water through a membrane from the side with lower solute concentration to the side with higher solute concentration

Osteoarthritis A chronic disease of one or more joints involving gradual degeneration of joint cartilage and causing pain, stiffness, deformities, and loss of joint function

Osteophytes Small outgrowths of bone that develop in joints with arthritis; Also called bone spurs

Osteoporosis A condition characterized by a decrease in bone mass, decrease in bone density, and bone fragility

Overweight A condition characterized by excess body fat, defined at the population level as a body mass index above 25.0 kg/m²

Ovum, *plural* ova Cell(s) produced by women that, when fertilized by a sperm cell, is capable of producing a new organism

Oxidation A chemical reaction in which a chemical loses electrons to another chemical (that is often but not always oxygen)

Oxycodone An opioid that is frequently prescribed, the active drug in OxyContin

P

p24 A protein that makes up the capsid of HIV

Pancreas An organ in the abdomen that secretes enzymes used for digestion into the gastrointestinal tract and insulin into the bloodstream

Pancreatic ductal adenocarcinoma Cancer arising from the epithelial cells in the ducts of the pancreas

Pancreatic intraepithelial neoplasia (PaIN) Microscopic neoplasms found in the ducts of the pancreas that are benign but that have the potential to become malignant

Panic disorder A mental disorder characterized by recurring, unexpected attacks of panic, including physical symptoms

Paranoid Characterized by extreme and irrational fear or distrust of others

Particulate matter Particles small enough to be inhaled into the small airways of the lung

Partner notification (for HIV) The process of identifying sex- and needle-sharing partners of persons with HIV infection and offering those partners education and HIV testing

Pathogen An infectious agent, like a virus, bacterium, or protozoan, that causes a disease

PCP A pneumonia caused by the fungus *Pneumocystis jirovecii* (formerly called *Pneumocystis carinii*) that is seen in people with immune deficiency

Perennial malaria chemoprevention Treatment of infants and children in the first two years of life with antimalarial drugs to prevent malaria or its adverse consequences

Periodontal disease Infection of the gums

Peripheral artery disease Insufficient blood flow to the arms or legs caused by atherosclerosis

Peripheral nervous system The group of nerves that connect the brain and spinal cord to other organs and tissues

Peritoneal dialysis Dialysis in which fluid is inserted into the abdomen and later removed, removing wastes and toxins with it

Permit-to-purchase laws Laws requiring a person to have a firearm owner's license or permit to purchase a firearm

Persistent depressive disorder A disorder characterized by persistently negative mood most of the time for at least two years (previously called dysthymia)

Persistent diarrhea An episode of diarrhea that lasts 14 days or longer

Personalized smart guns Guns that fire only if held by their owners

Phagocytosis The process by which one cell surrounds and then ingests another cell or a particle

PHQ-2 and PHQ-9 Two versions of brief questionnaires used to screen for depression

Physical activity domains Categorization of physical activity according to the circumstances under which it occurs—the four commonly used domains are occupational, household, transportation, and leisure-time

Physical activity paradox The observation that while leisure-time physical activity is associated with lower mortality, occupational physical activity is sometimes associated with higher mortality

Pit latrine A hole in the ground for safe deposition of human wastes, sometimes covered by a seat with a central hole for defecation and a small structure for privacy

Placenta The organ connected to the umbilical cord and implanted into the lining of the uterus that serves as the interface between the fetus and the mother

Plaque An abnormal accumulation of cholesterol and other substances underneath the lining of an artery

Plasmodium The genus of organisms that cause malaria

Plasmodium falciparum The species of *Plasmodium* that causes nearly all cases of malaria in Africa and is responsible for most deaths from malaria

Plasmodium malariae A less common species of *Plasmodium* that causes malaria

Plasmodium ovale A less common species of *Plasmodium* that causes malaria

Plasmodium vivax The second most common species of *Plasmodium* that causes malaria, seen mostly in tropical areas other than Africa

Plyometric exercises Exercises in which muscles contract quickly after having been stretched, for example, by jumping

PM$_{10}$, PM$_{2.5}$ Particles (also called particulate matter) less than 10 microns and less than 2.5 microns in size, respectively

Pneumococcal conjugate vaccine (PCV) A vaccine against the bacterium *Streptococcus pneumoniae*

Pneumococcus Another name for the bacterium *Streptococcus pneumoniae*

Pneumonia An illness caused by infection of the alveoli of the lung

Point sources (of air pollution) Large, stationary sources of air pollution such as factories, power plants, or other large industrial operations

Polychlorinated biphenyls (PCBs) Industrial chemicals that can accumulate in fish and that have been linked to various health problems

Polycyclic aromatic hydrocarbons A group of carcinogenic chemicals that contain multiple rings of carbon and that are produced by burning organic matter

Polyp A growth of tissue into the interior space of an organ, such as the colon

Polysaccharides Chains of more than two monosaccharides

Polysubstance use Use of more than one addictive drug, such as alcohol and marijuana

Polyunsaturated fatty acids Fatty acids in which two or more pairs of carbon atoms are double-bonded to each other

Portal vein The vein that receives blood containing nutrients from the intestines and directs it to the liver

Positive symptoms of schizophrenia Hallucinations and delusions

Post-traumatic stress disorder A mental disorder that occurs after experiencing or witnessing a terrifying event, characterized by symptoms of flashbacks, nightmares, or severe anxiety, as well as uncontrollable thoughts about the event

Potassium A positive ion (abbreviated K+) that has many central functions in biology; the main positive ion in body fluid that is inside of cells

Prediabetes A condition of altered glucose metabolism characterized by a HbA1c between 5.7% and 6.4% or a fasting blood glucose of 100 to 125 mg/dL or a glucose between 140 and 199 on a 2-hour oral glucose tolerance test

Pre-eclampsia An abnormal condition of pregnancy characterized by hypertension and proteinuria, often accompanied by signs of organ damage

Pre-exposure prophylaxis (PrEP) Treatment of an uninfected person with medications to prevent infection

Prefrontal cortex A region of the cerebral cortex involved in planning and executing complex behaviors

Premature (in an infant) Born before 37 weeks gestation

Preterm birth Birth before 37 weeks of gestation

Prevention paradox The observation that small differences in disease risk, if broadly shared across a population, can have a larger impact on that population's disease rate than large differences in disease risk in a high-risk subset of the population

Primary active tuberculosis A disease caused by an initial infection with *Mycobacterium tuberculosis* that is usually characterized by fever, night sweats, cough, and weight loss

Primary prevention Actions to prevent disease involving reducing risky exposures or behaviors before any biologic indicators of disease risk appear

Primer (in firearm ammunition) A small impact-sensitive explosive that ignites the propellant in an ammunition cartridge

Proenzymes Inactive forms of enzymes, which become activated by coming in contact with other enzymes

Progesterone A female sex hormone that helps regulate the menstrual cycle and pregnancy

Progesterone receptor (PR) A receptor on breast epithelial cells or cancer cells that fits progesterone

Proliferate Increase in number through repeated cell division

Propellant The powdered substance in an ammunition cartridge that explodes when ignited, propelling the bullet

Propylene glycol A small chemical that forms a clear liquid at room temperature and that is used in e-cigarette liquids

Protease An enzyme used by HIV to produce other enzymes

Protective factor A characteristic of an individual, group, or environment that reduces the likelihood that a disease will occur

Protein A molecule that is a long chain of amino acids which is twisted and folded to serve specific functions in cells

Proteinuria The presence in the urine of proteins that ordinarily circulate in the blood

Protozoa A type of complex single-celled organism

Psychoactive drugs Drugs that affect mental processes, such as perception, cognition, and mood

Psychological stress A response by the body to a threat that the person feels they cannot overcome or handle

Psychosis A mental illness characterized by hallucinations and delusions

Psychotic symptoms Hallucinations and delusions

Pulmonary artery Blood vessel that transports blood (with low levels of oxygen) from the heart to the lungs

Pulmonary circuit The section of the cardiovascular system that includes the pulmonary arteries, capillaries in the lungs, and pulmonary veins

Pulmonary function test Test that measures capabilities of the lungs

Pulmonary vein Blood vessel that transports blood (containing high levels of oxygen) from the lungs to the heart

Pupa, *plural* pupae The life stage of an insect that does not feed, that has a protective cover, and that undergoes metamorphosis

Purified protein derivative (PPD) A compound derived from *Mycobacterium tuberculosis* that is injected into the skin to test for immunity to the organism

Pyrethroid A type of insecticide used to kill *Anopheles* mosquitos for malaria control

Q

Quinine An antimalarial drug present in the bark of the cinchona tree

Quitline A service available through a toll-free phone number through which smokers can get nicotine replacement therapy and/or other help quitting

R

R21/Matrix-M A vaccine used in infants to prevent malaria or its adverse consequences

Racial discrimination The imposition of barriers to education, employment, income, and other aspects of society based on a person's race

Radon A radioactive gas that is naturally present underground in rock and soil

Reabsorption (in the kidney) The second step of cleansing body fluids carried out by the kidney, in which fluid, electrolytes, and small chemical compounds selectively flow from the tubule into the efferent arteriole

Reactivation tuberculosis A disease caused by a reactivation of a latent infection with *Mycobacterium tuberculosis* that is characterized by fever, night sweats, cough, and weight loss

Receptor A compound in the membrane of a cell that fits a specific hormone like a lock fits a key and that alters the cell's functioning

Rectum The final section of the large intestine, which extends from the colon to the anus

Red blood cells The cells that carry hemoglobin in the blood

Regional cancer stage Stage of cancer in which cancer cells have spread to nearby lymph nodes

Regulatory T lymphocytes Immune cells that suppress the activity of other immune cells

Renal tubule A microscopic tube in the nephron connected to Bowman's capsule through which glomerular filtrate flows

Replication (of DNA) The process by which an organism's DNA is copied

Respirator A mask that protects its user from contaminants in the air

Respiratory secretions Fluid that originates in the lung or respiratory tract

Respiratory syncytial virus (RSV) A virus that infects the cells in the lung and increases the risk of asthma

Respiratory tract The network of channels through which air enters and leaves the body, including the nose, throat, larynx, trachea, bronchi, bronchioles, and alveoli

Retrovirus A type of virus that carries its genes in the form of RNA but that "reverse transcribes" that RNA into DNA and inserts them into the DNA of host cells

Reverse transcriptase An enzyme used by retroviruses to "reverse transcribe" RNA into DNA

Revised NIOSH Lifting Equation An equation that helps employers determine the maximum weight of an object that workers can lift safely

Revolver A handgun with a cylinder of several chambers brought successively into line with the barrel

Reward circuit, reward pathway A network of neurons and neurotransmitters in the brain that provide a feeling of pleasure in response to actions that are important for life or reproduction

Reward neuron A neuron located in the ventral tegmental area with axon connections to the nucleus accumbens, which when stimulated produces euphoria

Rhinovirus A virus that infects the cells in the lung and increases the risk of asthma

Rifampin, rifampicin An antimicrobial drug commonly used in combination with other drugs to treat latent tuberculosis infection or active tuberculosis

Rifle A long firearm designed by be held against the shoulder that fires a rotating bullet

Risk factor A characteristic of an individual, group, or environment that increases the likelihood that a specific disease will occur

Risk marker A characteristic of an individual, group, or environment that is statistically associated with a disease but does not increase or decrease the likelihood that the disease will occur

Rotavirus A virus that is a common cause of diarrheal disease

Roundabout A circular intersection with design features that promote safe and efficient vehicle traffic flow

RTS,S/AS01 A vaccine used in infants to prevent malaria or its adverse consequences

Rubella A virus informally known as "German measles" that can cause congenital hearing loss if a woman is infected during pregnancy

Rumble strips A series of small road bumps that causes vibrations in a vehicle passing on top

S

Sacrum A triangular bone at the base of the spine just below the lumbar vertebrae and above the coccyx

Safe System Approach The approach to transportation planning that anticipates human errors and builds redundant systems to protect them from injury

Sanitation The disposal of human wastes in ways that reduce the spread of diseases

SARS-CoV-2 The type of coronavirus that causes the disease COVID-19

Saturated fats Triglycerides composed of glycerol and three saturated fatty acids

Saturated fatty acids Fatty acids that contain the maximum number of hydrogen atoms

Scar tissue Tissue that grows after an injury, consisting of generalized cells connected by fibers

Schizont The life stage of *Plasmodium* that has many nuclei and that appears inside hepatocytes or red blood cells

Schizophrenia Mental illness characterized by positive symptoms (hallucinations and delusions), negative symptoms (lack of interest and motivation, withdrawal from others), and impaired cognition, in the absence of unusually depressed or elevated mood

Screening, brief intervention, and referral to treatment (SBIRT) The process by which people seen in medical clinics or other settings are asked about alcohol and/or drug use, counseled if they report dangerous use, and if appropriate referred for more intense treatment

sDNA-FIT test A test for blood in feces that combines the fecal immunochemical test with a test that detects DNA found in colon cancer cells

Seasonal malarial chemoprevention Treatment of all children under 5 years of age with antimalarial drugs during the rainy season to prevent malaria or its adverse consequences

Secondary infection Infection by a second organism that occurs because infection by a first organism has increased the body's susceptibility

Secondary prevention Actions to prevent disease undertaken after biologic signs of damage first appear

Secondary tuberculosis A disease caused by a reactivation of a latent infection with *Mycobacterium tuberculosis* that is characterized by fever, night sweats, cough, and weight loss

Sedentary behavior Physical behavior that requires less than 1.5 METs

Selective mutism A mental disorder characterized by refusal to speak to persons other than those one is attached to, such as family members

Self-harm Intentional injury directed at the self

Semiautomatic pistol A handgun in which the chamber is integral to the barrel and that can fire more than one bullet without reloading

Sensitized (in the immune system) Primed to respond to exposure to a specific substance with inflammation

Separation anxiety disorder A mental disorder characterized by developmentally inappropriate attachment to another person, particularly attachment of children to a parent

Serotonin A neurotransmitter involved in regulating appetite, sex drive, concentration, and mood

Severe Acute Respiratory Syndrome (SARS) A respiratory illness caused by the SARS-CoV-1 coronavirus, which caused an outbreak in Asia in 2002

Severe malaria A severe illness caused by malaria that can lead to damage of many organs

SGLT-2 inhibitor A drug that reduces blood sugar by blocking the sodium-glucose co-transporter-2 protein in the kidneys

Short-chain fatty acids Fatty acids produced by metabolism of dietary fiber that may protect against cancer formation

Shotgun A long firearm that fires a packet of small pellets

Sickle cell disease A disease leading to anemia caused by two copies of a gene that codes for a malaria-resistant form of hemoglobin

Sigmoidoscope, sigmoidoscopy A flexible instrument (sigmoidoscope) that can be inserted through the anus as far as the sigmoid colon (the final section of the colon) to view the interior and to remove tissue; the procedure that involves using this instrument (sigmoidoscopy)

Silent stroke A stroke (that is, sudden damage to the brain and partial loss of brain function due to a rupture or obstruction of an artery) that is not noticed by a person or those around him or her

Single-use zoning Rules that allow only one type of land use within zones, for example, only single-family residential buildings

Sinusoids Specialized capillaries in the liver lobules that connect branches of the portal vein to the central vein

Skeletal muscles The specialized tissues that can shorten (contract) or lengthen (relax), giving the body the ability to move

Slide (on a pistol) A horizontal piece of a pistol that, when moved back and forth, loads a cartridge in the chamber

Small intestine The section of the gastrointestinal tract between the stomach and the large intestine, including the duodenum, jejunum, and ileum

Smear-positive Having sputum that shows acid-fast bacilli under a microscope, a marker for tuberculosis contagiousness

Smokeless tobacco Chewing tobacco, snus, or snuff

Smooth muscle cells Cells that wrap around the walls of the bronchi and bronchioles and that change the diameter of the airways by contracting or relaxing

Snus A form of tobacco that is sold in a pouch that is used by holding it inside the mouth

Sobriety checkpoints Stopping by police of all or a predetermined proportion of drivers at high-risk locations and times to identify alcohol- and drug-impaired drivers and stop them from driving

Social anxiety disorder A mental disorder characterized by fear or avoidance of interactions with other persons

Social cohesion The degree to which people in a social group trust each other, help each other, and work together to solve common problems

Social connection Having multiple, strong, helpful relationships with other persons

Social determinants of health Social factors that directly or indirectly influence rates of disease or mortality, including income, education, employment, housing, and racial discrimination. Some experts consider access to medical care to also be a social determinant of health.

Social disadvantage Having less resources, autonomy, and power than people in another group. For example, people with lower levels of income or education and people in groups subjected to racial discrimination have social disadvantage.

Social epidemiology A branch of epidemiology that studies the relationship of social factors like income, education, employment, neighborhood conditions, and racial discrimination to health

Sodium A positive ion (abbreviated Na+) that has many central functions in biology; the main positive ion in body fluid that is outside of cells

Sodium chloride Chemical compound made of sodium and chloride (abbreviated NaCl); table salt

Sodium-glucose co-transporter-1 (SGLT1) A protein embedded in the membrane of small intestine epithelial cells that actively transports sodium and glucose from the lumen into the cell

Sodium-glucose co-transporter-2 (SGLT2) A specialized protein embedded in the lining of the renal tubule that reabsorbs glucose and sodium

Specific phobias A mental disorder characterized by anxiety and avoidance of specific objects or situations

Speeding Driving faster than the legal speed limit

Spina bifida A neural tube defect in which the spinal cord does not fully close on the lower end

Spinal canal A hollow tube through the spine that surrounds and protects the spinal cord

Spinal cord A cord of tissue containing neurons and axons that extends from the brain stem through the spinal canal and that connects the brain to peripheral nerves

Spine The column of bones that supports the core, upper body, and skull and that protects the spinal cord

Spirometry A test of lung function that measures the volume of air that the lungs can hold and how quickly it can be expelled

Spontaneous preterm birth A preterm birth that occurs without being induced by a medical provider

Sporogenic cycle The cycle of reproduction of *Plasmodium* that takes place within mosquitoes

Sporozoite The life stage of *Plasmodium* that is carried by mosquitoes and that is transmitted to humans by a mosquito bite

Sprain A partial or complete tear of a ligament

Sputum Mucus that originates in the lung or respiratory tract and is expelled by coughing

Stage (of cancer) The degree to which a cancer has spread

Stage 1 hypertension A blood pressure with a systolic value between 130 and 139 mm Hg or a diastolic value between 80 and 89 mm Hg

Stage 2 hypertension A blood pressure with a systolic value of 140 mm Hg or higher or a diastolic value of 90 mm Hg or higher

Starch A long-chain carbohydrate that is abundant in plants (including their roots, fruits, stems, and seeds)

Statin A type of drug that reduces LDL cholesterol levels in the blood

Steato-hepatitis The combination of steatosis and inflammation of the liver

Steatosis The abnormal accumulation of fats in an organ

Stem cells Cells that have the ability to reproduce themselves and to differentiate into other specialized cell types

Stenosis Abnormal narrowing of an opening or tube

Stillbirth Death of a fetus between the 20th week of pregnancy and delivery

Stimulants Addictive drugs that stimulate brain activity, including amphetamine and methamphetamine

Stools Feces

Strain A partial or complete tear of a muscle or tendon

Straw purchase The purchasing of a firearm by a non-prohibited person on behalf of a prohibited person

Strengthening activity Physical activity in which muscles contract a small number of times against resistance

Stress (physical) A measure of the force applied per unit of cross-sectional area of an object (such as a biologic tissue)

Stress (psychological) A response by the body to a threat that the person feels he or she cannot overcome or handle

Stroke Sudden damage to the brain and partial loss of brain function due to a rupture or obstruction of an artery

Stunted, stunting Having a length or height that is more than two standard deviations below the median for age in the WHO growth standards

Substance use disorder A disorder characterized by recurrent use of alcohol and/or drugs that causes impairment, disability, and failure to meet major responsibilities at work, school, or home

Sudden Infant Death Syndrome (SIDS) Sudden and unexplained death of an infant between one month and one year of age

Sufficient cause A combination of component causes that leads to the occurrence of a disease

Suicide Fatal, intentional injury directed at self

Supplemental Nutrition Assistance Program (SNAP) A federal government program operated by the U.S. Department of Agriculture that provides financial benefits for low-income persons and families to purchase food (previously called Food Stamps)

Survival rate (relative) The number of people with a disease still alive at a specific interval after diagnosis divided by the number who would be expected to survive if they did not have the disease

Synapse The tiny gap between neurons through which chemical signals are passed from one neuron to another

Syndrome A group of symptoms that occur together and characterize a particular abnormal state of the body

Synovial fluid The fluid inside a synovial joint

Synovial joint A joint that is wrapped in a joint capsule filled with fluid

Synovium The interior lining of the joint capsule in a synovial joint

Syphilis A sexually transmitted disease caused by the bacterium *Treponema pallidum* that can cause sores, rash, and long-term damage to many organ systems; If a woman has syphilis during pregnancy, she can pass the infection to her infant, causing congenital syphilis

Systemic circuit The section of the cardiovascular system that includes the systemic arteries, capillaries in all organs other than the lungs, and systemic veins

Systolic blood pressure Maximum blood pressure in the pulse cycle

T

Tangles (in neurons) Another name for neurofibrillary tangles

Tau proteins Proteins that can accumulate in the brain and cause damage to neurons

TB Commonly used abbreviation for tuberculosis disease

Tendon A dense band of tissue that connects muscles to bones

Teratogen, teratogenic drug A substance that can cause congenital malformations

Tertiary prevention Actions to prevent further disease in persons who have already experienced a disease

Tetrahydrocannabinol (THC) The biologically active chemical in marijuana

Thalamus One of two oblong-shaped structures in the brain that are involved in processing sensory information and regulating sleep, among other functions

Thalassemia A disease leading to anemia caused by two copies of a gene that codes for a malaria-resistant form of hemoglobin

Thoracic Part of or relating to the thorax (chest)

Thyroid gland A gland in the neck that produces a hormone that regulates the speed of metabolism and that is essential for infants' growth and brain development

Tissue Cells of a single type grouped together to serve a biologic function

Tolerance The pattern in which, after repeated use of a drug, the drug has less biologic effect

Toxoplasmosis A disease caused by the protozoan parasite *Toxoplasma gondii*, which is carried by cats and can infect farm animals

Trachea The air-filled tube that connects the larynx (voice box) with the large airways in each lung. Commonly called the windpipe.

Traffic-calming devices Features built into roads to slow vehicle traffic

Trans fats Fats created by hydrogenation of oils that promote atherosclerosis

Treatment support (for tuberculosis control) The practice of providing both observation and various forms of support for persons prescribed a course of medical treatment to ensure that they take all medications as prescribed

Trigger (in a firearm) The part a firearm that, when pulled backward, releases a spring or a catch, causing the firearm to fire

Trigger lock A safety feature that requires a combination or key for a gun's trigger to be pulled

Triglycerides Organic compounds composed of glycerol bound to three fatty acids; Also called fats

Trimester One of three periods of a pregnancy, lasting approximately three months or 13 weeks

Triple-negative cancer Type of breast cancer that does not express ER, HER2, or PR

Trisomy A condition in which three chromosomes are present instead of a pair

Trisomy 21 A trisomy involving chromosome number 21, also known as Down Syndrome

Trophozoite The life stage of *Plasmodium* that grows in red blood cells

Tuberculin skin test (TST) A test that uses purified protein derivative injected into the skin to measure immunity to *Mycobacterium tuberculosis*

Tuberculosis A disease caused by infection with the bacterium *Mycobacterium tuberculosis*

Tumor An abnormal growth of tissue arising from a single cell that has acquired damage to its genes, also called a neoplasm

Tumor suppressor gene A gene that suppresses a cell's ability to become transformed into a tumor cell

Type 1 diabetes A disease characterized by high blood glucose and failure of the pancreas to produce insulin

Type 1 muscle fibers Muscle fibers that can contract repeatedly, also called "slow-twitch" fibers

Type 2 diabetes A disease characterized by high blood glucose levels and insulin resistance

Type 2 muscle fibers Muscle fibers that can provide power but tire quickly also called "fast-twitch" fibers

U

Ultra-processed foods Foods produced industrially from food components, such as wheat flour, corn syrup, and vegetable oils, which typically are high in fat, sugar, sodium, and energy density

Umbilical cord A cord connecting the fetus to the placenta, through which blood, oxygen, and nutrients flow

Undernutrition Impaired growth or illness caused by insufficient intake of energy, macronutrients, or micronutrients

Unintentional injury Injury that was not caused intentionally by a person, often referred to as an accident

Universal background check laws Laws requiring background checks for firearm sales regardless of the type or person or organization selling firearms

Unsaturated fat Triglycerides composed mainly of monounsaturated and polyunsaturated fatty acids

Upper respiratory infection (URI) Infection involving the epithelium of nose, throat, and trachea but not the lower respiratory tract

Uterus The organ in the pelvis of a female in which a fertilized egg develops into a fetus

V

Vascular dementia A disease that causes dementia through damage to and narrowing of the arteries supplying the brain

Vascular resistance The total resistance to blood flow from the heart created by all of the arteries combined

Vector (in infectious disease epidemiology) An organism that carries an infectious agent (such as a virus, bacteria, or one-celled parasite) and transmits it to another organism

Vector control Efforts to reduce the incidence of a disease by reducing the number of vectors present in an area

Vegetable glycerine A small chemical derived from vegetables that forms a clear liquid at room temperature and that is used in e-cigarette liquids

Vein A blood vessel that transports blood from organs and tissues to the heart

Ventral tegmental area A region of the midbrain where reward neurons are located

Vertebra, *plural* vertebrae Bone(s) in the spine between the sacrum and the skull

Vertebral body The round or oval-shaped front part of a vertebra

Very low-density lipoproteins (VLDL) Lipoproteins that carry cholesterol in the blood and that, like low-density lipoproteins, are associated with atherosclerosis

Vigorous physical activity Physical activity requiring 6.0 or more METs

Villus, *plural* villi Finger-like projections of tissue that extend from the wall of the intestines into the lumen

Violence interrupter programs Programs designed to prevent violence by mediating conflicts and providing services to people who have been shot and those around them

Viral hepatitis Infection of the liver by a virus

Viral load The number of viral particles per microliter of blood

Viral suppression Reduction of viral load to undetectable levels with the use of antiviral drugs

Virus A submicroscopic agent that infects living organisms and that replicates only by using the capabilities of a host cell

Vision Zero A strategy to eliminate all motor vehicle-related deaths and serious injuries

Vitamin A small organic compound that is essential in small amounts to health and that must be obtained from food

Vitamin A A vitamin that is any of several chemically related compounds (including retinol and beta-carotene) needed for cell growth, the immune system, maintaining healthy epithelium, and vision

W

Waiting period laws Laws requiring a delay between when a person requests a firearm and when he or she can receive it

WASH Abbreviation for safe water, sanitation, and hygiene

Wasted, wasting Having a weight that is more than two standard deviations below the median for length or height in the WHO growth standards

Wheeze A whistling sound produced by air going through narrowed airways in persons with asthma or other lung diseases

Withdrawal (from a drug) A group of negative symptoms caused by discontinuation of a drug (including alcohol) on which a person has become dependent through regular use

Work-related asthma Occupational asthma

Y

Years of (potential) life lost (YLL), YLL rate The number of years of potential life lost from a death occurring before estimated life expectancy, summed across a population; This can be expressed as the total number of years (YLL) or that number divided by the population (YLL rate)

Z

Zika A virus spread by mosquitos that can cause a fetal infection, which can lead to the child having microcephaly or other congenital malformations

Zoning Government rules that specify the type of buildings and activities permitted in each zone of a municipality

Zygote A cell formed by the fertilization of an ovum by a sperm cell

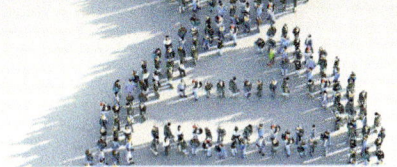

Index

Note: Page numbers followed by *b*, *f*, or *t* indicate material in boxes, figures, or tables, respectively.

A

Accelerometers, 389
ACE inhibitors, 182
Acetaldehyde, 64, 185, 335
Acid-fast/acid-fast bacilli (AFB), 263
Acini, 67
Acquired immunodeficiency syndrome (AIDS), 228
ACR. *See* Albumin-creatinine ratio
Active tuberculosis, 264
Acute bloody diarrhea, 238
Acute HIV infection, 227
Acute infection, 186
Acute low back pain, 85
Acute respiratory distress syndrome (ARDS), 251
Acute watery diarrhea, 238
Adaptive immunity, 224–226
Addiction, 354
Addictive drugs
　addiction, 354–355
　dependence, 354–355
　epidemiology of, 357–359, 358f, 359f
　pathophysiology of, 355–357, 356f, 356t
　preventive interventions, 360–363, 361f
　resources, 363
　reward circuit, 349–351, 350f, 351f
　　alcohol, 352t, 353, 353f
　　benzodiazepines, 352t, 353, 353f
　　cocaine, 351–352, 352t, 353f
　　nicotine, 351, 352t, 353f
　　stimulants, 352–353, 352t, 353f
　risk factors, 359–360, 360f, 361f
　tolerance, 354–355
Adenocarcinomas, 43, 60
Adenomas, 43, 60
Adenovirus types 40/41, 239
Adipocytes, 163, 186
Aerobic, 80
Aerobic activity, 388
Aerosols, 255
Afferent arterioles, 176
AIDS. *See* Acquired immunodeficiency syndrome

Air exchanges (or air changes) per hour, 261
Air pollution, 202, 299
Airways, 248
Albumin, 178
Albumin-creatinine ratio (ACR), 178
Alcohol use
　epidemiology of, 339–341, 340f, 341f
　ethanol, 333–334, 334f
　marketing of, 342, 343t
　neurotransmitters, 334
　pathophysiology of, 334–339, 334f, 335t, 336f–339f
　　attributable deaths, 339, 339f
　　brain, 334–335
　　cancer, 337
　　fetal alcohol syndrome, 337–338, 337f
　　heart disease, 338–339, 338f
　　infectious diseases, 336–337
　　liver, 335–336
　　non-traffic fatal injuries attributable, 336, 336f
　preventive interventions, 342–344, 343f
　resources, 345
　risk factors, 341–342, 342f
Alcohol use disorder, 335
Alcoholic hepatitis, 336
Alcoholic liver disease, 185
Allergens, 200
Allergy, 197, 199
Allostatic load, 411
Alveoli, 47, 53, 197, 197f, 248
Alzheimer's disease, 111
Ambient (outdoor) air pollution, 50, 202, 299
Amino acid, 176, 368
Amnion, 292
Amniotic fluid, 292
Amphetamine, 352
Amygdala, 101, 108, 351
Amyloid beta fragments, 112
Amyloid plaques, 112

Anaerobic, 294
Anaerobic physical activity, 388
Anemia, 272, 371
Anencephaly, 305
Anhedonia, 335, 354
Annulus fibrosus, 82, 83f
Anopheles mosquitoes, 272
Anopheles funestus, 273
Anopheles gambiae, 273
Anopheles stephensi, 273
Anthropogenic, 202
Antibiotic, 222, 246, 249
Antibody, 200, 224, 243, 259, 275
Antidepressants, 152
Antigenic drift, 251
Antigenic shift, 251
Antihypertensives, 30, 37
Antimalarial drugs, 275
Antioxidants, 377
Antipsychotic medications, 96
Antiviral medication, 251
Anxiety, 95, 108
　definition and description, 108
　epidemiology, 109
　pathophysiology of, 108–109, 109f
　primary prevention, 110, 110f
　resources, 111
　risk factors, 109–110, 110f
　secondary prevention, 110–111
Anxiety disorder, 101, 108, 324
ApoE4, 115
Apoptosis, 44
ARB antihypertensives, 182
ARDS. *See* Acute respiratory distress syndrome
Artemisinin, 275
Artemisinin-based combination therapy (ACT), 275
Arterial roads, 126
Arteries, 19, 20f, 175
Arterioles, 113, 175
Arthritis, 75
Articular cartilage, 76
ASCVD. *See* Atherosclerotic cardiovascular disease
Assault, 123